Psychiatry for Neurologists

CURRENT CLINICAL NEUROLOGY

Daniel Tarsy, MD, SERIES EDITOR

Psychiatry
for Neurologists

Edited by

Dilip V. Jeste, MD

*Departments of Psychiatry and Neurosciences, University of California,
San Diego and VA San Diego Healthcare System, San Diego, CA*

Joseph H. Friedman, MD

*Parkinson's Disease and Movement Disorders Center, NeuroHealth,
Warwick, RI and Brown University Medical School, Providence, RI*

HUMANA PRESS ✳ TOTOWA, NEW JERSEY

© 2006 Humana Press Inc.
999 Riverview Drive, Suite 208
Totowa, New Jersey 07512

humanapress.com

Due diligence has been taken by the publishers, editors, and authors of this book to assure the accuracy of the information published and to describe generally accepted practices. The contributors herein have carefully checked to ensure that the drug selections and dosages set forth in this text are accurate and in accord with the standards accepted at the time of publication. Notwithstanding, as new research, changes in government regulations, and knowledge from clinical experience relating to drug therapy and drug reactions constantly occurs, the reader is advised to check the product information provided by the manufacturer of each drug for any change in dosages or for additional warnings and contraindications. This is of utmost importance when the recommended drug herein is a new or infrequently used drug. It is the responsibility of the treating physician to determine dosages and treatment strategies for individual patients. Further it is the responsibility of the health care provider to ascertain the Food and Drug Administration status of each drug or device used in their clinical practice. The publisher, editors, and authors are not responsible for errors or omissions or for any consequences from the application of the information presented in this book and make no warranty, express or implied, with respect to the contents in this publication.

This publication is printed on acid-free paper. ∞
ANSI Z39.48-1984 (American Standards Institute) Permanence of Paper for Printed Library Materials.

Production Editor: Robin B. Weisberg

Cover design by Patricia F. Cleary.

For additional copies, pricing for bulk purchases, and/or information about other Humana titles, contact Humana at the above address or at any of the following numbers: Tel.: 973-256-1699; Fax: 973-256-8341; E-mail: orders@humanapr.com; or visit our Website: www.humanapress.com

Printed in the United States of America. 10 9 8 7 6 5 4 3 2 1

e-ISBN: 1-59259-960-5

Library of Congress Cataloging-in-Publication Data

Psychiatry for neurologists / edited by Dilip V. Jeste, Joseph H. Friedman.
    p. cm. -- (Current clinical neurology)
  Includes bibliographical references and index.
  ISBN 1-58829-483-8 (alk. paper)
 1. Neuropsychiatry. 2. Psychiatry. 3. Neurologists. I. Jeste, Dilip V.
II. Friedman, Joseph H. III. Series.
  RC341.P892 2005
  616.8--dc22

                                                          2005001928

Dedication

For *Susie*,
with love, admiration, and gratitude
for the many sacrifices,
great and small.

—JHF

To *Sonali, Shafali*, and *Neelum*,
for filling my life with fun and love.

—DVJ

Series Editor's Introduction

Psychiatry for Neurologists is an ambitious volume that was recruited for the Current Clinical Neurology series because of a perceived need to provide neurologists with a useful and convenient resource covering the areas of clinical psychiatry that impact the management of neurological disorders. Although it may be a cliché to reiterate that the disciplines of neurology and psychiatry concern the same organ, the fact is that long ago they unfortunately went their separate ways. The reasons for this and a description of the paths they followed are elegantly reviewed by Dr. Goetz in his chapter concerning the history of neurology and psychiatry in America. Curiously, although in this country neurology became more allied with internal medicine, it has continued to share its specialty board with psychiatry. Somehow, this alliance managed to survive the mid-20th century era when psychoanalytic theory and practice, founded by the neurologist Sigmund Freud, held sway.

Beginning in the 1950s, the arrival of effective antipsychotic drugs, antidepressants, lithium, and anxiolytic agents provided an alternative medical approach to the treatment of psychiatric disorders. The effects of these agents, many of which were originally discovered serendipitously, precipitated enormous interest into the biochemical underpinnings of psychiatric disorders. Thus, by the 1970s, the dopamine hypothesis of schizophrenia and norepinephrine and serotonin hypotheses of depression were born. The remarkable effects of hallucinogenic drugs gave further impetus to the field, driving a concept suggesting a possible "chemistry of the mind" that might unlock the secrets of all psychiatric disease. Although that somewhat overreaching promise has not been realized, even for the psychotic disorders, a new generation of biological psychiatrists is actively engaged in the study of the molecular and genetic basis of psychiatric disorders.

It is no accident that the editors, Drs. Jeste and Friedman, have spent much of their careers studying the neurological effects of antipsychotic drugs. The striking ability of antipsychotic drugs to mimic parkinsonism, tremor, dyskinesia, and dystonia was appreciated early on as a potential window into understanding the pathophysiology of organic movement disorders and paralleled the impact these drugs had on the understanding of psychotic disorders. Thus, in no small part, owing to the psychiatric and neurological effects of antipsychotic drugs, psychiatry and neurology began to share an area of common ground. The concept of a motor and limbic striatum and proposals concerning parallel cortical-subcortical motor and limbic circuits helped shape the understanding of both extrapyramidal and psychiatric disorders. With the advent of effective treatments for psychotic disorders and Parkinson's disease, together with their inevitable side effects (antipsychotics cause movement disorders and antiparkinson drugs cause psychosis), it became clear that psychiatrists and neurologists need each other. Now other areas of mutual interest and concern are being increasingly appreciated. This volume provides the comprehensive and useful overview needed to allow neurologists to feel comfortable managing the psychiatric aspects of the neurological disorders they treat. After all, it *is* the same organ!

Daniel Tarsy, MD
Parkinson's Disease & Movement Disorders Center
Beth Israel Deaconess Medical Center
Harvard Medical School
Boston, MA

Preface

Although one of the editors is trained in both psychiatry and neurology (DJ), the other, not originally interested in behavioral problems at all, has come, through long clinical practice, to be increasingly convinced of the broad overlap between the two disciplines. This means that the lack of an appreciation and understanding of the behavioral problems that are so common in neurological patients puts both the neurologist and the patient at a disadvantage in both diagnosis and treatment. And although there are texts on "neuropsychiatry" and "neurology for psychiatrists," we envisioned a resource that will acquaint clinical neurologists with "bread-and-butter" psychiatric issues that these physicians face with their neurological patients. Some patients will have behavioral problems as a result of their primary neurological problems, such as Huntington's disease or Tourette's syndrome, whereas others have primary psychiatric disorders and later develop neurological problems, such as persons with schizophrenia who develop seizures, strokes, Parkinson's disease, and the like. However, it becomes increasingly apparent with experience that it is the exceptional neurological patient who does not have some behavioral component as part of the illness.

In *Psychiatry for Neurologists*, we have focused on practical issues and mostly shied away from the theoretical. For example, we have favored the approach of describing depression and its treatment in Parkinson's disease rather than addressing the role of the basal ganglia in mood. We think the available neuropsychiatry texts address these theoretical issues quite well, but that these texts have mainly targeted psychiatric audiences who are looking for a grounding in neurophysiology and anatomy, seeking "hard" explanations for disorders that until recently have been considered "functional."

Neurology residency training only recently has mandated a rotation on the psychiatry service. This has resulted in a generation of neurologists who often have little direct experience with primary psychiatric disorders and have no intellectual foundation on which to interpret their findings. In the hospital, the liaison psychiatrists, themselves sometimes adrift in the world of neurological disorders, often prove unable to provide significant assistance in the interpretation or management of behavioral problems, leaving the neurologist without a true safety net. *Psychiatry for Neurologists* is intended to help the clinical neurologist interpret the behavioral problems in their patients themselves, not necessarily to manage the problems independently, but rather to understand the patient in a larger context. This will hopefully allow the neurologist to better interpret the psychiatric problems leading to improved interactions with psychiatric consultants, when they are needed.

When one editor (JHF) started working in Parkinson's disease 20 plus years ago, it was clear to him that it was a movement disorder, that the discussions over depression being intrinsic or reactive were akin to wondering about the number of angels that could dance on the head of a pin. With greater experience and increased sensitivity, he has come to realize that Parkinson's disease is really a "neurobehavioral disorder" defined clinically by its movement disorder. The most devastating aspects of Parkinson's disease are, in fact, the behavioral aspects, not the movement dysfunction. There is sometimes a tendency to regard psychiatry as a "different" type of medical practice because the patients don't get "sick" in the same way. The stigma against mental illness needs to be combated with education. There is an interesting "The Far Side" cartoon by Gary Larson. A patient is lying on a couch and a somewhat deranged appearing Sigmund Freud imitation is scribbling in his pad, "Just plain nuts." It is time to move beyond this image. As we learn more and more about emotional problems, we find "organic" explanations in genetic and physiological derangements. One gene problem creates tics, a "neurological" disorder, while a closely related mutation causes obsessive-compulsive disorder, a "psychiatric" disorder. Why these fall into separate categories owes more to accidents in history (*see* chapters by Goetz and Boller) than anything else. Alzheimer's disease and dementia with Lewy bodies are good examples of illnesses that fall clearly into both camps, with many successful collaborations. We believe that neurology and psychiatry are increasingly coming together after a long period of moving apart. We hope to help reduce this gap at least a little with this text.

Joseph H. Friedman, MD
Dilip V. Jeste, MD

Contents

Part V. Other Topics

Contributors

MARC E. AGRONIN, MD • Director of Mental Health Services, Miami Jewish Home & Hospital for the Aged; Department of Psychiatry, University of Miami School of Medicine, Miami, FL

KAREN E. ANDERSON, MD • Departments of Psychiatry and Neurology, University of Maryland Hospital, University of Maryland School of Medicine, Baltimore, MD

GIANFRANCO DALLA BARBA, MD • Department of Neurology, INSERM U549, Centre Paul Broca, Paris, France

FRANÇOIS BOLLER, MD, PhD • Department of Neurology, INSERM U549, Centre Paul Broca, Paris, France

CATHY BUDMAN, MD • Departments of Neurology and Psychiatry, North Shore University Medical Center, Manhasset, NY

JOHN C. M. BRUST, MD • Department of Neurology, Harlem Hospital Center, Columbia University School of Physicians and Surgeons, New York, NY

LAURA CAMPBELL-SILLS, PhD • Department of Psychiatry, University of California, San Diego, CA

ERIC J. CHRISTOPHER, MD • Departments of Internal Medicine and Psychiatry, Veterans Administration Hospital, Duke University Medical Center, Durham, NC

JEFFREY ALLEN COHEN, MD • Department of Medicine (Neurology), Dartmouth-Hitchcock Medical Center, Lebanon, NH

JODY COREY-BLOOM, MD, PhD • Department of Neurology, University of California, San Diego, CA

DARCY COX, PsyD • Department of Neurology, University of California, San Francisco, CA

CHRISTOPHER CHRISTODOULOU, PhD • Department of Neurology, State of New York at Stony Brook, Stony Brook, NY

DARIN D. DOUGHERTY, MD, MSC • Department of Psychiatry, Massachusetts General Hospital, Harvard Medical School, Boston, MA

COLIN A. DEPP, PhD • Department of Psychiatry, University of California, San Diego, CA

CHRISTIAN DOLDER, PharmD • Wingate University School of Pharmacy, Wingate, NC

LAURA DUNN, MD • Department of Psychiatry, School of Medicine, University of California, San Diego, CA

DAVID P. FOLSOM, MD • Department of Psychiatry, University of California, San Diego, CA

ADAM S. FLEISHER, MD • Department of Psychiatry, University of California, San Diego, CA

JOSEPH H. FRIEDMAN, MD • Parkinson's Disease and Movement Disorders Center, NeuroHealth, Warwick, RI; Department of Clinical Neurosciences, Brown University Medical School, Providence, RI

CHRISTOPHER G. GOETZ, MD • Departments of Neurological Sciences and Pharmacology, Rush University Medical Center, Chicago, IL

SANJAY GUPTA, MD • Department of Psychiatry, Olean General Hospital, Olean, NY; University of Buffalo School of Medicine and Biomedical Sciences, Buffalo, NY

ANSAR HAROUN, MD • Departments of Psychiatry and Pediatrics, School of Medicine, University of California, San Diego; University of San Diego School of Law; Superior Court of San Diego, San Diego, CA

COLIN HARRINGTON, MD • Department of Psychiatry, Rhode Island Hospital, Department of Psychiatry and Human Behavior, Brown Medical School, Providence, RI

SANDRA JACOBSON, MD • Department of Psychiatry, The Miriam Hospital and Department of Psychiatry and Human Behavior, Brown Medical School, Providence, RI

DILIP V. JESTE, MD • Departments of Psychiatry and Neurosciences, University of California, San Diego, and VA San Diego Healthcare System, San Diego, CA

ANDRES M. KANNER, MD • Department of Neurosciences, Rush-Presbyterian-St Luke's Medical Center, Chicago, IL

LAUREN B. KRUPP, MD • Department of Neurology, State of New York at Stony Brook, Stony Brook, NY

ROGER KURLAN, MD • Department of Neurology, University of Rochester School of Medicine and Dentistry, Rochester, NY

W. CURT LAFRANCE, JR., MD • Rhode Island Hospital, Division of Neuropsychiatry, Departments of Psychiatry and Neurology, Brown University Medical School, Providence, RI

ARIEL J. LANG, PhD • Department of Psychiatry, VA San Diego Healthcare System, University of California, San Diego, CA

BEATRIZ LUNA, PharmD • Wingate University School of Pharmacy, Wingate, NC

JEFFREY LYNESS, MD • Department of Psychiatry, Strong Memorial Hospital, University of Rochester School of Medicine and Dentistry, Rochester, NY

WILLIAM S. MACALLISTER, PhD • Department of Neurology, State of New York at Stony Brook, Stony Brook, NY

KAREN MARDER, MD, MPH • Department of Neurology, Neurological Institute of New York, Columbia University College of Physicians and Surgeons, New York, NY

RUSSELL L. MARGOLIS, MD • Departments of Psychiatry and Neurology, Johns Hopkins Hospital, Johns Hopkins University School of Medicine, Baltimore, MD

LAURA MARSH, MD • Departments of Psychiatry and Neurology, Johns Hopkins Medical Center, The Johns Hopkins University School of Medicine, Baltimore, MD

MICHAEL F. MAZUREK, MD • Department of Neurology, McMaster University Hospital, McMaster University Medical School, Hamilton, Ontario, Canada

JOHN R. MCQUAID, PhD• Psychology Service, VA San Diego Healthcare System; Department of Psychiatry, University of California, San Diego, CA

DAVID C. MOHR, PhD• Departments of Neurology and Psychiatry, VA Medical Center, University of California, San Francisco, CA

GRANT MORRIS, JD, LLM • University of San Diego School of Law; Department of Psychiatry, University of San Diego School of Medicine, San Diego, CA

DAVID NAIMARK, MD • Department of Psychiatry, School of Medicine, University of California, San Diego; Superior Court of San Diego, CA

DAVID W. OSLIN, MD • Department of Psychiatry, Philadelphia VA Medical Center, University of Pennsylvania, Philadelphia, PA

FRED OVSIEW, MD • Department of Psychiatry, University of Chicago Hospitals, University of Chicago School Pritzker School of Medicine, Chicago, IL

LAWRENCE T. PARK, MD • Department of Psychiatry, Massachusetts General Hospital, Harvard Medical School, Boston, MA

ANTON P. PORSTEINSSON, MD • Department of Psychiatry, Strong Memorial Hospital, University of Rochester School of Medicine and Dentistry, Rochester, NY

SCOTT L. RAUCH, MD • Department of Psychiatry, Massachusetts General Hospital, Harvard Medical School, Boston, MA

IRENE HEGEMAN RICHARD, MD • Departments of Neurology and Psychiatry, Strong Memorial Hospital, University of Rochester School of Medicine and Dentistry, Rochester, NY

ROBERT G. ROBINSON, MD • Department of Psychiatry, University of Western Australia and Fremantle Hospital School of Psychiatry and Clinical Neurosciences, Fremantle, Australia

PATRICIA I. ROSEBUSH, MD • Department of Psychiatry, McMaster University Hospital, McMaster University Medical School, Hamilton, Ontario, Canada

STEPHEN SALLOWAY, MD, MS • Department of Neurology, Butler Hospital and Departments of Clinical Neurosciences and Psychology and Human Behavior, Brown Medical School, Providence, RI

SERGIO E. STARKSTEIN, MD • School of Psychiatry and Clinical Neurosciences, Fremantle Hospital, University of Western Australia, Fremantle, Australia

MURRAY B. STEIN, MD, MPH • Department of Psychiatry, VA San Diego Healthcare System, University of California, San Diego, CA

DOROTHY E. STUBBE, MD • Department of Child and Adolescent Psychiatry, Yale Child Study Center, Yale–New Haven Hospital, Yale University School of Medicine, New Haven, CT

WARREN D. TAYLOR, MD • Department of Psychiatry, Duke University Medical Center, Durham, NC

RENEE MARIE VEBELL, RN, MA Department of Nursing, Colby-Sawyer College, New London, NH

DANIEL WEINTRAUB, MD • Departments of Psychiatry and Neurology, Philadelphia VA Medical Center, University of Pennsylvania School of Medicine, Philadelphia, PA

JULIE LOEBACH WETHERELL, PhD• Department of Psychiatry, VA San Diego Healthcare System, University of California, San Diego, CA

I Introduction

Historical Interfaces Between American Neurology and Psychiatry

Christopher G. Goetz

INTRODUCTION

Medical specialization evolved out of the burgeoning scientific advances of the 19th century *(1)*. This movement was an international one, but most pronounced in France, where the celebrated *Faculté de Médecine* in Paris developed numerous professorial chairs to honor and prioritize advances in selective medical fields *(2)*. Other countries echoed this movement, adapting the concept of specialization to their own medical cultures and working with the experts available in their universities. Some specialties related primarily to the emerging laboratory disciplines, such as microbiology, pathology, pharmacology, and physiology. In most instances, however, clinical specialties were based anatomically, dividing the human body by organ systems and leading to divisions like pulmonology, dermatology, cardiology, and others. Because each organ system was distinct, these specialties were largely autonomous from one another, integrating with each other only through their original base of internal medicine.

The brain posed a unique anatomical problem for specialization in being the organ system of focus for two very different evolving specialties, neurology and psychiatry. This chapter examines the early historical interfaces between these two specialties with an emphasis on 19th-century United States. As the author is a neurologist, the perspective admittedly focuses primarily on the history of American neurology and its relationship to psychiatry, rather than the reverse. As an introductory chapter to a book that emphasizes the currently close interface between the two disciplines, this chapter selects a number of topics to trace the origins of an often uneasy relationship that has been marked at times by elitism, controversy, and overt antagonism. It is not a comprehensive history, but rather a focused view of several early themes that became the historical infrastructure for the unstable, changing flux of relationship between the two disciplines during the 20th century. Whereas the two fields sometimes deferentially honored each other, they more frequently emphasized their differences with the most far-reaching polarization occurring during the mid-1900s when American psychiatry was largely dominated by psychoanalytic theory. As the 21st century opens, the emergence of a psychiatric emphasis on molecular biology and neurochemistry, as well as the increasing consciousness by neurologists of the impact on disability and impairment in neurological function by psychiatric co-morbidities, have helped to dissipate much of the dissonance that began in the 19th century. These

From: *Current Clinical Neurology: Psychiatry for Neurologists*
Edited by: D.V. Jeste and J.H. Friedman © Humana Press Inc., Totowa, NJ

new-found realizations are the anchors of the positive co-dependence between these two specialties that is the core of this current textbook.

AMERICAN NEUROLOGY'S ORIGINAL DUAL ALLIANCES WITH INTERNAL MEDICINE AND PSYCHIATRY

With no patronization, it is fair to state that American medicine largely modeled itself on 19th-century European models. Most prominent physicians of the 19th century studied in Europe, traveled extensively, and thereafter brought back to the United States the images of the large and well-established medical services in Vienna, Paris, London, and Berlin *(3)*. Europe, however, was not medically homogenous. In defining neurology in the second half of the 1800s, American physicians and universities faced two very different paradigms, the first anchored in France and the second in the Germanic medical centers of Austria and Prussia *(4)*. In France, psychiatry was an early medical specialty, and the term "alienists" designated physicians dealing with psychiatric problems of psychosis, delirium, insanity, and retardation. Because of their disruptive behaviors, psychiatric patients were usually housed in asylums that largely isolated them from general medical settings. As a result, medical specialties, including neurology, arose out of administrative subdivisions and specialty units within the major medical hospitals without a strong vying influence of psychiatric concerns. As the most salient example, the celebrated neurologist, Jean-Martin Charcot (1825–1893) developed his interest in neurology within the general medical wards of the large Parisian hospice of the Salpêtrière where the patient population was largely dominated by geriatric patients with chronic medical illness. Charcot's academic career started with studies of arthritic, hepatic, pulmonary, and renal diseases, but as specialty divisions in Paris drew these patients to other hospital units, the chronically disabled and largely unclassified neurological patients remained under his direct care. Out of this administrative shifting, Charcot developed a neurological wing of wide research proportions and in 1882 received the first European professorial chair of clinical diseases of the nervous system. His contact with other medical specialties remained close, but he had almost no association with alienists whose work occurred in entirely different administrative divisions. In the late 1880s, when Charcot reached the zenith of his influence, his neurological unit included a division of research psychology headed by Janet, but there were no alienists as psychiatric specialists on his staff *(5)*.

In contrast, the Germanic medical model emphasized the fusion of neurology and psychiatry, largely based on the influential leadership of Wilhelm Griesinger *(6)*. Writing of the Prussian concept of approaching the study of brain disorders, Griesinger articulated: "Psychiatry and neurology are not like closely connected fields, they are one field, ruled by the same laws, where everyone speaks the same language" *(7)*. As such, when Griesinger gained his professorial chair in Berlin (1865), the title was Professor of Psychiatry and Nervous Disease. Likewise, Wernicke, the celebrated clinician scientist whose name is linked to fluent aphasias, led both the psychiatric service and the polyclinic for nervous diseases in Breslau. The Prussian model anchored itself in laboratory studies and pathology, bringing substantive advances to organic concepts of dementias and psychosis.

Against this historical backdrop, the development of American specialties varied by region and time period, and, in the case of neurology and psychiatry, the models drew from both the French and Germanic traditions. The result was an ambiguous hybrid and uneasy peace between neurology and psychiatry in the 19th century that took a full century to stabilize. Studying early university professorships, 19th-century specialty journals, and local as well as national professional societies unveils several dimensions of the uncomfortable and unresolved relationship that embodied early American neurology and psychiatry.

EARLY UNIVERSITY PROFESSORSHIPS

Harvard Medical School was the first in the United States to conceptualize a professorship in neurological science *(8)*. In 1864, the dean initiated recruitment of CE Brown-Séquard under the title of

Professor of Physiology and Pathology of the Nervous System. The professorship was short-lived and unsuccessful, primarily because of Brown-Séquard's own indecisiveness and unreliable behavior. After Brown-Séquard left Harvard to return to Europe, the university turned to its own Department of Clinical Medicine for neurological staff. J. Putnam lectured on diseases of the nervous system in the 1870s and eventually was awarded a professorship designated exclusively to diseases of the nervous system. This chair was largely based on the French model of neurology as a division of internal medicine. The heritage of linkage between neurology and medicine remained instilled in the Boston program through the 20th century with a tradition of recruitment of neurology trainees who were already graduates of internal medicine programs.

In New York, the Bellevue Hospital Medical School developed a model much closer to the Prussian tradition. After the American Civil War, William Hammond, who would become one of the most distinguished American neurologists of the 19th century, moved to New York and joined the staff of the medical school. Hammond had been the surgeon general and was largely responsible for the organization of military hospitals for the Union campaign *(9)*. The combat style, weaponry, and grueling exposure that characterized the Civil War led to a vast medical experience with neurological and psychiatric diagnoses related to war trauma. The medical school post that he occupied was titled "lecturer of Diseases of the Mind and Nervous System," thereby fusing the responsibility for psychiatric and neurological teaching. Hammond's "Nerve Clinic" incorporated both psychiatric and neurological patients in the same service. In 1866, when the medical school awarded him a professorship, the title of Professor of Diseases of the Mind and Nervous System reflected this double responsibility. Hammond's introductory lecture, "The Proper Use of the Mind," drew upon examples of dementia, psychotic behaviors, and motor or sensory symptoms with equal emphasis *(4)*.

Both Brown-Séquard and Hammond had difficult and alienating personalities that caused significant disruption in the smooth administrative acceptance of neurology in American medical schools. From an administrative perspective, Hammond's demanding and antagonistic postures were as problematic as Brown-Séquard's restlessness, because both led to very short-lived neurological professorship that required full revamping. After a rift with the administration and faculty at Bellevue, Hammond resigned, and the medical school administration dissolved the chair altogether. The reorganization involved the naming of two separate chairs, one for diseases of the nervous system and the other for psychological medicine. Whether this solution was selected to limit the power of one man over too wide a discipline or to recognize inherent differences between neurology and psychiatry, the division of work was clearly stated as a departure from the earlier Prussian model and reinforced the separation of the two disciplines academically.

To search for a more clear understanding of issues between early neurology and psychiatry in 19th-century America without the confounding problems of troublesome personalities, the most respected of American neurologists should be studied. Although never a university professor, the Philadelphian, S.W. Mitchell was undoubtedly the most revered and senior of early American specialists dealing with neurological and psychiatric conditions. A celebrated clinician with national and international ties throughout the medical world, Mitchell trained in general medicine and was world renown for his studies of toxins, neuropathies, hysteria, and malingering. His detailed studies of nerve injuries, his extensive analyses of rattlesnake venom, and his interest in rehabilitation therapies in Sydenham's chorea stand along side his internationally respected rest therapy used for the treatment of hysteria and other behavioral impairments. Nonetheless, he was short tempered with psychiatric patients and harsh with psychiatric colleagues, establishing an American tradition, even in the early years of neurology that legitimized an attitude of condescendence by neurologists toward psychiatrists and psychiatric patients. As one example of patient treatment, his student, B. Tucker described Mitchell's assessment of a woman whose illness inexplicably precluded her from walking. As the team of doctors entered the hall after Mitchell examined the patient, Tucker recalled:

> "Will she ever be able to walk?" asked one of the doctors. "Yes, in a moment," said Dr. Mitchell.
> Then the door of the room flew open and the paralyzed patient in her nightgown rushed out and down

the hall. Smoke exuded from the room. "What on earth is the matter?" asked someone. "I set the bedclothes on fire," said Dr. Mitchell. (*10*, p. 343)

Mitchell publicly drew the lines between the two specialties in 1894 when he accepted an invitation to speak at a meeting of the American Medico-Psychological Association. Although a guest of his psychiatric colleagues, he vehemently criticized the lackluster progress in psychiatric research, the isolation of psychiatry from the rest of medicine, the lack of resident physicians in asylums, and the customs, bureaucracy, and politics that hampered research efforts. The shocking and alienating presentation led to defensive responses that set a new tone within American medicine and crystallized a tension that had been largely unarticulated before *(4)*. Neurologists rallied to the criticism, and the American Neurological Association (ANA) developed official position papers on the development of special neurological centers and the removal of neurological patients from the state and local asylums where they were deemed under inadequate expert care. The rift categorically fostered the placement of American neurology beside internal medicine and not beside psychiatry, although the reality of a shared patient population necessitated continuing interactions.

SCIENTIFIC JOURNALS

The *Journal of Nervous and Mental Disease* was the primary American journal of the 19th century that addressed the interface of early neurology and psychiatry *(11)*. Still an active journal today, it serves as an on-going record of the relationship between the two fields. Volume I appeared in 1876, and the journal's early years emphasized an even and respectful balance between articles on topics that would today be considered as neurological and psychiatric, ranging from neuroanatomical and neurophysiological studies to observations on hysteria, dementia, and melancholia and including open discussions of public health issues pertinent to large institutions, asylums, and government-affiliated hospitals. Toward the close of the 19th century, however, there was a clear indication of the journal's growing prioritization of neurology as the journal began publishing the proceedings of the ANA. Covertly and overtly, articles drew increasing attention to an opposition between the ANA and the American Association of Asylum Superintendents, forerunner of the American Psychiatric Association. As early as 1897, the ANA Executive Council minutes reflect discussions of the ANA's desire to control a journal specifically separate from psychiatric concerns, and discussions began thereafter with the American Medical Association (AMA) to create a new journal. This plan did not develop, but was reinitiated in 1919 at a time when the editorial pendulum had swung in the opposite direction, and the *Journal of Nervous and Mental Disease* was prioritizing psychiatric issues, specifically psychoanalysis, under the editorship of S.E. Jelliffe. The journal has survived these swings into the present, but did not maintain its premier status, being replaced by specialty journals in neurology and psychiatry. Even in the 20th century, when the AMA developed its specialties journals, it used the same tradition and started the *Archives of Neurology and Psychiatry*, but this effort was short-lived and the *Archives of Neurology* and *Archives of General Psychiatry* became separate journals *(4)*.

Other journals developed in the 19th century that capitalized on a readership with presumed shared interests in topics to cover neurological and psychiatric domains. *The Alienist and Neurologist* started in 1880 and remained in circulation for 40 years, offering readers a pragmatic venue for reading about new therapies. The journal title honored both fields in slightly different ways. Although it listed psychiatry first, the choice of alienist to describe psychiatric specialists was a marginally archaic designation even in the late 1880s. In contrast, neurologist was a very modern term, and its use is among the first in official settings. *The American Journal of Neurology and Psychiatry* developed in 1882, and although its title honors the two fields, the journal distinguished itself primarily as a venue for articles on the interface between neurology and internal medicine rather than between neurology and psychiatry *(4)*.

In distinctive ways, each journal adopted strategies to defining a proper niche of readership, although these efforts increasingly honored differences over similarities. The term "neuropsychiatrist" grew primarily out of administrative organizational documents during World War I and was not a well-formed 19th-century concept *(12)*. In parallel to the movement among neurologists to define their own journals, specialty journals devoted more specifically to psychiatry developed, including the *American Journal of Insanity* (1844) and the *American Journal of Mental Deficiency* (1876), among others. Efforts to realign the two fields in shared publication efforts would await the movement of détente that surrounded the development of a unified American Board of Psychiatry and Neurology for certification efforts in the 1930s. The panels and colloquia linked to this effort to save both specialties as distinct medical entities fostered co-authorships and collective writing efforts that had not been seen for decades. Although these efforts did not specifically lead to new journals, a re-appreciation of shared interests between neurology and psychiatry developed and led to several joint position papers and publications that helped in the establishment of government bodies including the National Institutes of Health.

PROFESSIONAL SOCIETIES

The ANA was founded in 1875 and is the oldest national neurological organization in the world *(4,12)*. Its original mission clearly included the establishing and fostering of an intellectual and structural forum for neurologists as distinct from other physicians. The argumentative William Hammond was the primary energy source behind the founding effort, and a transparent battle with the superintendents of mental asylums brewed even in the beginning meetings of the new organization. The ANA was very socially proactive in its early years, publishing position papers on public health issues and similar to Mitchell's 1894 edict, specifically attacked the mental asylum administrative systems. In this way, without ambiguity, the ANA positioned itself as an organization for neurologists, not psychiatrists, and although the qualifications and credentials of these two fields remained vague in the 19th century, a spirit of separatism was clearly articulated at an official level. Some neurological historians have suggested that the ANA's elitism was based as a reaction against the pre-existing exclusiveness of the American Association of Asylum Superintendents, but such arguments of precedence are less important than the reality of bipartisan antagonism.

An important distinction however merits emphasis in this growing polarization at an administrative level, because the alienation did not occur along diagnostic or disease lines. As only one example, George Beard, a prominent New York physician, was the first elected member of the ANA *(13)*. As part of the entry criteria, each new member presented a paper, and his presentation was on neurasthenia, a diagnosis he had studied extensively, and, as a result, was known internationally as Beard's disease. Although his contemporaries argued whether neurasthenia was a stress-related emotional condition without focal neurological signs, Beard nonetheless entered the ANA on the credibility of his work in this research area. His example emphasizes that although neurology and psychiatry evolved as separate fields, the distinction between a neurologist and psychiatrist remained poorly defined and, in a practice environment outside asylums, the two terms in fact largely embodied the same specialist.

At the local level within the United States, administrative antagonisms were less marked, and the reality of a limited number of colleagues interested in brain disorders forced more collegiality. A variety of different models were used for gathering physicians with neurological, psychiatric, or shared interests. In Boston, the original venue was the Boston Medico-Psychological Society, and this name was changed in 1901 to the Boston Society of Psychiatry and Neurology *(14)*. This local group gathered for case presentations and discussion, but was also important in steering social and government policies, especially in dealing with the rights of intellectually deficient patients. The Chicago Neurological Society, founded in 1898, may have sounded exclusive in its title, but was openly receptive to members and presentations from ophthalmology, psychiatry, surgery, and internal medicine *(15)*. The Philadelphia Neurological Society held a more neurological focus on the rules for membership, but regularly had combined or joint-sponsored meetings with psychiatric colleagues, usually in the form of partnership with the Medical Jurisprudence Society of Philadelphia, a group that focused on medico-legal aspects of insanity and mental deficiency *(16)*.

THE FRUITS AND PRICES OF DISTINCTION

The rise of specialism allowed the development of intellectual distinction and research focus at the scientific level, personal and financial independence for practitioners at the professional level, and administrative autonomy at university and government levels. With all these motivations, however, 19th-century American physicians who identified themselves by an interest in nervous system disorders did not have the advantage of a unified, systematic educational model for career development. The disjointed and volatile atmosphere that surrounded the budding areas of neurology and psychiatry created marked disparities in training credentials throughout the United States in the 19th and early 20th centuries. Against the threat of neurology's absorption into internal medicine in the 1920s and the reality of highly varying training programs across the United States in both neurology and psychiatry, the visionaries who formulated the American Board of Psychiatry and Neurology in 1934 sought to reduce the alienation of the past and work together to establish basic credentials in both fields *(17)*. The recognition of needed shared expertise and complementary educational guidelines allowed the first major step toward simultaneously honoring both fields and dissipating prior antagonism. More than any other administrative body, this board has fostered a liaison between the two fields that never existed in the 19th century and has stabilized a relationship to the mutual benefit of both fields.

In the author's view, however, the major source of reconciliation between neurology and psychiatry has been the evolution in scientific discoveries and the on-going reality that the distinction between a patient with psychiatric disease and neurological disease remains unequivocally difficult to define. The discoveries of genetic patterns in psychotic disorders, the specificity of dopamine receptor antagonists to the treatment of schizophrenia, and the increasing literature on the biochemistry of depression parallel similar axes of research in such neurological diagnosis as primary epilepsies and Parkinson's disease. Just as many of the techniques applied to neurological research have been adopted by psychiatric teams, pharmacogenomics, a field largely driven by psychiatrists in the past to define groups of patients most likely to respond to different medications, is increasingly being applied within neurology *(18)*. With the advent of medications that selectively treat psychiatric illness, neurological side effects, primarily in the form of movement disorders, have brought neurologists and psychiatrists into cross-consultation relationships. These interfaces are equally crucial to the care of subjects with dementias, chronic epilepsy, and conditions that have both motor and behavioral elements such as Huntington's disease and Gilles de la Tourette syndrome. Perhaps most importantly, the psychogenic neurological disorders, still a vague class of diagnoses, require an interface of combined specialties for accurate delineation and management *(19)*. New studies that demonstrate objective clinical neurological improvements during placebo treatments underscore the interface, overlap, and likely shared biochemical mechanisms between phenomena traditionally segregated with comfort into neurology or psychiatry *(20)*. These scientific and patient-based realizations by both neurologists and psychiatrists bridge a gap that was formulated very early in the fields' histories and could not be fully reconciled by administrators or official credentialing bodies. As such, the preparation of this volume is founded in medical science and justifies itself on a shared, mutually beneficial current working relationship between psychiatrists and neurologists. It is tempting to consider the historical antagonism and discomfort between American neurology and psychiatry as dissipated with these developments, but in the author's view, old traditions tend to show their residual effects in continuing although subtle ways. This chapter therefore is written not only as an historical backdrop for the other chapters of this volume but is offered so that neither the past is forgotten nor its traditions minimized.

REFERENCES

1. Rosen G. The Specialization of Medicine. New York, NY: Arno Press; 1972.
2. Ackerknecht IH. Medicine at the Paris Hospital 1794–1848. Baltimore: Johns Hopkins University Press; 1967.
3. Gardner AK. Old Wine in New Bottles: Or Spare Hours of a Student in Paris. New York: Francis Company; 1848.
4. Goetz CG. History of the American Neurological Association in celebration of the 125th anniversary: tempus et hora: time and the hour. Ann Neurol 2003;53(Suppl 4):S1–S45.

5. Goetz CG, Bonduelle M, Gelfand T. Charcot: Constructing Neurology. New York: Oxford University Press; 1995.
6. Hirschmuller A. The development of psychiatry and neurology in the nineteenth century. Hist Psychiatry 1999;10:395–423.
7. Griesinger W. Vorwort. Archiv für Psychiatrie und Nervenkrankheiten1868;1:i–viii.
8. Tyler HR, Tyler KL. Charles Edouard Brown-Séquard: professor of physiology and pathology of the nervous system at Harvard Medical School. Neurology 1984;34:1231–1236.
9. Goetz CG, Pappert EJ. Early American professorships in neurology. Ann Neurol 1996;40:258–263.
10. Tucker BR. Speaking of Weir Mitchell. Am J Psychiatry 1936;93:341–346.
11. Brody EB. The Journal of Nervous and Mental Disease: the first 100 years. J Nerv Ment Dis 1974;158:6–17 and 1974;159: 1–11.
12. Denny-Brown D. Centennial Anniversary Volume of the American Neurological Association. New York, NY: Springer; 1975.
13. Goetz CG. Poor Beard!! Charcot's internationalization of neurasthenia, the "American disease." Neurology 2001;57: 510–514.
14. Channing W. The history of the Boston Society of Psychiatry and Neurology for 25 years. Bost Med Surg J 1905;152: 387–393.
15. Mackay RP. The history of neurology in Chicago. J Int Coll Surg 1963;40:191–205.
16. Weisenburg TH. The founders and work of the Philadelphia Neurological Society. J Nerv Ment Dis 1915;42:419–440.
17. DeJong RN. A History of American Neurology. New York: Raven Press; 1982.
18. Hamon M, Gorwood P. Psychopharmacogenetics. New York: Klüwer; 2005.
19. Factor SA, Podskalny GD, Molho ES. Psychogenic movement disorders: frequency, clinical profile, and characteristics. J Neurol Neurosurg Psychiatry 1995;59:406–412.
20. De la Fuente-Fernandez R, Ruth TJ, Sossi V, Stoessl AJ. Expectation and dopamine release: mechanism of the placebo effect in PD. Science 2001;293:1164–1166.

2

The Evolution of Psychiatry and Neurology

Two Disciplines Divided by a Common Goal?

François Boller and Gianfranco Dalla Barba

INTRODUCTION

This chapter traces the evolution of psychiatry and neurology with special emphasis placed on the European scene. For a long time, there was hardly any distinction between these two disciplines that are now considered quite separate. They started together and they may well be in the process of reuniting, particularly in certain domains. We may see, and as the Germans say, *Zukunft in der Vergangenheit* (translation: the past is probably holding the key to the future.)

It is nearly impossible to state when neurology and psychiatry were "born," but most historians hypothesize that scientific interest in the brain and mind—which had always existed—developed and reached a critical mass in Europe in the late 18th and early 19th centuries. As pointed out elsewhere *(1)*, for much of the 19th and even parts of the 20th century, many persons practiced not only neurology and psychiatry including, in some cases, psychoanalysis—but also neuropathology. One could go even farther and extend the "boundaries" of the disciplines. For instance, the founders of neurosurgery in France, Thierry de Martel and Clovis Vincent—who was first trained as a neurologist and gained a special fame of sort for having operated on Ravel *(2)*—first developed their neurosurgical practice within the context of the Neurology service of the Salpêtrière, then directed by Joseph Babinski *(3)*. As for neuroradiology, some of its pioneers like Arthur Schueller in Vienna and Egas Moniz in Lisbon were neuropsychiatrists *(4)*. Many of the founders of psychiatry and neurology practiced both disciplines. Among some of those who come to mind is Jean-Martin Charcot, whom Sigmund Freud visited for a few months because of his interest in neuroanatomy and neurophysiology. Charcot is often considered one of the founding fathers of neurology, but a considerable portion of his activity related to conditions that are considered "typically" psychiatric such as hysteria. The famous painting representing the Master during one of his lectures *(5)*, shows a female patient, known by her first name (Blanche) and her nickname *Reine des hystériques* (Fig. 1). As stated by Wechsler *(6)*, Charcot's studies of hysteria laid much of the groundwork for Janet and Freud, both his pupils.

Alois Alzheimer, now best known for the clinical and neuropathological description of the disease that bears his name, was also a very versatile person with considerable achievements in both neurology and psychiatry *(7)*. Much of his work was dedicated to cerebrovascular diseases and neurosyphilis. Figure 2 shows Alzheimer and, next to him Emil Kraepelin, the then head of the laboratory. Kraepelin authored nine editions of a textbook, of psychiatry that was for many years the leading reference for the discipline. In addition to Alzheimer and Kraepelin, one also finds people who became famous in the fields of neurology and neuropathology, such as Gaetano Perusini and Friedrich Lewy (of Lewy

From: *Current Clinical Neurology: Psychiatry for Neurologists*
Edited by: D.V. Jeste and J.H. Friedman © Humana Press Inc., Totowa, NJ

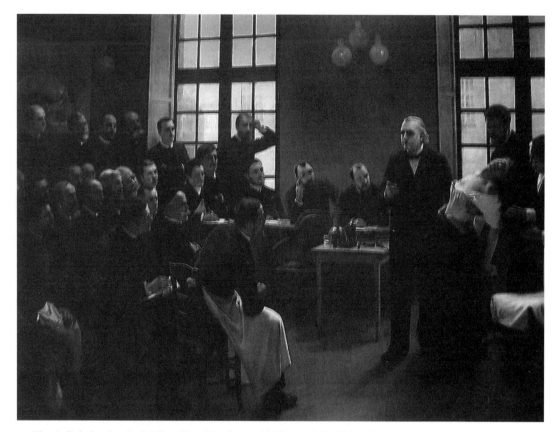

Fig. 1. Painting by André Brouillet: Une leçon de Charcot à La Salpêtrière. Contrary to what is sometimes stated, Freund does not appear in the painting.

bodies fame) (Fig. 2). There is also Ugo Cerletti, who was later to introduce, together with Luciano Bini, electroshock therapy. Much of Alzheimer's career developed in psychiatric institutions. In the early years of the *Zeitschrift fur Neurologie und Psychiatrie* (now the *Journal of Neurology*), the person in charge of the psychiatric section was Alois Alzheimer, whereas the neurology section was edited by M. Lewandowsky.

Henry Charlton Bastian, one of the founders of neurology in the United Kingdom, was a professor of pathologic anatomy and dedicated much of his work toward neuroanatomy and to finding ways of improving neurological diagnosis. He also worked on hysteria (which he called a "neurosis") and considered his book "the brain as an organ of mind" as his greatest work *(8)*. Throughout the years, many persons who considered themselves "alienists" sought an accommodation with neurology. Berrios *(9)* includes Wernicke, von Monakow, and Liepmann among these major figures. A very important step for both psychiatry and neurology took place when Julius Wagner von Jauregg introduced a physical treatment (malarial fever) for the treatment of "general paresis of the insane," a condition long thought to be psychiatric in nature. For that discovery he was awarded the Nobel Prize for Physiology and Medicine in 1927, the first of an extremely short list of psychiatrists to have received such distinction *(10)*.

There is a distinct difference in the historical relations between psychiatry and neurology in different parts of the world. In eastern and central Europe, the two were merged for a long time with often a predominance of psychiatry. For instance, in the mid-1970s, the head of the Neuropsychiatry Department of the famous Charité Hospital in Berlin was a psychiatrist. The young Sigmund Freud, before and even after his stay in Charcot's department had long been interested in basic neurosciences, in clinical neu-

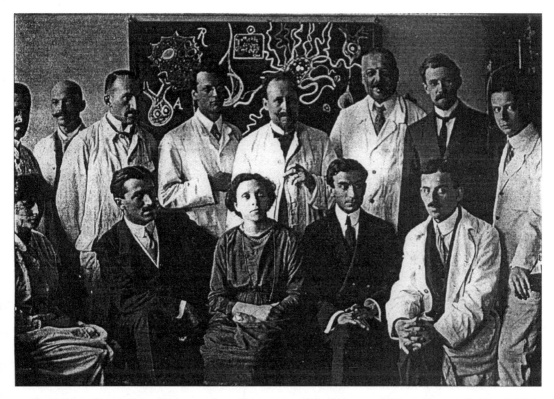

Fig. 2. Alois Alzheimer and his co-workers. Top row from left, F. Lotmar; N.N.; S. Rosenthal; Allers?; N.N.; A. Alzheimer; N. Achucarro; F.H. Lewy. Front row from left: Mrs. Grombach; U. Cerletti; N.N.; F. Bonfiglio; G. Perusini. This photograph was taken in Alois Alzheimer's laboratory on the second floor of the Nervenklinik Nussbaumstraße in Munich during 1909 or 1910, and not, as erroneously stated on the original legend, at the Deutsche Forschungsanstalt für Psychiatric which was founded only years later. It is often stated (even in this text) that the person in the center holding a cigar is Kraepelin. There is, however, no evidence that this is the case. (Courtesy of B. Lucci, MD and F. Vinci, MD.)

rology and even in neuropsychology and his "Essay on Aphasia" *(11)* is still very much worth reading. In Japan, on the other hand, the two disciplines did not develop together because neurology was for a long time a branch of internal medicine. The situations in Italy and France are considered below. Joseph Martin recently examined the historical basis for the divergence of neurology and psychiatry over the past century *(12)*. He states that neurology and psychiatry have, for much of the past century, been separated by "an artificial wall created by the divergence of their philosophical approaches and research and treatment methods." It can be argued, however, that this separation, in some cases, was also a result of opportunism and politics. In this respect, it is interesting to consider the way in which, in the United States, the *Archives of Neurology and Psychiatry* separated. In the first issue of the *Archives of Neurology*, editor Harold Wolff defined the aims of the journal without a word about the previous association. Roy Grinker Sr., editor of the *American Medical Association Archives of General Psychiatry* stated in the first issue *(13)* "that decision was based on realistic recognition that neuropsychiatry has become separated into neurology and psychiatry as distinct clinical specialties." He added, however, that the decision was also based on the need for both disciplines to be able to publish more papers.

It is certain that for a long time thereafter, in the Anglo-Saxon world, except for some exceptions reviewed by Goetz in the previous chapter, the two disciplines ignored each other, when they were not in open conflict. It is interesting in this respect to read the words written as recently as 1975 by MacDonald Critchley. Critchley was a British neurologist, for many years head of the National Institute for Neurological Diseases (known as Queen Square), and the author of many books related to neurology and neuropsychology *(14)*. In an essay in which he outlined the "training of a neurologist" *(15)* he wrote, among the recommendations to the proper neurologist (who of course could only be a male) that "if throughout his nine year apprenticeship, he could fit in a spell as a part-time clinical assistant in a psychiatric clinic, so much the better." He added, "personally, I do not feel that neurology should be oriented towards psychiatry. A neuropsychologist is far less of an anomaly than a neuropsychiatrist." In Italy, psychiatry and neurology were traditionally studied together and in some cases are still part of one department. When the chair of neurology position was created at the University of Padua in the early 1950s, it was attributed to Giovanni Battista Belloni who, up to that time, had mainly practiced psychiatry. Some of his assistants were encouraged to develop neurosurgery and one of them, Sergio Dalle Ore, was the co-author of Terzian in the first description of a human case of the Klüver-Bucy syndrome *(16)*. Franco Basaglia who, together with some colleagues, revolutionized the practice of psychiatry in Italy by opening up all the closed wards, was initially trained as a neurologist. In France, until the "cultural revolution" of May 1968, psychiatry and neurology had strong ties, but on the whole the field was very much dominated by neurology. Not uncommonly, one of the departments of Sainte Anne, the major psychiatric hospital in Paris, was chaired by a neurologist for whom no other position had been found. As a result, all of the psychiatrists who trained there had experience in both clinical neurology and neuropathology. That is why an early description of progressive supranuclear palsy is co-signed by the then young Jacques Lacan *(17)*. Psychiatry and neurology are now quite separate and autonomous disciplines, but their close ties remain. Pierre Pichot, who was president of the World Psychiatric Association in 1977, wrote several articles clearly related to neurology and neuropsychology, one of which *(18)* was intended to inspire further work *(19)*. Henry Hécaen, one of the founders of modern neuropsychology *(20)*, had initially been trained as a psychiatrist and worked at Sainte-Anne in close cooperation with psychiatrists, neurologists, and neurosurgeons. Similarly, Julian de Ajuriaguerra trained at Sainte-Anne and became an expert in both fields. Two international journals currently published out of Sainte-Anne show a clear distinction between the two disciplines. *L'Encéphale*, founded in 1906, was initially dedicated to both, but is now almost exclusively focused on psychiatry, as indicated by its subtitle—*Journal of Clinical, Biological, and Therapeutic Psychiatry*. The other journal, the *European Journal of Neurology (21)* has two psychiatrists on its editorial board, but the number of psychiatry-related articles submitted to the journal remains very small. A new journal, entitled *Psychologie & NeuroPsychiatrie du Vieillissement (22)*, edited by Christian Derouesné, aims to bridge the gap between neurology and psychiatry.

There are at least three areas of research where psychiatry and neurology are clearly coming together. The first is pharmacology. Since the 1950s, progress in neurotransmitter research has contributed significantly to a true convergence of the two disciplines *(23)*. Taking depression as an example, future research will require developing better animal models of mood disorders, identifying genetic determinants of normal and abnormal mood in humans and animals, discovering novel targets and biomarkers of mood disorders and treatments, and increasing the recruitment of investigators from diverse backgrounds to mood disorder research *(24)*. The second is physiology. The startling mood effects that deep brain stimulation sometimes has on people with Parkinson's disease, as well as the dramatic success ablative surgery has had in otherwise intractable cases of obsessive-compulsive disorder clearly underscores the "organicity" of behavior. The third is the overlap in the study of the dementias where behavioral aspects are so prominent, in addition to the memory and cognitive aspects. We have already seen that Hécaen and Ajuriaguerra, who are among the founders of modern neuropsychology, were initially trained as psychiatrists. In North America, the field was led by Norman Geschwind and was, for a long time, essentially in the hands of neurologists who, in fact, re-baptized the discipline "behavioral neurology." Now, however, people from different backgrounds are happily working together. The successes of societies such as the British Neuropsychiatry Association *(25)* and the Society of Child

Neuropsychiatry in Italy *(26)* are examples of that cooperation. One can predict that in years to come, there will be increasing collaboration and integration between the two fields and that other subdisciplines will join neuropsychology (behavioral neurology) and neuropharmacology as examples of this new entente.

REFERENCES

1. Boller F, Duyckaerts C. 1914 to 1917: the Great War years. Arch Neurol 1999;56:882–885.
2. Amaducci L, Grassi E, Boller F. Maurice Ravel and right-hemisphere musical creativity: influence of disease on his last musical works? Eur J Neurol 2002;9:75–82.
3. Poirier J. History of Neurosciences at La Pitié and La Salpêtrière 2004.
4. Alper MG. Three pioneers in the early history of neuroradiology: the Snyder lecture. Doc Ophthalmol 1999;98:29–49.
5. Signoret JL. "A Clinical Lesson at the Salpetriere" (1887) by Andre Brouillet. Rev Neurol (Paris) 1983;139:687–701.
6. Wechsler I. Jean Martin Charcot (1825–1893). In: Haymaker W, Schiller F, eds. The Founders of Neurology.) Springfield: Charles C. Thomas; 1970.
7. Maurer K, Maurer U, Levi N. Alzheimer: The Life of a Physician and the Career of a Disease. New York: Columbia University Press; 2003.
8. Kalinowsky L, Henry Charlton Bastian. In: Haymaker W, Schiller F, eds. The Founders of Neurology. Springfield: Charles C. Thomas;1970:405–407.
9. Berrios GE, Markova IS. The concept of neuropsychiatry: a historical overview. J Psychosom Res 2002;53:629–638.
10. Dattner B, von Jauregg JW. In: Haymaker W, Schiller F, eds. The Founders of Neurology. Springfield: Charles C. Thomas; 1970:528–531.
11. Freud S. Zur Auffassung der Aphasien: eine kritische Studie. Leipzig: Deuticke; 1891.
12. Martin JB. The integration of neurology, psychiatry, and neuroscience in the 21st century. Am J Psychiatry 2002;159:695–704.
13. Grinker R. Editorial. AMA Arch Gen Psych 1959;1:1–2.
14. Critchley M. The Parietal Lobes. New York: Hafner Publishing Company; 1966.
15. Critchley M. The training of a neurologist. Int J Neurol 1975;9:.
16. Terzian H, Dalle Ore S. Syndrome of Klüver and Bucy reproduced in man by bilateral removal of the temporal lobes. Neurology 1955;5:373–380.
17. Alajouanine T, Delafontaine P, Lacan J. Fixité du regard par hypertonie prédominant dans le sens vertical avec conservation des mouvements automatico-réflexes, aspect spécial de syndrome de Parinaud par hypertonie associée a un syndrome extrapyramidal avec troubles pseudobulbaires. Revue Neurologique 1926;2:410–418.
18. Pichot P. Language disturbances in cerebral disease. Arch Neurol Psych 1955;74:92–96.
19. Boller F, Vignolo AL. Latent sensory aphasia in hemisphere damaged patients: an experimental study with the Token Test. Brain 1966;89:815–830.
20. Boller F. History of the International Neuropsychology Symposium: a mirror of the evolution of a discipline. Neuropsychologia 1999;37:17–26.
21. European Journal of Neurology, 2004; Available at: http://www.blackwellpublishing.com/journal.asp?ref=1351-5101. 2004.
22. Psychologie & NeuroPsychiatrie du Vieillissement, 2004; Available at: http://www.john-libbey-eurotext.fr/fr/revues/medecine/pnv/sommaire.md
23. Carlsson A. A half-century of neurotransmitter research: impact on neurology and psychiatry (Nobel lecture). Chembiochem 2001;2:484–493.
24. Nestler EJ, Gould E, Manji H, et al. Preclinical models: status of basic research in depression. Biol Psychiatry 2002;52:503–528.
25. British Neuropsychiatry Association, 2004; Available at: http://www.bnpa.org.uk/Execcommittee.htm
26. Society of Child Neuropsychiatry, 2004; Available at: http://www.childneurology.it/

II Evaluation

3

Psychiatric Evaluation of the Neurological Patient

Stephen Salloway, Colin Harrington, and Sandra Jacobson

INTRODUCTION

Symptoms of anxiety, depression, and abnormal behavior are commonly seen in patients with neurological disorders. Screening for psychiatric symptoms is an important part of the evaluation of neurological patients. Many nonpsychiatric clinicians feel uncomfortable with psychiatric history-taking and examination. The goal of this chapter is to provide a concise overview of essential components of the psychiatric evaluation of neurological patients for practicing clinicians, residents, and medical students. This chapter discusses the process of taking a psychiatric history, the organization of the psychiatric examination, and the major psychiatric syndromes that should be reviewed as part of a comprehensive neuropsychiatric assessment.

PSYCHIATRIC HISTORY

Psychiatric history-taking and examination should be seen as a core part of the assessment of neurological patients. The history should be obtained from the patient and in most cases from one or more knowledgeable informants, as many patients will have difficulty reporting reliably on the extent and nature of their behavioral problems because of cognitive or emotional factors. The psychiatric history should be organized like that of any other medical-surgical specialty. The patient and any corroborating sources of history should be asked about the chief complaint. Onset, duration, and quality of symptoms should be determined. Triggering and exacerbating factors and associated symptoms should be explored. A detailed medication history should be obtained with special attention to current and prior treatment with psychoactive medications. The physical diagnosis maxim that directs the physician to "look, listen, and feel" is particularly relevant to the neuropsychiatric examination. The neuropsychiatric evaluation is marked by an important interplay between patient and examiner. When inquiring about the patient's mood, it is important to note not only the content of the patient's answer but the affect, speech, gesture, choice of words, and psychomotor speed used to convey his/her answer. When performing a cognitive assessment, it is important to note word-finding difficulties, confabulation, use of compensatory cognitive strategies, and pauses and delays in answering questions, as well as the content and correctness of the patient's answers. For example, when exploring symptoms of anxiety, it is crucial to note the quality of voice, the presence of tremor, fidgetiness, and compulsive or repetitive behaviors of the patient during the evaluation.

From: *Current Clinical Neurology: Psychiatry for Neurologists*
Edited by: D.V. Jeste and J.H. Friedman © Humana Press Inc., Totowa, NJ

Psychiatric syndromes are contextually bound by medical and developmental history. Possible relationships between the onset of psychiatric symptoms and past medical events should be explored. Past psychiatric history is of particular importance. The neurologist must be adept at eliciting psychiatric history and reviewing psychiatric symptoms. It is often helpful to establish the patient's premorbid baseline behavioral style or temperament. This allows a more accurate measurement of index behavior and symptoms as a change from this baseline. The examiner can ask, simply and unassumingly, "Are you basically a quiet (reserved, boisterous, talkative, garrulous, or guarded) person? Do you tend to stick to yourself? If so, would you call yourself shy or do you choose to be alone? Do other people know you as a social and outgoing person? Do you tend to be careful or a little on guard about interactions with other people? Would you or others say you have a temper? Does it ever get you into a bind or into trouble? Are you typically blue or do you see the glass as half empty? Would you say that you're the anxious type?" History of prior psychiatric evaluation and treatment must be explored. Past psychiatric diagnoses should be clarified. History of inpatient, as well as outpatient, treatment should be assessed. Psychotropic medication treatment trials, their indications, target symptoms, doses, duration, benefits, and side effects should all be documented. Suicidal thinking and attempts are encountered in many neurological diseases including stroke, multiple sclerosis, traumatic brain injury, amyotrophic lateral sclerosis, and dementia (especially Huntington's disease). Past psychiatric history and review of symptoms must therefore include an assessment of suicidal ideation and behavior. Patients should be asked forthrightly about symptoms of suicide. Violent behaviors directed against others can also be seen in these and other neurological diseases. The examiner should ask the patient, family, and significant others about erratic, disinhibited, and violent behaviors. If there is any question of significant violent behavior, the examiner should attend to his/her safety during the examination. Common safety measures include leaving the door slightly ajar, situating oneself between the patient and the door for egress as needed, arranging for security to be present, and using restraints when indicated.

Many psychiatric syndromes bear a relationship to developmental and social history. Developmental history should include information, if available, about pregnancy, delivery, prolonged hospital stays in infancy and childhood, and achievement of language and motor milestones. School performance, tutoring, special testing or education, and final grade completed should be documented. Peer-group interaction and social behavior should be assessed. Participation in hobbies, athletics, and other extracurricular activities can offer insight into social and cognitive abilities. Occupational history and, if appropriate, time spent in the armed services should be explored as they can provide insights into general function in adult life.

Marital and parental status should be documented. Composition of the home should be clarified including living arrangements and relationships with spouse, children, parents, siblings, grandparents, and extended family members. The patient should be asked about physical, verbal, and sexual abuse if it appears clinically relevant.

Illicit substances can have profound effects on mood, cognition, and behavior. For this reason, substance abuse and dependence must be assessed. Whereas patients may at times be ashamed of and/or reluctant to volunteer information about substance use, the examiner should have no compunction about reviewing this history. Patients should be asked directly about use and abuse patterns of illicit substances, both past and present. Types of drugs (cocaine and stimulants, opiates, ethanol, hallucinogens, cannabis, etc.) and routes of drug use should be documented. History of detoxification and other substance treatment should be reviewed. Indeed, prior alcohol detoxification is a risk factor for complicated alcohol withdrawal syndromes such as delirium tremens. Risk factors and prior testing for human immunodeficiency virus (HIV) such as sharing needles, multiple sexual partners, male homosexual contact, and exposure to HIV-positive individuals should be explored if clinically indicated.

Patients and physicians are often uncomfortable discussing sexual histories. Because patients are often reluctant to volunteer symptoms of sexual dysfunction, it is incumbent on the examiner to approach the sexual history in a confident and straightforward fashion. Patients are frequently pleased that the physician has broken the ice to discuss concerning but embarrassing sexual symptoms. Patients can be asked, "Many patients whom I see complain of problems with sexual function. Has this been a problem for you?" Once introduced as an area to be explored, the patient should be asked about sexual orientation, sexual abuse (if indicated) pain associated with sexual activity, libido, arousal, and orgasmic capacity. The timing of onset of sexual problems to the use of medications, such as serotonin reuptake inhibitors, should be determined because many psychotropic agents can cause decreased libido, erectile dysfunction, and orgasmic delay. Issues of safe sex can be discussed as well, providing a component of preventative medicine in the initial evaluation.

Many psychiatric and neurological diseases have a genetic component. Elaboration of family history of neuropsychiatric symptoms and disease can be very helpful in guiding differential diagnosis and treatment. Rates of dementia, depression, anxiety, and schizophrenia are increased in first-degree family members of patients with these disorders. Attention to familial patterns of mood, motor, cognitive, and behavioral symptoms can aid in the diagnosis of these and other neuropsychiatric disorders. Treatment response in genetic family members with similar symptoms or diagnoses should also be documented. Response to psychotropic medications of family members, with regard to both beneficial and adverse effects, can sometimes predict response of the patient to similar agents.

Mood disorders are marked by discrete episodes of depressive or manic spectrum signs and symptoms. Patients who experience only depressive spectrum symptoms are diagnosed as having a unipolar depressive disorder. Patients who experience both manic and depressive spectrum symptoms are diagnosed with bipolar disorder. Depressive symptoms include sad or depressed mood, lack of energy (anergia), reduced interest or involvement in pleasurable activities (anhedonia), constricted sense of the future, hopelessness, helplessness, feelings of guilt, changes in vegetative functions of sleep, appetite, and sexual behavior, and suicidal ideation. Aggressive, irritable, and labile affect and behaviors are accepted criteria in the diagnosis of child and adolescent depression. Patients must experience symptoms for at least 2 weeks to meet criteria for a major depressive episode. Patients who experience depressive symptoms that are chronic (>2 years) and subsyndromal are diagnosed as dysthymic.

Patients should be asked if they are depressed. If patients volunteer a history of depression, they should be asked what they mean by the use of the word "depression." Patients should be offered other terms that they or the examiner might equate with depression including sad, blue, or down. After establishing the patient's core mood state, the examiner should evaluate for the presence or absence of associated depressive symptoms such as loss of interest in usual activities, change in appetite or weight, difficulty sleeping, change in libido, and physical symptoms.

PSYCHOTIC DISORDERS

Psychosis is a syndrome comprised of symptoms of hallucinations, delusions, thought disorder, and disorganized behavior. Psychotic symptoms can occur across a wide range of neuropsychiatric syndromes ranging from schizophrenia in younger patients to dementia in the elderly. Perhaps more than any other psychiatric symptoms, those of psychosis need to be considered in the broader context of medical, neurological, and psychiatric illness to ensure accurate diagnosis and proper treatment. Although it is at times difficult to distinguish between normal and pathological mood and anxiety states, psychotic symptoms always represent aberrant experience.

New-onset psychotic symptoms should be approached as a mental status change. Generally speaking, psychotic symptoms in the elderly represent encephalopathy, delirium, or dementia, until proven otherwise. Psychotic symptoms occur commonly in dementia syndromes including Alzheimer's disease, Parkinson's disease, and Dementia with Lewy Bodies. Documentation of a history of cognitive dysfunction and/or functional decline is, thus, diagnostically very important. Clarification of baseline cognitive function is crucial in the evaluation of more acute onset psychotic symptoms that suggest a delirium.

Psychotic symptoms often generate significant fear, confusion, and agitation. When possible, especially in the patient with delirium or dementia, it is helpful to explain to the patient the nature of brain-based sensory misperception, cognitive misprocessing, and misattribution of cause and meaning of events in the environment that lead to hallucinations and delusions. This effort at education and appeal to patient insight can provide understanding, reassurance that the patient is "not crazy," and evidence that his/her otherwise strange and foreign experience is familiar to and treatable by the examiner.

Patients may report discrete episodes of abnormal behavior that range from panic attacks to dissociative episodes. Information about the frequency, duration, and pattern of these events and any known precipitants should be obtained from the patient and a knowledgeable informant. The neurologist should ask the patient to describe a typical event from beginning to end with corroboration from individuals who have witnessed the event. Patients with panic attacks may describe experiences of depersonalization where they feel disconnected from their body, or derealization, "spaciness" or altered perception where they feel disconnected from their surroundings. These symptoms are often difficult for the patient to describe and can be difficult to elicit as well. Patients can be asked, "When you get these episodes of anxiety do you ever feel weird or get the sense that things around you aren't 'quite right', distorted in size, too fast, or too slow?".

Neurologists and psychiatrists frequently encounter patients whose subjective complaints cannot be adequately explained by objective examination findings. A disparity between subjective symptoms and objective examination is common to a number of psychiatric diagnoses including somatoform disorders (somatization disorder, somatoform pain disorders, and hypochondriasis), conversion disorder, factitious disorder, and malingering. Patients with hypochondriasis are often very concerned with the meaning and significance of their symptoms. Hypochondriacal patients are preoccupied with the worry that they have a serious disease based on misinterpretation of symptoms. Conversion disorder patients typically present with neurological deficit symptoms such as numbness, weakness, blindness, mutism, and/or a change in level of consciousness that are either nonanatomic or unexplained by diagnostic studies. Disparity between patient complaints and diagnostic tests can cause frustration for the physician. The evaluation of symptoms that lack a clear physiological basis should be direct and thorough. A review of psychosocial stressors and evaluation for the presence of anxiety or depressive symptoms that may relate to the somatic presentation should be sought. The results of the evaluation should be reviewed sensitively and openly with the patient and the patient's family.

Patients should be asked directly about memory problems. Patients may have limited insight into cognitive dysfunction and it is important to query family about changes in the patient's memory and behavior and the degree to which these symptoms interfere with the patient's daily functioning. Families often describe a patient's excellent recall of remote events and thus report that the patient does not have problems with memory. Often, mild depression and irritability may be the first sign of a degenerative disorder such as Alzheimer's disease.

Axis II diagnoses, known as personality disorders, refer to long-standing maladaptive patterns of behavior that interfere with interpersonal relationships and general function *(1)*. A common feature of axis II personality disorders is an oversensitivity and vigilance to real or perceived interpersonal slight. Patients with a personality disorder are often on guard for any signal or suggestion of frustration, anger, mistrust, or other negative emotions on the part of the examiner. When these patients feel slighted or misunderstood, they frequently respond with anger, righteousness, defensiveness, and accusations of mistreatment. If a patient with a personality disorder responds angrily and with accusations to a perceived slight that was unintended or of which a physician is unaware, it may catch the physician off guard and the physician may reflexively respond with anger of his/her own. When this occurs, the patient with limited insight into his/her own proactive behavior may interpret the physician's angry response as further evidence of the earlier assumed mistreatment. It is important that the examiner be attentive to the patient's interpersonal style and resist provocation.

PSYCHIATRIC EXAMINATION

The components of the psychiatric examination include the following, in the order in which they are described in a formal case presentation:

- Appearance and behavior
- Motor activity
- Mood and affect
- Speech and language
- Thought content
- Perception
- Insight and judgment
- Attention and orientation
- Memory and other cortical functions

The following are important points for conducting and interpreting the psychiatric examination. First, the patient's level of arousal must be adequate for evaluating cognition and behavior. Second, the examiner must interpret cognitive results in light of the patient's level of education and socioeconomic background. Third, the patient's best response is the most valid. Therefore, the examiner must make every reasonable effort to ensure a proper environment for testing. The examination should be stopped if the patient becomes noticeably fatigued.

Appearance and Behavior

What the examiner observes about the patient in terms of appearance and behavior contributes significantly to the differential diagnosis. Observations begin the moment the examiner meets the patient, and continue throughout history-taking and examination. It is important that the examiner be able to clearly describe and communicate his/her observations.

Useful observations are those describing characteristics such as the following:

- *Body type:* for example, Pickwickian in the patient with obstructive sleep apnea, emaciated in the anorexic or cancer patient.
- *Physical stigmata:* "Bat" ears of Fragile X syndrome, wrist scars from self-injury in borderline patients.
- *Posture:* Stooped posture of subcortical dementia, rigid posture of PSP, slumped posture of the depressed patient.
- *Bearing:* Aggressiveness in the manic patient, haughtiness in the narcissistic patient, self-effacement of the phobic or avoidant patient.
- *Attire:* Disheveled appearance or inappropriate dress (coats in hot weather) can be characteristic of the schizophrenic or demented patient, outlandish or risqué dress of the manic patient, and bizarre appearance of the schizophrenic patient (corks in the ears, ties worn around the arms).
- *Grooming:* Unwashed, unshaved, uncombed, dirty appearance can be characteristic of the schizophrenic patient, or (to a lesser degrees) of the depressed or demented patient. Poor dentition can be characteristic of chronic mental illness.
- *Level of alertness or vigilance:* Can be decreased in acute confusional states, vigilance can be increased in patients with obsessive compulsive disorder.
- *Level of comfort:* Can be low in the anxious or psychotic patient.
- *Ambulation status:* Refusal to walk can be characteristic of geriatric depression, temporary paralysis is also seen in conversion syndromes.
- *Unusual or repetitive behaviors:* Head-banging in the autistic patient, overfamiliarity with the doctor in the patient with frontal lobe dementia or mania; frequent checking outside the exam room door in the paranoid patient.

Motor Activity

To supplement information obtained in the course of the neurological examination, observations regarding the patient's motor activity are made during the evaluation. Posture and gait are observed as the patient enters the examination room. Abnormal movements, including tremor, chorea, dystonia, tics, mannerisms, and stereotypic movements, which are repetitive, seemingly driven, nonfunctional motor behaviors (e.g., head-banging), are noted.

Motor activity exhibited can be unusually increased or decreased in amount. Increased motor activity may be manifest by distractibility, restlessness, fidgeting, changing positions, jumping, shouting, or screaming. Hyperactivity and agitation are terms often used to describe increased motor activity. Increased motor activity is seen in various psychiatric conditions, including delirium, acute psychosis, mania, agitated depression, and drug-induced states. Aggression is a more extreme form of increased motor activity that may be verbal or physical in nature. Often, verbal aggression is the harbinger of physical aggression. Physical aggression may be directed towards objects or toward people. Escalating aggression should never be ignored, even in a seemingly safe or benign medical setting.

Reduced motor activity may be manifest by stooped or slumped posture, bowed head, abnormal stillness, slowness, delay of initiation of movement, early stopping of a movement initiated by the examiner, averting gaze, closing eyes, turning head away, or turning back to the examiner. Reduced motor activity may be seen as a manifestation of the negative symptoms of schizophrenia, depression, delirium, catatonia, or drug-induced states.

Psychomotor retardation consists of slowness in speech, movement, and thinking. When echopraxia is present the patient spontaneously mimics the movements of the examiner. Extreme examples of decreased movements are catalepsy and waxy flexibility in which the patient maintains his/her limbs in postures initiated by the examiner for extended periods.

Tardive dyskinesia is a hyperkinetic syndrome commonly seen among patients with chronic psychiatric illness, particularly those who have had long-term treatment with conventional antipsychotic medications. Clinically, patients may present with mouthing, chewing, puckering, smacking, sucking, licking, or other orolingual movements. Choreic movements of limbs may also be seen, especially distally. Speech abnormalities can include slowed rate, loss of intelligibility, and impaired phonation. The presence of these abnormal motor findings may provide an important clue that a patient has a chronic psychiatric condition. Tardive dyskinesia can be rated using standardized scales such as the Abnormal Involuntary Movement Scale *(2)*.

Akathisia is a subjective feeling of restlessness with the irresistible urge to move. Observed behaviors consist of pacing, stomping, tapping, running, and crossing/uncrossing of the legs. It particularly affects the lower extremities. Akathisia is a common side effect of neuroleptic medications, and can occur acutely, subacutely, or as a tardive (late-appearing) syndrome.

Affect and Mood

Both affect and mood contribute significantly to the patient's mental status profile, and frequently form the core of the diagnostic impression. Mood refers to the patient's subjectively experienced emotional state, whereas affect is what is observable by others. The examiner makes observations about affect, and the patient is questioned directly about mood. In general, mood is more stable than affect. Congruence (agreement) between mood and affect is the rule, except in certain pathological conditions such as pseudobulbar states, or in some types of schizophrenic exacerbation. Patients differ in their ability to sense and report their own emotions or moods. The complete inability to do so is termed "alexithymia." The experienced clinician will use his/her own feelings as a gauge to help determine a patient's internal state. The hostile patient may engender anger, the depressed patient sadness, the chaotic patient disorganization, and the elated patient laughter.

Affect and mood are characterized by the following:

- *Range:* The degree to which affect varies from a baseline. Normal affect spans a range that includes positive (happy) and negative (sad) elements, depending on the content of speech. Using a visual analog scale of mood (happy–sad) is an easy way for patients to rate their mood *(3)*, especially for patients with aphasia.
     Common terms used to describe mood:
          depressed—pathological feeling of sadness.
          dysphoric—unpleasant
          elevated—more cheerful and confident than usual
          euphoric—intense elation, with feelings of grandeur
          expansive—feelings expressed without restraint; often associated with overestimation of one's importance
          euthymic—healthy, balanced mood (not depressed or elevated) with normal range

> dysthymic—persistence of low grade depressed mood that does not meet criteria for major depression
>
> melancholic—profoundly depressed mood state that is usually associated with vegetative symptoms of impaired appetite and sleep, and psychomotor slowing.

- *Intensity:* Describes how extreme the affect appears, from shallow to intense. Affect characterized by reduced intensity is said to be "blunted." Flattened affect denotes the absence of affective expression. Restricted or constricted affect describe a reduction in range and intensity of affect.
- *Stability:* Affect is stable in healthy individuals with normal variability in response to environmental demands. Labile affect, in contrast, is highly variable and rapidly shifting, often with minimal provocation from events in the patient's environment.
- *Appropriateness:* How well affect matches the content of speech or thought. Inappropriate affect can be found in patients with psychotic states, frontal lobe dysfunction, somatoform disorders (la belle indifference), or certain personality disorders such as antisocial personality. Relatedness: how the patient interacts with the examiner or others. Lack of relatedness characterizes disorders such as autism and paranoid states.

The depressed individual may present with one or more of the following features: distressed appearance of facial muscles (frowning, squinting, down-turned corners of the mouth), poor eye contact, stooped posture, tearfulness, choking up when talking, frequent sighing, irritability, oppositional behavior, and negative content of speech. It can be challenging to evaluate depressive symptoms in patients with neurological illnesses such as Parkinson's disease and myasthenia gravis because the expression of affect may be blunted by bradykinesia and facial weakness. It is important to ask these patients directly about their mood and symptoms of depression.

Depression can be distinguished from apathy by the presence of neurovegetative signs (insomnia, anorexia, loss of libido), dysphoria, and psychological symptoms (guilt, hopelessness, low self-esteem) in depression. The apathetic patient appears indifferent rather than distressed *(4)*. Apathy can be found in association with abulia, which is loss of spontaneity manifested by motor slowing, loss of initiative, and lack of effort. At times, abulic patients will not respond to questions or commands, or will respond only intermittently.

The manic patient is readily recognized by elevated, euphoric, expansive, or irritable mood, distractibility during the examination, history of decreased need for sleep, grandiosity, flight of ideas, agitation, pressured speech, and thoughtless disregard for the consequences of present actions. The hypomanic patient can present with a subtler array of symptoms that seem to suggest a diagnosis of narcissism (e.g., excessive self-absorption, egotism, and lack of regard for others). The anxious patient may exhibit increased vigilance, exaggerated startle response, tremor, tremulous voice, tachycardia, and hypertension. Content of speech may be notable for themes of threat or worry. Significant anxiety may exist as a primary disorder, or in association with depression.

Speech and Language

Observations about the quality of the patient's speech, language, and articulation can be very useful in the differential diagnosis of neuropsychiatric disorders. Observations about speech and language are made during the interview. Describe the patient's spontaneous speech. Is it fluent? Is the rate of speech output normal, increased or decreased? The amount, speed and volume of speech may be increased in the manic or the anxious patient. When asked to slow down, the manic patient may not be capable of doing so, in contrast to the anxious patient. A reduced quantity of speech output, as when the patient does not answer, does not volunteer information, or has to have questions repeated, may indicate the presence of major depression or the negative syndrome of schizophrenia. Is speech effortful? Is articulation clear or slurred? Speech articulation can be tested by having the patient enunciate selected sounds ("l-k-g") or phrases ("yellow lorry," or "baby hippopotamus"). Is there difficulty with phonation? Is it soft or hypophonic such as seen in Parkinsonian disorders? Are there neologisms, made up words that may be seen in schizophrenia or paraphasic errors characteristic of aphasia? Does the language content make sense or is it meaningless or even incomprehensible? Does the patient struggle to find names for objects or people? To what degree is the patient aware or frustrated by their speech or language difficulty? Is repetition intact? Ask the patient to repeat a simple phrase such as "I am in the hospital" and progress to "no if's, and's, or but's." Comprehension can be assessed with simple motor commands and move on to more complex questions until the limits of the patient's comprehension are discovered. Is speech prosody or the ability to use rhythm and inflection of speech to express emotion in tact? Can the patient comprehend the emotional expression of others?

Thought Content and Perception

Thought Content

Although the skilled examiner may make some observations during the interview that suggest abnormalities of thought content, in general, the patient must be asked directly about this part of the examination. Specific content covered includes suicidal thoughts or plans, homicidal thoughts or plans, delusions, obsessions, phobias, and health preoccupations.

It is important that the neurologist recognize that simple discussion of suicidal or homicidal thoughts does not "plant" such thoughts where they did not exist before. On the contrary, it is the unspeaking patient with a violent thought or plan (particularly if that patient is paranoid) who represents the greatest danger. Frank discussion of suicidality and homicidality can be initiated in any number of ways, depending on the issues the patient brings to the evaluation, as the following examples illustrate.

For the patient who reports depression, the examiner might use a graded series of questions:

- Some of my patients who tell me they are depressed also say that they get to the point where it feels like life is not worth living anymore. Is that true for you? If so, have you ever thought about ending it all? If so, have you thought about how you would do that? Do you have access to weapons/pills/etc. at home?

For the patient who appears hostile or angry about something:

- Is there anyone out there you are mad at? Are you mad enough to do something about it? What are you thinking about doing? Do you have a plan for that?

In general, past history of suicide attempt or legal incarceration for assault or attempted murder are predictors of whether such behavior will be exhibited in the future. In addition, alcohol intoxication or use of drugs associated with impairment of impulse control also increase the risk of these behaviors. If the examiner does uncover homicidal thoughts or plans directed against another named individual, it is the examiner's legal responsibility to notify that individual directly (the "Tarasoff" warning) and to document that this was done in the medical record.

Delusions are fixed false beliefs. The degree of conviction with which a false belief is held can vary from a feeling to a preoccupation to an overvalued idea, and finally to total conviction or delusion. In the latter extreme, the patient is said to have poor "reality testing," which means that they have lost contact with what is happening in the external world. Selected types of delusions are listed below. The category of paranoid delusions includes persecutory delusions, delusions of reference, delusions of grandeur, and delusions of control.

- *Control:* The belief that one's will, thoughts, or feelings are controlled by external forces. Specific beliefs may include thought withdrawal (thoughts are being removed from one's mind), thought insertion (thoughts are being planted in one's mind), or thought broadcasting (thoughts can be heard by others, as if being broadcast).
- *Erotomanic:* The patient's belief that someone, usually a prominent person, is in love with them (more common in women).
- *Gandeur:* An exaggerated conception of one's own importance, power, or identity.
- *Infidelity:* Belief that one's lover is unfaithful (also called delusional jealousy).
- *Persecutory:* Belief that one is being harassed, cheated, or persecuted.
- *Reference:* Belief that events, objects, or the behavior of other people refers to oneself. The reference usually represents a negative influence.
- *Somatic:* Belief that some body function or organ is diseased (e.g., that intestines are rotting).

Perceptual abnormalities can occur in different modalities, including auditory, visual, gustatory, olfactory, and tactile. Abnormalities can be positive, where sensation is added (an illusion or hallucination), negative, where sensation is removed or reduced (neglect), or distorted (e.g., micropsia, where the stimulus is perceived as smaller than actual size). Simple observation can sometimes reveal perceptual abnormalities such as auditory hallucinations, when the patient appears to talk to someone not present; visual hallucinations, when the patient reaches for something in the air above the bed; or unilateral neglect, when the patient has shaved only one side of his face. Usually, however, the patient has to be asked about these phenomena, or tested with simple tasks such as clock-drawing to uncover deficits. Normalizing statements such as the following can be useful in eliciting information regarding perceptual abnormalities:

- Some patients who tell me they are very depressed also say that sometimes they have unusual sensory experiences such as hearing voices that other people don't hear. Has this happened to you?
- Some patients who have a fever can become delirious, and for a short time they have strange experiences like seeing visions. Has this happened to you?

Insight and Judgment

Insight refers to the patient's ability to understand the actual cause and meaning of a situation such as an illness. To evaluate the patient's level of insight ask the patient to explain the circumstances of his/her illness. "Why are you in the hospital?" is a good leading question. Ask the patient how the illness has affected his/her family or workplace relationships. Judgment implies the ability to make reasonable decisions in light of circumstances. The patient may demonstrate intellectual insight by reciting facts (e.g., risks and benefits of a proposed procedure), but true insight involves the ability to assess a situation and take appropriate action. This can be assessed by determining how a patient handles day-to-day affairs such as paying bills on time or cooking a meal. Alternatively, standard probes such as the "stamped letter" or "fire in the theater" scenarios may be used.

Frontal Systems

Irritability, emotional lability, disinhibition, and apathy are frequently seen following frontal systems injury. Some patients, most commonly those with medial frontal lobe impairment, are subject to an overflow of emotions with little provocation, called *pseudobulbar affect*. Environmental dependency and utilization behavior may be seen (5,6). Judgment, insight, and social restraint are mediated in large part by systems in the dorsolateral prefrontal cortex. The dorsolateral prefrontal cortex integrates highly processed sensory information from multiple sensory modalities and is responsible for executive functions, which provides for mental flexibility and control of working memory. Injury to the dorsolateral prefrontal cortex may produce loss of abstraction, impaired maintenance of goal-directed behavior, decline in self-awareness and poor modulation of behavior as conditions change (7). In this regard, practical bedside self-questions for the examiner are: Is the patient able to monitor his/her own behavior? Is the patient aware of his/her own errors during the examination? Easy to administer, standardized ratings of behavioral disturbance in neurological patients have been developed (8,9).

Attention

Decreasing attention may be the first sign of an underlying encephalopathy. One can usually get a good impression of the patient's attentional ability by observing his or her attentiveness during the examination. There are a number of useful bedside tests of attention. Digit-span forward is simple and reproducible. The patient is asked to immediately recall a small group of numbers, and the size of the group is increased until errors are made consistently. Asking literate patients to spell a word forward and then backward or to recite the months of the year or days of the week backward and digit-span backward are other good tests of attention and concentration. Another variation is to call out letters at the rate of one per second and ask the patient to tap whenever he or she hears the letter A. Subtraction of serial 7s from 100 can be used to assess attention, but this test is influenced by memory and arithmetic abilities.

Patients should be oriented to time (day of the week, month, season, and year) and place (hospital, floor, city, and state). They should be familiar with leading public officials such as the president of the United States and have some awareness of key events in the news. The clock-drawing test and Trail Making Test A and B are other useful tests of attention and executive function *(10,11)*.

Memory and Other Higher Cortical Functions

Memory is not a unitary function and different brain systems subserve specific memory functions. Immediate recall or working memory refers to memory traces that decay in seconds without rehearsal. The digit-span test, just described as a test for attention, is also a useful approximation of working memory. Auditory digit-span testing is not valid in aphasic patients with repetition deficits. Asking the patient to register three items is a good test of working memory. Episodic memory involves forming a record of recent events. Episodic memory can be tested by asking the patient to describe either a recent event or what he/she had for breakfast. Asking the patient to recall three words after a 5-minute delay is another good test of episodic memory *(12,13)*. Paragraph-recall tests such as the Logical Memory Scale of the Wechsler Memory Test and the New York University Paragraph Test are reliable tests of episodic memory *(14,15)*. A number of standardized list learning tasks have also been developed to test episodic memory *(16)*. Nonverbal memory can be tested by asking the patient to reproduce shapes from memory or to find objects hidden in the room after a delay. For aphasic patients, one can present three objects and ask the patient to pick them out after an appropriate delay. Long-term memories refer to events that occurred days, weeks, months, or years in the past. The examiner can usually form an assessment of the patient's long-term memory function when compiling the history. To test long-term memory further, the patient can be asked about specific earlier personal life events or about past events in local or national history.

Damage to hippocampal-limbic memory circuits may produce amnesia. *Retrograde amnesia* refers to lost recollection of events before a specific event (e.g., head injury) and *anterograde amnesia* to the absence of memory for events thereafter. In retrograde amnesia, the patient has lost the brain's record of events that have already been registered, whereas in anterograde amnesia the brain is unable to record ongoing events. Patients with Alzheimer's disease will have trouble with registration and recall. Patients with subcortical dementia usually do fairly well on immediate recall and they may retrieve the three items after prompting.

Is there evidence of agnosia or the inability to recognize the meaning or use of a stimulus or object? Does the patient have apraxia or the inability to perform a requested motor act despite intact motor and sensory systems, adequate comprehension, and adequate cooperation and attention? Ideomotor praxis relates to the performance of a single motor act such as sticking out the tongue. A patient who can perform single actions but cannot do a series of them in sequence has ideational apraxia, suggesting a dominant parietal localization. This can be tested by asking the patient to demonstrate lighting a match and blowing it out. Is there evidence for neglect suggesting a right parietal deficit? Is the patient inattentive to the one side of the body or space? Is there active denial of illness or deficit suggesting anosognosia and raising the possibility of conversion disorder?

PSYCHIATRIC DIAGNOSIS

Psychiatric diagnoses are most commonly reported based on the diagnostic criteria of the Diagnostic and Statistical Manual IV (DSM IV-TR) *(1)*. Five different domains of information (axes) are used, with the intent of ensuring a more comprehensive evaluation, facilitating treatment planning, and generating prognostic information. The five axes are as follows:

Axis I: Clinical disorders
   Other conditions that may be a focus of clinical attention
Axis II: Personality disorders
   Mental retardation

Axis III: General medical conditions
Axis IV: Psychosocial and environmental problems
Axis V: Global assessment of functioning

Axis I disorders include most of the major psychiatric diseases and syndromes:

- Disorders usually first diagnosed in infancy, childhood, or adolescence
- Delirium, dementia, and amnestic and other cognitive disorders
- Mental disorders due to a general medical condition
- Substance-related disorders
- Schizophrenia and other psychotic disorders
- Mood disorders
- Anxiety disorders
- Somatoform disorders
- Factitious disorders
- Dissociative disorders
- Sexual and gender identity disorders
- Eating disorders
- Sleep disorders
- Impulse-control disorders not elsewhere classified
- Adjustment disorders
- Other conditions that may be a focus of clinical attention

Personality disorders and mental retardation are listed separately on axis II in an attempt to increase surveillance for these conditions, which may be co-morbid with axis I disorders. Axis II disorders are as follows:

- Paranoid personality disorder
- Schizoid personality disorder
- Schizotypal personality disorder
- Antisocial personality disorder
- Borderline personality disorder
- Histrionic personality disorder
- Narcissistic personality disorder
- Avoidant personality disorder
- Dependent personality disorder
- Obsessive-Compulsive personality disorder
- Personality disorder not otherwise specified
- Mental retardation

General medical conditions are listed on axis III. In some cases, axes I and III are linked physiologically, as in: *axis I: 293. 83 Mood Disorder Due to Hypothyroidism, With Depressive Features and axis III: 244. 9 Hypothyroidism*. In other cases, axis I and axis III are linked psychologically, as in: *axis I: 309. 0 Adjustment Disorder with Depressed Mood and axis III: Carcinoma of the Breast*. Other medical disorders listed on axis III can help guide pharmacotherapy for axis I disorders, as in diabetes mellitus in a patient with schizophrenia.

Axis IV is used to record psychosocial and environmental problems that affect the diagnosis, treatment, or prognosis of disorders listed on axes I and II. Often, multiple problems must be listed. Usually, the problems noted will be recent (i.e., present in the year prior to the current evaluation), but in some cases, it will be important to note significant earlier life events. An example would be combat experience in a patient with an axis I diagnosis of posttraumatic stress disorder. Problems noted on axis IV may be categorized as follows:

- Problems with a primary support group
- Problems related to the social environment

- Educational problems
- Occupational problems
- Housing problems
- Economic problems
- Problems with access to health care services
- Problems related to interaction with the legal system/crime
- Other psychosocial and environmental problems

Axis V is used to report the patient's overall level of functioning, using the Global Assessment of Functioning (GAF) scale. Function is rated only in terms of psychological, social, and occupational functioning. The GAF is divided numerically into 10 ranges of function (0 [low]–100 [high] level of function), with each 10-point range described by two parameters: symptom severity and functioning. The GAF score for a particular patient is determined by estimating where on the scale each of the two parameters fall. If the two parameters differ, the lower of the two is selected. For example, the GAF rating for a patient who represents a significant danger to him/herself but is otherwise functioning well would be below 20.

SUMMARY

The evaluation and treatment of psychiatric symptoms is a part of the routine care of neurological patients. Neurologists should approach this aspect of care knowledgeably and directly. Symptoms of psychosis, unusual behavior, suicidality, and substance abuse should be evaluated in a straightforward manner with information obtained from the patient, family, clinicians, and other reliable sources. Familiarity with psychiatric terminology and diagnoses is important for communicating with colleagues and developing an effective treatment plan.

REFERENCES

1. American Psychiatric Association. Diagnostic and Statistical Manual of Mental Disorders, Fourth Edition. Washington DC: Amer Psychiatric Pub; 2000.
2. Munetz MR, Benjamin S. How to examine patients using the Abnormal Involuntary Movement Scale. Hosp Community Psychiatry 1988;39:1172–1177.
3. Temple RO, Stern RA, Latham J, Ruffolo JS, Arruda JE, Tremont G. Assessment of mood state in dementia by use of the Visual Analog Mood Scales (VAMS). Am J Geriatr Psychiatry 2004;12:527–530.
4. Salloway S. Diagnosis and treatment of patients with "frontal lobe" syndromes. J Neuropsy Clin Neurosci 1994;6:388–398.
5. Lhermitte F, Pillon B, Serdaru M. Human autonomy and the frontal lobes. Part I: imitation and utilization behavior: a neuropsychological study of 75 patients. Ann Neurol 1986;19:326–334.
6. Lhermitte F. Human autonomy and the frontal lobes. Part II: patient behavior in complex and social situations: the "environmental dependency Symdrome." Ann Neurol 1986;19:335–343.
7. Malloy P, Richardson E. Assessment of frontal lobefunctions. J Neuropsy Clin Neurosci 1994;6:399–410.
8. Cummings J, Mega M, Gray K, Rosenberg-Thompson S, Carusi D, Gornbein J. The neuropsychiatric inventory: comprehensive assessment of psychopathology in dementia. Neurology 1994;44:2308–2314.
9. Grace J, Malloy P. Frontal Systems Behavior Scale (FrSBe): Professional Manual. Lutz: Psychological Assessment Resources Inc.; 2001.
10. Royall JR, Cordes JA, Polk M. CLOX: an executive clock drawing task. J Neurol Neurosurg Psychiatry 1998;64:588–594.
11. Reitan RM, Wolfson D. The Halstead-Reitan Neuropsychological Test Battery. Tucson: Neuropsychology Press;1985.
12. Folstein M, Folstein E, McHugh P. Mini-mental state exam: a practical method for grading the cognitive status of patients. J Psych Res 1975;12:189–198.
13. Malloy PF, Cummings JL, Coffey CD, et al. Cognitive screening instruments in neuropsychiatry: a report of the Committee on Research of the American Neuropsychiatric Association. J Neuropsych Clin Neurosci 1997;9:189–197.
14. Wechsler D. Wechsler Memory Scalerevised. San Antonio: Psychological Corp; 1987.
15. Kluger A, Ferris SH, Golomb J, Mittelman MS, Reisberg B. Neuropsychological prediction of decline to dementia in nondemented elderly. J Geriatr Psychiatry Neurol 1999;12:168–179.
16. Rosenberg SJ, Ryan JJ, Prifitera A. Rey Auditory-Verbal Learning Test performance of patients with and without memory impairment. J Clin Psychol 1984;40:785–787.
17. Guy W. ECDEU Assessment Manual for Psychopharmacology, revised. Washington DC: US Department of Health, Education, and Welfare; 1976.

III Major Psychiatric Disorders

4

An Overview of Depression

Irene Hegeman Richard and Jeffrey M. Lyness

INTRODUCTION

Depressed mood is a common part of normal as well as abnormal human experience. This ubiquity leads many to consider depressive illness as a benign, "functional" condition. As seen in this overview, such notions should be put to rest. We stress that depression is a disabling and potentially progressive condition, best conceptualized as an illness (or set of illnesses) affecting many aspects of brain function. Fortunately, depression is treatable, and there is clear evidence that early intervention and sustained treatment can ameliorate symptoms, reduce disability and vastly improve quality of life.

EPIDEMIOLOGY AND PHENOMENOLOGY

Depressive disorders are associated with disturbances in emotion, cognitive, autonomic, and motor functions. Depression may range in severity, and includes diagnostic constructs such as major depression, minor depression, dysthymic disorder, and so-called "subsyndromal depressions," as described here. The point prevalence of major depression is about 3–5% in males and 8–10% in females; lifetime prevalence figures are twice as high. Major depressive disorder can begin any time from childhood through old age, although the peak age at onset is probably in the fourth decade of life. Depression is a major public health problem (1,2), representing the leading correlate of disability and premature death among people 18–44 years of age and is the second leading correlate of disability for people of all ages. Depression is frequently co-morbid with systemic or neurological disorders (3). For example, depression is associated with increased rates of death and disability from cardiovascular disease, accounts for more disability than medical burden *per se* in some medical populations (e.g., low-vision elders), and is the biggest factor decreasing quality of life in many neurological conditions (e.g., Parkinson's disease [4]). Although major depression (*see* discussion below) is associated with the most severe morbidity and mortality, the cumulative functional morbidity is actually greater for the more common, less severe forms of depression. Functional disability can range from impaired school or work performance, social withdrawal, or in severe cases total lack of performing basic activities of daily living.

Depression is a syndrome reflecting alterations in several domains of brain functioning. By definition, patients experience lowered mood (such as dysphoria), or markedly decreased interests or anhedonia (inability to derive pleasure in things formerly deemed pleasurable). Often, patients experience

From: *Current Clinical Neurology: Psychiatry for Neurologists*
Edited by: D.V. Jeste and J.H. Friedman © Humana Press Inc., Totowa, NJ

other emotional symptoms, such as anxiety or irritability, which may be particularly prominent in children and older adults. The ideational symptoms of depression include thoughts of hopelessness, helplessness, worthlessness, guilt, and suicidal ideation. Cognitive symptoms include difficulty concentrating or making decisions (*see* "Cognitive Deficits in Depression" section). The depressive syndrome also includes alterations in somatic function (sometimes referred to as the "neurovegetative" symptoms), including changes in sleep, appetite, weight, psychomotor function, level of energy, and libido. Some patients (particularly those with neurovegetative symptoms) experience a diurnal variation in their symptoms. Abnormalities of sleep architecture associated with depression include sleep-continuity disturbances (prolonged sleep latency, increased intermittent wakefulness, early morning awakening), reduced non-rapid eye movement (REM) stages 3 and 4 (slow-wave) sleep and decreased REM latency. The neurovegetative changes may be the first symptom of a depressive episode and may persist after clinical remission. Neurovegetative (frequently referred to as "somatic") symptoms of depression are different than somatization symptoms, the latter of which may include worry about existing physical symptoms or (unconscious) generation of new physical symptoms. If this is the main way in which a patient's depression manifests itself, it may be referred to as a "masked depression."

DIAGNOSIS

The Diagnostic and Statistical Manual of Mental Disorders, fourth edition (DSM-IV *[5]*) provides criteria for various depressive diagnostic entities. The unipolar depressive disorders included in the body of DSM-IV are major depressive disorder (MDD), dysthymic disorder, and depressive disorder not otherwise specified (NOS). Minor depressive disorder is included in the appendix as set of criteria meriting further study. There are other diagnostic entities that can have depressed mood as a feature, but they are not classified as primary depressive disorders (e.g., adjustment disorder with depressed mood, substance-induced mood disorder, mood disorder caused by a general medical condition). Compared to MDD, the depressive symptoms associated with dysthymic disorder are less severe but more chronic. Minor depression is comparable to MDD with regard to symptom duration (episodes must last at least 2 weeks, and the "most of the day nearly every day" stipulation is maintained) but it is distinguished by having a lower severity, as fewer depressive symptoms are required to make this diagnosis. There is also an increasing literature on clinically significant depressive symptoms not meeting criteria for any of the above syndromically defined depression, which might be subsumed under the "Depressive Disorder NOS" rubric. Whereas the optimal approach to classifying such so-called lesser depressions is not known, it is clear that they are associated with considerable distress, and that, because of their great prevalence, their cumulative functional morbidity exceeds that of more traditionally defined depressions.

DSM-IV distinguishes between a major depressive episode and MDD (characterized by more than one major depressive episode). Symptoms associated with a major depressive episode are outlined in Table 1. In order to meet criteria for a major depressive episode, patients must have had five or more of nine potential symptoms present (in most cases, specified as most of the day, nearly every day) during the same 2-week period. These symptoms must represent a change from previous functioning and must cause clinically significant distress or functional impairment. At least one of the symptoms must be depressed mood, or loss of interest or pleasure. The other symptoms include weight change, sleep difficulties, psychomotor agitation or retardation, fatigue or loss of energy, feelings of worthlessness or guilt, decreased concentration or indecisiveness, and suicidal ideation.

DSM-IV provides specifiers that can be used to better characterize the depressive episodes which include the following: (a) mild, moderate, severe without psychotic features, or severe with psychotic features, (b) in full remission, in partial remission, or chronic, and (c) with catatonic features, with melancholic features, with atypical features or with postpartum onset. Melancholic depression is characterized by particular emotional and ideational symptoms (anhedonia, lack of reactivity to pleasurable stimuli, a distinct quality of the depressed mood, and excessive guilt), vegetative symptoms

Table 1
Symptom Overview for a Major Depressive Episode

Domain	DSM-IV symptoms	Other symptoms	Melancholic features	Atypical features
Emotional	1) Depressed mood 2) Interest/pleasure ("core" symptoms: at least one must be present)	Anxiety Irritability	Mood not reactive Mood distinct quality	Mood reactive
Vegetative	1) Weight loss/gain 2) Insomnia/hypersomnia 3) Fatigue/loss of energy	↓ Libido	Weight loss Early morning awakening Diurnal variation (morning worse)	Weight gain Hypersomnia
Ideational	1) Worthlessness/guilt 2) Suicidal ideation	Hopelessness Helplessness	Guilt	Rejection sensitivity
Cognitive	Concentration/indecisiveness	(text)		
Motor	Psychomotor retardation/agitation		Retardation/agitation	Leaden paralysis

(diurnal variation with symptoms generally worse in the morning, early morning awakening and diminished appetite), and motor features (marked psychomotor retardation or agitation). The distinctions drawn in the DSM-IV and the majority of reports in the literature support the notion that melancholic depression is best viewed as a distinct subtype. Atypical features include mood reactivity (capacity to be cheered up when presented with positive events), increased appetite or weight gain, hypersomnia, leaden paralysis (a feeling of heaviness in the limbs), and a long-standing pattern of extreme sensitivity to perceived interpersonal rejection. There is some evidence to suggest that these depressive subtypes may have different underlying causes and, more clearly, differential responses to treatment.

Dysthymia is characterized by a chronically depressed mood that occurs for most of the day, more days than not, for at least 2 years. In children, the mood may be irritable rather than depressed and the required minimum duration is only 1 year. During periods of depressed mood, patients must have at least two of the following symptoms present: poor appetite or overeating, insomnia or hypersomnia, low energy or fatigue, low self-esteem, poor concentration or difficulty making decisions, and feelings of hopelessness. The point prevalence of dythymic disorder is approx 3% and the lifetime prevalence approx 6%. Dysthymic disorder often has an early onset and a chronic course.

DIFFERENTIAL DIAGNOSIS

The differential diagnosis of depressive disorders includes other primary psychiatric disorders such as bipolar spectrum disorders (I, II, and III, etc., cyclothymic disorder) or adjustment disorder with depressed mood, cognitive disorders such as Alzheimer's disease that may initially be characterized by social withdrawal and apathy, bereavement, and metabolic problems such as vitamin B_{12} deficiency or hypothyroidism.

COGNITIVE DEFICITS IN DEPRESSION

MDD may be associated with cognitive deficits sometimes referred to as "pseudodementia" or the "dementia syndrome of depression" *(6–8)*. Subjective complaints of altered cognition may include a decreased ability to concentrate and memory impairment and be accompanied by impaired performance on objective testing. Such bedside cognitive examination, or more formal neuropsychological testing, when combined with other clinical information, can help with the diagnosis. In most depressed patients, objective cognitive performance is intact, or is limited solely by effort and motivation, as further evidenced by inconsistent effort or responses of exasperated, uncaring, or hopeless "I don't know" statements rather than incorrect responses. However, a substantial proportion of depressed patients, particularly those of older age or with more severe depression (e.g., with melancholic features) demonstrate objective cognitive deficits beyond those caused by inadequate effort. Whereas a wide range of deficits have been described over the years, often with mixed or conflicting findings, overall the pattern of cognitive impairment in depression suggests a functional disconnection between subcortical structures and the frontal lobes. Particular emphasis has been placed on prefrontal and cingulate cortical regions. Depressed patients may have impairments in attention, mental processing speed, spontaneous verbal elaboration, memory retrieval, and executive functions including planning, sequencing, organizing, and abstracting.

There is some evidence to suggest that white matter lesions may play a role in the vulnerability of some elderly patients to develop cognitive impairment during depressive episodes *(9)*. As well, an association between white matter lesions and executive dysfunction has been noted.

In addition to cognitive deficits as part of depressive illness, depressive symptoms may co-exist with dementias owing to neurodegenerative diseases. The precise nature of this co-existence remains to be determined. Although there is some evidence to suggest that depression may cause or contribute to dementia, there is substantial evidence to support the notion that depression may be an early manifestation of dementing illnesses such as Alzheimer's disease. Particularly in elderly persons and in those for whom detailed history is not available it may be difficult to determine whether cognitive deficits are due to depression alone or to a separate neurodegenerative disease process. Depressed patients often experience significant distress related to cognitive impairment and/or complain of cognitive impairment out of proportion to actual deficits. They may be more apt to have a history of previous depressive episodes and their current symptoms may have a more abrupt or subacute onset. Whereas motivational deficits can be associated with both depression and dementia, appetite disturbances and somatic complaints are more typical of depression. Depressed patients rarely experience the nocturnal worsening of cognitive functions ("sundowning") often seen in neurodegenerative dementias. The presence of prominent sadness or ideational symptoms (e.g., hopelessness, worthlessness, guilt, suicidality) suggests the likelihood of depression, but does not by itself distinguish whether the depression exists alone or co-morbid with a dementing disease.

CO-MORBIDITY

Depression is associated with substantial psychiatric co-morbidity including substance use disorders, personality disorders, primary anxiety disorders, eating disorders, as well as co-morbidity with medical and neurological illnesses (e.g., stroke, heart disease, Parkinson's disease *[10]*).

NEUROBIOLOGY

Depression is generally viewed as idiopathic and multifactorial. There appears to be a complex interplay of environmental stressors and individual diathesis toward symptomatic expression. Depression appears to be polygenic, although some family pedigrees may be traceable to a single locus. The concordance for depression in monzygotic twins is about 50%. MDD is 1.5–3 times more common among first-degree biological relatives of persons with this disorder than among the general population.

In the past, the leading theories of depression pathophysiology were relatively simplistic and suggested that deficiencies in one or more neurotransmitter systems were responsible for the condition. The main neurotransmitters invoked in the pathophysiology of depression include serotonin, norepinephrine, and (to a lesser degree) dopamine, with extensive literature supporting the notion that altered function in these aminergic systems is associated with the depressed state *(11)*. There is also ample literature on the altered function of the hypothalmic–pituitary axis (e.g., abnormal dexamethasone suppression test, blunted thyroid-stimulating hormone response to thyrotropin-releasing hormone), the immune system, neuropeptides, amino acids, and reproductive hormones. There is also a great deal of literature from "naturally occurring" lesions such as stroke, disease models, and neuroimaging studies devoted to brain localization. Newer functional imaging techniques, results of deep brain stimulation procedures, and sophisticated models of neural circuitry suggest that the prefrontal cortex, anterior cingulate cortex, and basal ganglia may have important roles in the pathogenesis of depression *(12)*.

More recently, researchers have proposed that genetic factors and life stress contribute not only to neurochemical alterations in depression, but also to impairments of cellular plasticity and resilience. Furthermore, it has become clear that depression is not localized to dysfunction of a single brain structure or system, but rather that there are disturbances in underlying neural circuits involving multiple brain regions and systems. This has led to drug development research targeting neurotrophic pathways, glucocorticoid signaling, phosphodiesterase activity, and glutamatergic activity. Perhaps surprisingly, the advances in molecular biology have only strengthened the notion that life experiences have a crucial impact on the development and course of depressive illnesses. Available data reinforce the concept of plasticity and suggests that experience contributes to the pathophysiology of depression and may influence response to treatment *(11,13,14)*.

PSYCHOLOGICAL AND PSYCHOSOCIAL FACTORS

It is important to recognize that considerable empirical evidence supports the role of a number of psychological and psychosocial factors in the pathogenesis of depression. As with neurobiological factors, it remains unclear which are truly causal or part of the disease process, and which are merely manifestations—epiphenomena—of depression. However, as discussed here, psychosocial interventions have clearly demonstrated efficacy for depression, and are important sole or co-treatments for many patients with depression.

Cognitive psychology perspectives focus on patterns of negativistic, distorted thinking (about the self, the future, and/or the environment) that confer risk for depression, and which become accentuated during acutely depressed states. Psychodynamic perspectives emphasize the roles of self-esteem regulation (as, e.g., in the narcissistic patient faced with rejections or other narcissistic injuries), failed defense and coping mechanisms, and the processing of losses. Indeed, early life stressors, particularly losses such as deaths of parents or other important figures, increase the risk for developing depression later in childhood or in adulthood. Current stressful life events or circumstances also play important roles for many patients—particularly so-called "exit" events, which include not only interpersonal losses and separations but also symbolic or actual bodily losses such as those produced by many neurological diseases. Couples, families, and other social support/social network factors may protect against or contribute to the development of depression, depending on the quantity, frequency, and qualitative nature of these relationships. Cultural factors often play important roles in the presentation of depression, and may strongly influence attitudes and behaviors determining help seeking or acceptance of treatment options.

COURSE AND PROGNOSIS

Symptoms of major depression usually develop over days to weeks. The major depressive episode may be preceded by a prodromal period lasting for weeks to months that includes anxiety and mild depressive symptoms. Untreated, most major depressive episodes in the community are associated with spontaneous and complete remission in about 6 months, although the spontaneous remission rate in clinical populations is much lower. In naturalistically followed clinical populations, as many as 20% of depressed patients may have persistent major depressive syndrome for months or years ("chronic"), whereas an additional one-third or more may have some improvement followed by persistent "subsyndromal" symptoms ("partial remission"). Even after achieving full remission, the lifetime risk for at least one recurrent episode is more than 50%. Individuals who have had two episodes have a 70% chance of having a third, and individuals experiencing three or more have a 90% probability of suffering another recurrent depressive episode *(15)*.

Kraepelin first emphasized that the long-term nature of affective illness is characterized by episode recurrence and that there is a general tendency for the evolution and progression of symptoms *(16)*. Research supporting the progressive nature of depressive disorders includes the following: depressive episodes increase in severity and treatment refractoriness over time, there is cycle acceleration (i.e., shorter well intervals between episodes) and whereas mood disorder episodes are often initially precipitated by psychosocial stressors, after a sufficient number of episodes they begin to emerge autonomously. It is often presumed by clinicians (the authors included) that treatment to reduce the number, severity, or duration of recurrent episodes will reduce the likelihood of subsequent worsening of depression course, although it must be admitted that direct empirical evidence to support this notion is modest. Similarly, clinical experience long has suggested that early intervention improves acute outcomes; it is paramount to teach patients about the risk of recurrence, need for early intervention, and thus the need to recognize early warning symptoms of a recurrence.

Proposed neurobiological models for the progressive nature of depression have included kindling, sensitization, and alterations in downstream second-messenger systems involved in neurotransmission and neurotrophism *(13)*. It has been suggested that the actions of these second-messenger systems may ultimately result in neuronal loss or alterations in neuronal sprouting and connectivity. In support of this notion are postmortem and neuroimaging studies demonstrating atrophy of various brain areas (hippocampus, frontal/cingulate cortex, basal ganglia). There is also evidence to suggest that mood stabilizers and antidepressants have effects on neuronal trophic factors.

TREATMENT OVERVIEW

There are several approaches to the treatment of depression and available modalities include psychotherapy, pharmacotherapy, electroconvulsive therapy (ECT) as well as several other less commonly used techniques (e.g., transient magnetic stimulation, light therapy). When considering the results of depression treatment studies, it is important to note that the placebo response rate in depression is fairly high (approx 30–40%). The presence of melancholia and/or psychosis may require pharmacological intervention *(17)*.

The treatment of depression can be divided into the acute phase (until patient is well), continuation phase (6 to 12 months after achieving remission) and maintenance (indefinite for those with two to three or more episodes or particularly destructive episodes).

Treatments (AHCPR Guidelines—from Depression in Primary Care www.ahrq.gov clinical practice guideline archive *[18]*) include the following:

1. Maintain high index of suspicion/evaluate risk factors
2. Detect depressive symptoms with clinical interview
3. Diagnose the mood disorder by history/interview (MSE)
4. Evaluate with complete medical history/physical examination
5. Identify and treat known causes of a mood disorder
6. Re-evaluate for mood disorder
7. Develop a treatment plan with the patient
8. Select an acute phase treatment
9. If medication is chosen, select type, drug, and dose
10. Evaluate treatment response
11. Proceed to continuation phase treatment
12. Evaluate the need for maintenance treatment
13. Seek consultation if needed

Nonpsychiatrists should consider referring the patient to a psychiatrist when the depression is severe (suicidality, psychosis), occurring in the context of another psychiatric illness (bipolar, schizoaffective, personality disorder, anxiety disorder), complicated by medical co-morbidity that complicates the diagnosis or management, or when it appears to be refractory to treatment.

PSYCHOTHERAPY

There are several types of focused and time-limited psychotherapies used to treat depression. Specific psychotherapies may have a 70–80% response. These include cognitive (correct cognitive distortions), interpersonal, (role transitions, grief, interpersonal conflicts, or deficits) and problem solving (identify, prioritize, solve). Psychotherapy may play an important role in the long-term treatment of recurrent depression and is particularly useful for those with obvious stressors, interpersonal difficulties, or low social support, or those who "can't" or won't take medications. Adjunctive psychosocial treatments may include couples or family therapy, socialization programs, psychiatric programs (day treatment, partial hospitals, inpatient), or change in residential setting or care level.

ELECTROCONVULSIVE THERAPY

ECT involves the use of electrical stimulation to induce a seizure in controlled and modified circumstances (anesthesia, muscle relaxation). ECT is remarkably safe and effective (80–90%) and is especially useful for severe, psychotic, or treatment-refractory depression.

PHARMACOTHERAPY

The main antidepressant drug classes in common use include the selective serotonin reuptake inhibitors (SSRIs), serotonin and norepinephrine reuptake inhibitors (SNRIs), tricyclic antidepressants (TCAs), monoamine oxidase (MAO) inhibitors, and other atypical agents (e.g., bupropion). An overview of these agents is provided in Table 2.

Several principles should be adhered to when using antidepressant medications. The patient should be seen every 1–2 weeks during the acute phase of treatment to re-educate, support, and monitor adherence, side effects, and treatment response. The maximum response may take 6 weeks or more but usually one sees the beginnings of a response in 1–2 weeks. If there is no response at all in 2–3 weeks, one should reassess the diagnosis and patient compliance. At this point, one can consider switching drugs (within class vs change class), pharmacological augmentation (i.e., addition of medications that are not powerful antidepressants when used as monotherapy, such as lithium, triiodothyronine, psychostimulants such as methylphenidate), or combination pharmacotherapy (i.e., two antidepressants from different drug classes, such as an SSRI plus a TCA, or bupropion plus mirtazapine).

When deciding which antidepressant to start, one should consider the side-effect profile, the history of response or nonresponse to a particular drug or class of drugs in the patient or patient's family, potential drug interactions, the presence of co-morbid psychiatric or medical conditions, and the age of the patient. Often with older patients, one must increase the dose slowly, although ultimate target doses may be similar to those in younger patients ("start low and go slow but go all the way"). Recent controversy about suicidality emerging with antidepressant treatment has received considerable attention in the lay media, particularly regarding children. Although data are conflicting and not fully available for review, at this time it is far from clear that antidepressant medications cause suicidal behavior in adults, and benefit-risk considerations favor treatment of diagnosable depression, although prudent clinical monitoring and patient-family education about suicidality are warranted.

One needs to be aware of a potential withdrawal syndrome when discontinuing the SSRIs (and paroxetine in particular). Withdrawal symptoms include dizziness, nausea, headache, tingling, fatigue, and irritability. Most symptoms are mild and short-lived and require no therapy. If symptoms occur, they generally occur a few days after stopping the medication and get better within a week. The gradual tapering of the study medication makes these symptoms less likely to occur.

Table 2
Overview of Antidepressant Medications

Agent	Mechanism	Comments
Citalopram	SSRI	Sexual dysfunction, few drug interactions
Escitalopram	SSRI	Sexual dysfunction, few drug interactions
Sertraline	SSRI	Sexual dysfunction, few drug interactions, ± stimulating
Paroxetine	SSRI	Sexual dysfunction, anticholinergic effects
Fluvoxamine	SSRI	Sexual dysfunction, marketed for OCD
Fluoxetine	SSRI	Sexual dysfunction, stimulating, long half-life
Venlafaxine	SNRI	SSRI at ↓ dosages, SNRI at ↑ dosages, Must be titrated, can ↑ blood pressure (clinically significant hypertension uncommon)
Mirtazapine	NE/5HT antagonist	Weight gain, sedation (often decreases at higher dosages)
Bupropion	Atypical (NE/DA)	Not anxiolytic, stimulating, no sexual dysfunction
Nefazodone	SSRI/5HT antagonist	Sedation, no sexual dysfunction, titration/BID dosing, hepatic toxicity, recently removed from US market
Trazodone	SSRI/5HT antagonist	Primarily used to treat insomnia
Nortriptyline Desipramine (and others)	TCAs (SNRIs)	Proven efficacy in severe, melancholic, psychotic depression, EKGs in older patients; relatively contraindicated in CAD (pro-arrhythmogenicity, risk of sudden death)
Phenelzine Tranylcypromine Isocarboxazid	MAOIs	Save for psychiatric specialists, potentially lethal drug and dietary interactions, require tyramine-free diet

SSRI, selective serotonin reuptake inhibitor; SNRI, serotonin and norepinephrine reuptake inihibitor; NE, norepinephrine; DA, dopamine; BID, twice a day; TCA, tricyclic antidepressant; EKG, electrocardiograph; CAD, coronary artery disease; MAOI, monoamine oxidase inhibitor.

REFERENCES

1. Charney DS, Reynolds CF 3rd, Lewis L, et al. Depression and bipolar support alliance. Depression and bipolar support alliance consensus statement on the unmet needs in diagnosis and treatment of mood disorders in late life. Arch Gen Psychiatry 2003;60:664–672.
2. Lebowitz BD, Pearson JL, Schneider LS, et al. Diagnosis and treatment of depression in late life. Consensus statement update. JAMA 1997;278:1186–1190.
3. Lyness JM, Bruce ML, Koenig HG, et al. Depression and medical illness in late life: report of a symposium. J Am Geriatr Soc 1996;44:198–203.
4. McDonald WM, Richard IH, DeLong MR. Prevalence, etiology, and treatment of depression in Parkinson's disease. Biol Psychiatry 2003;54:363–375.
5. American Psychiatric Association (DSM-IV Task Force). Diagnostic and Statistical Manual of Mental Disorders, Fourth Edition. Washington DC: Amer Psychiatric Pub; 1994.
6. Caine ED. The neuropsychology of depression: the pseudodementia syndrome. In: Grant I and Adams KM, eds. Neuropsychological Assessment of Neuropsychiatric Disorders. New York: Oxford University Press; 1986.
7. Post F. Dementia, depression, and pseudodementia. In: Benson DR, Blumer D, eds. Psychiatric Aspects of Neurologic Disease. New York: Grune & Stratton;1975.
8. Richard IH. Cognitive impairment in depression. In: Kurlan R, ed. Secondary Dementias. New York: Marcel Dekker; in press.
9. Kramer-Ginsberg E, Greenwald BS, Krishnan KRR, et al. Neuropsychological functioning and MRI signal hyperintensities in geriatric depression. Am J Psychiatry 1999;156:438–444.
10. Williamson GM, Shaffer DR, Parmelee PA. Physical Illness and Depression in Older Adults: A Handbook of Theory, Research, and Practice. New York: Kluwer Academic/Plenum; 2000.
11. Duman RS. The neurochemistry of mood disorders: preclinical studies. In: Charney DS, Nestler EJ, Bunney BS, eds. Neurobiology of Mental Illness. New York: Oxford University Press; 1999:333–347.
12. Sheline YI. Neuroimaging studies of mood disorder effects on the brain. Biol Psychiatry 2003;54:338–352.

13. Post RM, Weiss SRB. Neurobiological models of recurrence in mood disorders. In: Charney DS, Nestler EJ, Bunney BS, eds. Neurobiology of Mental Illness. New York: Oxford University Press; 1999:365–384.
14. Vaidya VA, Duman RS. Depression-emerging insights from neurobiology. Br Med Bull 2001;57:61–79.
15. Maj M, Veltro F, Pirozzi R, Lobrace S, Magliano L. Pattern of occurrence of illness after recovery from an episode of major depression: a prospective study. Am J Psychiatry 1992;149:795–800.
16. Kraepelin E. Manic-depressive insanity and paranoia.Edinburgh: E & S Livingstone; 1921.
17. Stahl SM. Essential Psychopharmacology: Neuroscientific Basis and Practical Applications, Second Edition. Cambridge: Cambridge University Press; 2000.
18. AHCPR Guidelines. Depression in Primary Care. Available at www.ahrq.gov clinical practice guideline archive.

5

Anxiety Disorders

Julie Loebach Wetherell, Ariel J. Lang, and Murray B. Stein

INTRODUCTION

The psychiatric disorders that are designated as anxiety disorders include the specific diagnoses of panic disorder with and without agoraphobia, agoraphobia without history of panic disorder, specific phobia, social phobia, obsessive-compulsive disorder (OCD), posttraumatic stress disorder (PTSD), acute stress disorder, generalized anxiety disorder (GAD), anxiety disorder due to a general medical condition, substance-induced anxiety disorder, and anxiety disorder not otherwise specified (NOS) *(1,2)*. An additional diagnosis, separation anxiety disorder, is reserved for children. This chapter is organized to include general information about the epidemiology, phenomenology, biology, and development of anxiety in adults, followed by disorder-specific information about epidemiology, signs and symptoms, diagnosis and differential diagnosis, familial and genetic influences, course and prognosis, and pharmacological and behavioral treatment. The chapter concludes with a discussion of the possible effects of anxiety on patients seen by neurologists.

EPIDEMIOLOGY OF ANXIETY

Anxiety disorders overall are the most common type of psychiatric disorder in adults, with a 12-month prevalence of 13.1 to 18.7% and a lifetime prevalence of more than 25% *(3,4)*. Mood disorders, by contrast, have a 12-month prevalence of 7.1 to 11.1% *(3)*. Prevalence rates for anxiety disorders peak in young adulthood (age 25 to 34) and decrease thereafter; they are 1.5 to 2 times higher in women than in men *(4)*. Anxiety disorders are highly chronic and are often co-morbid with mood disorders, other anxiety disorders, and substance use disorders *(3)*.

PHENOMENOLOGY OF ANXIETY

In general, anxiety and its disorders are characterized by subjective feelings of apprehension or fear and by somatic sensations characteristic of autonomic arousal such as increased heart and respiration rate, shortness of breath, dizziness, perspiration, flushing or pallor, dry mouth, pupillary dilatation, chest tightness, gastrointestinal distress, and incontinence *(3)*. Other physical symptoms of anxiety may include muscle tension, restlessness, hypervigilance or exaggerated startle response, sleep disturbance, and fatigue. These physiological changes, mediated by the autonomic nervous system, all serve in some way to prepare the organism to respond to threat or danger or result from such preparation. For example, perspiration cools the body during flight or defensive fighting; it also makes the skin more slippery to facilitate escape from a predator. A distinction is often made between state anxiety—transient levels of apprehension, fear, and physiological reactions to perceived threat—and trait

From: *Current Clinical Neurology: Psychiatry for Neurologists*
Edited by: D.V. Jeste and J.H. Friedman © Humana Press Inc., Totowa, NJ

anxiety—anxiety proneness—which is related to the personality trait neuroticism *(5)*. Trait anxiety may represent a vulnerability factor for the development of anxiety disorders.

Anxiety-related cognitions often involve an exaggerated sense of risk or danger and diminished sense of ability to cope *(6)*. Anxiety sensitivity describes individual differences in fear of the physical, psychological, and social manifestations of anxiety and may represent another risk factor for the development of anxiety disorders, particularly panic disorder with or without agoraphobia and PTSD *(7)*. Anxiety is often associated with threatening interpretations of ambiguous or even neutral situations. The evidence for an anxiety-related explicit memory bias for threatening events is mixed, with evidence for explicit memory bias in panic disorder, PTSD, and OCD, but not in social phobia or GAD *(8)*. Evidence is strong for the existence of implicit memory bias across disorders. Evidence is also strong for an attentional bias for threat cues, which operates at a preconscious level and appears to be a cause rather than a consequence of anxiety *(9)*. This bias may lead to distractibility and often results in poorer task performance at high levels of anxiety. In general, the relationship between anxiety and performance follows an inverse U-shaped curve, with highest levels of performance achieved at an intermediate level of anxiety.

Behavioral concomitants of anxiety typically involve escape or avoidance, which can include actually leaving or avoiding a feared object or situation, immobilization, procrastination, distraction, or self-medication with drugs or alcohol. Worry, a verbal process consisting of a chain of thoughts about actual or possible current or future dangers, may also serve as an avoidance mechanism by reducing aversive autonomic sensations associated with anxiety-provoking imagery *(10)*. Rituals, safety objects, or safety behaviors such as checking or seeking reassurance may be used as protection from harm.

BIOLOGY OF ANXIETY

Both the central and peripheral nervous systems are involved in anxiety. The brain structure most often implicated in anxiety and its disorders is the amygdala, which is believed to be the site of fear recognition, memory acquisition, and response. The amygdala receives input from the thalamus and the cortex and projects to the periaqueductal gray, lateral hypothalamus, periventricular hypothalamus, and the reticulopontis caudalis, which control the freezing, blood pressure, stress hormone, and startle reflex responses, respectively *(11)*. Other important central nervous system (CNS) structures include the locus coeruleus, which regulates arousal and attention; the hippocampus, which encodes contextual information involved in emotional memories; and the prefrontal cortex, which can inhibit or modify responses to anxiety-provoking stimuli *(12)*.

Gray has proposed another model of the anatomical correlates of anxiety. In this model, a behavioral inhibition system (BIS) *(13)* consisting of the septal area, hippocampus, and the Papez circuit, includes cortical and cholinergic inputs to the septo-hippocampal system, dopaminergic inputs to the prefrontal cortex, and noradrenergic input to the hypothalamus and the locus coeruleus. The BIS suppresses behavior and redirects attention to relevant stimuli after receiving signals of novelty, nonreward, or punishment. Anxiety is believed to be caused by a BIS that is overly reactive to novelty or punishment. In contrast, the behavioral approach system involving the medial forebrain bundle responds to signals of nonpunishment and rewards by facilitating approach. A third system, the fight-flight system, organized by the central periaqueductal gray, the medial hypothalamus, and the amygdala, responds to punishment, pain, and the omission of expected reward by facilitating defensive aggression or escape.

The BIS model is broadly consistent with Peter Lang's bioinformational theory of emotion, which holds that emotions, including anxiety, consist of stimulus (context), response (action tendencies), and meaning structures stored in memory *(14)*. Action tendencies include an appetitive system (similar to the behavioral approach system) and a defensive system (similar to the BIS and the fight-flight system). Evidence from the laboratory of Richard Davidson suggests that some aspects of these systems may be localized in the left and right anterior frontal cortex, respectively *(15)*.

Neurotransmitters involved in anxiety include the γ-aminobutyric acid (GABA), noradrenergic, serotonergic and dopaminergic systems, glutamate, and the corticotropin-releasing hormone pathway *(12)*. GABA, the principal inhibitory neurotransmitter, acts by opening neuronal chloride channels, leading to hyperpolarization that decreases the responsiveness of the nerve cell. The noradrenergic system is closely related to the activity of the locus coeruleus, which increases arousal and enhances the signal-to-noise ratio for detecting relevant environmental events. Depletion of serotonin is believed to increase response to punishment, impulsivity, and anxiety. Based on preclinical studies (including brain lesioning, genetic knockout techniques, and pharmacological probes), different serotonin receptors are believed to have different roles in the development and maintenance of anxiety: based on brain lesioning, genetic knockout, and pharmacological probe studies, activation of the $5HT_{1a}$ receptor presynaptically reduces anxiety-related behaviors, whereas activation of the postsynaptic $5HT_{1a}$ receptor and the $5HT_{1b}$, $5HT_{1c}$, $5HT_{2a}$, $5HT_{2c}$ and $5HT_3$ receptors increases anxiety-related behaviors. Serotonin also affects anxiety indirectly by altering noradrenergic and dopaminergic release, by stabilizing arousal through its effect on the locus coeruleus, and by attenuating prefrontal cortical activity. Although stress causes the release of dopamine in the prefrontal cortex, this release is not necessarily associated with anxiety. Rather, the dopaminergic system may serve to increase motivation and acquire coping responses. Glutamate, an excitatory neurotransmitter, is important for the acquisition of memories and the acquisition and extinction of conditioned emotional responses. One of the more exciting new developments in the treatment of anxiety disorders involves the use of *N*-methyl-D-aspartate (NMDA), a glutamate agonist that has been shown to facilitate extinction of fear-related behaviors, as an adjunct to exposure therapy *(16)*. Finally, corticotropin-releasing hormone stimulates the release of adrenocorticotropic hormone and activates the hypothalamic–pituitary–adrenal axis, which produces many of the physiological sensations associated with anxiety.

Endocrine changes reported to be associated with anxiety include increased release of epinephrine and norepinephrine, cortisol, growth hormone, and prolactin, as well as decreased testosterone in men *(12)*, although none of these has been consistently replicated across studies. Chronic anxiety is associated with diminished autonomic variability, probably caused by lower levels of parasympathetic nervous system activity, which leads to attenuated but longer lasting responses. This diminished autonomic variability appears to represent a vulnerability factor for chronic anxiety and perhaps for cardiovascular disease as well. Although anxiety is characterized by physiological responses, these changes are often nonspecific or subtle enough to preclude reliable psychophysiological assessment of anxiety. Thus, there are at present no "laboratory tests" to aid in the diagnosis of anxiety disorders.

DEVELOPMENT OF ANXIETY

Estimated heritability of anxiety disorders is 30 to 40%, lower than for schizophrenia or bipolar disorder *(17)*. Genes that have been associated with specific anxiety disorders are discussed below. Research by Jerome Kagan and colleagues has led to the identification of a temperament, "behavioral inhibition" (BI), that is found in 10 to 15% of infants and children and appears to be related to the subsequent onset of anxiety disorders, particularly social phobia *(18)*. Infants and children with BI react to novel situations with behavioral restraint and physiological differences such as high and stable heart rate, increased salivary cortisol and urinary catecholamines, pupillary dilation, and laryngeal muscle tension. These findings have led to the hypothesis that BI, which is likely genetically mediated, is related to a low threshold for arousal in the amygdala and hypothalamus.

PANIC DISORDER

Epidemiology

Almost 13% of the adult population experiences panic attacks *(19)*. Twelve-month and lifetime prevalence rates of panic disorder in the National Comorbidity Survey (NCS), an epidemiological study of mental disorders in a nationally representative sample of Americans age 15 to 54, were 2.3 and 3.5%, respectively *(4)*. Rates for men were 1.3 and 2.0%, whereas rates for women were 3.2 and 5.0%. These rates are somewhat higher than those found in the earlier Epidemiologic Catchment Area survey (ECA) *(20)*. Co-morbidity between panic disorder and other psychiatric syndromes is common, with as many as 65% of patients with panic disorder also meeting criteria for major depressive disorder (MDD), 15 to 30% meeting criteria for social phobia or GAD, 2 to 20% meeting criteria for specific phobia, and up to 10% meeting criteria for OCD or PTSD *(2)*.

Signs and Symptoms

Panic disorder is characterized by at least two unexpected panic attacks followed by at least 1 month of persistent apprehension about the possibility of another attack or by significant behavioral change resulting from the attacks (e.g., avoidance of situations associated with an attack) *(2)*. Panic attacks, which can occur in the context of any anxiety disorder as well mood disorders, substance-related disorders, and various general medical conditions, are sudden rushes of intense fear or discomfort in which at least four of the following symptoms develop abruptly and reach a peak within 10 minutes: palpitations or pounding or racing heart; sweating; trembling or shaking; shortness of breath or smothering sensations; feeling of choking; chest pain or discomfort; nausea or abdominal distress; dizziness, lightheadedness, unsteadiness, or faintness; derealization or depersonalization; fear of losing control or going crazy; fear of dying; numbness or tingling; and chills or hot flushes. Panic disorder may or may not be accompanied by agoraphobia, described below.

Diagnosis and Differential Diagnosis

Panic attacks are a common feature of many other psychiatric disorders and medical conditions. In some cases, this may represent a differential diagnosis (e.g., is it cardiac chest pain or panic disorder?) whereas in others it may represent the common co-occurrence of panic in patients with particular medical disorders (e.g., panic disorder and asthma) *(21)*. Panic disorder should not be diagnosed if the panic attacks are the direct physiological consequence of a general medical condition or substance or if the panic attacks are situationally bound or situationally predisposed. For example, if the panic attacks occur exclusively in the presence or anticipation of social situations, the diagnosis of social phobia is more appropriate than panic disorder. Likewise, panic attacks can be triggered by an object or situation in specific phobia, OCD, or PTSD, or by worry in GAD; in none of these instances, if the attacks were confined to those scenarios, would a diagnosis of panic disorder be applicable.

Familial and Genetic Influences

First-degree relatives of adult-onset panic disorder patients have up to eight times the risk of developing panic disorder, and relatives of childhood or adolescent onset panic disorder have up to 20 times the risk *(2)*. Twin studies indicate a genetic influence on panic disorder, with a heritability estimate of 48% and the rest of the variance owing to nonshared environmental influences *(17)*, as well as genetic influences on a trait believed to increase susceptibility to panic disorder–anxiety sensitivity *(22)*. Specific genes that, in preliminary studies, appear to be associated with panic disorder, particularly panic disorder with agoraphobia, include the catecholamine-*O*-methyltransferase gene on chromosome 22q11.2, the adenosine 2A receptor, and the 5-HT1A receptor gene polymorphism on chromosome 5q12.3 *(23–26)*.

Course and Prognosis

Onset of panic disorder is typically between late adolescence and the mid-30s, but onset in later life also occurs *(2)*. Course is typically chronic, with waxing and waning dependent on environmental stressors. Naturalistic follow-up studies in tertiary care settings suggest that approx 30% of individuals with panic disorder recover within 6–10 years of treatment, 40-50% improve but remain symptomatic, and 20–30% fail to improve. Relapse rates appear to be higher in women than in men *(27)*.

Treatment

The pharmacological treatments of choice for panic disorder are selective serotonin reuptake inhibitors (SSRIs); other efficacious treatments include high-potency benzodiazepines, reversible monoamine oxidase inhibitors, and tricyclic antidepressants *(28)*. Cognitive-behavioral therapy (CBT), including the elements of psychoeducation, breathing retraining, cognitive restructuring, and exposure to interoceptive panic-like sensations, is as effective for panic disorder as medications in the initial phase of treatment *(29)*. Short-term response to medications may be enhanced with adjunctive medication or CBT *(28,30,31)*.

AGORAPHOBIA

Epidemiology

One-year prevalence rates of agoraphobia with or without panic disorder range from 3.7 to 4.9%, with a best estimate on the higher end of that range *(3)*. Twelve-month and lifetime prevalence rates of agoraphobia without panic disorder are estimated at 2.8 and 5.3%, respectively *(4)*. Rates for men are 1.7 (12-month) and 3.5% (lifetime), whereas rates for women are 3.8 (12-month) and 7.0% (lifetime).

Signs and Symptoms

Agoraphobia is characterized by anxiety about situations from which escape might be difficult or embarrassing or help unavailable in the event of a panic attack or embarrassing panic-like symptoms *(2)*. These symptoms may include any of the symptoms of a panic attack as well as other potentially incapacitating or embarrassing symptoms (e.g., vomiting, pain). Typical situations associated with agoraphobia include being in a crowd or standing in a line, being outside the home alone, being on a bridge, or traveling in a bus, train, or automobile. The patient typically avoids these situations, endures them with marked distress, or requires the presence of a companion to face them.

Diagnosis and Differential Diagnosis

Agoraphobia should not be diagnosed when the anxiety or avoidance is more appropriately accounted for by another mental disorder. For example, avoidance related to social situations should be diagnosed as social phobia, avoidance limited to specific objects or situations should be diagnosed as specific phobia or OCD, and avoidance of stimuli associated with a traumatic stressor should be diagnosed as PTSD. Care should be taken to distinguish agoraphobic avoidance from the anhedonia and lack of energy seen in MDD. In certain medical conditions, anxiety or avoidance may be the result of realistic concerns (e.g., urinary incontinence) and should not be diagnosed as agoraphobia unless the anxiety or avoidance is clearly in excess of what would normally be associated with the condition.

Course and Prognosis

Agoraphobia usually develops within the first year of recurrent panic attacks *(2)*. The course of agoraphobia, however, is not always related to the course of panic disorder; for some patients, agoraphobia may become chronic regardless of the presence or absence of panic attacks. Little is known about the course of agoraphobia without history of panic disorder.

Treatment

Pharmacological treatment for agoraphobia is identical to treatment for panic disorder. In vivo exposure, or systematic desensitization to a hierarchy of real-life situations that evoke fear or avoidance, is the behavioral first-line treatment *(3)*.

SPECIFIC PHOBIA

Epidemiology

Specific and social phobias are the most common anxiety disorders. Twelve-month and lifetime prevalence rates of specific phobia are estimated at 8.8 and 11.3%, respectively *(4)*. Rates for men are 4.4 (12-month) and 6.7% (lifetime), whereas rates for women are 13.2 (12-month) and 15.7% (lifetime). The best estimate for 12-month prevalence based on both ECA and NCS data is 8.3% *(3)*. Co-morbidity with other disorders, particularly other anxiety disorders, mood disorders, and substance-related disorders, ranges from 50 to 80% in community samples *(2)*.

Signs and Symptoms

Anxiety reactions in specific phobia (formerly called simple phobia) are predictable and situationally bound or situationally predisposed *(2)*. Confrontation or anticipation of the anxiety-provoking stimulus evokes an immediate, intense anxious response, which can include a panic attack. The object or situation is avoided or endured with dread. The patient recognizes that the fear is excessive and unreasonable, and the fear or avoidance is associated with functional impairment or marked distress. Types of phobic stimuli include situations such as flying or being in enclosed places; objects in the natural environment such as heights or water; blood, injury, or injections; and animals or insects.

Diagnosis and Differential Diagnosis

Delusional disorder, rather than specific phobia, might be diagnosed if the patient does not recognize the fear as excessive and unreasonable (except in the case of children, where such insight—or the ability to express it—may be lacking). Specific phobia would also not be diagnosed if the fear is reasonable in a given context (e.g., fear of walking alone at night in a dangerous neighborhood), or if the fear or avoidance does not interfere with functioning or cause distress. Specific phobia can be differentiated from panic disorder with agoraphobia by the focus of the fear (e.g., the object or situation as opposed to the consequences of a panic attack) and whether or not panic attacks occur unpredictably.

Familial and Genetic Influences

Family members of individuals with specific phobias are at higher risk for developing specific phobias, and types of phobias tend to aggregate in families (e.g., animal phobias, although not necessarily of the same animal) *(2)*. Fears of blood, injury, or injections are associated with a particularly strong familial pattern, as well as marked biological reactivity (specifically, vasovagal responses such as fainting). One small twin study found a heritability of 47% for specific phobia of animals but no heritability for situational or environmental phobias *(32)*.

Course and Prognosis

Different types of specific phobias have different typical ages of onset, although onset is typically childhood or early adolescence and may be younger for women than for men *(2)*. Phobias involving animals or objects in the natural environment generally have an onset in childhood. Phobias involving situations have onsets either in childhood or in the mid-20s. Only 20% of phobias in adults remit spontaneously.

Treatment

According to one recent review, no pharmacological agent has been proven efficacious for specific phobia *(33)*. In vivo exposure-based behavioral treatments are effective, and preclinical studies suggest that enhanced efficacy may be possible by combining imaginal and in vivo exposure with NMDA receptor agonists such as D-cycloserine *(3,16)*.

SOCIAL PHOBIA

Epidemiology

Twelve-month and lifetime prevalence rates of social phobia are estimated at 7.9 and 13.3%, respectively *(4)*. Rates for men are 6.6 (12-month) and 11.1% (lifetime), whereas rates for women are 9.1 (12-month) and 15.5% (lifetime).

Signs and Symptoms

In social phobia, social or performance situations with the possibility of embarrassment or negative evaluation from others are the anxiety-evoking stimuli *(2)*. For some individuals, this phobia is relatively specific (e.g., public speaking), whereas others experience fear in a wide range of social situations. As is the case with specific phobia, exposure to the social or performance situation evokes an immediate anxious response, which can include a situationally bound or situationally predisposed panic attack. The social situation is usually avoided but may be endured with dread, the patient recognizes that the fear is excessive and unreasonable, and the fear or avoidance is associated with functional impairment or marked distress. Situations associated with social phobia include public speaking; eating, drinking, or writing in public or using a public restroom; initiating or maintaining conversations; speaking to strangers or meeting new people; participating in small groups; speaking to authority figures; attending social events; and meeting potential romantic partners. Generalized social phobia, or a fear of most social situations, is associated with severe social and occupational impairment.

Diagnosis and Differential Diagnosis

Social phobia should not be diagnosed if the fear or avoidance is limited to concern about the social impact of another mental disorder or general medical condition (e.g., body dysmorphic disorder, spinal cord injury). Individuals with panic disorder may avoid social situations out of fear of having a panic attack in public; such avoidance should not be diagnosed as social phobia. The situations avoided in social phobia are limited to those involving possible evaluation by other people. Avoidance of other people does not constitute social phobia in pervasive developmental disorders or schizoid personality disorder because individuals with these disorders lack interest in relating to others, whereas individuals with social phobia do not.

Familial and Genetic Influences

First-degree relatives of patients with social phobia are at higher risk for developing social phobia *(2)*. Generalized social phobia has a particularly strong familial component. Specific genes influencing social phobia may include chromosome 16 near marker D16S415 (possibly including the region encoding the norepinephrine transporter protein SLC6A2), chromosome 14 at marker D14S75, and areas on chromosomes 9 and 18 *(34,35)*.

Course and Prognosis

Typical onset of social phobia is in adolescence, although many individuals have a history of social inhibition or shyness as children *(2)*. Social phobia often precedes the development of other anxiety disorders, mood disorders, substance-related disorders, and eating disorders. The course of social phobia is often chronic, with lifelong duration *(27)*. It may also fluctuate with environmental stressors.

Treatment

Pharmacological treatments for social phobia include monoamine oxidase inhibitors, particularly phenelzine; SSRIs, particularly paroxetine; and clonazepam *(36,37)*. Behavioral treatments include social skills and assertiveness training, relaxation training, imaginal and in vivo exposure with behavioral experiments, video feedback, cognitive restructuring, and behavioral activation for co-morbid depressive symptoms *(3,38)*.

OBSESSIVE-COMPULSIVE DISORDER

Epidemiology

Community studies estimate a 12-month prevalence of 0.5 to 2.1% and a lifetime prevalence of 2.5% *(2)*. Prevalence of OCD was not evaluated in the NCS study.

Signs and Symptoms

OCD is characterized by recurrent, intrusive, inappropriate, or distressing ideas, thoughts, impulses, or images (obsessions) or repetitive behaviors or mental actions to reduce anxiety or distress (compulsions) *(2)*. These obsessions or compulsions are usually recognized by the patient as excessive or unreasonable and are either engaged in for more than 1 hour a day or cause marked impairment or distress. Typical obsessions involve contamination, doubts, order, religion, and aggressive, horrific, or sexual impulses. Compulsions are usually employed to neutralize the distress associated with the obsession or to prevent some feared event or situation. The most common compulsions include cleaning, counting, checking, seeking reassurance, repeating actions, and putting things in order. Tic disorders (including Tourette's Syndrome) are commonly co-morbid with OCD. A syndrome of early-onset OCD associated with tics and a history of streptococcal infection, termed pediatric autoimmune neuropsychiatric disorder associated with streptococcal infection, has been described *(39)*.

Diagnosis and Differential Diagnosis

OCD would not be diagnosed when the symptoms result from a general medical condition or substance. Repetitive, intrusive, distressing thoughts or behaviors caused by another mental disorder, such as preoccupation with perceived physical deformity in body dysmorphic disorder, apprehension about a feared object or situation in social or specific phobia, rumination in MDD, and worry about real-life circumstances in GAD should not be diagnosed as OCD. Patients with no insight into the excessiveness or unreasonableness of their thoughts or behaviors may receive an additional diagnosis of delusional disorder or psychotic disorder NOS. A belief that the thoughts are not the product of the patient's own mind (e.g., thought insertion) would typically lead to a diagnosis of a psychotic disorder rather than OCD. Neither stereotyped movements (e.g., tics, rocking) nor excessive engagement in behaviors that can give pleasure (e.g., eating, gambling) should be considered compulsions, although it should be noted that verbal and/or motor tics may frequently co-occur with OCD.

Familial and Genetic Influences

Genetic influences are significant for OCD *(40)*. The 5072T/G variant and the 5072G-5988T haplotypes of the glutamate receptor, ionotropic, NMDA 2B gene, the brain-derived neurotrophic factor gene, and the C516T 5HT2A gene polymorphism have been associated with OCD, although all these studies require independent replication *(41–43)*.

Course and Prognosis

OCD usually begins in adolescence or early adulthood, with earlier onset in males (where it is frequently co-morbid with attention deficit hyperactivity disorder) than in females *(2)*. Onset is typically gradual, with a waxing and waning course related to environmental stressors. Approximately 15% of patients show progressive deterioration in social and occupational functioning.

Treatment

CBT with exposure and response prevention is the treatment of choice for OCD and has demonstrated its superiority to SSRIs as well as to alternative psychotherapeutic approaches in well-controlled clinical trials *(44)*. SSRIs are the recommended first-line pharmacological treatment for OCD; clomipramine is also efficacious but has a less favorable adverse event profile *(45,46)*. There is some evidence for the efficacy of augmentation with clonazepam or buspirone. Studies comparing

CBT alone to CBT plus SSRI medications have yielded equivocal results as to whether or not the combination is superior to CBT alone.

POSTTRAUMATIC STRESS DISORDER

Epidemiology

The 12-month and lifetime prevalence rates of PTSD are 3.6 and 7.8%, respectively *(3,47)*. Although men have higher rates of exposure to trauma, women are twice as likely to develop PTSD *(48)*. The highest prevalence rates are typically found in survivors of rape, combat, prisoner of war or internment camps, and genocide *(2)*.

Signs and Symptoms

PTSD is diagnosed when a person who has been exposed to an event that involved actual or threatened death or serious injury and who reacted at the time with intense fear, helplessness, or horror exhibits the following symptoms: re-experiencing or reliving the trauma through intrusive memories, dreams, flashbacks, or intense distress or physiological reactivity during exposure to reminders of the event; emotional numbing or avoidance of trauma-related cues, including efforts to avoid internal and external reminders of the event, dissociative amnesia, anhedonia, feelings of detachment or estrangement from others, restricted affect, or sense of a foreshortened future; and increased arousal, including sleep disturbance, irritability or anger outbursts, difficulty concentrating, hypervigilance, or exaggerated startle response *(2)*. The symptoms must be present for at least 1 month and must cause functional impairment or significant distress. Traumatic events include combat, accidents, assault, natural or manmade disasters, and acute life-threatening illness (e.g., myocardial infarct; chronic or progressive illnesses such as cancer do not appear to be associated with PTSD, although medical interventions for cancer may be).

Diagnosis and Differential Diagnosis

Development of symptoms after a less severe stressor should be diagnosed as an adjustment disorder rather than PTSD. Acute stress disorder rather than PTSD should be diagnosed if symptoms include dissociation and develop and resolve within 4 weeks of exposure to a traumatic event. Flashbacks must be distinguished from hallucinations and other perceptual disturbances seen in psychotic disorders. Secondary gain (e.g., financial benefit, diminished responsibility for criminal behavior) may raise the suspicion of malingering.

Familial and Genetic Influences

First-degree relatives of patients with PTSD are at elevated risk for PTSD, and twin studies of male Vietnam veterans have showed heritability of 13 to 34% for various symptom clusters and 35% overall, with the remainder of variance accounted for by unique environmental factors *(49,50)*. Specific genes for PTSD have not yet been identified.

Course and Prognosis

Although PTSD can develop at any age, it usually arises in young adulthood, when exposure to traumatic events is most common. Symptoms typically begin within 3 months of the trauma, although delayed onset is possible *(2)*. Course is variable, with approx 50% of patients achieving recovery within 3 months and the rest experiencing chronic or fluctuating symptoms, often for years.

Treatment

SSRIs are the recommended first-line treatment for PTSD and the only class of medication that has shown effectiveness for all three clusters of symptoms *(51,52)*. Benzodiazepines do not appear to be effective in PTSD *(53)*. The behavioral treatment with the most empirical support is prolonged exposure, including repeatedly listening to audiotaped descriptions of the traumatic event, although some evidence exists for the efficacy of anxiety management training and eye movement desensitization and reprocessing *(54)*. Transcranial magnetic stimulation of the right dorsolateral prefrontal cortex has also shown efficacy for PTSD in one randomized, controlled trial *(55)*. Compared to pharmaceutical approaches to treatment, psychosocial interventions have lower attrition and appear to be more effective at symptom reduction, with some evidence for decreased risk of relapse following treatment discontinuation *(56,57)*.

ACUTE STRESS DISORDER

Epidemiology

Rates of acute stress disorder range from 14 to 33% in individuals exposed to a severe trauma *(2)*. Prevalence in the general population is unknown.

Signs and Symptoms

Because the diagnosis was developed to identify a precursor to PTSD, acute stress disorder and PTSD are quite similar in presentation. The chief difference is the time course; acute stress disorder must arise within 4 weeks of a traumatic event, whereas PTSD may have a delayed onset and is not diagnosed unless symptoms have persisted for at least 1 month. Additionally, in acute stress disorder, symptoms of dissociation such as numbing, detachment, reduced awareness of surroundings, derealization, depersonalization, or dissociative amnesia are prominent relative to symptoms of re-experiencing, avoidance, and arousal. The symptoms must last for at least 2 days and must cause functional impairment or distress.

Diagnosis and Differential Diagnosis

Acute stress reactions that last longer than 4 weeks should be diagnosed as PTSD. Brief psychotic disorder may be diagnosed instead of acute stress disorder if psychotic symptoms are experienced following exposure to a traumatic event. Exacerbations of pre-existing mental disorders following a stressor should not be diagnosed as acute stress disorder.

Course and Prognosis

Acute stress disorder develops within four weeks of exposure to a traumatic event and lasts at least 2 days. Most individuals with acute stress disorder go on to develop PTSD. There is some evidence that dissociative symptoms in acute stress disorder and lower baseline cortisol levels may be predictive of PTSD, although these findings are still controversial *(58,59)*.

Treatment

Single-session debriefing interventions designed to prevent PTSD after trauma exposure are controversial. A recent meta-analysis of such interventions indicated that they neither reduce distress nor prevent PTSD onset; risk for PTSD was actually significantly higher in the intervention participants than in controls at 1-year follow-up *(60)*. CBT to prevent PTSD in motor vehicle collision victims with acute stress disorder has been exceptionally successful *(61)*. Pharmacological interventions to prevent the onset of PTSD in patients with acute stress disorder are currently being tested.

GENERALIZED ANXIETY DISORDER

Epidemiology

Twelve-month and lifetime prevalence rates of GAD are estimated at 3.1 and 5.1%, respectively *(4)*. Rates for men are 2 (12-month) and 3.6% (lifetime), whereas rates for women are 4.3 (12-month) and 6.6% (lifetime). The best estimate for 12-month prevalence of GAD is 3.4% *(3)*. GAD is often co-morbid with mood disorders, other anxiety disorders, substance-related disorders, and general medical conditions such as gastrointestinal disorders or headaches.

Signs and Symptoms

The chief symptom of GAD is excessive and hard-to-control worry about several events or activities, accompanied by at least three of the following symptoms: restlessness or feeling keyed up or on edge, feeling easily fatigued, difficulty concentrating, irritability, muscle tension, and sleep disturbance *(2)*. Symptoms must be present more days than not for at least 6 months and must cause functional impairment or distress. GAD patients often worry about minor matters or very unlikely events. The specific topics of worry may change over the course of the disorder.

Diagnosis and Differential Diagnosis

If the focus of the worry is confined to features of another mental disorder, such as apprehension about a panic attack or fear of negative evaluation or social embarrassment, GAD should not be diagnosed. Anxiety that is the direct physiological result of a medical condition such as hyperthyroidism or diabetes or of a substance should be diagnosed as anxiety disorder due to a general medical condition or substance-induced anxiety disorder. Obsessions can be distinguished from GAD-related worry by the patient's perception of the thoughts as unrealistic. Functional impairment, intensity of and difficulty controlling worry, the number of worry topics, and the presence of physical symptoms may indicate GAD even in the presence of multiple real problems (e.g., serious medical condition, marital or job trouble).

Familial and Genetic Influences

Twin studies suggest that GAD and MDD share a genetic diathesis but different environmental influences *(62)*. Estimated heritability for GAD is approx 32%, with the remaining variance the result of nonshared environment in men but with shared environmental liability observed for women *(17)*. A recent study found an association of a T941G single nucleotide polymorphism in the monoamine oxidase A gene with GAD but not with panic disorder or MDD *(63)*.

Course and Prognosis

Many if not most individuals with GAD indicate that they have experienced anxiety since childhood, although onset is possible even in older adulthood *(64)*. Course is typically chronic with fluctuations owing to environmental stressors *(27)*.

Treatment

Pharmacological treatment of GAD may include venlafaxine extended-release, paroxetine, buspirone, and tricyclic antidepressants *(33,65)*. Pregabalin and tiagabine have also demonstrated efficacy for GAD in randomized controlled trials *(66–68)*. Benzodiazepines are not recommended for long-term treatment because of their side-effect profile, lack of efficacy for co-morbid depression, and potential for dependence. Behavioral treatments, particularly those that combine relaxation techniques and cognitive therapy, have demonstrated superior efficacy to nondirective approaches *(29)*.

ANXIETY DISORDER DUE TO A GENERAL MEDICAL CONDITION

Epidemiology

Many medical conditions may cause anxiety symptoms, including thyroid conditions, pheochromocytoma, hypoglycemia, congestive heart failure, pulmonary embolism, arrhythmias, chronic obstructive pulmonary disease, pneumonia, vitamin B_{12} deficiency, porphyria, dementia, stroke, encephalitis, and neoplasms *(2)*. The prevalence of anxiety disorders in community samples of patients with these disorders and the overall prevalence of anxiety disorder due to a general medical condition are unknown.

Signs and Symptoms

When evidence from the patient's history, physical examination, or laboratory findings suggests that prominent anxiety symptoms are the direct physiological consequence of a medical condition, the symptoms are not better accounted for by another mental disorder, symptoms do not occur exclusively during the course of a delirium, and symptoms cause functional impairment or distress, the patient meets criteria for anxiety disorder due to a general medical condition *(2)*. The clinical picture typically includes generalized anxiety, panic attacks, or obsessions or compulsions.

Diagnosis and Differential Diagnosis

If the disturbance occurs exclusively during the course of a delirium, anxiety disorder due to a general medical condition is not diagnosed. Substance-induced anxiety disorder would be diagnosed if the anxiety is secondary to a medication, toxin, or withdrawal from a substance. Adjustment disorder or a primary anxiety disorder would be diagnosed if the anxiety is a psychological reaction to a medical condition rather than a direct physiological consequence of the condition.

Course, Prognosis, and Treatment

The course and prognosis of anxiety disorder due to a general medical condition would depend on the underlying medical condition. Treatment should first involve addressing the medical condition. If no further improvement of the medical condition is possible, treatment of anxiety can involve symptomatic relief through pharmacological agents with low potential for medication interactions and favorable side-effect profiles (e.g., SSRIs rather than benzodiazepines). Behavioral treatments including relaxation training and cognitive techniques may reduce anxiety symptoms and excess disability.

SUBSTANCE-INDUCED ANXIETY DISORDER

Epidemiology

Anxiety disorders can be the consequence of intoxication from alcohol, amphetamines, caffeine, cannabis, cocaine, hallucinogens, inhalants, phencyclidine, and other substances or of withdrawal from alcohol, cocaine, sedatives, hypnotics, or anxiolytics, among others *(2)*. Medications such as analgesics, bronchodilators, anticholinergics, insulin, thyroid medication, contraceptives, antihistamines, corticosteroids, antihypertensives, anticonvulsants, antipsychotics, and antidepressants may also cause significant anxiety, as can exposure to heavy metals, gasoline, paint, insecticides, nerve gas, carbon monoxide, and carbon dioxide. Prevalence rates of substance-induced anxiety disorder are unknown.

Signs and Symptoms

Similar to anxiety disorder due to a general medical condition, substance-induced anxiety disorder is diagnosed when evidence from the patient's history, physical examination, or laboratory findings suggests that prominent anxiety symptoms developed within 1 month of substance intoxication or withdrawal or are caused by medication use or exposure to a toxin, the symptoms are not better accounted for by another mental disorder, symptoms do not occur exclusively during the course of a delirium, and symptoms cause functional impairment or distress *(2)*. The clinical picture typically includes generalized anxiety, panic attacks, obsessions or compulsions, or phobic symptoms.

Diagnosis and Differential Diagnosis

Substance-induced anxiety disorder is diagnosed rather than substance intoxication or substance withdrawal only when the anxiety symptoms are severe and in excess of those usually associated with intoxication or withdrawal syndrome. Substance-induced anxiety disorder is not diagnosed when symptoms only arise during the course of a delirium. If the substance in question is a medication used to treat a general medical condition, it must be determined whether the anxiety is related to the medication or to the underlying medical condition.

Course, Prognosis, and Treatment

Typically the anxiety symptoms arise and resolve within 4 weeks of discontinuation of the substance. Short-term pharmacotherapy, relaxation training, or cognitive techniques may be used to provide symptomatic relief.

ANXIETY DISORDER NOT OTHERWISE SPECIFIED

This residual category includes co-occurring symptoms of anxiety and depression not meeting full criteria for an anxiety or mood disorder, social phobic symptoms that do not meet criteria for social phobia because they are related to another mental disorder or a general medical condition, clinically significant anxiety symptoms that fail to meet criteria for another disorder, and cases in which it cannot be determined whether an anxiety disorder is primary, the result of a general medical condition, or substance-related. Treatment, which can include pharmacological or behavioral approaches, would depend on the clinical presentation.

ANXIETY AND THE NEUROLOGIST

Anxiety may affect patients seen by neurologists in several important ways. Because anxiety is associated with an attentional bias toward threat cues, anxious patients may selectively attend to symptoms and information that are consistent with a threatening interpretation of events. Asking patients specifically to monitor themselves for signs that would be consistent with alternative explanations or diagnostic rule-outs (e.g., stiff muscles elsewhere in the body might suggest tension rather than a brain tumor as an explanation for headaches) may be helpful in both achieving an accurate diagnosis and in reassuring an anxious patient.

An additional consequence of the attentional bias for threat associated with anxiety is that patients may have difficulty encoding other information. To address this problem, neurologists working with anxious patients should provide clear, written instructions for diagnostic and treatment procedures. Telephone or mailed reminders may be helpful, as may be enlisting the assistance of a family member or other support person. Patients can be encouraged to bring written lists of questions and to take notes during appointments to ensure that important information is communicated and understood. Some patients may benefit from additional time with a nurse or other staff member during scheduled appointments as well as from the availability of telephone support or advice between appointments.

Because of their hypervigilance for threat, some anxious patients may overreport symptoms. Psychiatric conditions involving physical symptoms suggestive of general medical conditions that may present as co-morbid or independent syndromes are called somatoform disorders and include somatization disorder, undifferentiated somatoform disorder, conversion disorder, pain disorder, and hypochondriasis. In contrast to factitious disorders and malingering, symptoms of these disorders are not under the patient's conscious control. Somatization disorder is diagnosed when a patient has a history of complaints of somatic symptoms in multiple organ systems for which no organic cause has been found despite appropriate diagnostic testing. At least one symptom, other than pain, must suggest a neurological condition (e.g., impaired coordination or balance, paralysis or localized weakness, loss of sensation, difficulty swallowing, aphonia, urinary retention, hallucinations, double vision, blindness, deafness, seizures, amnesia, or loss of consciousness other than fainting). Symptoms develop before the age of 30, and prevalence is estimated at less than 2% *(2)*. Co-morbidity with MDD, panic disorder, and substance-related disorders is common.

Undifferentiated somatoform disorder is characterized by one or more physical complaints that persist for at least 6 months and that cannot be fully explained by a general medical condition or substance. Conversion disorder is associated with one or more symptoms affecting voluntary motor or sensory function, suggesting a neurological or other general medical condition. Symptoms are initiated or exacerbated by psychological factors. Prevalence rates as high as 14% have been reported in medical inpatients, and as many as one-third of individuals with conversion symptoms have a current or past history of a neurological condition *(2)*. Pain disorder can be diagnosed when pain is the predominant focus of the clinical presentation and psychological factors play a significant role in the onset, severity, exacerbation, or maintenance of pain. Pain disorder is often associated with mood and anxiety disorders. Patients with hypochondriasis believe, over at least a 6-month period, that they have a particular disease despite reassurances from medical providers that they do not. Prevalence is estimated at 1 to 5% in the general population and 2 to 7% among primary care patients.

Somatic disorders that are often associated with anxiety are listed in the section describing anxiety disorders due to a general medical condition. Anxiety symptoms that can be mistaken for symptoms of neurological disorders include headache, dizziness, and blurred vision. Patients who present with these symptoms may benefit from a referral to a mental health professional after neurological, substance-related, and other medical conditions that could account for these symptoms have been ruled out. Referral to a behavioral health specialist may also be called for if a patient's anxiety is interfering with necessary diagnostic or treatment procedures (e.g., exposure therapy may be required before a claustrophobic patient will undergo magnetic resonance imaging).

Finally, even patients whose anxiety symptoms are related to neurological conditions may benefit from interventions to reduce excess disability caused by anxiety. Anxiolytic medications, particularly SSRIs or venlafaxine, can help anxious neurology patients. Relaxation training has been shown to provide symptomatic relief even in patients with dementia *(69)*. Guidelines for improving sleep hygiene, such as keeping a regular sleep and awakening schedule, not taking daytime naps, and not engaging in behaviors other than sleep or sex in bed, can reduce insomnia and related problems such as fatigue. Instructing patients to perform at least three pleasant activities per day can alleviate both anxiety and depressive symptoms, as well as help establish rapport.

REFERENCES

1. American Psychiatric Association (DSM-IV Task Force). Diagnostic and Statistical Manual of Mental Disorders, Fourth Edition. Washington DC: Amer Psychiatric Pub; 1994.
2. American Psychiatric Association (DSM-IV Task Force). Diagnostic and Statistical Manual of Mental Disorders, Fourth Edition, revised. Washington DC: Amer Psychiatric Pub; 2000.
3. BarlowDH. Anxiety and its Disorders: The Nature and Treatment of Anxiety and Panic, SecondEdition. New York: Guilford Press; 2002.
4. Kessler RC, McGonagle KA, Zhao S, et al. Lifetime and 12-month prevalence of DSM-III-R psychiatric disorders in the United States: results from the National Comorbidity Survey. Arch Gen Psychiatry 1994;51:8–19.
5. Spielberger CD. Anxiety, cognition, and affect: a state-trait perspective. In: Tuma AH, Maser JD, eds. Anxiety and the Anxiety Disorders. Hillsdale: Erlbaum; 1985.
6. Beck AT, Emery G, Greenberg RL. Anxiety Disorders and Phobias: A Cognitive Perspective. New York: Basic Books; 1985.
7. Taylor, S. Anxiety Sensitivity: Theory, Research, and Treatment of the Fear of Anxiety. Mahwah: Erlbaum; 1999.
8. Coles ME, Heimberg RG. Memory biases in the anxiety disorders: current status. Clin Pychol Rev 2002;22:587–627.
9. Mathews A, MacLeod C. Induced processing biases have causal effects on anxiety. Cognition and Emotion 2002;16: 331–354.
10. Borkovec TD, Alcaine OM, Behar E. Avoidance theory of worry and generalized anxiety disorder. In: Heimberg RG, Turk CL, Mennin DS, eds. Generalized Anxiety Disorder. Advances in Research and Practice. New York: Guilford; 2004:88–108.
11. LeDoux JE. Emotion: clues from the brain. Annu Rev Psychol 1995;46:209-235.
12. Noyes R, Hoehn-Saric R. The Anxiety Disorders. New York: Cambridge University Press; 1998.
13. Gray JA, McNaughton N. The neuropsychology of anxiety: reprise. Nebr Symp Motiv 1996;43:61–134.
14. Lang PJ, Bradley MM, CuthbertBN. Emotion, motivation, and anxiety: brain mechanisms and psychophysiology. Biol Psychiatry 1998;44:1248–1263.
15. Davidson RJ. Affective style, mood, and anxiety disorders: an affective neuroscience approach. In: Davidson RJ, ed. Anxiety, Depression, and Emotion. New York: Oxford University Press; 2000:88–108.
16. Davis M, Walker DL, Myers KM. Role of the amygdala in fear extinction measured with potentiated startle. Ann N Y Acad Sci 2003;985:218–232.
17. Hettema JM, Neale MC, Kendler KS. A review and meta-analysis of the genetic epidemiology of anxiety disorders. Am J Psychiatry 2001;158:1568–1578.
18. Kagan J. Temperamental contributions to affective and behavioral profiles in childhood. In: Hofmann SG, Marten P, eds. From Social Anxiety to Social Phobia: Multiple Perspective. Needham Heights: Allyn & Bacon; 2001:216–234.

19. Goodwin RD. The prevalence of panic attacks in the United States: 1980 to 1995. J Clin Epidemiol 2003;56:914–916.
20. Eaton WW, Dryman A, Weissman MM. Panic and phobia. In: Robins LN, Regier DA, eds. Psychiatric Disorders in America: The Epidemiological Catchment Area Study. New York: Free Press; 1991.
21. Goodwin RD, Eaton WW. Asthma and the risk of panic attacks among adults in the community. Psychol Med 2003;33:879–885.
22. Stein MB, Jang KL, Livesley WJ. Heritability of anxiety sensitivity: a twin study. Am J Psychiatry 1999;156:246–251.
23. Domschke K, Freitag CM, Kuhlenbäumer G, et al. Association of the functional V158M catechol-O-methyl-transferase polymorphism with panic disorder in women. Int J Neuropsychopharm 2004;7:1–6.
24. Hamilton SP, Slager SL, De Leon AB, et al. Evidence for the genetic linkage between a polymorphism in the adenosine 2A receptor and panic disorder. Neuropsychopharmacology 2004;29:558–565.
25. Rothe C, Gutknecht L, Freitag C, et al. Association of a functional -1019C>G 5-HT1A receptor gene polymorphism with panic disorder with agoraphobia. Int J Neuropsychopharmacol 2004;7:1–4.
26. Woo JM, Yoon KS, Yu BH. Catechol O-methyl-transferase genetic polymorphism in panic disorder. Am J Psychiatry 2002;159:1785–1787.
27. Yonkers KA, Bruce SE, Dyck IR, Keller B. Chronicity, relapse, and illness course of panic disorder, social phobia, and generalized anxiety disorder: findings in men and women from 8 years of follow-up. Depress Anxiety 2003;17:173–179.
28. Pollack MH, Allgulander C, Bandelow B, et al. World Council of Anxiety(WCA) recommendations for the long-term treatment of panic disorder. CNS Spectr 2003;8(Suppl. 1):17–30.
29. Barlow DH, Raffa SD, Cohen EM. Psychosocial treatments for panic disorders, phobias, and generalized anxiety disorder. In: Nathan PE, Gorman JM, eds. A Guide to Treatments That Work, Second Edition. New York: Oxford University Press; 2002:301–336.
30. Barlow DH, Gorman JM, Shear MK, Woods SW. Cognitive-behavioral therapy, imipramine, or their combination for panic disorder: a randomized controlled trial. JAMA 2000;283:2529–2536.
31. Doyle A, Pollack MH. Long-term management of panic disorder. J Clin Psychiatry 2004;65:24–28.
32. Skre I, Onstad S, Torgersen S, Philos DR, Lygren S, Kringlen E. The heritability of common phobic fear: a twin study of a clinical sample. J Anxi Dis 2000;14:549–562.
33. Roy-Byrne PP, Cowley DS. Pharmacological treatments for panic disorder, generalized anxiety disorder, specific phobia, and social anxiety disorder. In: Nathan PE, Gorman JM, eds. A Guide to Treatments that Work, Second Edition. New York: Oxford University Press; 2002:337–366.
34. Gelernter J, Page GP, Bonvicini K, Woods SW, Pauls DL, Kruger S. A chromosome 14 risk locus for simple phobia: results from a genomewide linkage scan. Mol Psychiatry 2003;8:71–82.
35. Gelernter J, Page GP, Stein MB, Woods SW. Genome-wide linkage scan for loci predisposing to social phobia: Evidence for a chromosome 16 risk locus. Am J Psychiatry 2004;161:59–66.
36. Davidson JR. Pharmacotherapy of social phobia. Acta Psychiatrica Scandinavica Suppl 2003;417:65–71.
37. Van Ameringen M, Allgulander C, Bandelow B, et al. World Council of Anxiety (WCA) recommendations for the long-term treatment of social phobia. CNS Spectr, 2003;8(Suppl 1):40–52.
38. Huppert JD, Roth DA, Foa EB. Cognitive-behavioral treatment of social phobia: new advances. Curr Psychiatry Rep 2003;5:289–296.
39. Snider LA, Swedo SE. Pediatric obsessive-compulsive disorder. JAMA 2000;284:3104–3106.
40. Nestadt G, Lan T, Samuels J, et al. Complex segregation analysis provides compelling evidence for a major gene underlying obsessive-compulsive disorder and for heterogeneity by sex. Am J Hum Genet 2000;67:1611–1616.
41. Arnold PD, Rosenberg DR, Mundo E, Tharmalingam S, Kennedy JL, Richter MA. Association of a glutamate (NMDA) subunit receptor gene (GRIN2B) with obsessive-compulsive disorder: a preliminary study. Psychopharmacology (Berl) 2004;174:530–538.
42. Hall D, Dhilla A, Charalambous A, Gogos JA, Karayiorgou M. Sequence variants of the brain-derived neurotrophic factor (BDNF) gene are strongly associated with obsessive-compulsive disorder. Am J Hum Genet 2003;73:370–376.
43. Meira-Lima I, Shavitt RG, Miguita K, et al. Association analysis of the catechol-o-methyltransferase (COMT), serotonin transporter (5-HTT) and serotonin 2A receptor (5HT2A) gene polymorphisms with obsessive-compulsive disorder. Genes Brain Behav 2004;3:75–79.
44. Franklin ME, Foa EB. Cognitive behavioral treatments for obsessive compulsive disorder. In: Nathan PE, Gorman JM, eds. A Guide to Treatments That Work, Second Edition. New York: Oxford University Press; 2002:367–386.
45. Dougherty DD, Rauch SL, Jenike MA. Pharmacological treatments for obsessive compulsive disorder. In: Nathan PE, Gorman JM, eds. A Guide to Treatments That Work, Second Edition.. New York: Oxford University Press; 2002:387–410.
46. Greist JH, Bandelow B, Hollander E, et al. World Council of Anxiety (WCA) recommendations for the long-term treatment of obsessive-compulsive disorder in adults. CNS Spectr 2003;8(Suppl 1):7–16.
47. Kessler RC, Sonnega A, Bromet E, Hughes M, Nelson CB. Posttraumatic stress disorder in the National Comorbidity Survey. Arch Gen Psychiatry 1995;52:1048–1060.
48. Kimerling R, Ouimette P, Wolfe J. Gender and PTSD. New York: Guilford Press; 2002.
49. Chantarujikapong SI, Scherrer JF, Xian H, et al. A twin study of generalized anxiety disorder symptoms, panic disorder symptoms and post-traumatic stress disorder in men Psychiatry Res 2001;103:133–145.

50. True WR, Rice J, Eisen SA, et al. A twin study of genetic and environmental contributions to liability for posttraumatic stress symptoms. Arch Gen Psychiatry 1993;50:257–264.

51. Stein DJ, Bandelow B, Hollander E, et al. World Council of Anxiety. (WCA) recommendations for the long-term treatment of posttraumatic stress disorder. CNS Spectr 2003;8(Suppl 1):31–39.

52. Yehuda R, Marshall R, Penkower A, Wong CM. Pharmacological treatments for posttraumatic stress disorder. In: Nathan PE, Gorman JM, eds. A Guide to Treatments That Work, Second Edition. New York: Oxford University Press; 2002:411–446.

53. Davidson JR. Use of benzodiazepines in social anxiety disorder, generalized anxiety disorder, and posttraumatic stress disorder. J Clin Psychiatry 2004;65(Suppl):29–33.

54. Rothbaum BO, Meadows EA, Resick P, Foy DW. Cognitive-behavioral therapy. In: Foa EB, Keane TM, Friedman MJ, eds. Effective treatments for PTSD: Practice Guidelines From the International Society for Traumatic Stress Studies. New York: Guilford Press; 2000, 60–83.

55. Cohen H, Kaplan Z, Kotler M, Kouperman I, Moisa R, Grisaru N. Repetitive transcranial magnetic stimulation of the right dorsolateral prefrontal cortex in posttraumatic stress disorder: a double-blind, placebo-controlled study. Am J Psychiatry 2004;161:515–524.

56. Sherman JL. Effects of psychotherapeutic treatments for PTSD: a meta-analysis of controlled clinical trials. J Trauma Stress 1998;1:413–435.

57. Van Etten ML, Taylor S. Comparative efficacy of treatments for post-traumatic stress disorder: a metaanalysis. Clin Psychol Psychother 1998;5:126–144.

58. Bryant RA. Acute stress reactions: can biological responses predict posttraumatic stress disorder? CNS Spectr 2003;8:668–674.

59. Marshall RD, Garakani A. Psychobiology of the acute stress response and its relationship to the psychobiology of posttraumatic stress disorder. Psychiatric Clin North Amer 2002;25:385–395.

60. Rose S, Bisson J, Wessely S. Psychological debriefing for preventing post traumatic stress disorder (PTSD) (Cochrane Review). In: The Cochrane Library, Issue 1, Chichester: Wiley; 2004.

61. Bryant RA, Moulds ML, Nixon RVD. Cognitive behaviour therapy of acute stress disorder: a four-year follow-up. Behav Res Ther 2003;41:489–494.

62. Roy MA, Neale MC, Pedersen NL, Mathe AA, Kendler KS. A twin study of generalized anxiety disorder and major depression. Psychol Med 1995;25:1037–1049.

63. Tadic A, Rujescu D, Szegedi A, et al. Association of a MAOA gene variant with generalized anxiety disorder, but not with panic disorder or major depression. Am J Med Genet 2003;117B:1–6.

64. Le Roux H, Gatz M, Wetherell JL. Age of onset of generalized anxiety disorder in older adults. Am J Geriatr Psychiatry 2005;13:23–30.

65. Allgulander C, Bandelow B, Hollander E, et al. World Council of Anxiety (WCA) recommendations for the long-term treatment of generalized anxiety disorder. CNS Spectr 2003;8(Suppl 1):53–61.

66. Feltner DE, Crockatt JG, Dubovsky SJ, et al. A randomized, double-blind, placebo-controlled, fixed-dose, multicenter study of pregabalin in patients with generalized anxiety disorder. J Clin Psychopharmacol 2003;23:240–249.

67. Pande AC, Crockatt JG, Feltner DE, et al. Pregabalin in generalized anxiety disorder: a placebo-controlled trial. Am J Psychiatry 2003;160:533–540.

68. Rosenthal M. Tiagabine for the treatment of generalized anxiety disorder: a randomized, open-label, clinical trial with paroxetine as a positive control. J Clin Psychiatry 2003;64:1245–1249.

69. Welden S, Yesavage JA. Behavioral improvement with relaxation training in senile dementia. Clin Gerontol 1982;1:45–49.

6
Schizophrenia

David P. Folsom, Adam S. Fleisher, and Colin A. Depp

EPIDEMIOLOGY

Schizophrenia affects approx 1% of the population. In the United States, somewhere between 2 and 4 million people have schizophrenia *(1)*. In addition, schizophrenia is widely considered to be the most severe and disabling of the psychiatric disorders. It is estimated that approx 30% of all hospital beds in the United States are occupied by persons with schizophrenia. In the Epidemiologic Catchment Area Study (ECA), the largest epidemiological study of psychiatric disorders, the lifetime prevalence of schizophrenic disorders (e.g., schizophrenia, schizoaffective disorder, delusional disorder) was 1.4%. However, in institutional settings, this prevalence was much higher; in mental hospitals the prevalence was 20.4%, in nursing homes it was 3.8%, and in prisons it was 6.7%. The prevalence of schizophrenia is highest in people aged 30–44 (2.3%) and lowest among those over age 65. Women were slightly more likely to have schizophrenia than men. African Americans had the highest rate at 2.1%, with Caucasians at 1.4%, and Latinos at 0.8% *(2)*.

Typically, the onset of psychotic symptoms is in the late-teens or early-20s. Many patients experience prodromal symptoms prior to full onset, particularly social withdrawal, worsening school performance, and declining personal hygiene *(3)*. In addition, there is evidence that many people who develop schizophrenia had subtle behavioral differences as children. In one study that compared childhood home movies of people who developed schizophrenia and their siblings who did not, blinded researchers were able to identify the pre-schizophrenic children *(4)*.

Overall, men and women are equally affected by schizophrenia, but in men the mean age of onset of the illness is 18–25 years of age vs 25–30 years of age for women. In addition, men tend to have a more severe course of illness with more severe negative symptoms (e.g., social withdrawal and flattened affect) and functional impairment, whereas women have more affective symptoms, delusions, and hallucinations *(5)*. Onset of schizophrenia often occurs in the teens or early-20s, when most people are completing their education, beginning to marry, and starting their careers; therefore, patients with schizophrenia have low rates of marriage and employment. One of the most striking signs of the impact of schizophrenia is the high rate of homelessness in persons with this disorder. One report found that 10% of homeless persons had a diagnosis of schizophrenia *(6)*, whereas a second study found 17% of the patients with schizophrenia treated in a public mental health system were homeless at least one time during a 12-month period *(7)*. Finally, the rates of substance abuse and dependence are elevated in people with schizophrenia, a total of 47% of the persons with schizophrenia in the ECA study also had a drug or alcohol use disorder *(8)*.

From: *Current Clinical Neurology: Psychiatry for Neurologists*
Edited by: D.V. Jeste and J.H. Friedman © Humana Press Inc., Totowa, NJ

SIGNS AND SYMPTOMS

Psychosis is one of the hallmark symptoms of schizophrenia. Although there is no universal definition of psychosis, the broad definition used by the fourth edition of the Diagnostic and Statistical Manual of Mental Disorders (DSM-IV) includes delusions (fixed false beliefs), hallucinations, disorganized speech, and disorganized behavior *(9)*. Psychosis occurs in disorders other than schizophrenia, including other psychotic disorders including schizoaffective disorder (characterized by both psychotic and mood symptoms), schizophreniform disorder (characterized by 1–6 months of schizophrenia-type symptoms), brief psychotic disorder (psychotic symptoms for 1 day to 1 month), psychosis as a result of a general medical condition, drug-induced psychosis, and psychosis caused by other central nervous system (CNS) disorders such as Alzheimer's disease.

The psychotic symptoms of schizophrenia are also called "positive" symptoms, and are the symptoms that most lay people associate with schizophrenia. In addition to the positive symptoms, many patients with schizophrenia also have negative symptoms and neurocognitive deficits. The negative symptoms of schizophrenia include avolition (a lack of initiative and persistence), flattened affect (decreased range of emotional expression), and alogia (paucity of speech). Although the negative symptoms are often not as dramatic as the positive symptoms, there is evidence that these symptoms cause more disability. For example, flattened affect and alogia make social interactions much more difficult for patients with schizophrenia, whereas avolition may make it harder for a patient with schizophrenia to obtain or keep a job. Neurocognitive deficits in patients with schizophrenia have become an area of increasing research interest in the past decade. Several neurocognitive deficits have been found to be associated with schizophrenia including verbal memory, immediate memory, and executive functioning. There is an increasing body of literature suggesting that these neurocognitive deficits are more strongly associated with functional impairments than positive or negative symptoms *(10,11)*. An important area of current research is studying the effect of second-generation antipsychotic medications and skills-training interventions on improving negative symptoms and neurocognitive functioning owing to schizophrenia.

The presentation of schizophrenia differs according to the age of onset of the illness. The most common age of onset is in the teens or early 20s. Childhood onset is classified as symptoms beginning before age 12. Late-onset schizophrenia is defined as symptoms starting after age 45. Patients with childhood-onset schizophrenia tend to a more chronic course and poorer outcome, with greater functional impairment. Patients with late-onset schizophrenia are more likely to be women, have more paranoid ideation, and less severe negative symptoms *(12)*.

BIOLOGICAL BASIS OF SCHIZOPHRENIA AND PSYCHOSIS

Despite much effort to understand the biological substrates of schizophrenia, there currently exists no biomarkers or definitive neuropathological signs that are sufficiently specific to this disorder. Some of the first insights into the biological basis of schizophrenia were derived from pharmacology. From the introduction of the first antipsychotic, chlorpromazine, in the early 1950s until the mid-1990s, the primary neuropharmacological explanation of schizophrenia was the dopamine hypothesis. Schizophrenia was hypothesized to be caused by a dysfunction of dopamine, primarily dopamine hyperactivity in the mesolimbic pathway. Evidence for this dopamine hypothesis of schizophrenia came from the fact that antipsychotic medications blocked the dopamine D_2 receptor, and that stimulants such as amphetamines (which increase dopamine) could cause psychotic symptoms. However, clozapine and other second-generation (or atypical) antipsychotics have a lower affinity for the D_2 receptor, and also bind to serotonin receptors (including the 5-HT 2A receptor), other dopamine receptors, and other neurotransmitter receptors *(13)*; these new medications have caused the dopamine hypothesis to be revised. It is currently believed that the psychotic (positive) symptoms of schizophrenia are primarily the result of dopamine hyperactivity in the mesolimbic pathway, whereas the neurochemical basis of the negative symptoms is still being worked out.

In addition to the advances in understanding schizophrenia based on the psychopharmacological profile of the newer medications, neuroimaging is providing significant advances in understanding the disorder. On magnetic resonance imaging (MRI) and computed tomography (CT) scans, brain changes in schizophrenia are not regionalized, nor are they as substantial as one would expect given the severity of impairment associated with this disorder. However, structural neuroimaging frequently demonstrates changes in both cortical regions, particularly the frontal and temporal cortices, and subcortical structures, including the hippocampus and thalamus *(14,15)*. Functional imaging studies using verbal or working memory tasks as probes have indicated abnormal connectivity between limbic and frontal regions, suggesting that schizophrenia may be due to disruptions in subcortical–cortical pathways *(14)*.

Most evidence indicates that schizophrenia is a neurodevelopmental disorder, rather than a neurodegenerative one. Evidence supporting this neurodevelopemental view incudes postmortem evidence from neuropathological examinations that show fewer dendritic projections in those with schizophrenia. Furthermore, neuroimaging studies have revealed that many of the brain changes associated with schizophrenia are present at the time of initial onset of symptoms, and perhaps even earlier. Studies of aging persons with schizophrenia conducted at University of California San Diego have revealed a surprising stability in their neurocognitive "deficits, with memory and executive functioning skills declining at about the same rate as associated with normal aging" *(16)*. In addition, as patients with schizophrenia age, their psychotic symptoms appear to become less severe *(17)*. Only a small subgroup of severely ill and chronically institutionalized patients exhibited progressively deteriorating cognitive functioning *(17)*. Conversely, a small portion of patients diagnosed with schizophrenia may have a complete remission of their illness *(18)*.

ETIOLOGY OF SCHIZOPHRENIA

Like all psychiatric disorders, there is no single cause of schizophrenia. Environmental factors and genetic predispositions are both important in the development of schizophrenia. Environmental factors that have been found to be associated with schizophrenia include being born in the winter months, maternal infections during gestation, being born in a city (vs a rural area), being born to a lower socioeconomic class, and severe life stresses. Genetic factors also play an important role in the development of schizophrenia. The concordance rate of schizophrenia in monozygotic twins is 33–78%, compared to 8–28% in dizygotic twins *(8,13)*. Possible chromosomal loci are on chromosomes 13, 8, 22, 6, and 10 *(15)*. The effects of genetics, prenatal infections, and environmental stress are likely each to be small but additive.

DIAGNOSIS AND DIFFERENTIAL DIAGNOSIS

The diagnostic criteria for schizophrenia are shown in Table 1. It is important to point out that there is no single symptom that is pathognomonic for schizophrenia. For a clinician first evaluating a patient who may be psychotic, the most important task is to rule out potentially life threatening conditions such as a delirium due to a systemic illness, toxins, drug withdrawal or toxicity, a CNS lesion, infection, neurodegenerative disorder, or another treatable medical illnesses that can either cause psychotic symptoms or make a person appear to be psychotic. Table 2 lists the differential diagnosis for a person who appears to be psychotic. Patients with schizophrenia can have "soft neurological signs," including abnormal sensory integration, motor coordination, and sequencing of complex tasks *(19)*. Although acute dystonia, psudoparkinsonism, and tardive dyskinesia are commonly seen in patients treated with antipsychotic medications, particularly the first-generation antipsychotics, focal neurological deficits are not seen in schizophrenia. Similarly, patients over age 45 can have new-onset schizophrenia (late-onset schizophrenia), but this is uncommon, and older patients with new-onset psychosis must have a careful workup to rule out medical and neurological causes of the psychosis *(20)*. The most common type of hallucinations found in schizophrenia are auditory hallucinations, although patients with

Table 1
DSM IV Diagnostic Criteria for Schizophrenia

A. *Characteristic symptoms:* Two (or more) of the following, each present for a significant portion of time during a 1-month period (or less if successfully treated):
   1. Delusions
   2. Hallucinations
   3. Disorganized speech (e.g., frequent derailment or incoherence)
   4. Grossly disorganized or catatonic behavior
   5. Negative symptoms (i.e., affective flattening, alogia, or avolition)
   Note: Only one Criterion A symptom is required if delusions are bizarre or hallucinations consist of a voice keeping up a running commentary on the person's behavior or thoughts, or two or more voices conversing with each other.
B. *Social/occupational dysfunction:* For a significant portion of the time since the onset of the disturbance, one or more major areas of functioning such as work, interpersonal relations, or self-care are markedly below the level achieved prior to the onset (or when the onset is in childhood or adolescence, failure to achieve expected level of interpersonal, academic, or occupational achievement).
C. *Duration:* Continuous signs of the disturbance persist for at least six months. This 6-month period must include at least 1 month of symptoms (or less if successfully treated) that meet Criterion A (i.e., active-phase symptoms) and may include periods of prodromal or residual symptoms. During these prodromal or residual periods, the signs of the disturbance may be manifested by only negative symptoms or two or more symptoms listed in Criterion A present in an attenuated form (e.g., odd beliefs, unusual perceptual experiences).
D. *Schizoaffective and Mood Disorder Exclusion:* Schizoaffective Disorder and Mood Disorder With Psychotic Features have been ruled out because either:(1) no major depressive, manic, or mixed episodes have occurred concurrently with the active-phase symptoms or (2) if mood episodes have occurred during active-phase symptoms, their total duration has been brief relative to the duration of the active and residual periods.
E. *Substance/General Medical Condition Exclusion:* The disturbance is not due to the direct physiological effects of a substance (e.g., a drug of abuse, a medication) or a general medical condition.
F. *Relationship to a Pervasive Developmental Disorder:* If there is a history of Autistic Disorder or another Pervasive Developmental Disorder, the additional diagnosis of Schizophrenia is made only if prominent delusions or hallucinations are also present for at least a month (or less if successfully treated).

From ref. 9.

schizophrenia can also have visual and tactile hallucinations. Visual hallucinations are more common than auditory ones in progressive dementias, a finding that can be useful in differential diagnosis. Finally, patients over age 45 can have new-onset schizophrenia (late-onset schizophrenia), but this is uncommon, and older patients with new-onset psychosis must have a careful workup to rule out medical and neurological causes of the psychosis *(21)*.

The initial workup for a person who appears to be psychotic is shown in Table 3; this workup typically includes laboratory studies looking for reversible causes of psychosis. Many psychiatrists obtain a CT or MRI in patients with new-onset psychosis, although a recent treatment guideline recommended this only if clinically indicated *(22)*. MRI or CT scan of the brain can reveal structural abnormalities associated with disorders that cause psychotic behavior. These may include a structural cause for temporal lobe epilepsy, evidence of CNS neoplasm, stroke, trauma, carbon monoxide poisoning, hydrocephalus, encephalitis, or Wernicke-Korsakoff syndrome, for example. In addition, further laboratory or diagnostic studies (such as lumbar puncture or electroencephalogram [EEG]) are often performed based on the findings of this initial evaluation. For example, an EEG may reveal psychosis associated with temporal lobe epilepsy or herpes encephalitis. Serology and cerebrospinal fluid testing can are important for ruling out treatable disease. If indicated, these studies may include erythrocyte sedimentation rate, heavy metal screen, ceruloplasmin, adrenal studies, or porphyria studies.

Table 2
Differential Diagnosis of a Patient Who Appears to be Psychotic

Psychiatric disorders
    Schizophrenia
    Schizoaffective disorder
    Mania
    Depression with psychotic features
    Severe personality disorder
    Posttraumatic stress disorder
Drugs of abuse
    Phencyclidine
    Lysergic acid diethylamide
    Amphetamine
    Cocaine
    Alcohol
    Ketamine/ecstasy/γ-benzene hexachloride (GBH)
    Barbiturate withdrawal
Neurodegenerative disorders
    Dementia with Lewy bodies
    Alzheimer's disease
    Frontal temporal dementia
    Huntington's disease
    Homocystinuria
    Metachromatic leukodystrophy
    Lafora's disease
    Cerebral lipidoses
    Fabry's disease
    Fahr's disease
    Hallervorden-Spatz
    Wilson's disease
Infectious diseases
    AIDS
    Neurosyphilis
    Herpes encephalitis
    Creutzfeldt-Jakob disease
Metabolic/nutritional disorders
    Thyroid disorders
    Adrenal disorders
    B_{12} deficiency
    Pellagra
Medication side effects
    Anticholinergics
    Levadopa
    Dopaminergics
    Deprenyl
    Glucocorticoids
Toxins
    Heavy metals
    Carbon monoxide
Structural disorders
    Trauma
    Neoplasm
    Normal pressure hydrocephalus
Other neurological disorders
    Epilepsy
    Cerebrovascular disease
    Autoimmune cerebritis

Table 3
Initial Workup for a Patient Who Appears to be Psychotic

Complete blood count
Chemistry panel
Vitamin B_{12}
Rapid plasma reagin (RPR)
Thyroid-stimulating hrmone
Urine drug screen

Other components to the initial assessment to consider depending on clinical presentation
and patient risk factors:
   HIV
   Neuroimaging (computed tomography or magnetic resonance imaging)
   Electroencephalogram
   Heavy metal screen

This initial workup can help rule out medical and neurological causes of psychosis. In addition, as Table 2 demonstrates, there are several other psychiatric disorders in addition to schizophrenia that include psychotic symptoms. In fact, it can be very difficult to determine on first presentation whether a person with psychosis resulting from a psychiatric illness has schizoaffective disorder, is manic, or has schizophrenia. Differentiating between schizophrenia and other psychiatric disorders can be difficult; careful attention to medical and psychiatric history (such as prior evidence of mood symptoms), as well as the use of available informants, is critical in making the diagnosis.

COURSE AND PROGNOSIS

Historically, schizophrenia has been thought of as the psychiatric disorder with the worst prognosis characterized by a gradual but progressive worsening of functioning. However, long-term follow-up studies indicate that the outcomes of patients with schizophrenia are more heterogeneous, with the majority of patients experiencing an initial drop in functioning, followed by a long-term stability of this poorer functioning. Neurocognitive deficits do not appear to worsen more than would be expected from normal aging even among elderly persons with schizophrenia *(16)*. A small minority of patients has progressive worsening of their illness, and a small minority also has remission of the disorder and a full return to premorbid level of functioning. Factors that have been found to be associated with better long-term outcomes include an older age of onset, abrupt onset of symptoms, female gender, response of symptoms to antipsychotic medications, and better premorbid functioning *(23,24)*. In addition, across all groups of patients with schizophrenia, exacerbations and relapses are common, are often the result of medication nonadherence, and are one of the main causes of psychiatric hospitalization. Patients with schizophrenia commonly attempt suicide, and up to 10% of patients with schizophrenia kill themselves.

TREATMENT

Antipsychotic medications are a critical component of treatment for schizophrenia, however these medications are primarily effective at treating the positive symptoms of schizophrenia, and are much less effective at treating the negative symptoms and neurocognitive deficits of the disorder. Table 4 lists the second-generation antipsychotic medications and one first-generation antipsychotic, haloperidol. As a class, the second-generation antipsychotics are less likely to cause movement disorders such as tardive dyskinesia and acute dystonia. In addition, many patients find these medications to have fewer side effects, and adherence to these medications may be higher than to the first-generation antipsychotics *(25)*. However, several of these newer antipsychotics have been associated with new-onset diabetes and increased risk of stroke *(20)*.

Table 4
Typical Maintenance Dose Ranges
of Antipsychotic Medications

	Typical maintenance dose
Haloperidol (Haldol)	2–10 mg
Clozapine (Clozaril)	100–900 mg
Risperidone (Risperdal)	2–6 mg
Olanzapine (Zyprexa)	5–20 mg
Quetiapine (Seroquel)	200–600 mg
Ziprasidone (Geodon)	40–160 mg
Aripiprazole (Abilify)	15–30 mg

Medications are a critical component of the treatment for schizophrenia, however, patients with schizophrenia often continue to have problems with cognitive functioning, social interactions, living independently, and getting and keeping a job. Programs that teach compensatory cognitive, social, and independent living skills and provide vocational rehabilitation are an important aspect of optimal treatment for many patients with schizophrenia *(26)*.

CONCLUSION

In evaluating a patient who may have a psychotic disorder, it is important to rule out medical and neurological causes for the patient's symptoms. This is especially true in patients with no prior history of mental illness, patients who are middle aged and older, patients hospitalized for a medical illness, and patients with evidence of delirium or focal neurological deficits. For complex patients, in whom it is difficult to differentiate between a psychotic disorder and a neurological disorder, close communication between the psychiatrist and neurologist is essential.

REFERENCES

1. Keith SJ, Regier DA, Rae DS. Schizophrenic disorders in psychiatric disorders in America. In: Robins LN, Regier DA, eds. The Epidemiologic Catchment Area Study. New York: Free Press; 1991.
2. Robins LN, Regier DA. Psychiatric disorders in America. In: Robins LN, Regier DA, eds. The Epidemiologic Catchment Area Study. New York: Free Press; 1991.
3. American Psychiatric Association. Diagnostic and Statistical Manual of Mental Disorders, Fourth Edition, revised. Washington DC: Amer Psychiatric Pub; 2000.
4. Schiffman J, Walker E, Ekstrom M, Schulsinger F, Sorensen H, Mednick S. Childhood videotaped social and neuromotor precursors of schizophrenia: a prospective investigation. Am J Psychiatry 2004;161:2021–2027.
5. Usall J, Haro JM, Ochoa S, Marquez M, Araya S. Needs of patients with schizophrenia group: influence of gender on social outcome in schizophrenia. Acta Psychiatr Scand 2002;106:337–342.
6. Folsom D, Jeste DV. Schizophrenia in homeless persons: a systematic review of the literature. Acta Psychiatr Scand 2002;104:1–10.
7. Folsom DP, Hawthorne W, Lindamer L, et al. Homelessness among patients with serious mental illness in a large public mental health system: prevalence, risk factors, and utilization of mental healthcare services among 10,340 patients. Am J Psychiatry 2005 162:370–376.
8. Norquist GS, Narrow WE. Schizophrenia: epidemiology. In: Kaplan A, Saddock BJ, eds. Schizophrenia. New York: Lippincott, Williams & Wilkins, 2004.

9. American Psychiatric Association. Diagnostic and Statistical Manual of Mental Disorders, Fourth Edition. Washington DC: Amer Psychiatric Pub;1994.
10. Green MF, Kern RS, Braff DL, Mintz J. Neurocognitive deficits and functional outcome in schizophrenia: are we measuring the "right stuff"? Schizophr Bull 2000;26:119–136.
11. Evans JD, Heaton RK, Paulsen JS, Palmer BW, Patterson T, Jeste DV. The relationship of neuropsychological abilities to specific domains of functional capacity in older schizophrenia patients. Biol Psychiatry 2003;53:422–430.
12. Eyler LT, Jeste DV. Schizophrenia in Encyclopedia of the Human Brain, Ramchandran VS, ed.. San Diego: Academic Press; 2002.
13. Freedman R. Schizophrenia. N Engl J Med 2003;349:1738–1749.
14. Tamminga CA, Thaker GK, Buchanan R, et al. Limbic system abnormalities identified in schizophrenia using positron emission tomography with fluorodeoxyglucose and neocortical alterations with deficit syndrome. Arch Gen Psychiatry 1992;49:522–530.
15. Krystal JH, D'Souza DC, Sanacora G, Goddard AW, Charney DS. Current perspectives on the pathophysiology of schizophrenia, depression, and anxiety disorders. Med Clin North Am 2001;85:559–577.
16. Heaton RK, Gladsjo JA, Palmer BW, Kuck J, Marcotte TD, Jeste DV. Stability and course of neuropsychological deficits in schizophrenia. Arch Gen Psychiatry 2001;58:24–32.
17. Jeste DV, Twamley EW, Eyler Zorrilla LT, Golshan S, Patterson TL, Palmer BW. Aging and outcome in schizophrenia. Acta Psychiatr Scand 2003;107:336–343.
18. Auslander LA, Jeste DV. Sustained remission of schizophrenia among community-dwelling older outpatients. Am J Psychiatry 2004;161:1490–1493.
19. Schubert EW, McNeil TF. Prospective study of neurological abnormalities in offspring of women with psychosis: birth to adulthood. Am J Psychiatry 2004;161:1030–1037.
20. Folsom DP, Nayak GV, Jeste DV. Antipsychotic medications and the elderly. Primary Psychiatry 2004;11:47–50.
21. McClure FS, Gladsjo JA, Jeste DV. Late onset psychosis: clinical, research, and ethical considerations [clinical conference]. Am J Psychiatry 1999;156:935–940.
22. American Psychiatric Association. Practice guidelines for the treatment of patients with schizophrenia. American Psychiatric Association 1997;154:1–63.
23. Fenton WS, McGlashan TH. Natural history of schizophrenia subtypes. II: Positive and negative symptoms and long-term course. Arch Gen Psychiatry 1991;48:978–986.
24. Breier A, Schreiber JL, Dyer J, Pickar D. National Institute of Mental Health longitudinal study of chronic schizophrenia: prognosis and predictors of outcome. Arch Gen Psychiatry 1991;48:239–246.
25. Dolder CR, Lacro JP, Dunn LB, Jeste DV. Antipsychotic medication adherence: is there a difference between typical and atypical agents? Am J Psychiatry 2002;159:103–108.
26. Patterson TL, McKibbin CL, Taylor MJ, et al. Functional Adaptation Skills Training (FAST): a pilot psychosocial intervention study in middle-aged and older patients with chronic psychotic disorders. Am J Geriatr Psychiatry 2003;11:17–23.

7

Hysteria in Neurological Practice

The Somatoform and Dissociative Disorders

Fred Ovsiew

The cases I speak of, some doctors like to call hysteria, but hysteria is the nosological limbo of all unnamed female maladies. It were as well called mysteria for all its name teaches us of the host of morbid states which are crowded within its hazy boundaries.

—Silas Weir Mitchell *(1)*

INTRODUCTION

The Somatoform and Dissociative Disorders* of the fourth edition of the Diagnostic and Statistical Manual of Mental Disorders (DSMIV) are the current representation of a disease known of old, hysteria; they amount to "hysteria split asunder," as one of the leaders of the nosological revolution in contemporary psychiatry put it *(2)*. Although the current diagnostic formulation is arguably a pale reflection of previous conceptualizations (the argument is made below), the disorder is certainly still a clinical presence. It has, as Sir Aubrey Lewis said, "outlive[d] its obituarists" *(3)*. In this chapter, I set the scene for understanding neurological presentations of Somatoform and Dissociative Disorders by pointing to a historical moment in the development of the understanding of hysteria; provide a review of the current diagnostic categories and describe the clinical features of patients fitting into those categories, with greatest emphasis on Conversion Disorder because of its importance in neurological practice; offer a summary of the known risk factors for somatization, as well as describing the limited information available on its neurobiology; and provide a set of recommendations for clinical management by the physician not specializing in psychological medicine.

THE HISTORY OF HYSTERIA

As everyone knows (and as textbook chapters commonly begin), hysteria was first recognized in Hippocratic times and so named because of the belief that movement of the uterus in the body led to the symptoms of the disease. Unfortunately, as is sometimes the case with what everyone knows, this account of the history of hysteria is mistaken, as Helen King conclusively showed *(4)*. Fortunately,

---

*The capitalization style is as given in the DSM and should be taken to mark the words as applying to those nosological categories. Readers skeptical of DSM-IV may want to see the capitals as equivalent to scare quotes. Individual citations for criteria or quotations are not provided in the text, but the reference should be clear from the context, because of the topical organization of the DSM.

From: *Current Clinical Neurology: Psychiatry for Neurologists*
Edited by: D.V. Jeste and J.H. Friedman © Humana Press Inc., Totowa, NJ

the error—which arose from reliance on secondary sources that suggested a categorical status not imagined by the Greeks for these symptoms purportedly of uterine origin—informatively points to the broader error of assuming that hysteria is a fixed entity, similar in all times and places and requiring merely the astuteness of present-day physicians to identify its occurrence retrospectively. This is arguably the case for epilepsy, for example, or for delirium among mental syndromes. However, the imbrication of hysteria in culture, especially the cultural position of women, makes it different from these other disorders. Unearthing and explicating the place of hysteria in Western thought and culture has been an active pursuit among nonclinical academics—the "new hysteria studies," as Mark Micale called the field in his historical survey *(5)*.

Greek medicine certainly embraced ideas about the movement of the womb, later about vapors arising from the womb, and described the symptoms presumed to result from these causes. Once a premodern idea of hysteria as a category of illness had developed, these beliefs were adopted as explanatory. Later, in the 17th century, the widely distributed nervous system was implicated as the cause of symptoms throughout the body. When, much later, even in the early part of the last century, doctors and the public referred to "shattered nerves" or a "nervous breakdown," they meant quite literally that the symptoms evinced pathology of the nervous system. This system of ideas, and the place of neurologists in treating "nerves," has been lucidly reviewed in the context of exposure to military combat— "shellshock"—by Ben Shephard *(6)*. For Jean-Martin Charcot, for example, hysteria was a *névrose*, a neurosis or condition of the nerves, like Parkinson's disease or other conditions without evident structural organic pathology. He believed that in describing the stages of hysterical convulsions, for example, he was delineating the course of an organic disease of the central nervous system, as he did so successfully with motor neuron disease or multiple sclerosis. Hysteria was, for Charcot, like other diseases of the nervous system, dependent on hereditary factors, and the environmental precipitants little more than *agents provocateurs (7)*. If the patient's father was a brute, this gave evidence of neuropathic heredity but did not raise the question what he did to her. The clinical features of hysteria were "perfectly legitimate pathological phenomena, in which the will of the patient counts for nothing, absolutely nothing" *(8)*. During the 19th century, much of the work of neurologists was the care of outpatients with these "nervous" complaints. To be sure, at least since Thomas Sydenham in the 17th century physicians had commented on the association between ideas or emotions and hysteria. True, some of the weakness of the nervous system was thought to be owing to modern civilization—an idea present at least from the 17th century. But the consequences of emotions and the stress of civilization were literally on the nerves, a weak or defective nervous system. Thus, treatment—such as rest and a diet including "porter [and] beef soup," as prescribed by Weir Mitchell *(1)*—was in the hands of the nascent neurological profession.

For clinicians, then, the inflection point in the trajectory of hysteria through the ages came toward the end of the 19th century, when Pierre Janet and Sigmund Freud provided accounts of hysteria proposedly deriving from ideas, memories, and emotions. When Charcot's sometime acolyte Joseph Babinski, after Charcot's death, rebelliously proposed considering hysteria to be in its essence a manifestation of suggestibility ("pithiatism"), the paper was headlined "the dismemberment *(démembrement)* of hysteria" *(9)*. Not until the late 19th century could the postulate be elaborated that the predisposition itself lay in the experience, not the nervous system, of the hysteric. Of course, no one is without predecessors. A line of British medical thought in the mid-19th century, in opposition to Charcot's approach in not assuming a defective nervous system, is represented by Reynolds' concept of "paralysis dependent on idea" *(10)*.

Janet and Freud began in concert, as Breuer and Freud acknowledged in 1893, in the paper taken to mark the very beginning of psychoanalysis:

> [T]he splitting of consciousness which is so striking in the well-known classical cases under the form of 'double consciousness' is present to a rudimentary degree in every hysteria, and . . . a tendency to such a dissociation, and with it the emergence of abnormal states of consciousness . . . is the basic phenomenon of this neurosis. In these views we concur with Binet and the two Janets [Pierre and his brother, Jules]. . . .

It will be noted that this starting point linked dissociation, as seen in the "somnambulistic" states of "double consciousness," and the conversion symptoms of the hysterical patients described in *Studies on Hysteria*. As Freud's ideas developed in the first decades of the 20th century, with increasing focus on the symbolic transformation of fantasies arising from inborn drives, he moved away from consideration of both constitutional predisposition and environmental trauma and equally away from a focus on dissociation. Janet, on the other hand, remained interested in the pre-existing weakness of the personality, a weakness that permitted dissociation *(désagrégation)*, as well as in the traumatic antecedents of symptom formation. Although both traditions have had important influence on psychological thinking about hysteria, in the 1970s and 1980s dissociation and trauma had a renaissance as topics of psychiatric concern, and Janet's work as well. Both constitutional predisposition and trauma are discussed further below.

SOMATOFORM DISORDERS

The characteristic feature of patients fitting into these diagnostic categories is the presence of somatic symptoms without discernable somatic cause. Obviously, our tools and astuteness in discerning causation are imperfect, and assignment of a patient to one of these categories should be undertaken with humility and an open mind. Somatoform Disorders, in which the presenting symptoms are felt to be genuine by the patient and are produced without conscious awareness of the psychological process, are to be distinguished from disorders in which the symptoms are deliberately feigned or produced. Patients in the latter categories are said to show malingering, if the purpose of the mimicry of medical illness is achievement of a practical end, such as financial gain; or factitious disorders, if the purpose is the achievement of the sick role. Here again, our capacity to recognize the motivation of our patients is limited. In fact, studies of the capacity of physicians to detect deception are chastening: physicians, like many other professionals for whom recognition of lying is of importance (e.g, police officers), perform poorly in experimental studies of the detection of deception.

A further caveat regarding the "somatoform" nature of these disorders is that patients with the disorder often produce accounts of symptoms in the psychological realm as well. Syndromes such as psychogenic amnesia cannot be called "somatoform" or "conversion" because the symptoms are mental, not somatic, yet the predisposition and mechanisms are likely similar. More broadly, somatizing patients give positive responses to questions regarding the mental symptoms of many psychiatric illnesses, illnesses they don't have *(11)*.

In contrast to DSM-IV, the 10th revision of the International Classification of Diseases (ICD-10), the European system of nosology, categorizes Conversion Disorder as one of the Dissociative Disorders, along with psychogenic amnesia and fugue. Whether this is a proper solution to the problem is taken up below.

Conversion Disorder

Patients with Conversion Disorder have sensory or motor symptoms suggestive of, but not explained by, an organic disorder; in contrast, clinical evidence suggests an association with psychological factors at least on the grounds that the "initiation or exacerbation of the symptom or deficit is preceded by conflict or other stressors." In some of the recent literature, these symptoms are referred to with intended neutrality as "medically unexplained." Many doctors call the symptoms "functional" or "psychosomatic" or "psychogenic."

Features commonly thought to characterize Conversion Disorder poorly identify the diagnosis. In practice, the association of the symptoms with stressors, although required by the criteria, can be hard to identify on initial evaluation, so the diagnosis is often made, at least in a tentative fashion, without definitive evidence of psychogenesis. In this sense, despite psychiatric claims to the contrary, it is often a diagnosis of exclusion. Moreover, many organic diseases are associated with stressful life events, and an association may be more apparent than real depending on the observer's threshold for establishing one. This situation—an insensitive and nonspecific criterion for the psychiatric diagnosis of

Conversion Disorder and a necessary reliance on the nonphysiological nature of the symptom—means that only a clinician comfortable with recognizing neurological symptoms as nonphysiological will be comfortable making the diagnosis. Thus arises the somewhat paradoxical result that the psychiatric diagnosis may be made by a neurologist with a neurologically inexperienced psychiatrist going along only reluctantly, perhaps suggesting yet more testing.

The presence of secondary gain—the benefits that flow to the patient from displaying symptoms—is common in organic disease, and the presence of primary gain—the reduction in emotional distress from the symbolic transformation of emotion and idea into somatic form—is hard to identify with confidence, especially in an initial consultation. *La belle indifférence*, the patient's obliviousness to impairments that appear to the doctor to deserve greater reactive distress, is a possible manifestation of organic anosognosia or of culturally or individually determined stoicism; moreover, patients with Conversion Disorder are often depressed or anxious rather than indifferent. The presence of ancillary nonorganic physical signs is nonspecific. Signs directly related to the complaint itself, such as entrainment of tremor frequency by voluntary tapping in a patient with psychogenic tremor or a Hoover sign in a patient with leg weakness, can be accepted as diagnostically helpful *(12)*. However, finding lateralized impairment of vibratory sensation on the sternum, for example—often the result of covert or overt suggestion by the examiner—is of no diagnostic utility *(13)*.

Conversion Disorder is common, although local referral patterns and specialty interests will play a role in any clinician's experience. In a prospective study in Scotland, 33 of 300 (11%) consecutively referred neurological patients were thought to have symptoms "not at all" explained by organic disease *(14)*. In a similar result from an entirely different setting, German investigators found that 9% of more than 4000 "inpatients presenting with typical neurological symptoms" had no organic cause for the symptoms *(15)*. Epilepsy monitoring units commonly report that about one-fifth of referrals prove to have pseudoseizures.

No extremity of severity is impossible. Pseudostatus epilepticus is well described and, according to some, common *(16)*. Administration of tissue plasminogen activator for pseudostroke occurs even in the best of hands *(17)*. Total disability of many years' duration is well known *(18)*.

The accuracy of diagnosis has been a subject of dispute at least since a provocative paper by the English psychiatrist Eliot Slater, who reported in 1965 that 22 of 85 (26%) patients diagnosed at the National Hospital, Queen Square, London, proved to have explanatory organic disease at long-term follow-up; he concluded that the diagnosis of hysteria is "a disguise for ignorance, and a fertile source of clinical error. It is in fact not only a delusion but a snare" *(19)*. Subsequent studies have been substantially more supportive of the clinical skills—and the advances in diagnostic technology—of neurologists. Two more recent reports from Queen Square showed rates of re-diagnosis as organic disease of 15% and 5% at follow-up *(20,21)*. A Dutch study found a rate of false-positive diagnosis of Conversion Disorder of 12% *(22)*, and a Scottish study found only one re-diagnosis in 48 patients at long-term follow-up *(23)*. Accounting for the differences among these studies on the basis of the nature of the patient populations or the initial evaluations does not tell individual clinicians how to make the diagnosis in a more secure fashion. Perhaps it is wise never to feel entirely secure in the diagnosis but always to keep an open mind, even if this means an open door, at least to re-examination if not re-investigation (*see* later). Despite my comment above that the diagnosis of Conversion Disorder in practice is often a diagnosis of neurological exclusion, probably the neurologist should be wary of a diagnosis of hysteria in the absence of confirmation of the plausibility of the diagnosis on psychiatric grounds (although I am not aware of data supporting this assertion).

The outcome of Conversion Disorder is not characteristically favorable. In many instances the presenting symptoms do not resolve. In a Scottish cohort, 35 of 42 (83%) patients still had sensorimotor conversion symptoms after more than a decade *(23)*. In a study of pseudoseizures, almost three-quarters of patients still had pseudoseizures 4 years after diagnosis (and more than a decade after presentation) *(24)*. Even when the presenting symptoms do resolve, other somatoform symptoms may develop.

Furthermore, when a broader view of outcome is taken, patients can be seen to have persisting psychological and interpersonal disturbances outside the somatoform realm. The rate of mood, anxiety, and personality disorders is very high. In particular, dissociative symptoms are common in patients with Conversion Disorder, even in comparison with other groups of psychiatrically ill patients *(25)*.

The pathogenesis of Conversion Disorder, and of somatization in general, is incompletely understood. Data suggest that early experience of painful medical procedures, parental illness in the patient's childhood, and a disturbed relation with parents are relevant risk factors *(26–28)*. A great deal of recent literature has stressed the relevance of trauma in childhood, such as physical or sexual abuse, to later Conversion Disorder *(29)*. This literature overlaps with the evidence for high levels of dissociative symptoms in patients with somatization, notably in patients with pseudoseizures *(30)*. However, the confounding factor is that childhood trauma predisposes to depression, anxiety, and a variety of other psychiatric syndromes; the evidence for this is compelling from a number of longitudinal and community studies that avoid the methodological problems of studying the issue by retrospective report in selected subjects in medical settings *(31–33)*. The mechanism of the association is not fully elucidated, but long-lasting or permanent biological consequences of early trauma are substantial and amount to "an environmentally induced complex developmental disorder" with neuroendocrine and structural and functional cerebral aspects *(34,35)*. The risk for somatization conferred by trauma may well be mediated largely or entirely by the presence of psychiatric illness. The concurrent presence of dissociation in some patients with Conversion Disorder may be a separate consequence of shared risk factors rather than part of the pathogenesis *(36)*. The issue is still open for study.

The older literature suggested—but the more recent cohort studies generally do not address—concurrent organic cerebral disease as a risk factor for hysterical states *(37)*. Slater believed the risk for developing conversion symptoms and the risk of a poor relation between (male) doctor and (female) patient were both attributable to organic brain disease, which "may bring about a general disturbance involving the personality. This personality change may then be a basis for hysterical conversion reactions, or by causing affective lability, hypochondriasis, attention-seeking, self-concern, suggestibility, variability of symptoms and so on, lead directly to an unfavorable reaction on the part of the clinician" *(19)*. This issue is badly in need of focused studies using contemporary techniques, including imaging and neuropsychological assessment.

Although by definition no organic disorder explains the pseudoneurological deficit, no one can doubt that some cerebral process corresponds to the behavioral findings. Functional imaging of a single patient with left-sided hysterical paralysis revealed excessive activation of right orbitofrontal and right anterior cingulate cortices with failure of activation of right primary motor cortex when the patient attempted to move the "paralyzed" leg. This was thought to indicate inhibition of primary motor areas in hysteria *(38)*. A study of hysterical sensory loss revealed reduction in activity of thalamic and basal ganglionic regions contralateral to the deficits despite normal cortical responses to sensory stimulation *(39)*. Another study of patients with nonorganic anesthesia revealed reduced responses in cortical sensory regions *(40)*. Whereas differences in method and patient characteristics may explain the discrepancies, further research will be needed to reach an integrated model.

Many authors have suggested that the reported lateralization of symptoms to the left reveals a disorder of lateralized cerebral function, with the right hemisphere "expressing itself" emotionally through the somatic symptom. However, whether conversion symptoms genuinely are more common on the left is uncertain *(41)*.

Somatization Disorder and Undifferentiated Somatoform Disorder

This category derives from an earlier construct, devised in the 1960s at Washington University, named Briquet's syndrome after the 19th-century French physician who cataloged the symptom picture of a large number of patients with hysteria. In its current use, Somatization Disorder refers to patients with the early onset—usually in childhood or adolescence but by criterion before the age of 30—of a chronic pattern of medical help-seeking and impairment because of a polysymptomatic condition. The criteria require multiple medically unexplained symptoms in multiple domains (*all* of these, not just one set or the other) over the course of the disorder: four pain symptoms, two gastrointestinal symptoms, one sexual symptom, and one conversion ("pseudoneurological") symptom. Although probably no one thinks that a patient who meets these criteria except for having only three pain symptoms is substantially different from a patient who fully meets the criteria, the point of the specification is to identify a chronic, severe disorder. Patients with somatization who fall short of the criteria for Somatization Disorder are considered by DSM IV to have Undifferentiated Somatoform Disorder. Other concepts, such as multisomatoform disorder or abridged somatoform disorder, have been applied in research studies to broaden the coverage beyond the most severe portion of the spectrum of somatization represented by Somatization Disorder. Evidence suggests that patients with somatization less narrowly defined share other psychopathological characteristics of patients with Briquet's syndrome.

The broad concept of somatization comprises a variety of syndromes, such as chronic fatigue syndrome, fibromyalgia, irritable bowel syndrome, multiple chemical sensitivities, and others; some would keep these separate, some see the somatization syndromes as overlapping *(42)*. Medical specialists, focusing on the nonorganic symptoms that resemble organic symptoms suggestive of "their" diseases, risk shaping the clinical picture to create simulacra of distinct syndromes. A further risk is that the symptoms, impairments, and psychiatric features beyond the bounds of the diagnosed syndrome will be ignored. In fact, mention of mental symptoms is curiously absent from the DSM account of Somatoform Disorders. In the classic work of the 19th-century neurologists, and then of Janet and Freud, characteristic disorders of affect and cognitive style were recognized and considered intrinsic to hysteria. In particular, affective dysregulation and a distortion or reduction of attention or the field of consciousness was stressed *(43)*. When hysteria was "split asunder," these observations were disregarded, even though every experienced clinician is aware of the disturbance of thought—vague, circumstantial, ego-centric, without direct replies to questions—frequently manifested by patients reporting somatization symptoms *(44)*. I have suggested that this thought disorder is related to the lack of coherence evident in the narratives of adults regarding their childhood relations with parents when those childhood experiences were characterized by disorganized attachment (i.e., a relation comprising an intolerable mixture of need with fear or confusion) and equally evinces a failure of maturation of representational or symbolic capacities *(45)*.

Medically unexplained symptoms and Somatization Disorders are common, impairing, and costly. The point prevalence of Somatization Disorder, the most severe form of this set of illnesses, is about 1%, with a female to male ratio of 5 : 1 *(46)*. The lifetime prevalence of somatoform disorders in the general population is estimated to be between 4 and 5%. However, doctors do not see the general population; they see patients who present for medical care, a subpopulation that obviously will be highly enriched for somatizers. Among people presenting for medical care, prevalence may vary substantially according to venue of care: primary vs specialty, psychiatric vs general medical, academic vs community, urban vs rural. A study in a Danish inpatient medical setting found that about one patient in five had one or another Somatization Disorder *(47)*. In a recent study, perhaps more reflective of the practice of some readers of this chapter, a group of investigators in New York City found that among patients in an American, urban, university-affiliated primary care practice serving a low-income population, 42 of 172 patients (24.4%) had multiple medically unexplained symptoms *(48)*. These patients were more likely to be female and unmarried, although other demographic measures such as ethnicity and income did not differentiate them from their nonsomatizing peers. They were two to three times more likely to have a mood or anxiety disorder and showed distinctly greater impairment on a range of measures of social and emotional functioning, in some cases even when concurrent psychiatric disorders were factored out. That is to say, somatization itself represented a substantial impairment of function apart from the defining somatic complaints.

Pain Disorder

The DSM IV diagnosis of Pain Disorder is divided into two subtypes, namely with or without an associated General Medical Condition; both subtypes are, by definition, "Associated with Psychological Factors." The pain must, by criteria, predominate in the clinical presentation and require clinical intervention by virtue of causing distress or impairment. More ambiguously, psychological determinants are judged to play a "major role" in "onset, severity, exacerbation, or maintenance" of the painful state. If a General Medical Condition is judged to play a similar major role, then the subtype "Associated with Both Psychological Factors and a General Medical Condition" is diagnosed. Duration is not specified in the criteria, but as a practical matter consideration of psychiatric factors usually takes place in patients with chronic pain.

Evaluation and treatment of pain require sensitivity to the cultural meanings and expressions of illness and pain. However, the patient's cultural background, even if different from the physician's, is in itself neither pathological nor a practical object of intervention (although the intervention may need to be attuned to the culture). Investigations of psychosocial risk factors in various painful states show a variable association of pain with pre-existing distress, personality disorder or cognitive styles, current life stressors, and childhood traumatic experience.

Many patients with chronic pain report depressed mood or show a full depressive syndrome. In most cases, the patient will assert that the depression results from the pain, a plausible claim that is certainly correct in many instances. Even if this is so treatment of depression has the potential to reduce suffering and alleviate functional impairment. Moreover, depression may be a risk factor for pain. In the interesting instance of migraine, a specific association is found such that each disorder increases the risk of incidence of the other, probably because of shared factors in pathogenesis *(49)*.

Hypochondriasis

This diagnosis applies to the patient whose preoccupation with disease produces impairment of function or clinically significant distress. The preoccupation, which by criteria must last more than 6 months, may take the form of worry or of belief short of full conviction. If the patient is considered to be delusionally convinced of the presence of disease, alternative diagnoses are Delusional Disorder and Depression with Psychotic Features. In a recent Danish study, 4.7% of medical inpatients met criteria for the DSM diagnosis *(47)*. The diagnosis of Hypochondriasis is unique in that it depends crucially on the nature of the doctor-patient interaction: the criteria specify that the preoccupation "persists despite appropriate medical evaluation and reassurance." An outside observer—such as a consulting psychiatrist—needs to be informed about what and how the patient was told in order to assess whether the patient's reaction is disordered.

Body Dysmorphic Disorder

In this condition, a patient is preoccupied with his or her physical appearance to a degree that causes impairment in function or substantial distress. Such patients may have no observable defect in the region that is the focus of preoccupation, or the defect may be slight in relation to the concern and impairment. Often, attention is focused on the face or skin. Patients characteristically look at themselves in a mirror continually; they imagine that others are equally attentive to the defects. Often, obsessive and compulsive features are present to the extent that an additional diagnosis of Obsessive-Compulsive Disorder is warranted; social avoidance may lead to an additional diagnosis of Social Phobia. Depression is common. The prevalence of the disorder is about 0.7% in the general population *(50)*. Not surprisingly, the prevalence in a group of patients seeking cosmetic surgery is much higher, as high as 18% in one report, and even higher in the men seeking cosmetic surgery *(51)*. Treatment is with serotonin reuptake inhibitors, even in patients without insight whose ideas about body defects are delusional *(52)*.

Psychiatric Treatment of the Somatoform Disorders

Many studies are available of treatment of Somatization Disorders with various psychotherapeutic methods. Good results have been reported with cognitive-behavioral therapy (CBT), group therapy, psychoeducational approaches, individual psychodynamic psychotherapy, hypnosis, and family intervention. For example, Barsky and Ahern recently reported a controlled clinical trial of CBT for Hypochondriasis, typically considered a treatment-resistant condition *(53)*. They reported significant benefit at 6- and 12-month follow-up in regard to not only hypochondriacal symptoms but also social functioning. Crucially, the results were based on an intent-to-treat analysis; analyzing only those patients, presumably with better prognosis, who come for treatment has vitiated many studies. Other drawbacks of the available data, such as short periods of follow-up and unimpressive effect sizes, also limit the confidence to be placed in psychotherapeutic intervention *(54)*. Nonetheless, most patients should have a trial of some form of psychotherapy, if possible.

Many patients with Somatization Disorders have prominent depressive and anxiety symptoms, potentially amenable to treatment with psychopharmacological agents. In some cases, conversion symptoms may resolve with reduction of abnormal mood. Treatment is along customary lines.

The problem with all of these approaches, however, is that although the neurologist feels the patient needs psychiatric treatment, and the psychiatrist may agree, the patient doesn't think so. The patient may refuse psychiatric consultation or, after an evaluation, may not appear for psychological or pharmacological treatment. For this reason, both pharmacological and psychological treatment may need to be conducted by the general physician or neurologist, or no treatment will happen at all. Suggestions for the psychological management of the somatizing patient outside the psychiatrist's office are outlined at the end of this chapter.

DISSOCIATIVE DISORDERS

Dissociation is defined by the DSM IV as "a disruption in the usually integrated functions of consciousness, memory, identity, or perception of the environment." Questionnaire studies of dissociative symptoms suggest that the construct comprises three factors: absorption (the capacity to "lose oneself" in an activity), amnesia (the tendency to put personal information out of mind), and depersonalization (*see* later discussion). Dissociation can be seen as a personality trait that varies along a dimension between normal and pathological. Normal dissociation is within the experience of most people, including neurologists. For example, after driving for a considerable time along a familiar route, one may "awake" to realize that one has no memory of the last few miles, even though during that period one obviously was performing complex motor tasks without error. One may have been "lost" in one's thoughts or in a piece of music on the radio. As is expectable for personality traits, the tendency to dissociation probably is under genetic control to a considerable degree *(55)*. One current, dominant hypothesis is that pathological dissociation arises when children with a tendency to use dissociation grow up in circumstances requiring them to take drastic measures to distance themselves from their experiences. Usually this means children exposed to abusive family environments, where literal escape from terror, pain, and confusion is impossible so that dissociated internal escape must be sought.

Dissociative Amnesia

Also called "psychogenic amnesia," this diagnosis refers to a nonorganic state of clinically significant inability to recall personal information. Of course, in organic disease anterograde amnesia virtually always predominates over the retrograde amnesia for personal information (one's own name, one's immediate and more remote circumstances, the identities of relatives, etc.). Whether true isolated retrograde amnesia of organic origin ever occurs is a matter of controversy *(56)*.

Amnesia for serious criminal behavior, such as murder, occurs in about one-fourth of offenders *(57)*. This high rate should be kept in mind when the question of epilepsy (or hypoglycemia, or rapid eye movement behavior disorder, or other organic cause of violent behavior) is raised; the presence of amnesia is not a strong pointer to organic disease. Although malingering (to seek exculpation or for other advantages within the forensic system) is doubtless an important factor in some cases, alcohol or drug intoxication at the time of offending and dissociative psychological mechanisms, as part of a reaction to acute stress, may play a role as well *(56)*.

Dissociative Fugue

When the inability to recall one's personal past is coupled with abrupt, unplanned travel, the diagnosis of Dissociative Fugue is made, unless the phenomenon occurs in the broader context of Dissociative Identity Disorder, described next, or an organic state. The ICD criteria make it clear that "travel" is to be distinguished from wandering. Fugue-like behavior in a post-ictal state or resulting from drug intoxication and wandering in dementia are potential aspects of the differential diagnosis. The British neurologist Sir Charles Symonds, basing his conclusions largely on wartime experience, believed that "all so-called hysterical fugues are examples of malingering" *(58)*. He reported good results from approaching the patient thus: "I know from experience that your pretended loss of memory is the result of some intolerable emotional situation. If you will tell me the whole story I promise absolutely to respect your confidence, will give you all the help I can and will say to your doctor and relatives that I have cured you by hypnotism."

Other clinicians have noted that depressive mood and a past history of organic amnesia, in the context of an acute psychosocial stressor, are characteristic features of Dissociative Fugue *(56)*. The condition is rare, at least at present; the 19th-century epidemic of fugue was described in its historical and medical context by Hacking *(59)*.

Dissociative Identity Disorder

Formerly known as Multiple Personality Disorder, this diagnosis is given when a person has "two or more distinct identities or personality states" and also shows psychogenic amnesia, characteristically of at least one state for the actions of another (although there may be a state aware of the actions of others). The background is thought almost always to be severe childhood abuse. The picture can be dramatic, with sudden changes of state in the clinical interview, or much more obscure, with a history of "lost time" and the presence of symptoms mistaken as psychotic (such as the thoughts of alters— the other personality states—being reported as "hearing voices"). This diagnosis has been controversial, some clinicians believing that it is common and missed or misdiagnosed, others believing that it is an artifact of overzealous clinicians whose very belief in the state induces it in suggestible patients. The dispute became politicized, with the former group accusing the latter of minimizing or denying the reality of child abuse, and the issue became bound up with the broader dispute over the question of "recovered memory," itself enormously controversial. Whereas the psychological debate over memory for trauma remains active (but is beyond the scope of this chapter), the vogue for the diagnosis of Multiple Personality Disorder, at its peak in the 1980s, seems to have largely passed.

A number of cases of Dissociative Identity Disorder of putative organic origin have been described (reviewed by Lambert et al. *[60]*). In most epilepsy is the key neurological feature.

Depersonalization Disorder

The symptom of depersonalization (a feeling of personal unreality and detachment), often accompanied by derealization (a feeling of the unreality of the external world), is common and can occur in the context of Panic Disorder, Schizophrenia, Acute Stress Disorder, and other psychiatric syndromes. Depersonalization Disorder refers to the state in which the symptom is persistently and significantly distressing or impairing but not part of one of these other clinical states. Although the diagnosis is listed under the Dissociative Disorders, concurrent dissociative symptoms are not as common as depressive and anxiety symptoms. The prevalence of Depersonalization Disorder is undetermined but may be higher than usually assumed *(61)*.

The most common organic cause of depersonalization is epilepsy, with migraine and other conditions also in the differential *(60)*. The literature suggests a left-sided predominance for focal lesions, although the phenomenologically related state of autoscopy is linked to dysfunction in the temporal-parietal junction on either side *(62,63)*.

NEUROLOGICAL MANAGEMENT OF SOMATOFORM AND DISSOCIATIVE DISORDERS

The first concern of neurologists encountering a patient with a Dissociative or Somatoform Disorder is to rule out organic disease explanatory of the patient's complaint or dysfunction. The current literature suggests that this can be done with adequate although not perfect accuracy. The need to review the patient's medical record should be stressed, for, as will come as a surprise to no experienced clinician, somatizing patients do not give accurate histories *(64)*.

Often, the work-up of a conversion symptom is undertaken with the expectation on the part of the neurologist that no organic disease will be found. It is the opinion of this physician, that, under such circumstances, the neurologist should discuss the psychiatric considerations at the outset and initiate psychiatric consultation at the outset as well. The physician can say, more or less, "symptoms like this can be caused by inflammation in the nervous system, or by epilepsy, or rarely by a brain tumor; or, very commonly, they can be related to stress. So I'm going to arrange for an imaging study of the brain, a brain wave test, a spinal fluid examination, and a psychiatric consultation. When we're done we'll have touched all the bases and I can sit down with you and tell you what I think." The alternative is to do all those tests, implicitly suggesting to the patient that the symptoms must be caused by some organic cause—after all, the doctor is looking so hard! When the suggestion for psychiatric consultation is made after obtaining the expected negative results—"The tests didn't show anything, so I want you to see a psychiatrist"—the patient may seek a smarter neurologist, one who will find what the first one was obviously looking for, or simply feel devalued and ignore the referral for psychiatric evaluation. If the psychiatric consultation occurs before a surprise positive result, leading to an organic diagnosis, the worst that has happened is that the psychiatrist has learned something about neurological disease, hardly a negative outcome.

Further, as mentioned above, concurrent organic disease, such as remote traumatic brain injury or concurrent epilepsy, may be present. Delineating the nature, extent, and neurological and neuropsychological consequences of such disease, which is not directly explanatory of the presenting symptom but plausibly a factor in the personality impairment underlying the disorder, is an important contribution to the understanding and care of the patient. Ideally, the consulting psychiatrist will collaborate in this formulation.

Once a diagnosis of Somatization Disorder is made, or more rarely of a Dissociative Disorder with neurological features, the neurologist may be faced with the continuing psychological management of the patient. Even if the patient's psychopathology is evident clinically, the patient may not be amenable to undertaking psychiatric treatment. How to proceed?

Advice can be partly based on controlled trial evidence, which is in accord with clinical experience *(65)*. Patients should be seen regularly, that is on a scheduled basis, rather than urgently, on an as-needed basis. The reason is that the relationship with the physician is important to many somatizing patients, and if necessary they will generate—perhaps unconsciously—symptoms that "require" consultation. To avoid this incentive for somatization, they should be seen regularly, irrespective of "need." The physician should keep an open mind about the diagnosis and should listen and examine attentively. However, investigations should be limited, if possible to situations in which they are indicated by signs rather than symptoms. This reduces the cost of medical care and, in the case of invasive procedures, its risk. In addition, it avoids the psychologically suggestive effect of test-ordering: "If the doctor thinks I need the test, then the doctor must think there is something seriously wrong."

In the meantime, what to say to the patient? No blanket advice can be offered, because the "right" thing to say depends on the patient and, to a considerable extent, on what the doctor is personally comfortable with. Many doctors talk with patients about "stress"; some talk about how the mind may interpret normal body sensations in an abnormal fashion because of the effect of emotions. In any event, the doctor should recognize that the patient often has little voluntary control over the process generating the symptom, so that exhortation or even encouragement may play little beneficial role in management.

A difficult and controversial issue is the use of placebo. Many neurologists customarily either elicit psychogenic symptoms with placebo (such as using saline injections to evoke pseudoseizures) or attempt to treat psychogenic symptoms with placebo, often an "active placebo" in the form of a relatively benign medicine that has some plausible relation to the medical condition that the patient doesn't have (but would have if the complaint were organically based). At least two arguments against this practice must be considered. One is ethical: it is impermissible to give agents to patients without explaining what they are and obtaining informed consent. Although this can be finessed with placebos, finesse is not the same as an honest doctor–patient relationship. The second point is that, just as an inactive agent can have a placebo effect, so it can have a negative ("nocebo") effect based on psychological mechanisms. No *a priori* reason guarantees a positive effect from a somatic intervention in a patient with a tendency to somatization, even an intervention that is allegedly harmless.

CONCLUSIONS

Somatization Disorders are common in medical practice, Dissociative Disorders rare, although the two sets of disorders have significant pathogenic and phenomenological commonalities as well as common roots in the history of medical thinking. Awareness of the psychiatric elements of the purportedly somatoform disorders should help the neurologist in an attempt to make confident diagnoses and provide effective treatment.

REFERENCES

1. Weir Mitchell S. Rest in nervous disease: its use and abuse. In: Seguin EC, ed. A Series of American Clinical Lectures. New York: G. P. Putnam's Sons; 1876:83–102.
2. Hyler SE, Spitzer RL. Hysteria split asunder. Am J Psychiatry 1978;135:1500–1504.
3. Lewis A. The survival of hysteria. Psychol Med 1975;5:9–12.
4. King H. Once upon a text: hysteria from Hippocrates. In: Gilman SL, King H, Porter R, Rousseau GS, Showalter E, eds. Hysteria Beyond Freud. Berkeley: University of California Press; 1993:3–90.
5. Micale MS. Approaching Hysteria: Disease and its Interpretations. Princeton: Princeton University Press; 1995.
6. Shephard B. A War of Nerves: Soldiers and Psychiatrists in the Twentieth Century. Cambridge: Harvard University Press; 2001.
7. Gelfand T. Charcot's response to Freud's rebellion. J Hist Ideas 1989;50:293–307.
8. Charcot JM, Harris R. Clinical Lectures on Diseases of the Nervous System. London, New York: Tavistock/Routledge; 1991.
9. Micale MS. On the "disappearance" of hysteria: a study in the clinical deconstruction of a diagnosis. Isis 1993;84:496–526.
10. Reynolds JR. Paralysis, and other disorders of motion and sensation, dependent on idea. Brit Med J 1869;ii:483–485.
11. Lenze EJ, Miller AR, Munir ZB, Pornnoppadol C, North CS. Psychiatric symptoms endorsed by somatization disorder patients in a psychiatric clinic. Ann Clin Psychiatry 1999;11:73–79.
12. Stone J, Zeman A, Sharpe M. Functional weakness and sensory disturbance. J Neurol Neurosurg Psychiatry 2002;73:241–245.
13. Gould R, Miller BL, Goldberg MA, Benson DF. The validity of hysterical signs and symptoms. J Nerv Ment Dis 1986;174:593–597.
14. Carson AJ, Ringbauer B, Stone J, McKenzie L, Warlow C, Sharpe M. Do medically unexplained symptoms matter? A prospective cohort study of 300 new referrals to neurology outpatient clinics. J Neurol Neurosurg Psychiatry 2000;68:207–210.
15. Lempert T, Dieterich M, Huppert D, Brandt T. Psychogenic disorders in neurology: frequency and clinical spectrum. Acta Neurol Scand 1990;82:335–340.

16. Reuber M, Pukrop R, Mitchell AJ, Bauer J, Elger CE. Clinical significance of recurrent psychogenic nonepileptic seizure status. J Neurol 2003;250:1355–1362.

17. Scott PA, Silbergleit R. Misdiagnosis of stroke in tissue plasminogen activator-treated patients: characteristics and outcomes. Ann Emerg Med 2003;42:611–618.

18. Allanson J, Bass C, Wade DT. Characteristics of patients with persistent severe disability and medically unexplained neurological symptoms: a pilot study. J Neurol Neurosurg Psychiatry 2002;73:307–309.

19. Slater ET, Glithero E. A follow-up of patients diagnosed as suffering from "hysteria". J Psychosom Res 1965;9:9–13.

20. Crimlisk HL, Bhatia K, Cope H, David A, Marsden CD, Ron MA. Slater revisited: 6 year follow up study of patients with medically unexplained motor symptoms. Br Med J 1998;316:582–586.

21. Mace CJ, Trimble MR. Ten-year prognosis of conversion disorder. Br J Psychiatry 1996;169:282–288.

22. Moene FC, Landberg EH, Hoogduin KA, et al. Organic syndromes diagnosed as conversion disorder: identification and frequency in a study of 85 patients. J Psychosom Res 2000;49:7–12.

23. Stone J, Sharpe M, Rothwell PM, Warlow CP. The 12 year prognosis of unilateral functional weakness and sensory disturbance. J Neurol Neurosurg Psychiatry 2003;74:591–596.

24. Reuber M, Pukrop R, Bauer J, Helmstaedter C, Tessendorf N, Elger CE. Outcome in psychogenic nonepileptic seizures: 1 to 10-year follow-up in 164 patients. Ann Neurol 2003;53:305–311.

25. Spitzer C, Spelsberg B, Grabe HJ, Mundt B, Freyberger HJ. Dissociative experiences and psychopathology in conversion disorders. J Psychosom Res 1999;46:291–294.

26. Grunau RV, Whitfield MF, Petrie JH, Fryer EL. Early pain experience, child and family factors, as precursors of somatization: a prospective study of extremely premature and fullterm children. Pain 1994;56:353–359.

27. Hotopf M, Mayou R, Wadsworth M, Wessely S. Childhood risk factors for adults with medically unexplained symptoms: results from a national birth cohort study. Am J Psychiatry 1999;156:1796–1800.

28. Craig TK, Bialas I, Hodson S, Cox AD. Intergenerational transmission of somatization behaviour: 2. Observations of joint attention and bids for attention. Psychol Med 2004;34:199–209.

29. Fleisher W, Staley D, Krawetz P, Pillay N, Arnett JL, Maher J. Comparative study of trauma-related phenomena in subjects with pseudoseizures and subjects with epilepsy. Am J Psychiatry 2002;159:660–663.

30. Prueter C, Schultz-Venrath U, Rimpau W. Dissociative and associated psychopathological symptoms in patients with epilepsy, pseudoseizures, and both seizure forms. Epilepsia 2002;43:188–192.

31. Fergusson DM, Horwood LJ, Lynskey MT. Childhood sexual abuse and psychiatric disorder in young adulthood: II. Psychiatric outcomes of childhood sexual abuse. J Am Acad Child Adolesc Psychiatry 1996;35:1365–1374.

32. Molnar BE, Buka SL, Kessler RC. Child sexual abuse and subsequent psychopathology: results from the National Comorbidity Survey. Am J Public Health 2001;91:753–760.

33. Mulder RT, Beautrais AL, Joyce PR, Fergusson DM. Relationship between dissociation, childhood sexual abuse, childhood physical abuse, and mental illness in a general population sample. Am J Psychiatry 1998;155:806–811.

34. De Bellis MD. Developmental traumatology: the psychobiological development of maltreated children and its implications for research, treatment, and policy. Dev Psychopathol 2001;13:539–564.

35. De Bellis MD, Keshavan MS, Shifflett H, et al. Brain structures in pediatric maltreatment-related posttraumatic stress disorder: a sociodemographically matched study. Biol Psychiatry 2002;52:1066–1078.

36. Reuber M, House AO, Pukrop R, Bauer J, Elger CE. Somatization, dissociation and general psychopathology in patients with psychogenic non-epileptic seizures. Epilepsy Res 2003;57:159–167.

37. Reuber M, Fernandez G, Helmstaedter C, Qurishi A, Elger CE. Evidence of brain abnormality in patients with psychogenic nonepileptic seizures. Epilepsy Behav 2002;3:249–254.

38. Marshall JC, Halligan PW, Fink GR, Wade DT, Frackowiak RS. The functional anatomy of a hysterical paralysis. Cognition 1997;64:B1–B8.

39. Vuilleumier P, Chicherio C, Assal F, Schwartz S, Slosman D, Landis T. Functional neuroanatomical correlates of hysterical sensorimotor loss. Brain 2001;124(Pt 6):1077–1090.

40. Mailis-Gagnon A, Giannoylis I, Downar J, et al. Altered central somatosensory processing in chronic pain patients with "hysterical" anesthesia. Neurology 2003;60:1501–1507.

41. Stone J, Sharpe M, Carson A, et al. Are functional motor and sensory symptoms really more frequent on the left? A systematic review. J Neurol Neurosurg Psychiatry 2002;73:578–581.

42. Wessely S, White PD. There is only one functional somatic syndrome. Br J Psychiatry 2004;185:95–96.

43. Meares R. Towards a psyche for psychiatry. Aust N Z J Psychiatry 2003;37:689–695.

44. North CS, Hansen K, Wetzel RD, Compton W, Napier M, Spitznagel EL. Nonpsychotic thought disorder: objective clinical identification of somatization and antisocial personality in language patterns. Compr Psychiatry 1997;38:171–178.

45. Ovsiew F. Psychogenic movement disorders: an overview of the psychiatric approach to conversion disorder. In: Hallett M, ed. Psychogenic Movement Disorders; in press.

46. Karvonen JT, Veijola J, Jokelainen J, Laksy K, Jarvelin MR, Joukamaa M. Somatization disorder in young adult population. Gen Hosp Psychiatry 2004;26:9–12.

47. Fink P, Hansen MS, Oxhoj ML. The prevalence of somatoform disorders among internal medical inpatients. J Psychosom Res 2004;56:413–418.

48. Feder A, Olfson M, Gameroff M, et al. Medically unexplained symptoms in an urban general medicine practice. Psychosomatics 2001;42:261–268.
49. Breslau N, Lipton RB, Stewart WF, Schultz LR, Welch KM. Comorbidity of migraine and depression: investigating potential etiology and prognosis. Neurology 2003;60:1308–1312.
50. Veale D. Body dysmorphic disorder. Postgrad Med J 2004;80:67–71.
51. Aouizerate B, Pujol H, Grabot D, et al. Body dysmorphic disorder in a sample of cosmetic surgery applicants. Eur Psychiatry 2003;18:365–368.
52. Phillips KA. Psychosis in body dysmorphic disorder. J Psychiatr Res 2004;38:63–72.
53. Barsky AJ, Ahern DK. Cognitive behavior therapy for hypochondriasis: a randomized controlled trial. JAMA 2004;291:1464–1470.
54. Allen LA, Escobar JI, Lehrer PM, Gara MA, Woolfolk RL. Psychosocial treatments for multiple unexplained physical symptoms: a review of the literature. Psychosom Med 2002;64:939–950.
55. Becker-Blease KA, Deater-Deckard K, Eley T, Freyd JJ, Stevenson J, Plomin R. A genetic analysis of individual differences in dissociative behaviors in childhood and adolescence. J Child Psychol Psychiatry 2004;45:522–532.
56. Kopelman MD. Disorders of memory. Brain 2002;125(Pt 10):2152–2190.
57. Cima M, Nijman H, Merckelbach H, Kremer K, Hollnack S. Claims of crime-related amnesia in forensic patients. Int J Law Psychiatry 2004;27:215–221.
58. Symonds C. Hysteria. In: Merskey H, ed. The Analysis of Hysteria. London: Balliere Tindall; 1979:258–265.
59. Hacking I. Mad Travelers: Reflections on the Reality of Transient Mental Illnesses. Charlottesville: University Press of Virginia; 1998.
60. Lambert MV, Sierra M, Phillips ML, David AS. The spectrum of organic depersonalization: a review plus four new cases. J Neuropsychiatry Clin Neurosci 2002;14:141–154.
61. Baker D, Hunter E, Lawrence E, et al. Depersonalisation disorder: clinical features of 204 cases. Br J Psychiatry 2003;182:428–433.
62. Blanke O, Landis T, Spinelli L, Seeck M. Out-of-body experience and autoscopy of neurological origin. Brain 2004;127 (Pt 2):243–258.
63. Maillard L, Vignal JP, Anxionnat R, TaillandierVespignani L. Semiologic value of ictal autoscopy. Epilepsia 2004;45:391–394.
64. Schrag A, Brown RJ, Trimble MR. Reliability of self-reported diagnoses in patients with neurologically unexplained symptoms. J Neurol Neurosurg Psychiatry 2004;75:608–611.
65. Dickinson WP, Dickinson LM, deGruy FV, Main DS, Candib LM, Rost K. A randomized clinical trial of a care recommendation letter intervention for somatization in primary care. Ann Fam Med 2003;1:228–235.

8

Catatonia

Clinical Features, Differential Diagnosis, and Treatment

Patricia I. Rosebush and Michael F. Mazurek

INTRODUCTION

Catatonia is a clinical syndrome characterized by a range of psychomotor abnormalities. It was first described in 1875 by Kahlbaum *(1)* who reported 25 patients with a "brain disease" characterized by four of the following signs: long periods of immobility, mutism alternating with verbigeration, staring, withdrawal and refusal to eat or drink, negativism, posturing and grimacing, echolalia, echopraxia, stereotypy, and waxy flexibility (*see* Table 1). Kahlbaum observed that these otherwise immobile patients could become very agitated or excited and were often found to have extremes of mood disturbance in the form of "melancholy" or "mania." This phenomenon of marked, polar alterations in the predominant psychomotor state eventually led to division of the syndrome into *retarded* and *excited* types *(2)*. The excited form has been much more difficult to characterize and distinguish from mania *(3)*. In rare instances, patients with severe motor excitement develop fever, autonomic disturbances, stupor, and rhabdomyolysis and may succumb to cardiovascular collapse. This clinical state has been referred to as lethal or malignant catatonia *(4,5)* and the clinical and laboratory similarities to neuroleptic malignant syndrome (NMS) has generated considerable interest and discussion *(6,7)*.

This chapter focuses on retarded catatonia including clinical, laboratory and autonomic features, diagnosis, complications, treatment, and underlying diagnoses.

THE CURRENT STATUS OF CATATONIA

Whereas catatonia seemed to "disappear" from the clinical landscape for many years *(8,9)* recent studies reported the incidence to be between 9 and 15% of admissions to acute-care psychiatric units *(10–13)*. This suggests that the term may simply have fallen into disuse and that the clinical phenomenon of immobile, mute, staring, withdrawn, and rigid patients has been with us all the time. Whether or not one used the term *catatonia* to describe this particular constellation of signs may, at one time, have been of only academic interest, but the situation changed once it became clear that the syndrome is exquisitely responsive to treatment with benzodiazepines (BZPs) *(14)*. This ability to treat the condition easily and effectively is, perhaps, the most compelling reason for "re-awakening" physicians to a "forgotten disorder" *(15)*. This is particularly true for neurologists who are often called on to assess patients with catatonic signs.

From: *Current Clinical Neurology: Psychiatry for Neurologists*
Edited by: D.V. Jeste and J.H. Friedman © Humana Press Inc., Totowa, NJ

Table 1
Catatonic Signs Described by Kahlbaum in 1874

Sign	Definition
Immobility	Paucity or absence of spontaneous movements
Staring	Decreased frequency of blinking
Mutism	Inaudible whisper or absence of spontaneous speech
Rigidity	Increased muscle tone during passive movement of limbs
Withdrawal and refusal to eat	Turning away from examiner, avoidance of eye contact, refusal of food or drink when offered
Posturing	Voluntary assumption and maintenance of an inappropriate or bizarre posture
Grimacing	Unusual or exaggerated spontaneous facial expressions; Kahlbaum also referred to these as "snout spasms," "convulsive-type spasms," and "tics"
Negativism	Active resistance to instruction, e.g., patient asked to close or open eyes or mouth does the opposite
Waxy flexibility (catalepsy)	The maintenance of a limb in any position in which it is placed by the examiner
Echolalia or echopraxia	The repetition or mimicking of the examiner's actions or words
Stereotypy	Aimless repetitive movements, often bizarre in nature
Verbigeration	The continuous and directionless repetition of single words or phrases

MAKING THE DIAGNOSIS OF CATATONIA

The first and most essential step in recognizing catatonia is to think of the diagnosis when presented with a particular constellation of clinical signs. The most common catatonic signs are immobility, staring, mutism, and withdrawal with refusal to eat or drink, each of which has been observed in more than 75% of patients who presented to either our acute-care inpatient psychiatric unit or our consultation-liaison service. The diagnosis in these cases was based on the following: the presence of four or more of the catatonic signs described by Kahlbaum, and the resolution of the catatonia in response to treatment with BZP medication. The frequency of individual signs in 165 consecutive cases is shown in Fig. 1.

In contrast to the core catatonic features of mutism, immobility, staring, withdrawal, and refusal to eat, the more bizarre signs are comparatively less common. Patients are often incontinent and, depending on the duration of untreated illness, may be cachectic and dishevelled as well. Catatonic immobility can be so profound that at times it is difficult to see respirations. Whereas the absence of meaningful responses to those around them suggests a disturbance of consciousness, these patients are typically hyper-alert, aware of their surroundings, and able to recall their catatonic state in detail once recovered. Awareness and consciousness are reflected in the finding of normal electroencephalograms (EEGs) in almost all catatonic patients, a quality of gaze that belies unawareness, and the "ability" of these patients to do the exact opposite of what is requested (negativism) or to engage in echoing another's words or gestures.

CONDITIONS ASSOCIATED WITH CATATONIA

The majority of patients who develop catatonia do so in the context of another illness. In fact, catatonia has been described in association with a wide range of conditions, which often become apparent only after the catatonia resolves. A final common pathway for the wide spectrum of disorders and

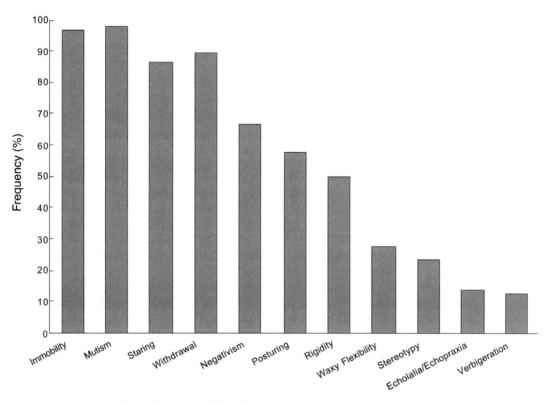

Fig. 1. Frequency of individual signs in 165 episodes of catatonia.

diseases said to cause or give rise to catatonia has not yet been identified. One possible unifying mechanism is the experience of overwhelming anxiety and preoccupation with death, reported by many patients who have been catatonic *(11,16)*. One suspects, for example, that this might have been operative in reports of catatonia occurring in the context of severe burns *(17)*. A minority of individuals appears to simply have catatonia and no other underlying disorder.

Underlying Diagnoses

Despite Kahlbaum's original observation that his catatonic patients suffered from disturbances of mood, Kraepelin, and later Bleuler, considered catatonia to be a subtype of schizophrenia. In his *Lectures on Clinical Psychiatry*, Kraepelin wrote that "the descriptions of disease summed up by [Kahlbaum] as katatonia are only special forms of dementia praecox" and he emphasized the difference between catatonia and manic-depressive illness *(18)*. For many years to follow, the subject of catatonia could be found only in reference to schizophrenia. Then, in the 1970s, the sole association of catatonia with schizophrenia was questioned as studies revealed that these patients ultimately enjoyed a more favorable outcome than generally expected with schizophrenia *(19,20)*. Later, prospective studies found that the majority of catatonic patients admitted to acute-care psychiatric units had mood disorders *(20,21)*, confirming Kahlbaum's impression. These findings are reflected in the inclusion of catatonia in the fourth edition of the Diagnostic and Statistical Manual of Mental Disorders (DSM-IV) as a modifier of certain mood disorders and general medical conditions in addition to being a subtype of schizophrenia *(22)*.

In our prospective study and 15-year follow-up of more than 100 patients admitted to our inpatient psychiatry service or seen on the medical units in a catatonic state, both unipolar and bipolar affective disorders have been the most common underlying diagnoses, accounting for approx 44% of cases.

Table 2
**Underlying Neurological and Medical Disorders
Found in 16 of 137 Prospectively Studied Patients
With Catatonia Presenting to a Psychiatry Service**

Neurological/medical disorder	N
Brain tumor (Posterior Fossa $n = 2$, Frontal $n = 1$)	3
AIDS	2
Viral encephalitis	2
Spongiform encephalopathy (CJD)	2
GM$_2$ gangliosidosis	1
Mitochondrial disorder (Kearne-Sayres)	1
Paraneoplastic syndrome (limbic encephalitis)	1
Frontal lobe dementia	1
Multi-infarct dementia	1
Normal pressure hydrocephalus	1
Temporal lobe dysrythmia	1

This is followed in frequency by schizophrenia (17%), other psychoses (e.g., brief reactive psychosis, atypical psychosis, paranoid disorders [7%]), cocaine intoxication (7%), and identifiable medical or neurological conditions (9%) (*see* Table 2). The vast majority of patients with catatonia are found to be psychotic once they are treated and able to speak.

Except for the patient with normal pressure hydrocephalus and one of the individuals with a posterior fossa tumor, all these patients responded to treatment with lorazepam.

A very important and readily treatable cause of catatonia, which accounted for 16% of our cases, is BZP withdrawal. Our first case is a striking illustration of the phenomenon. One of us was called on an emergency basis to admit an 88-year-old man who was thought by his physician to be suffering from the consequences of an apparent brainstem stroke. The patient was, until a few days earlier, cognitively intact and in semi-independent living because of blindness resulting from glaucoma. He had no other medical history. Because of his age, his family did not want him transferred to the hospital and subjected to investigations so we assessed him at the retirement home. On examination, he was found to be mute, staring, immobile, extremely rigid, and incontinent. He had not taken anything by mouth for several days and appeared very dehydrated. We learned that his clonazepam, which he had been taking at a dose of 1.5 mg for 15 years for sleep, had been tapered and finally discontinued just days before his deterioration. His family declined blood work or other investigations but gave permission for the intramuscular administration of 2 mg of lorazepam. Within 45 minutes he began to speak and take fluids by mouth. His rigidity lessened. Another 2 mg was given 6 hours later at bedtime and by the morning he had recovered fully. On a maintenance regimen of lorazepam he lived for another 6 years without any medical events.

Patients admitted to the hospital for any reason are often reluctant to report their use of this commonly prescribed agent. Shortly after, they experience withdrawal, one manifestation of which can be catatonia. Hauser *(23)* described catatonia precipitated by BZP withdrawal in 1989 and in 1996 we reported five patients in our series whose catatonia had occurred in this context *(24)*. Since that time, other similar reports have appeared in the literature *(25,26)*.

Neurological Conditions That Can Mimic Catatonia

Parkinsonism

We have been asked to see patients with a tentative diagnosis of catatonia who, upon examination, are found to be parkinsonian. In 1998 *(27)*, we described a 37-year-old woman who had been hospitalized at another center with a diagnosis of catatonia. On examination, she had profound psychomotor retardation with a stare and flat facial expression. Her "posturing" consisted of periods of freezing—a very stooped posture and flexed arms. She had no spontaneous speech and on further examination was found to have a shuffling gait, cogwheel rigidity, and micrographia. We subsequently learned that, prior to hospitalization, she had been treated with high-dose antipsychotic agents for anxiety and insomnia. We therefore diagnosed parkinsonism secondary to these drugs and she eventually recovered, albeit slowly, from their withdrawal.

The most common causes of parkinsonism in the patients we see are either idiopathic disease or extrapyramidal side effects secondary to antipsychotic drug treatment. Wilson's disease, a disorder of copper metabolism that results in copper deposition in the eye, liver, and basal ganglia, should always be considered in patients who present with any form of movement disorder at a young age and have concomitant psychiatric disturbances.

Unlike catatonic patients, those suffering from parkinsonism are usually cooperative and eager to interact with the physician rather than withdrawn and negativistic. Mutism, a key feature of catatonia, is uncommon with parkinsonism, although patients may be hypophonic. Rigidity characterizes both conditions, but parkinsonian patients often have a tremor, which is not part of the syndrome of catatonia. Furthermore, the bizarre behavioral features of catatonia, such as posturing and echophenomena, are absent. It is important to be alert to the possibility that a patient with parkinsonism can have superimposed catatonia, a situation we have observed a number of times.

Akinetic Mutism (28)

Akinetic mutism refers to patients who are fully aware but appear to have a profound lack of drive or motivation to speak or move. Rigidity and staring are typically absent, as are the more bizarre clinical features of catatonic state. A key point of differentiation from catatonia is the absence of negativism in patients with akinetic mutism. Despite this, the two conditions can be difficult to distinguish, as illustrated by an anecdote reported by Fisher *(29)* regarding a case of disulfuram-induced catatonia. He described a conference at the Massachusetts General Hospital in Boston during which 90 neurologists were presented with a mute, immobile patient who had, 2 weeks earlier, suffered rupture of an anterior communicating artery aneurysm. According to Fisher, the neurologists on hand were equally divided as to whether the patient should be regarded as having catatonia or akinetic mutism.

"Locked-In" Syndrome (30)

In locked-in syndrome, which typically reflects pontine pathology, patients are aware but unable to move, speak, or respond to their environment because of interruption of motor pathways and sparing of the reticular-activating system. Their alert gaze is similar to that observed in patients with catatonia. An important difference is that once the "locked-in" patient learns to use blinking to respond to questions, there is almost invariably a desire to communicate. As with catatonic patients, the EEG is typically normal and sleep–wake cycles are preserved.

Neuroleptic Malignant Syndrome (31,32)

This serious and life-threatening reaction to dopamine D_2-blocking agents is characterized by immobility, staring, rigidity, and mutism. The presence of diaphoresis, fever, and a labile blood pressure, as well as the absence of negativism, echolalia, echopraxia, grimacing or posturing, distinguishes NMS from catatonia. Additionally, NMS is typically associated with leukocytosis, low serum iron, and high levels of creatine phosphokinase not found in most cases of uncomplicated catatonia.

Persistent Vegetative State (33–35)

In persistent vegetative state, which typically follows a severe cerebral injury, patients are inattentive and mute with no apparent awareness of their surroundings. Whereas patients with catatonia may, at first blush, appear unaware of what is going on around them, the quality of their staring gaze indicates intense awareness and vigilance. The EEG in vegetative states is almost always abnormal in contrast to the normal results found in catatonic patients who also generally have excellent recall of events that took place when they were catatonic.

Nonconvulsive Status Epilepticus (36–39)

Patients with absence or partial complex status epilepticus (SE) can present in a state that is clinically indistinguishable from catatonia. They are immobile, mute, unresponsive, often rigid, and unable to eat, drink, or cooperate with an examination. Myoclonic jerking, automatisms, or semi-purposeful movements, eyelid fluttering or rhythmic twitching of the eyes, face, or jaw, if present, can be clues to the diagnosis. The EEG, which we believe is an important investigative tool in the diagnostic work-up of catatonia, is crucial in distinguishing nonconvulsive SE from catatonia.

Stiff-Man Syndrome (40,41)

This uncommon condition, now referred to as "stiff-*person* syndrome" (SPS), appropriately so given that women are affected more often than men, is very frequently misdiagnosed as a psychiatric condition such as conversion or catatonia. The clinical presentation of SPS often appears bizarre and exaggerated. Exacerbations or episodes can be triggered by emotional stress and the disorder is responsive to BZPs. Patients with SPS develop extensor muscle spasms of the spine and legs that can render them immobile and cause catatonia-like dystonic "posturing." The rigidity can be extremely severe and has been described as "stony," "board-like," and "rock-hard" *(40)*. In contrast to the mute state of catatonic patients, however, these individuals will indicate that they are in extreme pain. It now appears that SPS may be an autoimmune disease resulting from antibodies directed against glutamic acid decarboxylase, the rate-limiting enzyme in the production of γ-aminobutyric acid (GABA) *(42)*. Other autoimmune diseases such as diabetes and thyroiditis often afflict these individuals and in this respect, the medical history can alert one to the possible presence of the condition. The diagnosis of SPS is strongly supported by the presence of high serum levels of glutamic acid decarboxylase antibodies. The EEG in these patients will be normal and electomyographic studies will typically show continuous motor unit activity *(40)*.

EXAMINATION AND INVESTIGATION OF THE CATATONIC PATIENT

The very nature of catatonia means that the patient is unable to cooperate with many aspects of a physical examination, especially a detailed neurological assessment. The parts of the neurological exam that can usually be carried out on the catatonic patient and that can be helpful in differentiating catatonia from other conditions, include the pupillary reaction, ocular movements, the corneal reflex, reaction to pain, the presence of drooling, blink response to threat, reactions to light or sound, frontal release signs, assessment of tone, deep tendon reflexes, and the plantar responses *(29)*.

All patients with catatonia should have an EEG. Frequent determination of vital signs can assist in the early detection of infection or incipient NMS. In uncomplicated catatonia, patients are afebrile and normotensive, although they often have tachycardia. Hematological investigations should include a complete blood count, blood urea nitrogen, creatinine, muscle and hepatic enzymes, electrolytes, blood glucose, and urinalysis, all of which should be normal unless the patient is markedly dehydrated or has an intercurrent infection or illness. Fever and an elevated white blood cell count in a patient with apparent catatonia should raise concerns about possible encephalitis or, if antipsychotics have been administered, NMS.

COMPLICATIONS OF CATATONIA

Catatonia can be associated with considerable morbidity, particularly if the immobility, poor oral intake, and muscle rigidity are prolonged and develop in a patient who is alone and in a warm environment. Complications that can quickly arise under such circumstances include dehydration, malnutrition, pneumonia, deep vein thrombosis, pulmonary embolism, skin breakdown, contractures, and acute renal failure *(43)*.

There is evidence that patients are at increased risk of developing NMS if antipsychotic drugs (APDs) are administered when they are catatonic *(7,44,45)*. This is of considerable clinical relevance, given that catatonia affects approx 10% of patients hospitalized with acute psychiatric illness, the majority of whom are psychotic and in apparent need of APDs. The three patients on our inpatient unit who have developed NMS over the past 15 years were all catatonic prior to the administration of APDs. How then, is one to proceed with such patients? We recommend treating the catatonia with BZPs before APDs are prescribed. If this proves ineffective, electroconvulsive therapy (ECT) may be considered. It is our experience that once the catatonic syndrome has resolved, APDs may be introduced without undue risk of precipitating NMS. If a patient is judged to require APDs prior to resolution of the catatonia, we feel it is prudent to maintain BZPs during treatment with the APDs.

Lethal or malignant catatonia *(4)* is an extreme form of excited catatonia that bears remarkable similarity to NMS both in its clinical features and high mortality if untreated. Indeed it may be indistinguishable except for the absence of antecedent use of APDs and the history of rapidly increasing psychomotor activity. Early descriptions indicate that these patients develop psychosis, followed by uncontrollable motor activity. Fever, diaphoresis, dehydration, tachycardia, labile blood pressure, alterations in consciousness, and eventually cardiovascular collapse ensue.

TREATMENT

In 1990, following a number of individual case studies *(46–48)*, we reported that catatonia of the retarded type is exquisitely responsive to the administration of low-dose BZPs *(11)*. These agents have a paradoxical effect of rapidly activating the mute, immobile patient, making the treatment of catatonia one of the more memorable clinical experiences, akin to that of treating Parkinson's disease with L-dopa. Within a matter of hours of receiving the medication, a patient who previously may have been mistaken for dead, begins to move, talk, and eat. Yassa *(49)* described 10 patients, all of whom responded to low-dose lorazepam either by mouth or intramuscular injection. Seven had dramatic resolution of their catatonic state within hours of receiving BZP treatment. Immobility or severe psychomotor retardation, mutism, and withdrawal with refusal to eat or drink were the most common clinical features. Ungvari et al. *(50)* used low-dose lorazepam to treat 18 patients with catatonia that had been present for 2–22 days. Fifteen (83%) of these patients had virtually complete resolution of their catatonic state within hours. A literature review of 72 episodes of catatonia treated with BZPs *(51)* found a response rate of almost 80%. More recently, Lee et al. reported that 16 of 24 catatonic patients (73%) remitted fully with either lorazepam or clonazepam. In our ongoing prospective study that now involves 165 episodes of catatonia, predominantly of the retarded type *(52)*, we have continued to observe a robust response in approx 85% of patients following treatment with lorazepam. In our study, all catatonic patients admitted to the psychiatry unit are observed for 24 hours prior to treatment, in order to exclude those who recover spontaneously. The median duration of the catatonia has been 3 days with a range of 1–180 days. Catatonia had been present for 10 days or more in 19 cases.

The one diagnostic subgroup that does not enjoy a robust response to lorazepam is schizophrenia. In our prospective study, patients suffering from an underlying schizophrenic process responded 20–30% of the time, compared with an overall response rate of approx 90% in the other diagnostic subgroups, including those with underlying medical and neurological disorders *(53)*. Ungvari et al. *(54)* observed a similar lack of responsiveness in catatonic patients with underlying schizophrenia. In a randomized double-blind, placebo-controlled, crossover study of lorazepam 6 mg per day for 6 weeks in 17 patients with chronic schizophrenia and chronic catatonia, no significant differences were found on any measure between those who received lorazepam or those who received placebo, in contrast to the 83% response rate to lorazepam they had observed in their original study of patients with acute catatonia. Lee et al. *(13)* reported that patients who responded only *partially* to lorazepam were invariably schizophrenic. This poor responsiveness to BZPs, in patients with underlying schizophrenia, may be related to the nature of the core illness with more prominent psychosis and less anxiety, the nature of the particular catatonic symptoms that were present at the time of treatment or the chronicity that characterizes both the catatonia *and* the primary illness.

In the unresponsive schizophrenic patients studied by Ungvari et al., the typical catatonic signs included posturing, grimacing, stereotypy, and waxy flexibility; whereas in our series, in which there has been a high rate of response, the most frequent findings were immobility, mutism, staring, and withdrawal.

It is well recognized that chronic symptoms of any kind generally respond less robustly to treatment than do acute symptoms. The less robust effect of BZPs observed in patients with chronic catatonia should not, however, preclude a trial of therapy. Gaind et al. *(55)* reported success in a 29-year-old man with chronic schizophrenia and chronic severe catatonia, who responded slowly but completely to monotherapy with low-dose lorazepam. This patient went from a state of prolonged and profound incapacitation that lasted 5 years and required continuous hospitalization, to semi-independent living, which he had maintained at 8-year follow-up. We have also reported the effectiveness of lorazepam in the treatment of a long-standing catatonic state in a patient with late-onset Tay Sachs disease *(56)*.

The ideal treatment of any condition is one that is easily administered, produces a rapid response, and has a wide margin of safety. BZPs meet all three requirements and can be given orally, intramuscularly, or intravenously *(57)*. Low-dose lorazepam, which has been the most well studied BZP, produces a response within 1–3 hours and has a wide margin of safety even at high doses. Its speed of action decreases the time during which a patient is at risk of the complications that result from poor oral intake and immobility. The rapid response of catatonia to BZPs results in patients being able to cooperate with a full examination and any required investigations. It could be argued that, unless there is a clear contraindication to the use of BZPs, all mute, rigid, and immobile patients should be given a trial of this agent as a way to differentiate catatonia from clinically similar conditions. Even if another primary diagnosis is suspected, the patient may also be catatonic *(58)*. Davis and Borde *(59)* described a 12-year-old boy who presented with immobility, mutism, severe rigidity, double incontinence, reduced blinking, way flexibility, and "posturing." He was eventually diagnosed with Wilson's disease and treated with penicillamine. His "catatonia," however, improved little over 2 months until diazepam was administered. Within 2 days he was eating, speaking, and walking. To take another case in point, an 86-year-old woman was sent to the hospital from her nursing home with a tentative diagnosis of rapidly deteriorating Parkinson's disease. Over 1 month she had become mute, immobile, rigid, and appeared frightened. We considered catatonia in the differential and prescribed lorazepam 1 mg. Within 1 hour of the first dose, the patient had a "miraculous" full recovery from her worsening "parkinsonism."

Although ECT is also an effective treatment of catatonia, it is a more complicated intervention and requires clear consent from either the patient or a designated surrogate. By virtue of their mutism and withdrawal, catatonic patients are unable to engage in a discussion of ECT or consent to its administration. Surrogate consent is usually much more difficult to obtain for ECT because of the associated stigma. Furthermore, surrogate caregivers may not have full knowledge of the patient's medical history or medication use, making it difficult for them to be fully apprised of the risk–benefit ratio of anesthesia and the procedure itself. Often, a knowledgeable family member or caretaker is not available. Given that an initial dose of lorazepam is completely effective in quickly resolving catatonia in 85% of cases, it should be the first line of treatment. ECT should be considered after several days of lorazepam administration have been ineffective and the conditions for accepting consent from a fully competent, informed surrogate have been met *(60)*.

In the case of lethal catatonia, high doses of a BZP or ECT are the safest and most effective forms of treatment *(60)*.

RECOMMENDED TREATMENT REGIMEN

We recommend that most patients be treated initially with 2 mg of lorazepam intramuscularly. In the young, elderly, obese, or medically compromised patient, we suggest reducing each dosage to

1 mg. The possibility that lorazepam may be more effective than other BZPs such as Oxazepam *(48,61)* may relate to the fact that GABA-A receptors are made up of varying combinations of 16 different subunits, resulting in some diversity among the GABA-A receptors themselves. The different BZPs may differentially affect these various GABA-A receptor subtypes, thereby potentially producing "pharmacological diversity" and heterogeneity of response *(62)*. Whereas lorazepam can be given orally or sublingually, patient negativism is often manifested in a refusal to open the mouth, making oral administration impractical. Even when the patient appears to have accepted the tablet, it is often difficult to ascertain whether it has been ingested. The dehydration that is often present further reduces a patient's ability to absorb or swallow medication. For all these reasons, intramuscular injection is the preferred route of administration for the initial dose. Response to the initial injection usually occurs within 1–3 hours. If there is no response or only minimal change, the same dosage should be repeated after 3 hours and again after another 3 hours if the catatonia has not resolved. Although the intravenous route is effective, as well as practical if a patient is being rehydrated with intravenous fluids, the duration of action is very short unless the medication is given in the form of a continuous infusion.

BZPs not only bring about rapid resolution of the presenting catatonic state but seem to be required for maintenance of this effect until treatment of the primary disorder has been instituted. Discontinuation, immediately after the initial response, appears to put the patient at high risk of relapse. Once treatment of the patient's underlying illness has been established, BZPs can be tapered and discontinued in most cases. We have encountered a small subset of patients in whom long-term use of BZPs appears to be required. These individuals have responded robustly to acute treatment but appear to relapse into a catatonic state whenever the drugs are discontinued, despite the use of antidepressant medication or mood stabilizers. They appear to require long-term maintenance treatment with a BZP, raising the interesting question of whether catatonia in such cases might be considered a diagnosis in its own right and not simply a manifestation of another underlying disorder.

COMPLICATIONS OR SIDE EFFECTS OF BZP TREATMENT

Unsteadiness of Gait Following BZP Administration

This is a concern in the elderly or anyone with an underlying gait disturbance, especially when the therapeutic goal of treatment is motoric activation. Staff should be advised that treatment often takes effect rapidly and consideration should be given to using bed-side rails, making a walker available, and providing close supervision for vulnerable patients during the initial period of mobilization when they are up and about.

Respiratory Depression With BZP Use

BZPs depress alveolar ventilation and reduce hypoxic drive. These effects are more marked in patients with chronic obstructive pulmonary disease (COPD). At lower dosages, BZDs may worsen any sleep-related respiratory disorders like obstructive sleep apnea secondary to their effects on the upper airway musculature. This may result in reduced ventilatory response to carbon dioxide. One should, therefore, use a lower dosage of lorazepam and carry out more frequent monitoring of vital signs in any catatonic individual who is obese or known to have COPD or sleep apnea. Measurement of oxygen saturation is appropriate in these situations and provides an easy, noninvasive, and readily available tool for monitoring.

Precipitation of Agitation or Excitement Following Treatment

BZPs have the potential to disinhibit behavior, although this is felt to occur uncommonly. Patients with retarded catatonia, especially those with an underlying bipolar affective disorder, may become markedly agitated or excited following resolution of the catatonia. This can be associated with destruction of property and aggression toward others. It is, therefore, important for staff to be aware of, and prepared for, this eventuality. This would include maintaining the patient on close observation, being attentive to the rapidity and degree of activation following treatment, and having provisions for restraint or seclusion. Importantly, higher doses of the same BZP used to treat the catatonic immobility can be used to quell patients who become agitated. In our experience, this is a very uncommon event.

POTENTIAL MECHANISMS BY WHICH BENZODIAZEPINES MIGHT TREAT CATATONIA

The pharmacological properties of BZPs result from their relationship to the amino acid GABA, the primary inhibitory neurotransmitter in the central nervous system (CNS). BZPs act by binding to an allosteric site on the GABA-A receptor, resulting in the potentiation of GABA-mediated chloride conductance and inhibition of neuronal firing. GABA-A receptors are widely distributed in the CNS, ,allowing multiple potential sites of action for the BZP drugs *(63)*. The therapeutic actions of BZPs in catatonia can be understood in a number of ways, depending on how the disorder is conceptualized, including those discussed here *(14,16,64)*.

Catatonia As a Movement Disorder

We have previously proposed that catatonia can perhaps be best understood as a movement disorder. The clinical features of catatonia closely parallel those of parkinsonism *(27)*, which is known to arise from dysfunction of the basal ganglia. At least four major projection pathways in the basal ganglia use GABA as a neurotransmitter: (a) the so-called "direct" pathway from the striatum to the internal part of the globus pallidus (GPi) and the reticular part of the substantia nigra (SNr), (b) the "indirect" pathway from the striatum to the external segment of the globus pallidus (GPe), (c) the projection from GPe to the subthalamic nucleus, and (d) the projections from GPi and SNr to the ventral-anterior and ventral-lateral nuclei of the thalamus. BZPs may potentiate GABA signaling in any or all of these pathways, thereby alleviating the immobility, rigidity, and staring that characterized retarded catatonia. We have had patients with catatonia report that they felt better *because* they were able to move following treatment with lorazepam, supporting the notion that the basal ganglia might be one of the primary sites of action of the drug.

Catatonia As an Expression of Extreme Anxiety

In our ongoing study of 165 episodes of catatonia, a large majority of the patients reported having felt extremely anxious to the point that approx 15% actually believed they were dead or going to die. The experience of anxiety may be an important final common pathway for catatonia given that it can occur in the context of diverse conditions, including medical/neurological disorders, primary psychiatric illnesses, and BZP withdrawal. The potent anxiolytic properties of BZPs may explain their efficacy in treating catatonia in so many different clinical situations.

Catatonia As a State of Extreme Inhibition

The concept of behavioral disinhibition is of interest given that a small minority of individuals describe their catatonic immobility and mutism as defences against aggression or other actions that they find unacceptable. Furthermore, the resolution of retarded catatonia with BZPs can be followed by extreme agitation and aggression albeit rarely. Although there is considerable controversy about whether or not behavioral disinhibition is a real clinical consequence of BZP drug use in humans, studies in animals have repeatedly shown that BZPs have the potential to "release suppressed behaviors" and reduce the fear of negative consequences that would otherwise be attendant on certain actions. Indeed, BZPs are developed according to whether they induce feeding, drinking, and locomotor behaviors that have previously been decreased in response to punishment *(65)*.

CONCLUSIONS

1. Catatonia of the retarded type is present in approx 9% of all admissions to an acute psychiatric service.
2. The majority of patients admitted to an acute psychiatric service with catatonia have an underlying mood disorder.

3. BZP withdrawal can precipitate catatonia.
4. A wide range of underlying medical and neurological diagnoses may be associated with catatonia.
5. Catatonia has the potential to produce considerable morbidity from severe dehydration, contractures, deep vein thrombosis, pulmonary embolus, and skin break down.
6. Catatonia of the retarded type is exquisitely responsive to low-dose lorazepam.
7. The administration of antipsychotic agents to patients while catatonic may increase the risk of inducing NMS.
8. Except in a small subgroup of patients, BZPs can be discontinued once the catatonia resolves and treatment of the underlying disorder is established.
9. BZP represents a very safe, effective and easy to use treatment for catatonia.
10. For cases that do not respond to treatment with BZP, ECT is often effective.

REFERENCES

1. Kahlbaum KL. Catatonia. Baltimore: Johns Hopkins University Press; 1874.
2. Morrison JR. Catatonia. Retarded and excited types. Arch Gen Psychiatry 1973;28:39–41.
3. Taylor MA, Fink M. Catatonia in psychiatric classification: a home of its own. Am J Psychiatry 2003;160:1233–1241.
4. Mann SC, Caroff SN, Bleier HR, Welz WK, Kling MA, Hayashida M. Lethal catatonia. Am J Psychiatry 1986;143:1374–1381.
5. Mann SC, Carroff SN, Fricchione GL, et al. Malignant catatonia. In: Caroff SN, Mann SC, Francis A, Fricchione GL, eds. Catatonia: From Psychopathology to Neurobiology. Arlington: American Psychiatric Publishing; 2004:105–119.
6. Lee JW. Serum iron in catatonia and neuroleptic malignant syndrome. Biol Psychiatry 1998;44:499–507.
7. White DA, Robins AH. An analysis of 17 catatonic patients diagnosed with neuroleptic malignant syndrome. CNS Spectr 2000;5:58–65.
8. Stompe T, Ortwein-Swoboda G, Ritter K, Schanda H, Friedmann A. Are we witnessing the disappearance of catatonic schizophrenia? Compr Psychiatry 2002;43:167–174.
9. Mahendra B. Where have all the catatonics gone? Psychol Med 1981;11:669–671.
10. Lohr JB, Wisenewski AA. Movement Disorders: A Neuropsychiatric Approach. New York: Guilford Press; 1987.
11. Rosebush PI, Hildebrand AM, Furlong BG, Mazurek MF. Catatonic syndrome in a general psychiatric inpatient population: frequency, clinical presentation, and response to lorazepam. J Clin Psychiatry 1990;51:357–362.
12. Bush G, Fink M, Petrides G, Dowling F, Francis A. Catatonia. I. Rating scale and standardized examination. Acta Psychiatr Scand 1996;93:129–136.
13. Lee JW, Schwartz DL, Hallmayer J. Catatonia in a psychiatric intensive care facility: incidence and response to benzodiazepines. Ann Clin Psychiatry 2000;12:89–96.
14. Rosebush PI, Mazurek MF. Pharmacotherapy. In: Caroff SN, Mann SC, Fricchione G, eds. Catatonia: From Psychopathology to Neurobiology (), Arlington: American Psychiatric Publishing; 2004:141–150.
15. Rosebush PI, Mazurek MF. Catatonia: re-awakening to a forgotten disorder. Mov Disord 1999;14:395–397.
16. Rosebush PI, Mazurek MF. A consideration of the mechanisms by which lorazepam might treat catatonia. J Clin Psychiatry 1991;52:187–188.
17. Zarr ML, Nowak T. Catatonia and burns. Burns 1990;16:133–134.
18. Kraepelin E. Lectures on Clinical Psychiatry. New York: William Wood;1913.
19. Abrams R, Taylor MA. Catatonia: prediction of response to somatic treatments. Am J Psychiatry 1977;134:78–80.
20. Morrison JR. Catatonia: prediction of outcome. Compr Psychiatry 1974;15:317–324.
21. Abrams R, Taylor MA. Catatonia. A prospective clinical study. Arch Gen Psychiatry 1976;33:579–581.
22. American Psychiatric Association. Diagnostic and Statistical Manual of Mental Disorders, Fourth Edition. Washington DC: Amer Psychiatric Pub; 1994.
23. Hauser P, Devinsky O, De Bellis M, Theodore WH, Post RM. Benzodiazepine withdrawal delirium with catatonic features. Occurrence in patients with partial seizure disorders. Arch Neurol 1989;46:696–699.
24. Rosebush PI, Mazurek MF. Catatonia after benzodiazepine withdrawal. J Clin Psychopharmacol 1996;16:315–319.
25. Glover SG, Escalona R, Bishop J, Saldivia A. Catatonia associated with lorazepam withdrawal. Psychosomatics 1997;38:148–150.
26. Deuschle M, Lederbogen F. Benzodiazepine withdrawal-induced catatonia. Pharmacopsychiatry 2001;34:41–42.
27. Mazurek MF, Saver JL, Bodda RS, Garside S, Rosebush PI. Persistent loss of tyrosine hydroxylase immunoreactivity in the substantia nigra after neuroleptic withdrawal. J Neurol Neurosurg Psychiatry 2004;64:799–801.
28. Muqit MM, Rakshi JS, Shakir RA, Larner AJ. Catatonia or abulia? A difficult differential diagnosis. Mov Disord 2001;16:360–362.
29. Fisher CM. "Catatonia" due to disulfiram toxicity. Arch Neurol 1989;46:798–804.
30. Bauer G, Gerstenbrand F, Rumple E. Locked-in syndrome. J Neurol 1979;221:77–99.
31. Rosebush PI, Stewart T. A prospective analysis of 24 episodes of neuroleptic malignant syndrome. Am J Psychiatry 1989;146:717–725.

32. Rosebush PI, Mazurek MF. Neuroleptic malignant syndrome: differential diagnosis, treatment, and medical-legal implications. Essent Psychopharmacol 2003;5:187–215.
33. Ropper AH. Unusual spontaneous movements in brain-dead patients. Neurology 1984;34:1089–1092.
34. The Multi-Society Task Force on PVS. Medical aspects of the persistent vegetative state (1). N Engl J Med 1994;330: 1499–1508.
35. Kennard C, Illingworth R. Persistent vegetative state. J Neurol Neurosurg Psychiatry 1995;59:347–348.
36. Walls MJ, Bowers TC, Dilsaver SC, Swann AC. Catatonia associated with depression secondary to complex partial epilepsy. J Clin Psychiatry 1993;54:73.
37. Kirubakaran V, Sen S, Wilkinson CB. Catatonic stupor: unusual manifestation of temporal lobe epilepsy. Psychiatr J Univ Ott 1987;12:244–246.
38. Lim J, Yagnik P, Schraeder P, Wheeler S. Ictal catatonia as a manifestation of nonconvulsive status epilepticus. J Neurol Neurosurg Psychiatry 1986;49:833–836.
39. Primavera A, Fonti A, Novello P, Roccatagliata G, Cocito L. Epileptic seizures in patients with acute catatonic syndrome. J Neurol Neurosurg Psychiatry 1994;57:1419–1422.
40. Murinson BB. Stiff-person syndrome. The Neurologist 2004;10:131–137.
41. Meinck HM, Thompson PD. Stiff man syndrome and related conditions. Mov Disord 2002;17:853–866.
42. Solimena M, Folli F, Denis-Donini S, et al. Autoantibodies to glutamic acid decarboxylase in a patient with stiff-man syndrome, epilepsy and type 1 diabetes mellitus. N Engl J Med 1988;318:1012–1020.
43. McCall WV, Mann SC, Shelp FE, Caroff SN. Fatal pulmonary embolism in the catatonic syndrome: two case reports and a literature review. J Clin Psychiatry 1995;56:21–25.
44. White DA. Catatonia and the neuroleptic malignant syndrome—a single entity? Br J Psychiatry 1992;161:558–560.
45. Rosebush PI, Mazurek MF. Risk of Neuroleptic Malignant Syndrome in Patients with Catatonia. Proceedings of 149th annual meeting of the American Psychiatric Association, New York, 1996:30.
46. Fricchione GL, Cassem NH, Hooberman D, Hobson D. Intravenous lorazepam in neuroleptic-induced catatonia. J Clin Psychopharmacol 1983;3:338–342.
47. Barnes MP, Saunders M, Walls TJ, Saunders I, Kirk CA. The syndrome of Karl Ludwig Kahlbaum. J Neurol Neurosurg Psychiatry 1986;49:991–996.
48. Wetzel H, Heuser I, Benkert O. Benzodiazepines for catatonic symptoms, stupor, and mutism. Pharmacopsychiatry 1988; 21:394–395.
49. Yassa R, Iskandar H, Lalinec M, Cleto L. Lorazepam as an adjunct in the treatment of catatonic states: an open clinical trial. J Clin Psychopharmacol 1990;10:66–68.
50. Ungvari GS, Leung CM, Chiu HM. Lorazepam in stupor. Br J Clin Pract 1994;48:165–166.
51. Hawkins JM, Archer KJ, Strakowski SM, Keck PE. Somatic treatment of catatonia. Int J Psychiatry Med 1995;25:345–369.
52. Rosebush PI, Mazurek MF. Underlying diagnosis and response to lorazepam. 150th annual meeting of the American Psychiatric Association, 1997.
53. Mazurek MF, Rosebush PI. The treatment of catatonia: response to benzodiazepine medication is dependent on the underlying diagnosis. Psychogenic Movement Disorders Workshop, 2003.
54. Ungvari GS, Chiu HF, Chow LY, Lau BS, Tang WK. Lorazepam for chronic catatonia: a randomized, double-blind, placebo-controlled cross-over study. Psychopharmacology (Berl) 1999;142:393–398.
55. Gaind GS, Rosebush PI, Mazurek MF. Lorazepam treatment of acute and chronic catatonia in two mentally retarded brothers. J Clin Psychiatry 1994;55:20–23.
56. Rosebush PI, MacQueen GM, Clarke JT, Callahan JW, Strasberg PM, Mazurek MF. Late-onset Tay-Sachs disease presenting as catatonic schizophrenia: diagnostic and treatment issues. J Clin Psychiatry 1995;56:347–353.
57. Rosebush PI, Hildebrand AM, Mazurek MF. The treatment of catatonia: benzodiazepines of ECT? Am J Psychiatry 1992; 149:1279–1280.
58. Sternbach H, Yager J. Catatonia in the presence of mid-brain and brainstem abnormalities. J Clin Psychiatry 1981;42: 352–353.
59. Davis EJ, Borde M. Wilson's disease and catatonia. Br J Psychiatry 1993;162:256–259.
60. Fink M, Taylor MA. Catatonia: A Clinician's Guide to Diagnosis and Treatment. Cambridge: Cambridge University Press; 2003.
61. Scamvougeras A, Rosebush PI. AIDS-related psychosis with catatonia responding to low-dose lorazepam. J Clin Psychiatry 1992;53:414–415.
62. Cherubini E, Conti F. Generating diversity at GABAergic synapses. Trends Neurosci 2001;24:155–162.
63. Cooper JR, Bloom FE, Roth RH. The biochemical basis of neuropharmacology. New York: Oxford University Press; 2003.
64. Rogers D. Catatonia: a contemporary approach. J Neuropsychiatry Clin Neurosci 1991;3:334–340.
65. Charney DS, Mihic JS, Harris RA. Hypnosis and sedatives. In: Hardman JG, Limbird L E, Gilman AG, eds. The pharmacological basics of therapuetics. New York: McGraw-Hill; 2001:399–427.

9

Addictions

David W. Oslin

INTRODUCTION

Alcohol and drug dependence are two of the leading causes of disability and mortality worldwide; however, these problems are often not appreciated and are often unrecognized in primary and specialty medical settings *(1)*. Past drug or alcohol use has also been recognized as important in the care of patients, as past periods of abuse or dependence can increase vulnerability to subsequent medical and neuropsychiatric problems. Perhaps more importantly, recent research has demonstrated the efficacy of both psychosocial and pharmacological treatments for substance dependence and there is evidence that treatment can lead, not only to reductions in substance use and associated social problems, but also to substantial improvements in the physical and mental health of patients. This chapter highlights some of the recent advances in understanding and treating substance use and abuse, with a particular emphasis on the identification of patients, consequences of use, and methods for motivating patients to engage in treatment.

DIAGNOSIS AND TERMS

Substance dependence refers to a medical disorder characterized by loss of control, preoccupation with the substance, continued use despite adverse consequences, and physiological symptoms such as tolerance and withdrawal *(2)*. The current definition of *substance dependence* in the fourth edition of the Diagnostic and Statistical Manual of Mental Disorders (DSM-IV) is outlined in Table 1 *(2)*. The term *dependence*, as used in the official DSM-IV manual, often leads to semantic confusion with *dependence* in the pharmacological sense, which is a normal response to repeated use of many different types of medications, including drugs for the treatment of hypertension, depression, and pain. Thus, many clinicians prefer the term *addiction* when referring to dependence as defined in DSM-IV. In addition to the syndrome of addiction, some adults engage in *problem, abusive*, or *at-risk* substance use in which use of a substance is at a level that either has already resulted in adverse medical, psychological, or social consequences or substantially increases the likelihood of such problems, but not to a degree that meets the criteria of dependence. Because at-risk use often does not lead to some of the classic symptoms of addiction, such as employment or legal problems, individuals and practitioners may underestimate the risks associated with at-risk use. However, because of the risks, problem and at-risk use do represent an appropriate target for interventions.

In addition to these categories of problematic substance use, individuals may also consume substances at levels of *low risk* or be considered *abstainers*. Abstinence typically refers to no use of a substance in the previous year. Approximately 30–40% of adults are abstinent for alcohol use *(3)*. If

From: *Current Clinical Neurology: Psychiatry for Neurologists*
Edited by: D.V. Jeste and J.H. Friedman © Humana Press Inc., Totowa, NJ

Table 1
DSM IV Criteria for Substance Abuse and Dependence

Abuse

A. A maladaptive pattern of substance use as leading to clinically significant impairment or distress, as manifested by one or more of the following, occurring within a 12-month period.
 1. Failure to fulfill social, educational, or occupational roles
 2. Recurrent use in situations which are physically hazardous
 3. Recurrent substance related legal problems
 4. Continued use despite having persistent or recurrent social or interpersonal problems caused or exacerbated by the effects of the substance's adverse consequences

B. The symptoms have never met the criteria for Substance Dependence for this class of substance.

Dependence

A. A maladaptive pattern of substance use, leading to clinically significant impairment or distress, as manifested by three (or more) of the following, occurring at any time in the same 12-month period.
 1. Tolerance as defined by either of the following:
    a. a need for markedly increased amounts of the substance to achieve intoxication or the desired effect
    b. markedly diminished effect with continued use of the same amount of the substance
 2. Withdrawal, as manifested by either of the following:
    a. the characteristic withdrawal syndrome for the substance
    b. the same substance is taken to relieve or avoid withdrawal symptoms
 3. Increasing amounts over time when not intended
 4. Persistent desire or attempts to cut down or control substance use
 5. Great deal of time spent in activities necessary to obtain the substance or recover from its effects
 6. Important social, occupational, or recreational activities are given up or reduced
 7. Continued use despite adverse consequences

From ref. *2.*

a patient is abstinent, it is useful to ascertain why substances are not used or if there is a previous history of use. Some individuals are abstinent because of a previous history of alcohol or drug problems. Some are abstinent because of recent illness, whereas others have lifelong patterns of low-risk use or abstinence. Patients who have a previous history of alcohol or drug problems may require preventive monitoring to determine if any new stresses could exacerbate an old pattern. In addition, a previous history of abuse or dependence may increase the risks for developing other mental health problems in late life, such as depressive disorders or cognitive problems. Low-risk or moderate use is mostly related to the consumption of alcohol that falls within the recommended guidelines for consumption and is not associated with problems. Adults in this category drink within recommended drinking guidelines are able to employ reasonable limits on alcohol consumption, and do not drink when driving a motor vehicle or boat, or when using contraindicated medications. Low-risk use is rarely associated with illicit substances, except for some adults who smoke marijuana on limited occasions.

Although any repeated use of nicotine or illicit substances such as cocaine, heroin, and marijuana can be considered harmful and carries a high risk for addiction, alcohol use can be both problematic as well as socially and medical appropriate when consumed responsible. Thus, guidelines endorsed by the National Institute on Alcohol Abuse and Alcoholism (NIAAA) recommend that women drink no more than 10 standard drinks per week, that men drink no more than 14 standard drinks per week and that all persons age 65 and older consume no more than 7 standard drinks per week *(3,4)*. In addition, all adults should eliminate binge drinking, as defined by drinking more than five standard drinks on any drinking day. These drinking-limit recommendations are consistent with data regarding the relationship between heavy consumption and alcohol-related problems *(5)*. As discussed here, these recommendations are also consistent with the current evidence for a beneficial health effect of low-risk drinking *(6,7)*.

ADDICTION AS A NEUROPSYCHIATRIC DISORDER

A large body of basic and clinical neuroscience research supports the notion that addiction is a neuropsychiatric illness that disrupts brain pleasure centers *(8)*. Unfortunately, the biological bases of addiction are often forgotten or misunderstood, leading to views that alcohol and drug problems are purely behavioral and morally intolerable. Nevertheless, the disease concept of addiction is supported by the neuronal basis for many of its prominent clinical features *(9)*, the presence of genetic vulnerability *(10)*, and a characteristic chronic, relapsing course that resembles that of many medical illnesses.

At the core of understanding the neuroscience of addiction, investigators have determined that drug- or alcohol-induced euphoria is linked to the same reward pathways that are influenced by food and sex *(9)*. These reward pathways include both mesolimbic and mesocortical projections and involve several different neurotransmitter systems, including dopamine, serotonin, and opioid neurotransmission. The changes necessary to lead to addiction are hypothesized to be influenced both by genetic vulnerability and learned behavior from the chronic use of drugs. The clinical features of craving, loss of control, and impaired hedonic function, also have linkages with the dysregulation of brain reward centers *(9,11)*. This biological model assumes that there is a fundamental change in brain functioning that leads to increased consumption of alcohol or another substance. Simplistically, this represents either an upregulation of craving or disinhibition of normal controls or limits on drinking. Without abstinence, the disease is regarded as progressive and often fatal. Treatment focuses on addiction as the primary problem rather than on a lack of willpower, lack of self-control, or mental health disorder. Newer innovations in treatment focus on pharmacological treatments to improve craving or disinhibition.

Whereas neurobiology plays a substantial role in addiction other factors are also important and contribute to the chronic relapsing nature of this disease. Social learning may result from learning maladaptive habits through environmental, cultural, social, peer, and family influences *(12)*. It is also a product of external forces (e.g., poverty, family dysfunction). In some individuals, self-medication of another primary mental disorder or as a coping mechanism may support an addictive pattern of use *(13)*. Finally, the family and support network may be both beneficial for success in treatment and rehabilitation but also a source of toxicity and conflict leading to difficulties in reducing drug and alcohol use.

EXTENT OF THE PROBLEMS

The field of epidemiology offers a description of the nature and extent of problems associated with the use of alcohol, tobacco, illicit drugs, and other psychoactive drugs. In this section, we briefly describe trends and offer estimates for the prevalence of different forms of drug-taking, as well as the occurrence of the clinically defined syndrome of addiction. There are many caveats to this work and many problems with understanding the epidemiology of these problems. Many studies lack sufficient participation to truly understand racial, ethnic, and gender differences in addiction. Moreover, clinical samples likely reflect substantial bias toward patients motivated to seek help and with at least a modest insight for the need for help. Finally, there are almost no estimates of addictive disorders in outpatient neurological and medical subspecialty settings.

Alcohol abuse and dependence are the most well studied addictive disorders in the community. Overall, 1-year prevalence rates of alcohol abuse have risen during the last 10 years to 4.65% of the population (11.1 million Americans) *(14)*. Alcohol dependence has declined slightly with a 1-year prevalence of 3.81% (9.1 million Americans). There are substantially more men with alcohol abuse or dependence and prevalence rates appear to decline with advancing age. However, from 1991 to 2001, the elderly had the greatest increase in prevalence rates compared with all other age groups, suggesting a marked cohort effect with the baby-boom generation continuing to be at high risk for alcohol problems despite advancing age. Minorities, with the exception of Native Americans, have similar rates of alcohol dependence but lower prevalence rates of alcohol abuse compared with Caucasians.

Recent studies estimated that drug dependence costs approx $67 billion annually in crime, lost work productivity, foster care, and other social problems *(8)*. In the 2002 National Survey on Drug Use and Health, an estimated 7.1 million Americans 12 years of age or older were considered to meet criteria for drug dependence or abuse (3% of the total population) *(15)*. Of these, 4.3 million were dependent on or abused marijuana (1.8% of the population), 1.5 million were dependent on or abused cocaine (0.6% of the population), 1.5 million were classified with dependence on or abuse of pain relievers (0.6% of the population), and 200,000 were classified with dependence on or abuse of heroin (0.1% of the population). An additional 12.4 million Americans (5.3% of the population) acknowledged using drugs but did not meet criteria for abuse or dependence. Marijuana was the most frequently used substance among the nonabusive/dependent-user group. Rates of current illicit drug use vary significantly among the major racial/ethnic groups. The rate is highest among Native Americans/Alaska Natives (10.1%) and persons reporting two or more races (11.4%). The prevalence rate of drug use for Caucasians is approx 8.5%, for Hispanics 7.2%, for African Americans 9.7%, and for Asians 3.5%.

Tobacco continues to be the most commonly abused substance. An estimated 71.5 million Americans reported current use (past month use) of a tobacco product in 2002, a prevalence rate of 30.4% for the population 12 years of age or older *(15)*. The majority of tobacco use is cigarettes and the peak age of use is approx 21 years of age, in which 46% of this age group had smoked a cigarette in the last month. As with alcohol and drug use, males are more likely to smoke than females and Native Americans and Alaska Natives were more likely than any other racial/ethnic group to report the use of tobacco products.

A growing and perhaps unique problem for older adults is the misuse of prescription and over-the-counter (OTC) medications. This includes the misuse of substances such as sedative/hypnotics, narcotic and non-narcotic analgesics, diet aids, decongestants, and a wide variety of other OTC medications. For medications, definitions of misuse and addiction are somewhat more difficult to conceptualize. Some medications are abused in the true meaning of an addiction. Typically, these medications include psychoactive medications such as benzodiazepines (BZPs) and opioid-containing pain medications. An estimated 1.5 million Americans (0.6%) are dependent on pain relievers *(15)*.

A more common problem with medications is the inappropriate and indiscriminant use of products with limited documentation of demonstrated effectiveness within an individual and the use of multiple medications. Although not considered a disorder by DSM-IV, there is a growing body of literature on the increase in morbidity and mortality associated with misusing prescription and nonprescription medications. To highlight the issue, 32% of community-dwelling elderly are taking an analgesic, 8.9% are taking an antidepressant, and 10.4% are taking a BZP *(16)*. Many medications used by the elderly have the potential for inducing tolerance, withdrawal syndromes, and harmful medical consequences, such as cognitive changes, renal disease, and hepatic disease.

The use of multiple medications is also problematic and increases with age. One study found that the mean number of medications used in 2 weeks prior to the survey by persons over the age of 65 is 3.5 (2.2 prescriptions and 1.3 OTC) *(17)*. The use of multiple medications greatly increases the risk of drug–drug interactions, the chances of developing side effects, noncompliance, and the risk for inadvertently taking medications at the wrong time or dosage. Physicians and pharmacists should monitor medication use carefully, avoiding dangerous combinations of drugs, medications with a high potential for side effects, and ineffective or unnecessary medications.

CONSEQUENCES

Low-risk alcohol use is often cited as having beneficial effects, especially related to cardiovascular disease (CVD). There is a substantial body of epidemiological evidence to support the claim that, among otherwise healthy adults, particularly middle-aged adults, moderate alcohol use may reduce CVD, may reduce the risk of some dementing illnesses, and may have benefits in reducing cancer risk when compared to risk in abstainers (18–26). Low-risk alcohol use also may enhance subjective feelings of well-being or increased relaxation, especially during social situations (27). It should be noted that the drinking limits in these epidemiological studies have suggested benefits for drinking up to two standard drinks per day with increased morbidity and mortality above this limit. Clinicians should be mindful that nearly all of these studies have been done in middle-aged men and the drinking limits for older adults or women of all ages is no more than one standard drink per day. Another important concept is the recognition that past alcohol or drug use can also increase the vulnerability to central nervous system (CNS) disease as one ages. This is highlighted in the findings from the Liverpool Longitudinal Study demonstrating a fivefold increase in psychiatric illness among elderly men who had a lifetime history of 5 or more years of heavy drinking (28). Similarly, Vaillant found that the use of tranquilizers prior to the age of 50 was the most powerful negative biopsychosocial predictor of physical and mental health at age 65 (29). Recent case reports in former cocaine abusers also suggest long-lasting effects as some of these patients have developed parkinsonian-like symptoms (30). Thus, substance abuse in all ages may have profound effects on the incidence and course of diseases of the CNS and other organs in one's later years, despite nonuse of the substance.

NEGATIVE EFFECTS

The health-related consequences of alcohol use and other drugs of abuse have been articulated in many articles and reviews. Alcohol dependence is associated with increased morbidity and mortality from disease-specific disorders such as acute pancreatitis, alcohol-induced cirrhosis, or alcohol-related cardiomyopathy, as well as increasing the risks for such diseases as hypertension and increasing the risks of trauma from falls or motor vehicle accidents. At-risk and problem drinking have also been demonstrated to impair driving-related skills, may lead to other problems such as falls, depression, memory problems, liver disease, CVD, cognitive changes, and sleep problems (31–33). Of particular importance to clinicians are the interactions between alcohol and both prescribed and OTC medications, especially psychoactive medications such as BZPs, barbiturates, and antidepressants. Alcohol use is one of the leading risk factors for developing adverse drug reactions and is known to interfere with the metabolism of many medications, such as digoxin and warfarin (34–36). Illicit drug addiction is associated with increased risk of developing sexually transmitted disease such as hepatitis C and death from homicides, suicides, and accidents. Moreover, cocaine and other stimulant use increase the risk of acute cardiovascular events. The withdrawal from opioids and cocaine, although extremely unpleasant, is not typically life-threatening.

Substance abuse and dependence are also strongly associated with other behavioral disorders, such as depression and anxiety. Data from the Epidemiologic Catchment Area (ECA) study has underscored the notion that there is a link between alcohol use and abuse and the development of other psychiatric illnesses (37). Subjects with a lifetime diagnosis of alcohol abuse or dependence were 2.9 times more likely to have a lifetime diagnosis of another mental disorder. Co-morbid disorders associated with an increased likelihood included anxiety disorders, affective illness, schizophrenia, and antisocial personality disorder. Co-morbid depressive symptoms in particular are common and are an important factor in the clinical course and prognosis for patients. Depressed alcoholics have been shown to have a more complicated clinical course of depression with an increased risk of suicide and more social dysfunction than nondepressed alcoholics (38–40). Moreover, they seek more treatment leading to higher treatment costs.

The link between cognitive deficits, including dementia and alcohol or drug use, deserves special attention. Although the rates of alcohol-related dementia in late life differ according to diagnostic criteria used and the nature of the population studied, there is agreement that alcohol contributes significantly to the acquired cognitive deficits of late life *(41)*. In the ECA study, among subjects over the age of 55, the prevalence of a lifetime history of alcohol abuse or dependence was 1.5 times greater among persons with mild and severe cognitive impairment than those with no cognitive impairment *(42)*. In addition to alcohol-related dementia, alcohol use is also directly correlated with other potential causes of cognitive impairment including trauma, cerbrovascular events, and the development of Wernicke's-Korsakoff's syndrome. The recognition and treatment of Wernicke's-Korsakoff's syndrome is important, as this is a potentially preventable complication of alcohol use that leads to cognitive impairment *(43)*. Wernicke's-Korsakoff's syndrome is clinically characterized by cognitive deficits (especially anterograde memory deficits), gait apraxia, and nystagmus. The pathophysiology of Wernicke's-Korsakoff's syndrome involves the lack of the vitamin, thiamine. Giving alcoholic patients thiamine supplementation early in treatment can potentially prevent the dementing process.

Sleep disorders and sleep disturbances represent another group of co-morbid disorders associated with excessive alcohol use. Alcohol causes well-established changes in sleep patterns, such as decreased sleep latency, decreased stage IV sleep, and precipitation or aggravation of sleep apnea *(44)*. There are also age-associated changes in sleep patterns, including increased rapid eye movement (REM) episodes, a decrease in REM length, a decrease in stage III and IV sleep, and increased awakenings. The age-associated changes in sleep can all be worsened by alcohol use and depression. Moeller and colleagues demonstrated in younger subjects that alcohol and depression had additive effects on sleep disturbances when occurring together *(45)*. Wagman and colleagues also demonstrated that abstinent alcoholics did not sleep well because of insomnia, frequent awakenings, and REM fragmentation *(44)*.

SCREENING AND DIAGNOSIS

To be able to practice prevention and early intervention with older adults, clinicians need to screen for alcohol and drug use (frequency and quantity), consequences, and alcohol/drug–medication interaction problems. An important aspect of assessment is understanding the concept of standard drinks. It is generally accepted that the negative effects of alcohol are related to the alcohol content of a beverage. In order to improve assessment outcomes, clinicians should quantify alcohol in terms of standard alcohol drinks (one standard drink approximates 12 oz of beer, 1.5 oz of distilled spirits, and 4.5 oz of wine). It is neither important to be exact in the ascertainment of quantity nor is it helpful to engage in debates with patient over exact amounts consumed, however, ascertaining standard drinks do provide a method of standardization. Illicit drug use is more difficult to quantify do to the variability in purity of the drug, the route of administration, and the often practiced use of talc or other agents to dilute the drug in order to increase profitability.

Screening for alcohol and drug use is recommended by the US Preventive Task Force and can be done as part of routine mental and physical health care and should be updated annually, before beginning any new medication, or in response to problems that may be alcohol- or drug-related *(46)*. Screening questions can be asked by a verbal interview, by a paper-and-pencil questionnaire, or by a computerized questionnaire. All three methods have equivalent reliability and validity. The Alcohol Use Disorders Identification Test version C is recommended by the NIAAA as a screen for alcohol problems *(47,48)*. Any positive responses can lead to further questions about consequences. To successfully incorporate alcohol (and other drug) screening into clinical practice, it should be simple and consistent with other screening procedures already in place *(49)*. In addition to routine screening, certain clinical situations may warrant added suspicion and further inquiry. These situations include obvious clinical situations related to the particular drugs of abuse such as a patient with unexplained sleep problems; frequent falls; liver, gastrointestinal, or pancreatic symptoms; or cognitive impairment related to alcohol or unexplained cardiac palpitations or chest pain for patients abusing cocaine. Other opportunities for identifying addictive problems include careful attention to misuse of prescriptions (e.g., frequent lost prescriptions, unusual requests for samples, etc.) and close monitoring of chronic pain treatment.

Clinicians can follow-up the brief questions about consumption with a few more in-depth questions about consequences, health risks, and social/family issues. To assess dependence, questions should be asked about alcohol-related problems; a history of failed attempts to stop or to cut back; or withdrawal symptoms such as tremors, nausea, sleep problems, and autonomic hyperactivity. Self-report of alcohol use remains the principal method of ascertaining history with biomarkers such as liver function tests and carbohydrate-deficient transferrin only having modest specificity in the most alcohol-dependent patients and overall low sensitivity. However, urine drug screens or serum samples can be an effective way of screening and monitoring for most prescription and illicit drug use. Suggesting the use of a urine or serum drug screen can also be a mechanism for discussion about drug use and may open up further discussions. If the clinician is highly suspicious that drugs are being used and the patient denies the use, the clinician can suggest a urine drug screen as a way to confirm the patient's report.

ASSESSING THE PATIENT AND MANAGING AMBIVALENCE

Resistance or ambivalence can happen at any point during an assessment or intervention and can manifest itself in many different ways. In general, the best way of responding to resistance is with nonresistance. Acknowledging the patient's disagreement, emotion, or perception allows for further exploration and discussion. For patients who directly challenge the accuracy of what the clinician has said or assessed, it may be helpful for the clinician to reiterate his/her clinical impressions and to provide a little more detail to address the patients' questions or challenges. For example, if a patient suggests that the clinician is exaggerating risks or dangers and that it "really isn't so bad," it is important for the clinician to let the patient know that it is up to him/her to decide what information is relevant. This can be helpful in reducing disputes about minor details. If the patient expresses hostility toward the clinician, it is important that the clinician acknowledge the patient's anger, and expresses openness to the patient's concerns and feelings. Reflective listening on the part of the clinician can help diffuse anger and hostility. The clinician may also wish to inform patients that he or she does not want the patient to be angry, and that he or she is very interested in both what the patient agrees and disagrees with. It is possible that patients may become angry and state something like: "You're saying I'm an alcoholic," or "I'm not an alcoholic, and this is none of your business." In these situations, it is still important for the clinician to acknowledge patient anger, to be open to patient concerns, and to use reflective listening. However, it is also important to de-emphasize labels because they tend to increase resistance. The clinician should let the patient know that he or she is not concerned with labeling the patient in any way, and the clinican should reflect patient concerns. Finally, it is important that the clinican avoid arguing with patients especially over minor details such as whether the patient drank three or five times in a particular week.

TREATMENTS

Detoxification and Stabilization

Once the diagnosis of addiction has been made, it is important to note that each individual often presents with different treatment needs. The first step in treating any patient with a substance use disorder is breaking down the denial of the problem. The failure to do so usually results in patients leaving treatment when the factors that coerce them into treatment are no longer present. Social contacts including family, friends, and co-workers should be engaged early in the patient's treatment. Supportive family and friends can offer support as well as continual pressure to keep a patient in compliance with the treatment plan. Indeed, Gomberg and associates found that positive social and family support predicted treatment success *(50)*.

The assessment of any substance abuser starts with a thorough history, physical, and laboratory examination. Once the decision to treat substance abuse or dependence is made and accepted, the clinician must decide on the level of care necessary to achieve and maintain the individual treatment goals. The American Society of Addiction Medicine has established criteria for placing patients in various levels of treatment based on the severity of the patient's withdrawal potential, medical complications, emotional stability, and relapse potential *(51)*. Patients with high-relapse or withdrawal potential and patients with severe medical or psychiatric co-morbidity require inpatient hospitalization. Inpatient hospitalization not only provides the opportunity to begin detoxification under controlled conditions while attending to issues of medical and psychiatric co-morbidity, but it also helps break the cycle of addiction by temporarily removing patients from the environment in which they are using. In cases of alcohol-use problems, patients should receive thiamine, folate, and multivitamins. Patients should also be hydrated as necessary and have their vital signs and objective symptoms of withdrawal monitored regularly. Intermediate or long-acting BZPs (i.e., chlordiazepoxide, oxazepam, and lorazepam), are used as detoxification agents as alcohol-addcited patients are cross-tolerant to these substances. Use of oxazepam or lorazepam is warranted in patients with severe liver disease, as metabolism of these BZPs does not depend on hydroxylation by the liver and thus they will not accumulate and cause adverse effects *(51)*. The BZP dosage is decreased daily over the course of the detoxification. Clonidine and methadone should be used for opiate withdrawal and phenobarbital for barbiturate withdrawal. Evidence-based strategies for managing cocaine withdrawal have not been established, although β-blockers may be of some benefit *(52)*. In addition to detoxification and management of co-morbid medical or psychiatric conditions, the inpatient program provides an opportunity for early engagement of patients and families in addiction treatment. Furthermore, educational groups and group therapy can provide patients with the basic tools to develop recovery skills that will be necessary if treatment is to be successful.

Brief Interventions/Therapies

Low-intensity, brief interventions, or brief therapies have been suggested as cost-effective and practical techniques that can be used as an initial approach to problem drinking and those with alcohol dependence in various clinical settings including primary care and specialty medical clinics *(53)*. Studies of brief interventions for alcohol problems have employed various approaches to change drinking behaviors. Strategies have ranged from relatively unstructured counseling and feedback to more formal structured therapy using patient-oriented workbooks *(54–56)*. A number of large, randomized controlled trials of brief alcohol interventions have demonstrated efficacy among younger adults in a variety of clinical settings *(53)*. It is worth noting that brief interventions are likely most effective outside of addiction centers and can be effective in helping patients reduce use but can also be an effective strategy for referral management. Thus, brief interventions can be a relatively low-cost mechanism for primary and specialty medical care clinics to engage patients in treatment and increase adherence to specialty treatment as well as enhancing an ongoing dialogue between the addiction clinic staff and primary care staff.

Outpatient Management

Patients with less withdrawal or relapse potential and with less severe psychiatric and medical co-morbidity can be initially managed in an outpatient setting. Structured outpatient treatment generally includes supportive group psychotherapy and encouragement to attend regular self-help group meetings such as Alcoholics Anonymous, Alcoholics Victorious, Rational Recovery, or Narcotics Anonymous. Outpatient rehabilitation, in addition to focusing on active addiction issues, usually needs to address issues of time management. Abstinence reduces the time spent in maintaining the substance use disorder. The management of this time, which is often the greater part of a patients day, is critical to the prognosis of treatment. Social services, such as financial support and vocational rehabilitation, are often needed to stabilize the patient in early recovery. Supervised living arrangements such as halfway houses, group homes, nursing homes, and residing with relatives should also be considered.

To demonstrate the value of treatment, a comparison of those in treatment to those not in treatment is informative. Booth and colleagues studied 4000 intravenous drug users seeking HIV testing in 15 cities. Subjects were randomly assigned to either standard HIV testing alone or to standard testing plus three sessions of motivational counseling similar to a brief intervention. At 6-month follow-up, those who received additional counseling showed half the rate of drug injection (20 vs 45%), four times the likelihood of abstinence (confirmed by urinalysis), and significantly lower arrest rates (14 vs 24%) than those assigned to HIV testing alone *(57)*.

PHARMACOTHERAPY OF ADDICTION

Although not usually considered as part of relapse prevention, pharmacotherapy is increasingly becoming an important aspect of treatment of alcohol, opioid, and nicotine addiction. A complete review of this topic can be found in a recent review by the Institute of Medicine *(58)*.

For opioid dependence, the agonist methadone hydrochloride can be used in either detoxification or in the long-term as a maintenance regimen. Double-blind, placebo-controlled trials *(59,60)* have shown methadone to be effective in both inpatient and outpatient detoxification. As a maintenance medication, methadone has been effective in reducing opiate use, crime, and the spread of infectious diseases, as was recently validated by a National Institutes of Health Consensus Conference *(61)*. Most recently, the partial agonist buprenorphine hydrochloride plus naloxone hydrochloride has been shown to reduce opiate use to a level comparable with methadone but with fewer withdrawal symptoms on discontinuation *(62,63)*. Importantly, this combination can be prescribed by any physician after a brief training.

ALCOHOL DEPENDENCE

Naltrexone has been found effective at 50 mg per day for reducing drinking among alcohol-dependent patients *(64)*. It works by blocking at least some of the "high" produced by alcohol's effects on μ-opiate receptors. Although a positive family history of alcohol problems may be an important predictor of naltrexone response, Oslin and colleagues have suggested that response is mediated through a specific genetic polymorphism of the μ-opioid receptor *(65,66)*. Thus, naltrexone may be most effective in patients with dysregulation of the opioid system at the level of the opioid receptor. Recently, acamprosate has been studied as a promising agent in the treatment of alcohol dependence. Although the exact action of acamprosate is still unknown, acamprosate is thought to reduce glutamate response *(67)*. The clinical evidence favoring acamprosate is impressive. Sass and colleagues studied 272 alcohol-dependent subjects in Europe for up to 48 weeks using a randomized, placebo-controlled study of acamprosate. Forty-three percent of the acamprosate-treated group was abstinent at the conclusion of the study compared with 21% in the placebo group *(68)*.

SUMMARY

Over the past several years, there has been a growing awareness that addictive disorders are a common public health problem. Epidemiological studies suggest that alcohol dependence is present in up to 5% of community-dwelling adults *(32,69)*. Moreover, problem or hazardous drinking is estimated to be even more common than alcohol dependence *(32,70)*. However, there continues to be a gap in the number of adults who are referred for treatment or who receive treatment for addictive disorders. Although there are many reasons for patients not to be engaged in treatment, recommending treatment is partially based on the availability of effective treatment. Toward this end, there needs to be better dissemination of information regarding currently available and efficacious treatments for alcohol abuse and dependence and other addictive disorders, as well as continued development of more effective treatments. There is also a clear need to conduct research and clinical training beyond the problems of alcohol use. Current and past nicotine dependence as well as illicit drug and medication abuse, are similarly recognized for their impact and will need continued focus in treatment trials, epidemiology, and neuroscience.

REFERENCES

1. Murray C, Lopez A. The global burden of disease: a comprehensive assessment of mortality and disability from diseases, injuries, and risk factors in 1990 and projected to 2020. In: Murray C, Lopez A, eds. The global burden of disease and injury series, Vol. 1. Boston: Harvard University Press; 1996.
2. American Psychological Association. Diagnostic and Statistical Manual of Mental Disorders, Fourth Edition. Washington DC: Amer Psychiatric Pub; 1994.
3. Blow F. Substance abuse among older Americans. In: C.f.S.A. Treatment, ed. Treatment Improvement Protocol. Washington DC: US Government Printing Office; 1998.
4. National Institute on Alcohol Abuse and Alcoholism. Diagnostic criteria for alcohol abuse. Alcohol Alert 1995;30(PH 359):1–6.
5. Chermack ST, Blow FC, Hill EM, Mudd SA. The relationship between alcohol symptoms and consumption among older drinkers. Alchohol Clin Exp Res 1996;20:1153–1158.
6. Klatsky AL, Armstrong A. Alcohol use, other traits and risk of unnatural death: a prospective study. Alcohol Clin Exp Res 1993;17:1156–1162.
7. Poikolainen K. Epidemiologic assessment of population risks and benefits of alcohol use. Alcohol Alcohol 1991;1:27–34.
8. McLellan AT, Lewis DC, O'Brien CP, Kleber HD. Drug dependence, a chronic medical illness: implications for treatment, insurance, and outcomes evaluation. JAMA 2000;284:1689–1695.
9. Dackis C, O'Brien C. The neurobiology of addiction. In: Asbury A, McDonald I, Goadsby PJ, McArthur JC, eds. Diseases of the Nervous System. Cambridge: Cambridge University Press; 2003:431–444.
10. Vanyukov MM, Tarter RE. Genetic studies of substance abuse. Drug Alcohol Depend 2000;59:101–123.
11. Dackis C, O'Brien C. Cocaine dependence: a disease of the brain's reward centers. J Subst Abuse Treat 2001;21:111–117.
12. Beigel A, Ghertner S. Toward a social model: an assessment of social factors which influence problem drinking and its treatment. In: Kissin B, Begleiter H, eds. The Biology of Alcoholism: Vol. 5 Treatment and Rehabilitation of the Chronic Alcoholic. New York: Plenum Press; 1979.
13. Khantzian EJ. The self-medication hypothesis of addictive disorders: focus on heroin and cocaine dependence. Am J Psychiatry 1985;142:1259–1264.
14. Grant BF, Dawson DA, Stinson FS, Chou SP, Dufour MC, Pickering RP. The 12-month prevalence and trends in DSM-IV alcohol abuse and dependence: United States, 1991–1992 and 2001–2002. Drug Alcohol Depend 2004;74:223–234.
15. Substance Abuse and Mental Health Services Administration. Results from the 2002 National Survey on Drug Use and Health: National Findings In: NHSDA Series H-22, DHHS Publication No. SMA 03-3836, Rockville: Office of Applied Studies; 2003.
16. Moxey E, O'Connor JP, Novielli KD, Teutsch S, Nash DB. Prescription drug use in the elderly: a descriptive analysis. Health Care Financ Revi 2003;24:127–144.
17. Hanlon JT, Filenbaum GG, Burchett B, et al. Drug-use patterns among black and nonblack community-dwelling elderly. Ann Pharmacother 1992;26:679–685.
18. Scherr PA, LaCroix AZ, Wallace RB, et al. Light to moderate alcohol consumption and mortality in the elderly. J Am Geriatr Soc 1992;40:651–657.
19. Thun MJ, Peto R, Lopez AD, et al. Alcohol consumption and mortality among middle-aged and elderly US adults. N Eng J Med 1997;337:1705–1714.
20. Broe GA, Creasey H, Jorm AF, et al. Health habits and risk of cognitive impairment and dementia in old age: a prospective study on the effects of exercise, smoking and alcohol consumption. Aust N Z J Public Health 1998;22:621–623.
21. de Labry LO, Glynn RJ, Levenson MR, Hermos JA, LoCastro JS, Vokanas PS. Alcohol consumption and mortality in an American male population: Recovering the U-shaped curve—findings from the normative aging study. J Studies Alcohol 1992;53:25–32.
22. Klatsky AL, Armstrong MA, Friedman GD. Risk of cardiovascular mortality in alcohol drinkers, ex-drinkers and non-drinkers. Am J Cardiol 1990;66:1237–1242.
23. Orgogozo JM, Dartigues JF, Lafont S, et al. Wine consumption and dementia in the elderly: a prospective community study in the Bordeaux area. Rev Neurol 1997;153:185–192.
24. Shaper AG. Alcohol and mortality: a review of prospective studies. Br J Addict 1990;85:837–847.
25. Stampfer MJ, Colditz GA, Willett WC, Speizer FE, Hennekens CH. A prospective study of moderate alcohol consumption and the risk of coronary disease and stroke in women. N Engl J Med 1988;319:267–273.

26. Gunzerath L, Faden V, Zakhan S, Warren K. National Institute on Alcohol Abuse and Alcoholism report on moderate drinking. Alcohol Clin Exp Res 2004;28:829–847.

27. Dufour MC, Archer L, Gordis E. Alcohol and the elderly. Clin Geriatr Med 1992;8:127–141.

28. Saunders PA, Copeland JR, Dewey ME, et al. Heavy drinking as a risk factor for depression and dementia in elderly men. Br J Psychiatry 1991;159:213–216.

29. Vaillant GE, Vaillant CO. Natural History of Male Psychological Health, XII: a 45 year study of predictors of successful aging at age 65. Am J Psychiatry 1990;147:31–37.

30. Rodnitzky RL, Keyser DL. Neurologic complications of drugs. Tardive dyskinesias, neuroleptic malignant syndrome, and cocaine-related syndromes. Psychiat Clin North Am 1992;15:491–510.

31. Gambert S, Katsoyannis K. Alcohol-related medical disorders of older heavy drinkers. In: Beresford T, Gomberg E, ed. Alcohol and Aging. New York: Oxford University Press; 1995:70–81.

32. Liberto JG, Oslin DW, Ruskin PE. Alcoholism in older persons: a review of the literature. Hosp Comm Psychiatry 1992;43:975–984.

33. Kivela SL, Nissinen A, Ketola A. Alcohol consumption and mortality in aging or aged Finnish men. J Clin Epidemiol 1989;42:61–68.

34. Onder G, Pedone C, Landi F, et al. Adverse drug reactions as cause of hospital admissions: results from the Italian Group of Pharmacoepidemiology in the Elderly (GIFA). J Am Geriatr Society 2002;50:1962–1968.

35. Fraser AG. Pharmacokinetic interactions between alcohol and other drugs. Clin Pharmacokinet 1997;33:79–90.

36. HylekEM, Heiman H, Skates SJ, Sheehan MA, Singer DE. Acetaminophen and other risk factors for excessive warfarin anticoagulation. JAMA 1998;279:657–662.

37. Regier DA, Farmer ME, Rae DS, et al. Comorbidity of mental disorders with alcohol and other drug abuse: results from the epidemiologic catchment area (ECA) study. JAMA 1990;264:2511–2518.

38. Waern M. Alcohol dependence and misuse in elderly suicides. Alcohol Alcohol 2003;38:249–254.

39. Cook B, Winokur G, Garvey MJ, Beach V. Depression and previous alcoholism in the elderly. Br J Psychiatry 1991;158:72–75.

40. Conwell Y. Suicide in elderly patients. In: Schneider LS, Reynolds CF, Lebowitz BD, Friedhoff AJ, eds. Diagnosis and Treatment of Depression in Late Life. Washington DC: American Psychiatric Press Inc; 1991:397–418.

41. Oslin D, Atkinson RM, Smith DM, Hendrie H. Alcohol related dementia: proposed clinical criteria. Int J Geriatr Psychiatry 1998;13:203–212.

42. George LK, Landerman R, Blazer DG, Anthony JC. Cognitive impairment. In: Robins LN, Regier DA, eds. Psychiatric Disorders in America: The Epidemiologic Catchment Area Study. New York: The Free Press; 1991:291–327.

43. Victor M. Persistent altered mentation due to ethanol. Neurol Clin 1993;11:639–661.

44. Wagman AM, Allen RP, Upright D. Effects of alcohol consumption upon parameters of ultradian sleep rhythms in alcoholics. Adv Exp Med Biol 197;85A:601–616.

45. Moeller FG, Gillin JC, Irwin M, Golshan S, Kripke DF, Schuckit M. A comparison of sleep EEGs in patients with primary major depression and major depression secondary to alcoholism. J Affect Disord 1993;27:39–42.

46. Whitlock E, Polen MR, Green CA, et al. Behavioral counseling interventions in primary care to reduce risky/harmful alcohol use by adults: a summary of the evidence for the US Preventive Services Task Force. Ann Intern Med 2004;140:557–568.

47. Barry K, Fleming M. Computerized administration of alcoholism screening tests in a primary care setting. J Am Board Fam Prac 1990;3:93–98.

48. Greist J, Klein MH, Erdman HP, et al. Comparison of computer- and interviewer-administered versions of the Diagnostic Interview Schedule. Hosp Community Psychiatry 1987;38:1304–1311.

49. Barry KL, Oslin DW, Blow FC. Prevention and management of alcohol problems in older adults. New York: Springer Publishing; 2001.

50. Gomberg ESL, Nelson B, Hill EM. Treatment of Alcoholism in Elderly Persons: Preliminary Report. Marco Island, FL: Research Society of Alcoholism, 1991.

51. American Society of Addiction Medicine Patient Placement Criteria. Washington DC: Amer Psychiatric Pub; 1992.

52. Kampman KM, Volpicelli JR, Mulvaney F, et al. Effectiveness of propranolol for cocaine dependence treatment may depend on cocaine withdrawal symptom severity. Drug Alcohol Depend 2001;63:69–78.

53. Center for Substance Abuse Treatment (SAMHSA). Brief interventions and therapies in substance abuse treatment. In: Barry K, ed. Treatment Improvement Protocol. Washington DC: US Government Printing Office, 2001.

54. Chick J, Lloyd G, Crombie E. Counseling problem drinkers in medical wards: a controlled study. Brit Med J Clin Res Ed 1985;290:965–967.

55. Persson J, Magnusson PH. Early intervention in patients with excessive consumption of alcohol: a controlled study. Alcohol 1989;6:403–408.

56. Fleming M, Mundt MP, French MT, Manwell LB, Stauffacher EA, Barry KL. Brief physician advice for problem alcohol drinkers: a randomized controlled trial in community-based primary care practices. JAMA 1997;277:1039–1045.

57. Booth RE, Crowley TJ, Zhang Y. Substance abuse treatment entry, retention and effectiveness: out-of-treatment opiate injection drug users. Drug Alcohol Depend 1996;42:11–20.

58. Fulco C, Liverman C, Earley, L. The development of medications for the treatment of opiate and cocaine addictions: issues for the government and private sector. Committee to Study Medication Development and Research at the National Institute on Drugs. Institute of Medicine, 1995.

59. Gossop M, Johns A, Green L. Opiate withdrawal: inpatient versus outpatient programmes and preferred versus random assignment to treatment. Br Med J (Clin Res Ed) 1986;293:103–104.

60. Mattick RP, Hall, W. Are detoxification programmes effective? Lancet 1996;347:97–100.

61. National Consensus Development Panel on Effective Medical Treatment of Opiate Addiction. Effective medical treatment of opiate addiction. JAMA 1998;280:1936–1943.

62. Mattick RP, Ali R, White JM, O'Brien S, Wolk S, Danz C. Buprenorphine versus methadone maintenance therapy: a randomized double-blind trial with 405 opioid-dependent patients. Addiction 2003;98:441–452.

63. O'Connor PG, Oliveto AH, Shi JM, et al. A randomized trial of buprenorphine maintenance for heroin dependence in a primary care clinic for substance users versus a methadone clinic. Am J Med 1998;105:100–105.

64. Pettinati H, O'Brien CP, Wortman S, Oslin DW, Kampman KM, Lynch KG. The status of naltrexone in the treatment of alcohol dependence: specific effects on excessive drinking. under development.

65. Oslin DW, Berrettini W, Kranzler HR, et al. A functional polymorphism of the mu-opioid receptor gene is associated with naltrexone response in alcohol-dependent patients. Neuropsychopharmacology 2003;28:1546–1552.

66. Monterosso JR, Flannery BA, Pettinati HM, et al. Predicting treatment response to naltrexone: the influence of craving and family history. Am J Addiction 2001;10:258–268.

67. Pelc I, Verbanck P, Le Bon O, Gavrilovic M, Lion K, Lehert P. Efficacy and safety of acamprosate in the treatment of detoxified alcohol-dependent patients. A 90-day placebo-controlled dose-finding study. Br J Psychiatry 1997;171:73–77.

68. Sass H, Soyka M, Zieglgansberger W. Relapse prevention by acamprosate: results from a placebo-controlled study in alcohol dependence. Arch Gen Psychiatry 1996;53:673–680.

69. Osterling A, Berglund M. Elderly first time admitted alcoholics: a descriptive study on gender differences in a clinical population. Alch Clin Exp Res 1994;18:1317–1321.

70. Barry KL, Blow FC, Walton MA, et al. Elder-specific brief alcohol intervention: 3-month outcomes. Alch Clin Exp Res 1998; 22:32A.

10

Personality Disorders

Marc E. Agronin

INTRODUCTION

Personality disorders (PDs) represent some of the most insidious and challenging psychiatric conditions that clinicians encounter, and often create unwarranted and unwanted conflicts in clinical settings. The reasons for these conflicts lie at the core of the PD pathology, namely, a fundamental impairment in interpersonal relationships that leads to a variety of maladaptive, inappropriate, or outrageous behaviors that the affected person seems incapable of fully understanding and controlling. Consider these examples:

1. Vincent P. is a 78-year-old retired professor of English literature who is seen in an outpatient VA clinic. He has a consistent pattern of meeting a new doctor, asking repetitively for help with chronic headaches, and then cursing out and vilifying the doctor for failing to help him. On a regular basis he angrily demands meetings with the hospital administrator to complain about his current physician.
2. Susan R. is a 24-year-old graduate student who presents to a neurology clinic complaining of muscle twitches, headache, paresthesias, and nervousness. The clinic's staff notice numerous linear scars on her arms consistent with self-inflicted cutting. A thorough examination is unrevealing, and Susan is told that she should consider seeing a psychiatrist to help deal with stress. She becomes enraged at the neurologist, and accuses him of insensitivity and ignorance. She storms out of the office, cursing the physician and staff for misleading her.
3. John D. is a 34-year-old man with multiple sclerosis who lives with his mother. He has never been married and has few friends. He has worked at odd jobs in the past but is currently on disability. He presents to a neurology clinic intermittently for follow-up, but is minimally communicative with staff and rarely compliant with treatment. During previous hospitalizations, nurses have described him as aloof, distant, and odd.

Each case involves an individual with dysfunctional interpersonal behaviors that worsen under stress, and that have pervaded most of their relationships for many years. Clinicians often find such individuals unpleasant or difficult to work with, and as a result PD diagnoses are often conferred on such patients as pejorative labels rather than as clearly thought-out diagnoses.

Under current psychiatric classification, PDs are defined in the fourth edition (revised) of the Diagnostic and Statistical Manual of Mental Disorders (DSM-IV-TR) by the presence of a pervasive pattern of specific chronic, inflexible, and maladaptive behaviors (1). These behaviors are typically rooted in early development and thus should be detected since at least young adulthood, although in the elderly such history is often not available. The maladaptive patterns associated with PDs involve significant disruptions in four areas of function: interpretation and perception of self and others, affective expression, interpersonal relations, and impulse control. General diagnostic criteria appear in Table 1.

There are 10 official DSM-IV-TR personality disorders, grouped into three clusters based on phenomenological similarities. Two other PDs, depressive and passive-aggressive (also called negativis-

From: *Current Clinical Neurology: Psychiatry for Neurologists*
Edited by: D.V. Jeste and J.H. Friedman © Humana Press Inc., Totowa, NJ

Table 1
General Diagnostic Criteria for Personality Disorders

Personality disorders are characterized by the following:
A. An enduring pattern of inner experience and behavior that deviates markedly from the expectations of the individual's culture. This pattern is manifested in two or more of the following:
    (1) cognition (ways of perceiving and interpreting self, others, and events),
    (2) affective or emotional response,
    (3) interpersonal functioning,
    (4) impulse control
B. The enduring pattern is inflexible and pervasive across a broad range of personal and social situations.
C. The enduring pattern leads to clinically significant distress or impairment in social, occupational, or other important areas of functioning.
D. The pattern is stable and of long duration, and its onset can be traced back at least to adolescence or early adulthood.
E. The enduring pattern is not better accounted for as a manifestation or consequence of another mental disorder.
F. The enduring pattern is not due to the direct physiological effects of a substance or a general medical condition.

Adapted from ref. *1*.

tic), have empirical support but have been kept are in the appendix of DSM-IV-TR as provisional categories requiring further study. Each personality disorder has 8 to 10 diagnostic criteria, and an individual must meet a specified number of them in any combination in order to qualify for a diagnosis. The PDs are listed by cluster in Table 2. More detailed descriptions are provided later.

EPIDEMIOLOGY

Overall estimates of PDs in community-dwelling adults range from 10 to 22% *(2)*, with much higher rates seen in psychiatric outpatients and inpatients, especially in the setting of co-morbid psychiatric disorders such as depression *(3–5)*. Data from the 2001–2002 National Epidemiologic Survey on Alcohol and Related Conditions found an overall prevalence rate of PDs of 14.79% in a representative sample of more than 43,000 individuals in the United States *(6)*. This rate would mean that more than 30 million Americans would meet diagnostic criteria for at least one PD. As seen in Fig. 1, the sample looked at 7 of 10 PDs and found the most common ones to be obsessive-compulsive PD (7.88%), paranoid PD (4.41%), and antisocial PD (3.63%). Most estimates of personality disorders in elderly community-dwelling individuals are lower, ranging from 5 to 10%, although it is not clear whether there is an actual decline in the true prevalence rate, or whether this difference is owing more to problems with diagnosis *(3,7)*. To date, there is no data on the prevalence rates of PDs in association with specific neurological disorders.

DIAGNOSIS OF PDS

Accurate diagnosis of PDs requires a cooperative and reliable patient or informant, a reasonably detailed and accurate longitudinal history, and knowledge of diagnostic criteria. The first encounter with a patient with potential PD highlights several challenges, in that the patient's very pathology may interfere with his/her willingness to provide sufficient history. It can be difficult to ask any patient or informant to provide substantial personal history, going back many years, for a diagnosis that is socially undesirable. Psychiatric records rarely provide sufficient detail or longitudinal information, and previous records may contain outdated or inaccurate terms for personality disorders.

Without a complete and reliable longitudinal history it is difficult to distinguish acute symptoms from more chronic behavioral patterns. For example, the odd thinking and unusual perceptual experi-

Table 2
The DSM-IV-TR Personality Disorders

Odd cluster disorders
    Paranoid personality disorder
    Schizoid personality disorder
    Schizotypal personality disorder
Dramatic cluster disorders
    Antisocial personality disorder
    Borderline personality disorder
    Histrionic personality disorder
    Narcissistic personality disorder
Anxious cluster disorders
    Avoidant personality disorder
    Dependent personality disorder
    Obsessive-compulsive personality disorder
Provisional disorders
    Depressive personality disorder
    Passive-aggressive (negativistic) personality disorder

ences seen in schizotypal PD may resemble an acute psychosis, whereas the emotional lability seen in borderline or histrionic PDs may mimic a manic or hypomanic state. Many elderly psychiatric patients also have chronic medical conditions that will interfere with diagnosis. Degenerative and vascular dementias may cause or exacerbate many of the maladaptive behaviors seen in PDs, especially when frontal or temporal regions of the brain are involved. Chronic pain and disability can lead to excessive patterns of dependent or avoidant behaviors that resemble those seen in PDs. In such situations, clinicians must rely more on informants to provide a longitudinal history of premorbid personality characteristics. The third requirement of a solid PD diagnosis lies with the clinician's responsibility to be aware of current diagnostic criteria. This is difficult given the fact that there are 12 potential PDs comprised of more than 100 criteria—a database that few clinicians have memorized.

NEUROPSYCHIATRIC PERSPECTIVES ON PDS

Current neuropsychiatric theories for both personality development and PDs focus on the role of neurotransmitters and underlying genes for specific personality traits. Cloninger proposed four basic personality traits that are related to specific monoamine neurotransmitters: novelty-seeking (dopamine), harm avoidance (serotonin), reward dependence (norepinephrine), and persistence *(8,9)*. A similar model proposes four dimensions of personality that are mediated by monoamine pathways: cognitive-perceptual organization, affective regulation, impulse control, and anxiety modulation *(10)*.

In both models, impairment in neurotransmitter function can lead to pathological personality functioning. For example, there is strong evidence linking serotonergic dysfunction to compulsive behaviors, impulsive aggression, and suicidality seen in many PDs *(11– 13)*. Empirical research has not only identified genetic factors that generate monoamine metabolism, but has revealed that the impact of the genetic expression can be modulated by the environment *(14,15)*. For example, a longitudinal study of children who suffered from abuse found that those with low monoamine metabolism demonstrated more antisocial behaviors as they grew into young adulthood *(16)*. These findings do not, however, indicate that discrete behaviors or personality traits can be linked to a specific neurotransmitter or gene *(17)*. By extension, neither genetic testing nor a more general neurological workup will yield a PD diagnosis, or even shed much light on a particular PD or on dysfunctional personality traits.

In contrast, neurological and neuropsychological assessment can be tremendously helpful in assessing individuals who have demonstrated changes in personality owing to brain damage. The term

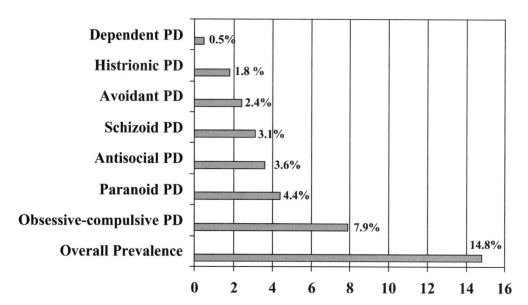

Fig. 1. The prevalence of personality disorders in the United States: The 2001–02 national epidemiologic survey on alcohol and related conditions (NERAC) of 43,000 American adults. (From ref. 6.)

organic personality disorder that appeared in earlier diagnostic schemes is now referred to as *personality change owing to a general medical condition or dementia* in the DSM-IV-TR, with common etiologies such as traumatic brain injury (TBI), stroke, endocrine dysfunction, encephalitis, and Alzheimer's disease (AD). Specified types of personality change disorder include labile, disinhibited, aggressive, apathetic, and paranoid. In older individuals, the most common cause of personality change is AD. Symptoms are often seen early on, and include apathy (withdrawal, passivity, decreased interest, and initiative), egocentricity, and increased irritability, aggression, and impulsivity *(18–20)*. TBI is more often the culprit in causing personality change in younger individuals. The following is an example of this type of patient:

> Vivian P is a 48-year-old woman who comes to a comprehensive pain center complaining of diffuse neck, back, hip, and leg pain for many years, with acute exacerbation after lifting a heavy box at work. She has a history of a skull fracture and frontal lobe contusion from a motor vehicle accident 5 years prior. She has lived alone for the past few years, functioning independently and working at a supermarket. However, ever since the accident she has had significant difficulty getting along with family members. During her initial interview, she talked incessantly about her life story and her relationship with her dog. At several points she imitated the dog's bark and the inflection in her voice when giving him commands. When asked about her pain she began sobbing for a few moments, but then quickly regained her composure and started laughing, stating that her crying had nothing to do with her pain but was in response to thinking about her dog being alone. She then began cursing out the squirrels in her yard that bother her dog: "those son-of-a-bitch squirrels better be happy that I don't have any bullets for my gun, I tell you!" she yelled, adding in a child-like voice, "but I love nature and all of God's creatures, believe me doc."

Frontal lobe injury is associated with two syndromes depending on where the lesion occurs: orbitomedial damage is characterized by affective lability, lack of judgment and forethought, jocularity, irritability, and disinhibition, and dorsolateral damage is characterized by apathy, behavioral slowing, and lack of affective range and spontaneity. Damage to either region can lead to impairments in executive function, including impulse control, insight, abstract reasoning, attention, and planning *(21)*. In the case just described, Vivian suffered damage to orbitomedial regions of her frontal lobes, and demonstrated a very labile, impulsive, and often irritable personality, quite different from her baseline personality prior to the injury. Besides TBI, neurological conditions associated with frontal lobe impairment include AD, frontotemporal dementia (e.g., Pick's disease), Parkinson's disease, and thyroid disease.

The temporal lobes of the brain mediate memory processing and language function, and contain the limbic structures in which sensory input is interpreted and assigned emotional significance *(21)*. In addition to memory impairment and aphasia, temporal lobe damage has been associated with overly dependent behaviors, avoidance, irritability, aggression, lability, paranoia, and depression *(21)*. Temporal lobe epilepsy is associated with a "sticky" or "viscous" personality (sometimes referred to as an "interictal personality disorder" or Geschwind syndrome), characterized by affective deepening, verbosity, hypergraphia, hyposexuality, and preoccupation with religious, moral, and cosmic issues.

TREATMENT

The first step in treatment of PDs must be to establish some form of working alliance with the patient, especially given the fact that interpersonal relationships quickly become a focus of the maladaptive behaviors. For all clinicians, a number of communication strategies can serve to engage patients and minimize conflict, while at the same time setting limits on behaviors that threaten to disrupt the alliance or that pose a danger to the patient or clinician. Many of these strategies are outlined in the following section. The second step is to set realistic goals based on both the PD diagnosis and the case formulation (i.e., the clinical theory of why the patient might be acting in certain ways). The overall goal is not to cure the individual of his/her PD because, by its very nature, a PD is both chronic and pervasive, and not subject to rapid change. Instead, the central goals are to reduce the intensity and frequency of maladaptive behaviors, avoid behavioral crises, and slowly move the patient toward more adaptive thought patterns and behaviors.

Several barriers to treating PDs usually emerge quite early. The greatest challenge is often how to engage individuals with a PD in treatment when they deny that a problem exists and have little insight or motivation to seek treatment. Such individuals often experience their interpersonal conflicts as *egosyntonic*, meaning that they see them as justified and congruent with their own beliefs and emotional responses. Avoidance of clinical contact is particularly relevant to schizoid, schizotypal, and paranoid individuals who have fundamental deficits in seeking out and building relationships. Individuals with borderline PD (BPD) and antisocial PD (ASPD) may demonstrate sufficiently disruptive behaviors to bring them to clinical evaluation unwillingly or unwittingly. Given the nature of PDs, some affected individuals may refuse to see mental health clinicians and only agree to see another clinician, and only for a circumscribed medical problem. As a result, it may fall to the family practitioner or a consulting neurologist to provide or recommend treatment.

Treatment of presumed PD must address co-morbid medical and psychiatric disorders that generate acute symptoms. Several key conditions include untreated pain syndromes, mood and anxiety disorders, substance abuse, adult attention deficit hyperactivity disorder, TBI, and mood or cognitive changes associated with subacute or chronic neurological illnesses such as multiple sclerosis, HIV-associated dementia, Lyme encephalopathy, and seizure disorders, particularly temporal lobe epilepsy. Symptomatic improvement in any of these acute co-morbidities may reveal a different baseline personality style. Clinicians should also look for acute psychological stresses or losses that may be overwhelming normal coping skills, such as the death of a key social support, or a traumatic experience. In these circumstances, a more adaptive baseline personality style may emerge under the direction of therapeutic counseling, after an appropriate period of grief, or simply with the tincture of time.

Various forms of psychotherapy are used to treat individuals with PDs, assuming that the individual has some degree of insight into the need for treatment and is willing to come on a regular basis. In general, real progress in psychotherapy requires long-term treatment, and many individuals present repeatedly over the years for short-term treatment of acute problems or behavioral crises. One particular form of cognitive-behavior therapy that has garnered a significant amount of attention in terms of both clinical use and empirical research is dialectical behavioral therapy (DBT) *(22–24)*.

Table 3
**Common Complications and Forms of Resistance in the Pharmacological Treatment
of Personality Disorders**

Noncompliance with medications
- Refusing to take medications
- Frequent forgetting of doses
- Experiences of repetitive, suspect, idiosyncratic, and/or inconsistent side effects that derail treatment
- Excessive or unrealistic fear of side effects
- Angry, belligerent response to side effects

Poor relationship with prescribing clinician
- Difficulty forming stable working relationship
- Distrust of clinician's intentions or recommendations
- Repetitive questions, complaints, or demands

Abuse of medications
- Polypharmacy/abusive patterns of use
- Self-injurious or suicidal use of medications
- Unsupervised and/or unwarranted use of medications

DBT was developed for BPD, but its use has been extended to other PDs and adapted for elderly individuals with depression and co-morbid PD *(25)*. DBT focuses on several domains of dysregulation: emotions, relationships, self, behavior, and cognitions *(23,24)*. The overall goal of therapy is to educate and retrain these patients to be more aware of both adaptive and maladaptive behaviors, to understand and learn to modulate the consequences of their behaviors, and to identify and avoid triggers *(26)*. Empirical research indicates that DBT can successfully reduce the incidence of self-injurious and suicidal behaviors; decrease the degree of depression, anxiety, and hopelessness; and decrease the number and length of hospitalizations *(22,24)*.

The problematic and disruptive behaviors seen with each PD often extend into the use of pharmacological agents for psychiatric and medical or neurological conditions. Some of the most common complications and forms of resistance to psychopharmacological treatment are listed in Table 3. The table divides these problems into three areas: noncompliance, poor treatment relationships, and abuse of medications. On the basis of these issues, it might be prudent not to use medications as part of treatment, especially when there is suspected abuse of the medication, self-injurious use, or use of the medication to maintain dependency and gain excess attention from the clinician. When concerns about medication use arise, the treating clinician must be prepared to discuss them with the patient and modulate treatment appropriately. Treatment failure is likely if the clinician does not recognize these disruptive patterns and provide adequate time and energy to intervene.

Several literature reviews of specific studies on pharmacological treatments of PDs since 1984 indicate a limited number of studies, with the majority focusing on three disorders: BPD, schizotypal PD, and ASPD *(17,27,28)*. For example, Soloff *(17)* was only able to locate 83 abstracts in a search of Medline for a 10-year period of time between 1984 and 1995. Of these abstracts, 77% looked at treatment of BPD and 12% looked at schizotypal PD, leaving only 9 abstracts on other categories. The majority of these studies looked at treatment for co-morbid symptoms of anxiety, depression, or psychosis instead of treatment for specific maladaptive traits.

INDIVIDUAL PDS: PHENOMENOLOGY AND TREATMENT

Paranoid Personality Disorder

Tony S. is a 55-year-old man with chronic lower back pain. He was seen in a neurology clinic for an electromyogram (EMG) study. He presented with a very serious expression and quiet demeanor, and seemed annoyed by small talk from the nurse. When the neurologist asked Tony how he had injured himself, he became angry and asked the doctor in return why he assumed he had done anything wrong to hurt himself. The neurologist tried to explain but to no avail: Tony pulled out the EMG needles during the procedure and left the appointment, accusing the doctor of being "just like every other quack—always blaming the patient."

Individuals with paranoid PD are characterized by a tendency to view other people with suspiciousness and distrust. As a result, benign behaviors by others may be interpreted as demeaning, threatening, or malevolent. In day-to-day interactions, these individuals may sometimes appear rather serious and rational. However, their pervasive distrust and sensitivity to perceived insults frequently leads to irritability, hostility, accusations, and grudges. Not surprisingly, such behaviors result in a history of occupational and marital problems in middle age, and can severely impair relationships with caregivers in late life. Differential diagnosis is important, because the paranoid stance of paranoid PD must be distinguished from paranoid psychosis. The paranoia of a delusional disorder is more fixed, severe, and resistant to therapeutic intervention. Paranoid ideation in schizophrenia may be more bizarre or fragmented, and is often accompanied by other delusions and hallucinations. Paranoid PD is believed to have a relatively chronic course, and symptoms may be exacerbated later in life as a result of changes in location or reliance on strangers for assistance *(29,30)*.

The patient with suspected paranoid PD should always be screened for an underlying paranoid psychosis, which may result from another psychiatric or medical disorder, or from transient decompensation of the PD. Treatment of acute psychotic symptoms with an appropriate antipsychotic medication, along with treatment of an underlying medical illness, may diminish the intensity of paranoia, agitation, and belligerence. Antianxiety and antidepressant medications may play a role in reducing the intensity of rage and belligerence that may erupt secondary to perceived slights and insults. Psychotherapy is limited by difficulty establishing trust with a therapist, and so a more supportive and less probing approach is necessary.

Compliance with treatment is a major difficulty with the paranoid personality. Medications may be viewed as a hostile extension of the physician or psychiatric system, and thus rejected. The paranoid individual often dismisses the need for medication because his or her suspiciousness is viewed as perfectly justified. It is important for the prescribing physician to recognize the intense fear and anger experienced by the paranoid individual, and attempt to empathize with these feelings. It is possible to acknowledge the paranoid person without having to accept the paranoid accusation, perhaps by wondering aloud to the patient how difficult it must be for them to face such worries. The physician can then present the medication as a way for the patient to reduce stress and worry. Overt and rapid attempts should be made to identify and treat side effects that may aggravate distrust of the prescribing physician.

It is never wise to challenge paranoid ideas outright, unless they are leading to behaviors that pose imminent risk of danger to the patient or others. Overly solicitous or friendly approaches, on the other hand, may be interpreted as patronizing or manipulative. A straightforward, honest, and businesslike description of treatment will minimize such reactions. Commitments made to the patient should be met promptly. An apology or honest admission made to the patient when he or she feels slighted will minimize conflict.

Schizoid and Schizotypal Personality Disorders

John D. is an example of schizoid PD, and was described in the opening section.

Henry P. is a 72-year old man recently diagnosed with Parkinson's disease. He was admitted to the hospital with chest pain and subsequently diagnosed with severe gastroesophageal reflux disease. A psychiatric consultation was ordered because the patient was refusing to let nurses examine him. His explanation was that they were disrupting his bodily energies that were aligned by his multiple body piercings. He refused to see the psychiatrist, stating that he was a male witch and it was against his creed to have mental health treatment. He was otherwise rational and fully oriented, and was noted to have brought numerous books on witchcraft with him to the hospital. He was seen by a neurologist because he was also refusing to take his Sinemet on a regular basis. He insisted that the Sinemet was less powerful than a potion that he was attempting to make.

Schizoid individuals are often seen by others as isolated, eccentric, or lonely. They appear uncomfortable or aloof in social situations, and demonstrate a constricted, flat, and detached affect. Their inner experience, however, is characterized less by loneliness and anxiety and more by a lack of desire for social relationships. As a result, they do not usually have close ties with friends, caregivers, or relatives outside of immediate family. To maintain their isolation, they may work odd hours in solitary jobs or pursuits, or spend time with their own fantasies or imaginary friends. It is important to distinguish such behaviors from the acute social withdrawal and constricted affect of schizophrenia, schizoaffective disorder, and mood disorders, and from the more profound deficits in social relatedness seen in pervasive developmental disorder (autism). It is also important to distinguish them from individuals with avoidant PD (APD), who may appear equally isolative, but because of fears of embarrassment and social scrutiny that are not characteristic of schizoid individuals.

Schizotypal individuals, as seen in the case of Henry R., typically come across as odd or eccentric, and demonstrate a lack of close friends and social relationships. In contrast with schizoid behaviors, however, schizotypal behaviors are more bizarre and inappropriate, and may manifest in paranoid ideation, ideas of reference, superstitious or supernatural beliefs, and odd speech. These cognitive and perceptual distortions are less extreme forms of psychotic behaviors seen in schizophrenia, but may increase in intensity during periods of stress. Solomon *(29)* has suggested that schizoid and schizotypal individuals become more eccentric, withdrawn, and anxious as they age, and often develop secondary psychopathology. However, many of these individuals marry and have children, and have better outcomes than individuals with schizophrenia *(31)*.

Establishing a therapeutic relationship on which to start treatment can be extremely difficult, and must be based on clearly problematic behaviors that both clinician and patient can recognize. For example, psychotropic agents can help treat co-morbid symptoms of psychosis, anxiety, or depression that the schizoid or schizotypal individual will agree are painful. Several studies have found both conventional and atypical antipsychotics to be useful in treating individuals with schizotypal personality disorder, particularly psychotic symptom clusters *(32–35)*. Antidepressants may play a beneficial role for schizotypal individuals in terms of reducing anxiety and depression *(36,37)*.

Antisocial Personality Disorder

Joseph S. is a 25-year-old man seen for a neurology consult while comatose, following a drinking binge and high-speed motor vehicle accident in which he suffered a head injury. He emerged from the coma after 4 days, and made a rapid recovery. Nurses described him as a slick character who denied having been drunk during the accident and refused substance abuse counseling. He insisted on being wheeled outside frequently to smoke, and on one occasion he got into a fight with another patient who refused to give him a cigarette. He signed himself out of the hospital against medical advice after several weeks of therapy, and refused to follow-up with the neurologist despite frequent complaints of headache.

The antisocial individual has a long-standing inability to conform to social norms, illustrated by a history of aggressive, reckless, irresponsible, impulsive, deceitful, and criminal behaviors. In fact, it is estimated that up to three-fourths of the prison population suffers from ASPD. Substance abuse is a common co-morbid disorder. Men are more frequently diagnosed with ASPD than women. The antisocial patient may initially come across in a deceptively charming manner. However, beneath this facade lies an angry and hostile personality, with little anxiety or remorse over the consequences of behaviors directed toward other people or their property. These individuals rarely seek psychiatric treatment for antisocial traits, and when they do it is often ineffective. When they do seek treatment it is usually for substance abuse or symptoms of depression and anxiety.

Longitudinal research of ASPD reveals a decreasing prevalence with age *(38,39)*, with more than one-third of individuals demonstrating improvement in antisocial traits, including declines in impulsivity, aggression, and violent crime *(29)*. Despite the potential for improvement, many antisocial individuals suffer from chronic symptoms of substance abuse, anxiety, and depression *(40)*.

The first step in treatment is to rule out acute causes of apparent antisocial behaviors, such as substance abuse, manic or psychotic states, or more chronic states associated with impulse control disorders or dementia. A history of neurological impairment resulting from stroke, head injury, or dementia with frontal or temporal lobe damage may also be associated with antisocial behaviors. Numerous psychotropic medications can then be used to target aggressive, impulsive, or disinhibited behaviors that are common to antisocial individuals, including antipsychotic agents *(41)*, antidepressants *(42)*, and mood stabilizers (e.g., lithium carbonate, divalproex sodium, and carbamazepine). It is imperative to take note of co-morbid substance abuse that might interfere with psychotropic medications, or increase the chances of medication-seeking behaviors, polypharmacy, or medication abuse *(43)*.

Noncompliance is a common problem with antisocial individuals, and clinicians rarely have much leverage. In both hospital and outpatient settings, staff should respond to antisocial behaviors that disrupt treatment with firm limit setting. This process may require a meeting between the patient and a figure of authority, such as a medical director or administrator. Patients should understand clearly what the rules are, that they are not arbitrary but apply to all patients, are mandated by the facility's highest authority, and are meant not as punishment but for the patient's protection. Rules may need to be written out for the patient, perhaps in the form of a signed contract. A behavioral contract may also be helpful, in which compliance with medication regimens and the absence of antisocial behaviors entitles the patient to desired privileges (such as cigarettes, or passes).

Borderline Personality Disorder

The case of Susan R. from the opening section illustrates BPD.

Individuals with BPD are characterized by their intense, unstable interpersonal relationships, poor emotional control, impulsive behaviors, and unstable self-image. Disruptive relationships with family, friends, lovers, or caregivers can lead to feelings of abandonment, depression, and rage. The borderline patient frequently appears to be in a state of crisis, which may culminate in brief episodes of agitation, rage, self-injurious or suicidal behaviors, or even psychosis. In clinical settings, such behaviors often prompt negative reactions from clinicians, who may dislike the borderline patient, viewing them as difficult and hateful.

Short-term follow-up studies of individuals with BPD have found persistence of symptoms *(44–46)*. More long-term follow-up, however, suggests decreased expression of borderline and depressive symptoms, improved occupational functioning, but persistence of impaired social relations and suicide risk *(47,48)*. Although these studies have shown selective decreases in symptoms throughout middle age, several researchers have suggested that there is eventually a re-emergence of symptoms in late life, but with age-adjusted manifestations *(49–51)*.

As described in the previous section, cognitive-behavioral psychotherapy in the form of DBT has become a mainstay of effective management for BPD. When dealing with borderline patients in clinical settings, it is important to coordinate a consistent treatment approach among all clinicians in order to avoid splits between staff that the patient has befriended and those the patient has labeled as foes. Anger toward the patient for outrageous behaviors should not be vented at the patient but instead discussed in team meetings or individual supervision. Otherwise, it may be highly reinforcing for the patient to see staff acting out their inner feelings of anger. Suicidal or self-injurious threats should be acknowledged, taken seriously, and responded to with compassion and yet firm limit-setting.

Psychopharmacological treatment should be considered early on for symptom clusters of BPD such as depression, anxiety or panic, and impulsivity, especially during periods of crisis. Although numerous studies have looked at the psychopharmacological treatment of BPD and found a variety of medications to be useful, there is no single medication of choice, and little research to support the long-term efficacy of any agent *(27,28,52)*. A variety of antidepressants have demonstrated efficacy in treating impulsive, aggressive, self-injurious, and depressive behaviors *(53–59)*. Selective serotonin reuptake inhibitors (SSRIs) are usually first-line agents *(60)*.

Antipsychotic medications may be helpful for transient paranoia, impulsive aggression, agitation, and self-injurious behaviors *(32,61–63)*. Atypical antipsychotic agents that have demonstrated efficacy with these symptoms include clozapine *(62,64)*, risperidone *(65)*, olanzapine *(66)*, and quetiapine *(67)*. In one study, olanazapine and floxetine alone and in combination substantially reduced symptoms of chronic dysphoria and impulsive aggression in a sample of women with BPD, although olanazapine alone and the combination were superior to fluoxetine alone for both symptoms *(68)*. Mood stabilizers such as divalproex sodium, carbamazepine, and lithium carbonate have reduced symptoms of anxiety and agitation *(69–73)*. Benzodiazepines with short half-lives should be used with caution: one study found increased behavioral dyscontrol in borderline patients treated with alprazolam *(74)*.

Histrionic Personality Disorder

> Jane R. is a 45-year-old married woman with two teenage daughters. She was admitted to the hospital after being stopped by the police for following a co-worker in her car, and then appearing to have a seizure. She was emotionally hysterical in the emergency room, and continued to have dramatic episodes of wailing while on the electroencephalogram (EEG) unit. During her hysterics, no seizure activity was measured on the EEG. The neurologist noted that when seen on rounds Jane would lie in bed wearing a pink, frilly negligee, with her breasts partially exposed. She admitted that she had been following a co-worker because he had spurned her flirtations, but she emphatically and dramatically denied that she was having marital problems.

Individuals with histrionic personality disorder (HPD) are extroverted, seductive, and provocative, and demonstrate excessive and dramatic expressions of emotion. These emotional displays are brief and lacking in depth, and not accompanied by much insight or consistency. The lability, impulsivity, and provocative nature of histrionic emotional displays may mimic those seen in BPD. Histrionic and narcissistic individuals are similar in their desire for attention, approval, and reassurance, and in the superficial nature of their relationships. In contrast, histrionic individuals are more trusting, sometimes to the point of gullibility, and are more reactive to a lack of attention and gratification than to narcissistic injury. Excessive and dramatic affective expression can also reflect more acute states of mania, agitation, and intoxication. Given its historical relationship to the hysterical personality, HPD may include symptoms of conversion and/or somatization disorder—a relationship quite relevant to neurology clinics.

Clinicians and staff members may feel overwhelmed by the dramatic emotional expressiveness, and exhausted by the attentional needs of HPD. The histrionic individual can benefit from participation in group activities, which provide attention along with constructive feedback and appropriate limits. Psychotherapy may help them clarify their true feelings. There have been virtually no studies of pharmacologic treatment of HPD. One study found that patients with HPD had an increased number of hypochondriacal complaints, and that these complaints decreased after treatment with fluoxetine *(75)*. It is not clear whether this decrease represented a true change in a personality trait (in this case, a decreased tendency to focus on bodily symptoms) vs an improvement in more acute depressive symptoms that, in turn, resulted in fewer somatic complaints. The study does suggest a role for SSRIs and perhaps other antidepressants for HPD.

Narcissistic Personality Disorder

> Vincent P. is an example of narcissistic PD (NPD), and was described in the opening section.
> Healthy narcissism is critical to the development of personality; it underlies self-esteem, and helps an individual adapt to losses. In NPD, however, narcissism manifests in a grossly exaggerated sense

of entitlement, grandiosity, and arrogance. Such individuals have a strong need for admiration, success, and power, and often demand special treatment. Like antisocial individuals, they often lack empathy for others, but more out of a sense of superiority than lack of conscience. Like the paranoid individual, they may be acutely sensitive to slights or rejection, but this results from a fragile sense of self that requires constant stroking, rather than from paranoid fears. Individuals with NPD may be especially devastated by age-related losses in physical function and attractiveness, occupational opportunities, independence, self-esteem, and self-identity. Their maladaptive attempts to cope with such losses may include excessive entitlement, hostility, rage, paranoid ideation, controlling behaviors, and depression *(76)*.

Clinicians on the frontline of care often feel inadequate, devalued, and angry when dealing with the narcissistic individual's inappropriate entitlement and angry sensitivity to perceived slights. They may feel put off by the narcissistic individual's attempts to manage their own medications, or by their impatience and angry responses to medication side effects or therapeutic failure. It is important, however, for clinicians to identify the losses that are especially devastating to the patient, and acquire an understanding of the fragile personality underlying the patient's attitudes. Supportive and friendly interactions with the patient will bolster their self-esteem and need for admiration. At the same time, prompt attention to fulfilling treatment-related commitments (e.g., appointments, prescription refills, requests for information) will prevent a patient from feeling unimportant. When complaints arise, extra attention such as phone calls may defuse anger by gratifying narcissistic needs. If available, the narcissistic patient can benefit from psychotherapy. As with histrionic individuals, there has not been research into pharmacological treatments of NPD in later life. Clinical experience has shown, however, that antianxiety, antidepressant, and antipsychotic medications may be needed to treat the individual in frequent crisis from narcissistic blows.

Avoidant and Dependent Personality Disorders

Jose M. is a 28-year-old single man who was referred to a pain clinic through worker's compensation after suffering recurrent back spasms while working on the night shift at a packing plant. Jose was described as a quiet and shy worker who avoided his foreman and was extremely uncomfortable with periodic performance reviews. After a neurological assessment, Jose was referred to a physical therapist in the office. The therapist noted that Jose became very uncomfortable when the therapist would critique his posture or offer suggestions on the exercises. Jose stopped coming to physical therapy and later it was learned that he quit his job.

Individuals with APD have a sense of inadequacy, coupled with a pervasive fear of exposure and rejection. As a result, they appear timid and inhibited, and avoid social situations. Avoidant and schizoid individuals are similar in that both have few friends and spend their time alone or with trusted family members. However, avoidant individuals genuinely desire companionship, but are too afraid.

Natalie W. is a 32-year-old single woman who was seen for a neurology consult after being admitted to a hospital for the sudden onset of leg weakness and incontinence. After the neurology attending examined her, he suggested the need for a brain scan and a spinal tap. Natalie stated that she wasn't sure and needed to ask her mother. When the neurologist indicated that Natalie was able to decide for herself, she became anxious and began to cry, insisting that her mother come to see her immediately. Her mother arrived later and agreed to the procedures. Despite her severe state of impairment, Natalie had no questions for the neurologist, but went along with all procedures as long as someone told her what to do.

As with APD, individuals with dependent personality disorder (DPD) are also afraid of rejection, but they cling to relationships instead of avoiding them. Their dependency makes it difficult for them to be alone, make decisions, or take initiatives without constant advice and nurturance from other people. In order to avoid such losses, they are often exceptionally cooperative and submissive. When dependency needs are frustrated, however, they can react with anger, clinging, and urgent demands, or become hopeless, depressed, apathetic, and withdrawn *(77)*.

Differential diagnosis can be complicated for avoidant and DPDs. Diagnostic criteria for DPD such as allowing other people to make decisions, difficulty initiating projects, feeling uncomfortable or help-less when alone, and fears of being abandoned are common after illness- or age-associated decreases in physical and cognitive ability, or after losses of social supports. Individuals who have experienced some of these losses might become exceptionally dependent on family members who are willing to be invested in their care, and display many symptoms of a DPD. Likewise, an individual restricted or embarrassed by physical constraints (e.g., amputation, arthritis, hemiparesis) or symptoms (e.g., incontinence, shortness of breath, visual loss) may display avoidant traits such as avoiding social or occupational activities with significant interpersonal contact, reticence in social situations, fears of being embarrassed, or seeming exaggeration of the risks or difficulties in ordinary tasks. These exam-ples illustrate how an individual could develop behaviors consistent with a diagnosis of a PD without a longstanding history of pervasive, maladaptive behaviors. The diagnosis of *personality change* might be appropriate in such circumstances.

A first step in treatment is to identify legitimate losses and fears that may result in avoidant and dependent behaviors. Many of these factors can be addressed by providing appropriate medical and rehabilitative support. Avoidant individuals will need consistent reassurance and encouragement. Chastising them or calling attention to their isolative or timid behaviors may only reinforce their sense of inadequacy and fear of rejection. Several antidepressants have been found to decrease avoidant behaviors *(78)*. Antidepressants can also be used to treat co-morbid major depression or anxiety dis-orders, in particular social phobia, which has shown significant overlap with APD *(79,80)*.

Once dependent individuals gain a sense of trust and hence dependence on a clinician, they can sometimes irritate the clinician with excessive questions and requests. As noted, failure to obtain enough nurturance can create a feeling of helplessness, and elicit more clinging behaviors, perhaps in the form of frequent somatic complaints. One way to pre-empt such behaviors while at the same time meeting dependency needs is to provide the patient with brief, supportive, regularly scheduled clinic contacts. In response to excessive demands, clinicians should explain limits in their ability to provide care, while also conveying their willingness to help and offering reasonable concessions *(77)*. Pharmacological treatment of DPD should focus on co-morbid symptoms of anxiety and depression, and antidepressants are usually the agents of choice.

The longitudinal courses of APD and DPD are not known, although both are felt to be chronic dis-orders *(81)*. Prevalence studies of PDs in elderly inpatients have found high incidences of DPD and APD and traits, in particular with co-morbid major depression *(82–84)*. These findings suggest that major depression may be a common endpoint for both disorders.

Obsessive-Compulsive Personality Disorder

> Edward M. is a 52-year-old man seen in a neurology outpatient clinic for an EMG study. He showed up 30 minutes early for the appointment, and checked in with the receptionist every 10 minutes until he was seen. He first asked to discuss the procedure, and began reading from a four-page, typewritten, color-coded list that he had prepared ahead of time. Afterward, he asked when the results would be available, who would call him, and how he could review them with the physician. He provided the receptionist with a card list-ing his several phone numbers and the best times of day to reach him at each one. The receptionist became annoyed when Edward returned several minutes later and insisted that he had several more questions for the neurologist.

Obsessive-compulsive behaviors are quite common, and often considered a necessity for success-ful professionals. The individual with obsessive-compulsive personality disorder (OCPD), however, has taken them to an extreme. Preoccupation with orderliness and perfectionism, coupled with a rigid and overly conscientious approach to activities, can be maddening for family members and other caregivers who must submit to such zealous control. Interpersonal relations are hampered when the obsessive-compulsive person is unable to compromise or act spontaneously. Such behaviors serve as defense mechanisms to control anxious and aggressive impulses. This pattern of behavior must be distinguished from obsessive-compulsive disorder (OCD), in which an individual has specific irresistible, intrusive thoughts (obsessions) or behaviors (compulsions) that are performed to ward off intense anxiety.

Symptoms of OCPD may be exacerbated by changes in daily routine and environment that disrupt an individual's sense of control and self-continuity. As a result, these individuals may redouble their efforts at control, leading to marked inflexibility, hesitation, doubting, and indecisiveness *(77)*. In late life, obsessive-compulsive individuals are especially vulnerable to a loss of self-worth and integrity provided by occupational activities *(85)*. The loss of control over their environment and personal space in hospitals and nursing homes is an even more noxious stress. As a result, individuals with OCPD are thought to become more rigid and demanding in late life *(29)*, and more vulnerable to depression, secondary physical illness, and psychosomatic disorders *(81)*. The presence of cognitive impairment can unleash many impulsive and disruptive behaviors if the patient is unable to remain in control of a daily routine.

Treatment strategies for obsessive-compulsive individuals must recognize this need for control. In clinical settings, it may manifest itself in repeated requests for detailed descriptions of disease states, medication actions, and side effects. Obsessive-compulsive individuals might insist on precise routines for scheduling, ingesting, and managing medication regimens. It is often difficult for clinicians to perfectly accommodate these demands. Instead, clinicians should attempt to focus the energies of obsessive-compulsive individuals on tasks in which they can invest time and have a sense of control. All medications, doses, and scheduling suggestions should be explained with sufficient detail, and with plenty of advance preparation *(77)*. Instructions should be written out in simple language, without ambiguity, especially when prescribing as-needed medications. Ample time for questions and provisions for follow-up phone calls should be provided. All of these efforts can prove fruitless when individuals with OCPD are overwhelmed by major medical or psychiatric illness, especially when mental status changes are involved. In those cases, antidepressant medications can treat depressive symptoms, and antipsychotic and antianxiety medications can ameliorate symptoms of belligerence and agitation. Pharmacological agents used to treat OCD, in particular the SSRI antidepressants, have not yet been established as efficacious in treating OCPD.

Passive-Aggressive and Depressive Personality Disorders

> Claude P. is a 36-year-old man with a seizure disorder. The neurologist who follows Claude notes that his divalproex sodium levels are frequently subtherapeutic, and he reminds him every appointment not to skip doses. Claude agrees to the neurologist's requests, but complains that the pharmacy provides him with confusing instructions. Clause misses his next appointment, and shows up 1 month later without having gotten his blood drawn. He complains to the neurologist that the lab forgot to remind him, and that when he tried to go there in the morning he couldn't find it because the directions given to him were faulty.

Passive-aggressive PD was included as a formal diagnostic entity in DSM-III-TR *(86)*, but has been classified (with the added title of "negativistic personality disorder") in the appendices of DSM-IV *(87)* and DSM-IV-TR *(1)* as a provisional disorder requiring further study. It is characterized by a pattern of resistance to demands placed on the individual, and manifested by complaining, half-hearted efforts, noncompliance, criticism and resentment of authority, and procrastination. When provided with treatment plans, these individuals will slow or derail progress, and frustrate and anger staff with their complaints and noncompliance. Psychotherapy can provide an opportunity for these individuals to verbalize their true feelings, rather than by indirectly acting them out. Similarly, passive-aggressive behaviors can sometimes be diminished by the patience of a staff member who is willing to listen to the individual and acknowledge their feelings of dissatisfaction or frustration. Pharmacological treatment frequently focuses on co-morbid anxiety and depression, or on chronic somatic complaints.

Wendy J. is a 48-year-old divorced woman with a diagnosis of fibromyalgia. She has been seeing the same neurologist for nearly 10 years. She has never suffered from actual major depression, and continues to work full time as an accountant. She spends much of the visit with the neurologist putting down her ex-husband and complaining about her kids. She describes herself as too heavy and unattractive to date again, and feels that she has a black cloud over her head. She describes her tissue pain as reflecting the poor state of her life and the world. No relationship has lasted more than several months since her dates tire of her gloomy demeanor and pessimistic comments.

Depressive PD is characterized by a gloomy, pessimistic, and critical outlook on life and others, guilt-proneness, and a sense of personal inadequacy or lack of self-esteem. Depressive PD is also classified in the appendix of DSM-IV-TR as a disorder requiring further study. Although there has not been much research on this current conceptualization, there have been many similar concepts throughout the psychiatric literature *(88)*. The main diagnostic concern has been whether this PD can be distinguished from major depression and dysthymic disorder, but data have supported its distinct phenomenology *(89)*. The disorder may, however, be more common than realized: one study of elderly psychiatric outpatients in a VA hospital found that 23% of those with PDs had depressive PD, representing roughly 2% of the clinic population *(90)*.

Target symptoms for depressive PD might include the characteristic gloomy or dysphoric mood and the tendency to worry or brood. Antidepressants would be the obvious pharmacological treatment for these traits. Engaging depressive individuals in pharmacologic treatment might be challenged by their pessimistic and critical attitudes towards the efficacy of medications. It is likely that patients will cooperate with pharmacotherapy, but that medications will bring only modest benefit at best. As a result, prescribing clinicians often end up switching to alternate agents or using augmentation strategies. It is more likely that the most beneficial use of antidepressants will be in treating more acute depressive symptoms that have developed on top of chronic depressive traits. Ultimately, psychotherapy may play a key role for these individuals, especially for target symptoms such as pessimistic and critical attitudes, and low self-esteem.

REFERENCES

1. American Psychiatric Association. Diagnostic and Statistical Manual of Mental Disorders, Fourth Edition, revised (DSM-IV-TR). Washington DC: Amer Psychiatric Pub; 2000.
2. Weissman MM. The epidemiology of personality disorders: a 1990 update. J Personal Disord 1993;7:44–62.
3. Abrams RC, Horowitz SV. Personality disorders after age 50: a meta-analysis. J Personal Disord 1996;10:271–281.
4. Kunik ME, Mulsant BH, Rifai AH, et al. Personality disorders in elderly inpatients with major depression. Am J Geriatr Psychiatry 1993;1:38–45.
5. Oldham JM, Skodol AE, Kellman HD, et al. Comorbidity of Axis I and Axis II disorders. Am J Psychiatry 1995;152: 571–578.
6. Grant BF, Hasin DS, Stinson FS, et al. Prevalence, correlates, and disability of personality disorders in the United States: results from the national epidemiologic survey on alcohol and related conditions. J Clin Psychiatry 2004;65:948–958.
7. Agronin ME, Maletta G. Personality disorders in late life: understanding and overcoming the gap in research. Am J Geriatr Psychiatry 2000;8:4–18.
8. Cloninger CR. A systematic method for clinical description and classification of personality variants. Arch Gen Psychiatry 1987;44:573–588.
9. Cloninger CR, Svrakic DM, Przybeck TR. A psychobiologic model of temperament and character. Arch Gen Psychiatry 1993;50:975–990.
10. Siever LJ, Davis KL. A psychobiological perspective on the personality disorders. Am J Psychiatry 1991;148:1647–1658.
11. Coccaro EF, Siever LJ, Klar HM, et al. Serotonergic studies in patients with affective and personality disorders: correlates with suicidal and impulsive aggressive behavior. Arch Gen Psychiatry 1989;46:587–599.
12. Stein DJ, Trestman RL, Mitropoulou V, Coccaro EF, Holander E, Siever LJ. Impulsivity and serotonergic function in compulsive personality disorder. J Neuropsychiatry Clin Neurosci 1996;8:393–398.
13. New AS, Siever LJ. Neurobiology and genetics of borderline personality disorder. Psychiatr Ann 2002;32:329–336.
14. Higley JD, Linnoila M. Low central nervous system serotonergic activity is traitlike and correlates with impulsive behavior. A nonhuman primate model investigating genetic and environmental influences on neurotransmission. Ann NY Acad Sci 1997;836:39–56.

15. Olds D, Henderson CR, Cole R, et al. Long-term effects of nurse home visitation on children's criminal and antisocial behavior: 15-year follow-up of a randomized controlled trial. JAMA 1998;280:1238–1244.

16. Caspi A, McClay J, Moffitt TE, et al. Role of genotype in the cycle of violence in maltreated children. Science 2002;297:851–854.

17. Soloff PH. Psychobiologic prespectives on treatment of personality disorders J Personal Disord 1997;11:336–344.

18. Rubin EH, Morris JC, Berg L. The progression of personality changes in senile dementia of the Alzheimers type. J Am Geriatr Soc 1987;35:21–25.

19. Petry S, Cummings JL, Hill MA, Shapria J. Personality alterations in dementia of the Alzheimers type. Arch Neurol 1988; 45:118–190.

20. Bozzola FG, Gorelick PB, Freels S. Personality changes in Alzheimer's disease. Arch Neurol 1992;49:297–300.

21. Miner JH. Neuropsychological contributions to differential diagnosis of personality disorders in old age. In: Rosowsky E, Abrams RC, Zweig RA, eds. Personality Disorders in Older Adults. Emerging Issues in Diagnosis and Treatment. Mahwah: Erlbaum; 1999:189–204.

22. Linehan MM, Armstrong HE, Suarez A, Allmon D, Heard HL. Cognitive-behavioral treatment of chronically suicidal borderline patients. Arch Gen Psychiatry 1991;48:1060–1064.

23. Linehan MM. Cognitive-Behavioral Treatment of Borderline Personality Disorder. New York: Guilford Press; 1993.

24. Robins CJ. Dialectical behavior therapy for borderline personality disorder. Psychiatr Ann 2002;32:608–616.

25. Lynch TR. Treatment of elderly depression with personality disorder comorbidity using dialectical behavior therapy. Cog and Beh Practice 2000;7:447–456.

26. Livesley WJ. Treating the emotional dysregulation cluster of traits. Psychiatr Ann 2002;32:601–607.

27. Markovitz PJ. Pharmacotherapy. In: Lively WJ, ed. Handbook of Personality Disorders. New York: Guilford Press; 2001: 477–493.

28. Markovitz PJ. Recent trends in the pharmacotherapy of personality disorders. J Personal Disord 2004;18:90–101.

29. Solomon, K. Personality disorders and the elderly. In: Lion JR, ed. Personality Disorders, Diagnosis and Management. Baltimore: Williams & Wilkins; 1981:310–338.

30. Straker, M. Adjustment disorders and personality disorders in the aged. Psychiatr Clin North Am 1982;5:121–129.

31. McGlashen TH. Schizotypal personality disorder. The Chestnut Lodge follow-up study: IV. Long-term follow-up perspectives. Arch Gen Psychiatry 1986;43:329–334.

32. Goldberg SC, Schulz SC, Schulz PM, Resnick RJ, Hamer RM, Freidel, RO. Borderline and schizotypal personality disorders treated with low-dose thiothixene vs placebo. Arch Gen Psychiatry 1986;43:680–686.

33. Hymowitz P, Frances A, Jacobsberg LB, Sickles M, Hoyt R. Neuroleptic treatment of schizotypal personality disorder. Compr Psychiatry 1986;27:267–271.

34. Schulz SC. The use of low-dose neuroleptics in the treatment of "schizo-obsessive" patients. Am J Psychiatry 1986;143: 1318–1319.

35. Koenigsberg HW, Reynolds D, Goodman M, et al. Risperidone in the treatment of schizotypal personality disorder. J Clin Psychiatry 2003;64:628–634.

36. Jensen HV, Anderson J. An open, comparative study of amoxapine in borderline disorders. Acta Psychiatr Scand 1989;79: 89–93.

37. Markovitz PJ, Calabrese JR, Schulz SC, Meltzer HY.. Fluoxetine treatment of borderline and schizotypal personality disorders. Am J Psychiatry 1991;148:1064–1067.

38. Robins LN, Helzer JE, Weissman MM, et al. Lifetime prevalence of specific psychiatric disorders in three sites. Arch Gen Psychiatry 1984;41:949–958.

39. Blazer DG, George LK, Landerman R, et al. Psychiatric disorders, a rural/urban comparison. Arch Gen Psychiatry 1985; 42:651–656.

40. Black DW, Baumgard CH, Bell SE. A 16- to 45-year follow-up of 71 men with antisocial personality disorder. Compr Psychiatry 1995;36:130–140.

41. Hirose S. Effective treatment of aggression and impulsivity in antisocial personality disorder with risperidone. Psychiatry Clin Neurosci 2001;55:161–162.

42. Penick EC, Powell BJ, Campbell J, et al. Pharmacological treatment for antisocial personality disorder in alcoholics: a preliminary study. Alcohol Clin Exp Res 1996;20:477–484.

43. Arndt IO, McLellan AT, Dorozynsky L, Woody GE, O'Brien CP. Desipramine treatment for cocaine dependence. Role of antisocial personality disorder. J Nerv Ment Dis 1994;182:151–156.

44. Gunderson JG, Carpenter WT, Strauss JS. Borderline and schizophrenic patients: a comparative study. Am J Psychiatry 1975;132:1257–1264.

45. Masterson JF. From Borderline Adolescent to Functioning Adult: The Test of Time. New York: Brunner/Mazel; 1980.

46. Pope HG, Jonas JM, Hudson JI, Cohen BM, Gunderson JG. The validity of DSM-III borderline personality disorder. Arch Gen Psychiatry 1983;40:23–30.

47. McGlashen TH. The Chestnut Lodge follow-up study: III. Long-term outcome of borderline personalities. Arch Gen Psychiatry 1986;43:20–30.

48. Paris J, Brown R, Nowlis D. Long-term follow-up of borderline patients in a general hospital. Compr Psych 1987;2: 530–535.
49. Reich J, Nduaguba M, Yates W. Age and sex distribution of DSM-III personality cluster traits in a community population. Compr Psych, 1988;29:298–303.
50. Rosowsky E, Gurian B. Borderline personality disorder in late life. Int Psychogeriatr 1991;3:39–52.
51. Agronin M. Personality disorders in the elderly: an overview. J Geriatr Psychiatry 1994;27:151–191.
52. Soloff PH. Is there any drug treatment of choice for the borderline patient? Acta Psychiatr Scand Suppl 1994;379:50–55.
53. Cowdry RW, Gardner DL. Pharmacotherapy of borderline personality disorder. Alprazolam, carbamazepine, trifluoperazine, and tranylcypromine. Arch Gen Psychiatry 1988;45:111–119.
54. Coccaro EF, Astill JL, Herbert JL, Schut AG. Fluoxetine treatment of impulsive aggression in DSM-III-R personality disorder patients. J Clin Psychopharmacol 1990;10:373–375.
55. Links PS, Steiner M, Boiago I, Irwin D. Lithium therapy for borderline patients: preliminary findings. J Personal Disord 1990;4:173–181.
56. Soloff PH, Cornelius J, George A, Nathan S, Perel JM, Ulrich RF. Efficacy of phenelzine and haloperidol in borderline personality disorder. Arch Gen Psychiatry 1993;50:377–385.
57. Kavoussi RJ, Liu J, Coccaro EF. An open trial of sertraline in personality disorder patients with impulsive aggression. J Clin Psychiatry 1994;55:137–141.
58. Salzman C, Wolfson AN, Schatzberg A, et al. Effect of fluoxetine on anger in symptomatic volunteers with borderline personality disorder. J Clin Psychopharmacol 1995;15:23–29.
59. Markovitz PJ, Wagner SC. Venlafaxine in the treatment of borderline personality disorder. Psychopharmacol Bull 1995;31: 773–777.
60. Rinne T, van den Brink W, Wouters I, van Dyck R. SSRI treatment of borderline personality disorder: a randomized, placebo-controlled clinical trial for females with BPD. Am J Psychiatry 2002;159:2048–2054.
61. Leone N. Response of borderline patients to loxapine and chlorpromazine. J Clin Psychiatry 1982;43:148–150.
62. Frankenburg FR, Zanarini MC. Clozapine treatment of borderline patients: a preliminary study. Compr Psychiatry 1993; 34:402–405.
63. Khouzam HR, Donnelly NJ. Remission of self-mutilation in a patient with borderline personality during risperidone therapy. J Nerv Ment Dis 1997;185:348–349.
64. Chengappa KN, Ebeling T, Kang JS, Levine J, Parepally H. Clozapine reduces severe self-mutilation and aggression in psychotic patients with borderline personality disorder. J Clin Psychiatry 1999;60:477–484.
65. Rocca P, Marchiaro L, Cocuzza E, Bogetto F. Treatment of borderline personality disorder with risperidone. J Clin Psychiatry 2002;63:241–244.
66. Zanarini MC, Frankenberg FR. Olanazapine treatment of female borderline patients: a double-blind, placebo-controlled pilot study. J Clin Psychiatry 2001;62:849–854.
67. Adityanjee, Schulz SC. Clinical uses of quetiapine in disease states other than schizophrenia. J Clin Psychiatry 2002;63: 32–38.
68. Zanarini MC, Frankenburg FR, Parachini EA. A preliminary, randomized trial of fluoxetine, olanazapine, and the olanazapine-fluoxetine combination in women with borderline personality disorder. J Clin Psychiatry 2004;65:903–907.
69. Gardner DL, Cowdry RW. Positive effects of carbamazepine on behavioral dyscontrol in borderline personality disorder. Am J Psychiatry 1986;143:519–522.
70. Stein DJ, Simeon D, Frenkel M, Islam MN, Hollander E. An open trial of valproate in borderline personality disorder. J Clin Psychiatry 1995;56:506–510.
71. Wilcox JA. Divalproex sodium as a treatment for borderline personality disorder. Ann Clin Psychiatry 1995;7:33–37.
72. Townsend MH, Cambre KM, Barbee JG. Treatment of borderline personality disorder with mood instability with divalproex sodium: series of ten cases. J Clin Psychopharmacol 2001;21:249–251.
73. Frankenburg FR, Zanarini MC. Divalproex sodium treatment of women with borderline personality disorder and bipolar II disorder: a double-blind, placebo-controlled pilot study. J Clin Psychiatry 2002;63:442–446.
74. Gardner DL, Cowdry RW. Alprazolam induced dyscontrol in borderline personality disorder. Am J Psychiatry 1985;142: 98–100.
75. Demopulos C, Fava M, McLean NE, Alpert JE, Nierenberg AA, Rosenbaum JF. Hypochondriacal concerns in depressed outpatients. Psychosom Med 1996;58:314–320.
76. Goldstein EG. Narcissistic personality disorder. In: Turner FJ, ed. Mental Health and the Elderly. New York: The Free Press; 1992.
77. Kahana RJ, Bibring GL. Personality types in medical management. In: Zinberg N, ed. Psychiatry and Medical Practice in a General Hospital. New York: International University Press; 1964.
78. Deltito JA, Stam, M. Psychopharmacological treatment of avoidant personality disorder. Compr Psych 1989;30:498–504.
79. Schneier FR, Chin SJ, Hollander E, Liebowitz MR. Fluoxetine in social phobia. J Clin Psychopharmacol 1992;12:62–64.
80. Fahlén T. Personality traits in social phobia, II: changes during drug treatment. J Clin Psychiatry 1995;56:569–573.
81. Vaillant GE, Perry JC. Personality disorders. In: Kaplan HI, Sadock B, eds. Comprehensive Textbook of Psychiatry, Fifth edition, vol. 2. Baltimore: Williams & Wilkins; 1990:1352–1387.

82. Abrams RC, Alexopoulos GS, Young RC. Geriatric depression and DSM-III-R personality disorder criteria. J Am Geriatr Soc 1987;35:383–386.

83. Mezzich JE, Fabrega H, Coffman GA, Glavin Y. Comprehensively diagnosing geriatric patients. Compr Psychiatry 1987; 28:68–76.

84. Thompson LW, Gallagher D, Czirr R. Personality disorder and outcome in the treatment of late-life depression. J Geriatr Psychiatry 1988;21:133–153.

85. Bergmann K. Neurosis and personality disorder in old age. In: Isaacs AD, Post F, eds. Studies in Geriatrics Psychiatry. New York: Wiley; 1978:41–76.

86. American Psychiatric Association Diagnostic and Statistical Manual of Mental Disorders, Third Edition, revised (DSM-III-R). Washington DC: Amer Psychiatric Pub; 1987.

87. American Psychiatric Association Diagnostic and Statistical Manual of Mental Disorders, Fourth Edition (DSM-IV). Washington DC: Amer Psychiatric Pub; 1994.

88. Phillips KA, Gunderson JG. Personality disorders. In: Hales RE, Yudolsky SC, Talbott JA, eds. Textbook of Psychiatry, Second Edition. Washington DC: Amer Psychiatric Pub; 1994:701–728.

89. Klein DN. Depressive personality: reliability, validity, and relation to dysthymia. J Abnorm Psychol 1990;99:412–421.

90. Agronin ME, Orr WB. Personality disorders in a geriatric psychiatry outpatient clinic. American Association for Geriatric Psychiatry—Abstracts. Annual Meeting, March 8–11, 1998, San Diego, CA.

IV Psychiatry of Major Neurological Disorders

11

Psychiatric Complications in Dementia

Daniel Weintraub and Anton P. Porsteinsson

INTRODUCTION

Psychiatric complications are very common in all dementias, which are best conceptualized as neuropsychiatric diseases. The most common complications involve disturbances in emotions (depression, anxiety, apathy, affective lability, irritability, and euphoria), psychosis (delusions and hallucinations), and behavior (restlessness and aggression). These complications are quite heterogeneous and can be difficult to categorize because of fluctuations in symptoms over time and the frequent occurrence of subsyndromal symptoms. Psychiatric co-morbidity is very common in dementia, and most of these symptoms or syndromes are associated with excess functional disability. In addition, psychiatric disturbances in the context of dementia are associated with poorer outcomes, decreased quality of life, increased institutionalization, and caregiver distress. Our understanding of the etiology and pathophysiology of behavioral and psychological signs and symptoms in dementia is limited. Screening instruments are available to assist in clinical evaluation and there are a variety of treatment options, both psychopharmacological and psychosocial. This chapter covers the neurobehavioral complications of common dementias not covered elsewhere in this book, specifically Alzheimer's disease (AD), vascular dementia (VaD), and frontotemporal dementia (FTD).

EPIDEMIOLOGY

Emotional Disturbances

Depression is the best studied of the emotional changes occurring in AD, but the relationship between depression and AD is complex, and research findings on the epidemiology of depression in AD have been inconclusive. There is evidence that both early- and late-onset depression frequently precede the clinical presentation of dementia *(1)*, suggesting that depression either is a risk factor for or a prodromal phase of dementia in some cases. *Vascular depression* is a term that has been coined to describe nondemented depressed patients with subcortical ischemic disease, and these patients may also be predisposed to subsequently develop dementia *(2)*. Depression is common in the earliest stages of AD, but it is not clear if it becomes more common as the disease progresses, and because of symptom fluctuation, there is little agreement about the natural course of depression in this population *(3,4)*. There is preliminary data that depression may slightly increase morbidity and mortality *(5)*. Gender and psychosocial factors may play less of a role in depression of AD than in primary depression *(6)*.

Studies in clinical settings have found the prevalence of depression (major and minor) in AD to be 30–50%. These findings have been confirmed by population studies reporting 1-month prevalence and

From: *Current Clinical Neurology: Psychiatry for Neurologists*
Edited by: D.V. Jeste and J.H. Friedman © Humana Press Inc., Totowa, NJ

18-month incidence rates of approx 20% for depressive symptoms. Studies from long-term care estimate the annual incidence of depression to be at least 6% in that setting.

The source of information affects depression estimates in AD, as informed others (e.g., spouses, family members, and other caregivers) are more likely to report depressive symptoms for the patient than patients themselves, either as a result of better appreciation of depressive symptoms or to overestimation of depression by attributing signs and symptoms of dementia (e.g., apathy) to a mood disturbance. Depressed AD patients have been reported in some studies to have greater impairment in activities of daily living (ADLs), more rapid cognitive decline, worse quality of life, earlier institutionalization, increased mortality, and greater caregiver depression than nondepressed AD patients *(4)*.

Examining other types of dementia, studies in general have found more emotional changes, including depression, anxiety, and apathy, in patients with VaD compared with AD *(7,8)*, whereas psychotic symptoms may be more common in AD than VaD *(9)*. An important point to make is that there appears to be considerable overlap between AD and VaD, and many patients diagnosed with either AD or VaD likely have "mixed" dementia. One study reported a 1-month prevalence of 19% for major depression in VaD, with 36% of patients having experienced an episode of major depression since the onset of dementia. In this study, older age was associated with both the presence and persistence of depression, and no patients with a Mini-Mental State Examination score of more than 20 had major depression, the latter a finding that may help distinguish depression in VaD from depression in AD *(7)*. Concerning FTD, although behavioral disturbances and personality alterations are the most common psychiatric manifestations, depression is also reported *(10)*. One study found that FTD patients, compared with AD patients, had greater total Neuropsychiatric Inventory (NPI) scores and higher scores on most emotional subscales, depression excluded *(11)*.

Anxiety is also common in AD, occurring in approx 20–50% of patients, and is frequently comorbid with depression. It also becomes more common as the disease progresses and is associated with excess disability for ADLs *(3)*. Anxiety is also reported to be common at all stages in VaD, but particularly in advanced dementia. One clinical study found generalized anxiety in 53% and panic attacks in 4% of VaD patients *(7)*. Compulsive-like behaviors are common presenting symptoms in FTD, but they are not linked to intrusive thoughts or to overt anxiety as in obsessive-compulsive disorder *(10)*. Generalized anxiety in FTD may be as common as in AD *(11)*.

Apathy is another common, complex emotional and behavioral syndrome in AD, with prevalence rates between 40 and 80% and an 18-month incidence rate of 20%. Although loss of interest is also commonly a symptom of depression and the two disorders can occur simultaneously, apathy frequently presents in the absence of depression. Similar to the other emotional changes described here, apathy also becomes more common as the disease progresses and leads to excess functional impairment *(3)*. Apathy is considered a core feature of FTD *(10)* and reported to be even more common in this disorder than in AD *(11)*. Three common behavioral presentations for FTD have been proposed, one of which is an apathetic subtype characterized by inertia, aspontaneity, loss of volition, unconcern, mental rigidity, and perseveration. One study found that 70% of a sample of FTD patients had early withdrawal from usual activities and decreased initiative, although frank emotional withdrawal was less common in the initial stages of the illness *(10)*. Anecdotally, family members often believe that the inactivity and aspontaneity in FTD represent a form of depression.

Irritability is another common (prevalence rates of 30–50%) emotional change in AD that is best understood as a secondary symptom of other neuropsychiatric changes. For instance, irritability may be an atypical symptom of depression, as has been reported in non-AD elderly patients. In addition, it commonly occurs in conjunction with behavioral changes and psychosis. In a comparison study of FTD and AD, irritability was equally common in the two disorders *(11)*.

There are other, less common emotional changes that can occur in dementias. Although mania is relatively rare in AD (<5% of patients), transient euphoria occurs in up to 10% of patients. Euphoria and frank mania is reported to be even more common in FTD than AD, affecting up to one-third of patients *(10,11)*. "Affective lability" (akin to the syndrome of "pseudobulbar affect") represents short-lived changes in affect, typically crying but sometimes laughing episodes, that either are unprovoked or minimally provoked and are disconnected from the underlying mood state. Finally, "catastrophic reactions," which are severe short-lasting emotional outbursts, occur in approx 15% of AD patients.

There is significant overlap in psychiatric symptoms in neuropsychiatric diseases, both within the emotional realm and between emotional, behavioral, and psychotic domains. For instance, applying Latent Class Analysis to the NPI, AD patients were classified into three groups: (a) those with no or little psychiatric symptoms; (b) those with primarily affective symptoms (depression, irritability, anxiety, and apathy); and (c) those with primarily psychotic symptoms (hallucinations and delusions). However, delusions and aberrant motor behavior also were common in the affective group *(12)*. In a separate study applying factor analysis to the NPI, a three-factor solution was generated. One was a mood factor with anxiety and depression; another a psychosis factor including agitation, hallucinations, delusions, and irritability; and the third was a frontal factor characterized by disinhibition and euphoria *(13)*.

Psychosis and Behavioral Disturbances

Psychotic symptoms and behavioral dyscontrol are common in dementia and can occur throughout its clinical course *(14)*, although they tend to be less common in the early stages. Delusions (frequently persecutory in nature), wandering, and agitation are common symptoms in moderate stages. In the advanced stages of dementia, socially inappropriate or disinhibited behavior, repetitive purposeless actions, and aggression can be present. Longitudinal studies have suggested that although depressive features tend to fluctuate over time, psychotic features are more persistent, and agitation persists in 60–80% of patients.

Psychosis has been described in all types of dementia but is best studied in AD. The prevalence of specific psychotic symptoms varies greatly depending on the type of dementia, which may reflect different neuropathologic origins. Up to one-half of patients with AD may develop a psychotic syndrome and/or agitation at some point during their illness, and isolated psychotic symptoms may be even more common. Studies of VaD report prevalence of psychotic symptoms on par with AD, but such symptoms are uncommon in FTD. Common psychotic symptoms associated with dementia include hallucinations, delusions, and misperceptions. The prevalence of hallucinations and delusions varies with the stage of dementia, becoming most prominent in the moderate to severe stages of illness. Essential questions remain about the nature of these symptoms in patients with more severe cognitive impairment, which limits accurate self-reporting of symptoms and interpretation of events in the environment.

Agitation also is common in dementia, occurring with similar frequency in AD and VaD. Incidence rates in patients with mild-moderate AD are 20–40% after 1 year and up to 50–60% after 2 years. Agitation becomes more common as dementia progresses *(15,16)*. Agitation, overactivity, and disinhibition are even more common in FTD than AD. A particularly troubling form of agitation is inappropriate sexual behavior, which has been reported to occur in 15% of patients with dementia.

SIGNS AND SYMPTOMS

Emotional Disturbances

It has been reported that depression in both AD and VaD is typically milder (i.e., minor as opposed to major depression, less suicide ideation, fewer melancholic features, more waxing and waning) than that seen in primary depression, meaning a decreased number, severity, or persistence of symptoms. In addition, depressive and dementia symptoms can be confounded. For instance, anhedonia (defined as a loss of interest or pleasure and a core symptom of depression in the fourth edition of the Diagnostic and Statistical Manual [DSM–IV]) may overlap with apathy. Also, neurovegetative disturbances (e.g., insomnia, decreased appetite), psychomotor changes, and problems with attention and concentration are common in depression, in AD itself, and in commonly co-occurring medical conditions. There is some evidence that irritability is a common symptom of depression in AD. For the reasons listed previously, it is important to establish the accuracy of a depression diagnosis by also inquiring if the patient is experiencing a sad mood and has typical cognitive symptoms of depression (e.g., thoughts of worthlessness, guilt, and life not being worth living) *(6)*.

Anxiety symptoms in AD typically are generalized in nature, although discrete anxiety attacks are possible. The generalized worrying is sometimes so extensive as to be perserverative in nature and difficult to ameliorate. Anxiety is often accompanied by motor restlessness, and patients with worsening neuropsychiatric symptoms in the late afternoon and evening (i.e., sundowning) often demonstrate increased anxiety at these times.

Apathy is commonly defined as a loss of interest, or more specifically as a decrease in goal-directed emotions, behavior, and speech. The emotional changes in FTD are characterized by both the loss of capacity to demonstrate both primary (e.g., happiness, sadness, and fear) and social emotions (e.g., embarrassment, sympathy, and empathy) *(17)*. Apathy is more typically observed by informed others as opposed to reported by patients, as lack of self-awareness can be a core component of this syndrome. Patients, if unprompted, will remain in a passive and introverted state for extended periods of time. It remains controversial if apathetic patients are able to achieve and maintain their premorbid emotional state if sufficiently engaged. Although it seems contradictory, both AD and FTD patients with apathy can present with a mixture of inertia and overactivity, demonstrating variability in symptomatology. Irritability usually manifests itself as short-temperedness and criticalness that is out of character or in excess of what would have been expected for the given individual. It may be completely unprovoked or an excessive reaction to a minor provocation.

Euphoria in AD and FTD commonly presents as inappropriate and disinhibited social behavior, including overfamiliarity, sexually inappropriate behavior or comments, and jocularity. Excessive spending with a lack of awareness of its implications has also been reported. The mood may be irritable as opposed to the classically described mood elevation, and motor restlessness is common. Pressured speech may occur in frank mania, which is more common in FTD than AD. There usually is a striking loss of insight and lack of concern over the problematic behavior.

Affective lability usually presents as short, tearful outbursts that are unprovoked or unexpected given the circumstances. A common example is crying over a particular scene in a movie, when this would not have previously occurred. Patients and family members are frequently puzzled by this behavior, which is short-lived, uncontrollable, and usually not associated with persistent changes in mood. It has been reported that affective lability may cluster with irritability and aggression rather than with depressive symptoms *(5)*.

Catastrophic reactions may be precipitated by a sudden awareness of cognitive impairment and may clearly signify the presence of dementia. For instance, a common scenario is someone with questionable memory deficits who becomes disoriented and emotionally distraught.

Psychosis and Behavioral Disturbances

Delusions in dementia are typically simple, nonbizarre, and focus on fear of theft, infidelity, or abandonment. Misperceptions are also prevalent in dementia. Examples include visual agnosia and believing that characters on television are real. Hallucinations are usually visual or auditory in nature.

It is uncommon for patients with dementia to have a sustained and well-developed delusional syndrome, which is common in schizophrenia. More often, delusions and hallucinations are intermediate in persistence. In many cases, the only obvious manifestation of psychosis is a behavioral change, such as agitation. Delusions and hallucinations are often associated with aggression and prominent caregiver burden.

Agitation is a descriptive term applied to a heterogeneous group of inappropriate verbal, vocal, or motor behaviors that may or may not be explained by apparent needs or confusion. It is perhaps the most troublesome form of behavioral dyscontrol in dementia. Agitated behaviors may be classified into four dimensional factors: physical nonaggressive, verbal nonaggressive, physical aggressive, and verbal aggressive. Features of agitation include: aggressive behaviors, such as hitting, kicking, cursing, biting, and spitting; motor agitation, such as pacing, aimless wandering, and repetitious mannerisms; and verbally agitated behaviors, such as screaming, incessant complaining, and repeating word, sentences, or sounds. Inappropriate sexual behavior usually manifests itself either as increased libido, a change in sexual orientation, or disinhibition.

NEUROBIOLOGY AND OTHER ETIOPATHOLOGICAL FACTORS

Although our understanding of the underlying neurobiology of AD is advancing rapidly, the etiology and pathophysiology of behavioral and psychological signs and symptoms is far less well understood. The literature is inconsistent, partly a result of the lack of consensus over phenomenology and the fleeting nature of behavioral symptomatology. The neurobiological changes of behavior likely are dynamic, involving biochemical, structural, genetic, and environmental factors that are in flux. It is also probable that certain behaviors reflect either unmet needs or emotions, or misapprehension of the behavior of others or of the environment on the basis of cognitive impairment. Specific dementia diagnosis may also be an important factor, as evidence mounts that patients with AD, VaD, FTD, Lewy body dementia, and Parkinson's disease dementia have varying clinical presentations.

Emotional Disturbances

Imaging studies have found a relationship between depression in AD and white matter hyperintensities on magnetic resonance imaging , particularly in the frontal lobes. Using functional imaging, depression patients are reported to have decreased cerebral blood flow and metabolism, including in the frontal, temporal, and parietal areas. Depression in AD has also been associated with selective loss of noradrenergic cells in the locus ceruleus and with a reduction in dorsal raphe serotonergic nuclei and cortical serotonin reuptake sites. No clear association between apolipoprotein E or serotonin transporter gene status and depression in AD has been found *(4)*. Concerning VaD, an interesting study finding requiring replication was that depressed patients were less likely to have experienced a major cerebrovascular accident than nondepressed subjects with VaD *(7)*.

Apathy in both AD and FTD has been associated with decreased cerebral blood flow and metabolism in the frontal lobes, particularly in the medial frontal/anterior cingulate regions and extending into the dorsolateral frontal cortex. Euphoria has also been associated with reductions in frontal cerebral perfusion *(3)*.

Findings from neuropsychological tests represent a surrogate biological marker in neuropsychiatric diseases. Apathy in AD and FTD has been associated with diminished executive function, including tests involving set shifting and verbal fluency. Similar findings have been reported for patients with euphoria *(3)*.

Affective lability, particularly symptoms meeting criteria for pseudobulbar affect, is thought to reflect a disruption in the cortical-brainstem pathways. As a result, the bulbar neurons are released from cortical modulation, resulting in tearful and laughing episodes previously described.

Psychosis and Behavioral Disturbances

Certain factors have been found to be associated with visual hallucinations in AD, such as older age, decreased visual acuity, greater occipital lobe atrophy, and presence of visual agnosia. Delusions have been associated with metabolic and perfusion abnormalities in the frontal and temporal cortex, areas that have a marked cholinergic deficit in AD. There also is evidence for a role in changes in aminergic neurotransmitter systems and temporolimbic structures in the development of hallucinations, delusions, and delusional misidentification.

Agitation has been associated with cholinergic and serotonergic dysfunction, norepinephrine hyperactivity, temporal and frontal lobe hypometabolism, and frontal lobe tangles and tau pathology.

Common genetic polymorphisms in serotonin and dopamine receptor genes, previously showing associations with other neuropsychiatric conditions characterized by florid psychopathology, may play a role in psychosis and behavioral dyscontrol in AD.

DIAGNOSIS

Emotional Disturbances

Diagnosing depression in AD can be difficult because of symptom overlap with the underlying disease state or with other neuropsychiatric disorders. For instance, neurovegetative symptoms, concentration and attention impairment, and psychomotor changes are all DSM-IV depression symptoms, yet they also commonly occur in AD without depression. Also, the syndrome of apathy may be confounded with depression, as it is natural to assume that lack of activity and emotional expression is a manifestation of depression. In such cases, it is important to inquire if the patient is aware of a sad mood or is unable to experience pleasure; without one of these additional symptoms, depression is unlikely. Other symptoms that are thought to be more specific to depression include guilt or negative thinking and suicide ideation. Although psychotic and depressive symptoms can overlap, episodes of psychotic depression, with delusions of guilt or nihilism, are rare in AD.

For the reasons outlined here and to facilitate clinical and pharmacological research in this area, a National Institute of Mental Health-sponsored work group recently drafted provisional consensus diagnostic criteria for depression of AD (6). The criteria, which emphasize depressed mood or inability to experience pleasure instead of loss of interest, eliminate decreased concentration or attention, and introduce irritability and social isolation or withdrawal as depressive symptoms, require fewer symptoms (a minimum of three) and less persistence than needed to achieve a DSM-IV diagnosis of major depression, thus capturing the larger number of AD patients who experience less severe forms of depression.

To assess severity of depression in dementia using a rating scale, it is recommended that self-report scales such as the Geriatric Depression Scale or the Beck Depression Inventory be used only in patients with no more than mild to moderate impairment (18). A commonly used rater-administered tool is the Cornell Scale for Depression in Dementia (CSDD), which is the only instrument validated specifically for the assessment of depression in dementia. One advantage to this instrument is that the assessor interviews both the patient and an informed other before making a rating, allowing for useful collateral information to be incorporated, and there is some evidence that the CSDD may be more sensitive than other instruments to changes in depression severity over time (4). As mood symptoms in dementia can fluctuate and occur at any stage of the illness, it was recently recommended that screening for depression in patients with dementia should occur every 6 months in nursing home settings (18).

Apathy sometimes is a presenting symptom of AD. Informed others will report a significant change in the patient's activity level, communication, or emotional state, and typically assume it is depression. These patients usually do not respond to antidepressants and are labeled as having treatment-resistant depression. Only by obtaining a careful history, assessing mood and cognitive symptoms, and administering neuropsychological testing focused on memory is it possible to establish that such patients are in the early stages of AD. Apathy is a core symptom of FTD and can be useful in distinguishing it from AD and VaD, particularly when depression is absent (11).

Because there is a common overlap between depression and anxiety, it is important to ask if anxiety symptoms are present even when depressed mood or other symptoms of depression are not. Inquiry should focus on specific, excessive concerns that a patient has, and whether they reach the threshold for anxiety or panic attacks, which are discrete, time-limited states of extreme worry accompanied by significant somatic distress.

Episodes of affective lability are distinguishable from depression, as the former are time-limited, relatively infrequent, and not accompanied by an underlying depressed mood. Likewise, the signs and symptoms of euphoria are not sustained the way they are in a true manic episode.

Psychosis and Behavioral Disturbances

In order to improve diagnosis and treatment of psychosis and behavioral disturbances related to dementia, a recent consensus conference *(14)* proposed criteria for Psychosis of AD in the format of DSM-IV. The criteria, which have been provisionally accepted by the Food and Drug Administration, include a primary diagnosis of AD, the presence of either hallucinations or delusions that begin after the onset of dementia, are present for at least one month, and are associated with disruption in the patient's and/or others' functioning. In addition, exclusion criteria are other causes for psychosis (e.g., schizophrenia, delirium, or other general medical condition). A similar consensus could not be reached for the definition of agitation in AD. Thus, in the absence of both consensus in the field and a better understanding of the pathoetiology of these symptoms, one must utilize a systematic approach to the evaluation and management of a dementia patient with psychosis and/or behavioral dyscontrol. The key general elements in this approach are: (a) clarification of target symptoms; (b) ruling out underlying medical conditions, drug effects and interactions, and occult major psychiatric diagnoses; and (c) creatively using social, environmental, and behavioral strategies. Only in emergent situations or when these nonpharmacological interventions have failed should medications be utilized.

Most behavioral rating scales designed for dementia have a broad focus that allows for ratings of various domains of behavior. The Brief Psychiatric Rating Scale, NPI, and Behavioral Pathology in Alzheimer's Disease Rating Scale are three commonly used tools. Of the rating scales that have specifically focus on agitation, the Cohen-Mansfield Agitation Inventory is the best known.

TREATMENT

Emotional Disturbances

Most medical treatment for depression is delivered by non-psychiatrist physicians. This is appropriate, given the relatively safe and uncomplicated first-line antidepressants that are now available. In general, it recommended that patients with suicide ideation, psychotic symptoms or other psychiatric co-morbidity, and nonresponders to at least 6 weeks of an adequate dosage of an antidepressant should be referred to a mental health professional for evaluation and treatment *(18)*.

First-line antidepressant treatment for depression in AD is a selective serotonin reuptake inhibitor (SSRI) or another newer antidepressant (e.g., mirtazapine or venlafaxine), which is similar to recommendations for the elderly in general *(19)*. Overall, results from antidepressant treatment studies in AD have been equivocal, partly as a result of heterogeneity in study designs, small sample sizes, and the inclusion of patients with milder forms of depression in many studies *(4,5)*. A recent, double-blind, placebo-controlled study for major depression in AD found an SSRI to be superior to placebo despite a small sample size *(20)*. Depression reduction has not consistently been associated with improvement in function, cognition, or other psychiatric symptoms in treatment studies, partly owing to small sample sizes and insensitive measures *(5)*.

Although all newer antidepressants are thought to have equal efficacy, there are slight differences between them in side effect profiles and drug–drug interactions. For instance, mirtazapine tends to promote sleep and weight gain, which might be desirable in some patients; citalopram and escitalopram appear to have very limited drug–drug interactions and a relatively benign side-effect profile, which may be useful in patients with co-morbid medical conditions who are taking numerous other medications.

As there have been very few treatment studies of depression in VaD (other than post-stroke depression) and FTD, treatment recommendations are similar to those for depression of AD. It has been reported that depressed patients with subcortical vascular lesions and frontal lobe syndromes have a poorer response to antidepressant treatment than nondemented elderly depressed patients. One small open-label study of antidepressants in FTD did report a decrease in depressive and other psychiatric symptoms with SSRI treatment *(21)*.

In general, it is best not to use tricyclic antidepressants in patients with dementia, as the anticholinergic side effects can worsen cognition. Trazodone is not commonly used as an antidepressant any longer, but is commonly used for sleep disturbances in dementia. Concerning nonantidepressant medications, several trials of cholinesterase inhibitors have found that in addition to their cognitive-enhancing effects they may also lead to improvement in depressive symptoms, anxiety, and apathy in both AD and VaD *(3)*.

Nonpharmacological treatments for depression of AD have not been well studied. However, if the level of cognitive impairment is mild, it is appropriate to consider psychotherapy that utilizes cognitive-behavioral, supportive, and problem-solving techniques, particularly for patients who have a significant cognitive or psychological component to their depression (e.g., trouble coping with a recent diagnosis of AD). For milder forms of depression, psychotherapy can be considered instead of antidepressant treatment; for major depression it is appropriate to consider psychotherapy in combination with an antidepressant *(18)*. It is often helpful to involve informed others when using psychotherapy for patients with dementia, and a nonpharmacological intervention study demonstrated the efficacy of two caregiver interventions in reducing both caregiver and patient depression. Other recommended nonpharmacological interventions include increasing social activities and providing meaningful activities, such as day programs, volunteering, religious activities, or activities that aim to incorporate the patient's particular skills or interests *(18)*.

Newer antidepressants are typically used as the first-line treatment for anxiety disorders in AD, and there is some evidence that atypical antipsychotics have antianxiety effects. Sometimes it is necessary to use benzodiazepines (BZPs) on a scheduled or as needed basis, but they should be used cautiously because of their potential to worsen cognition, impair gait, and cause sedation. When used, lorazepam is a common choice, as it does not require oxidative metabolism by the liver or have active metabolites. Although there is some evidence that buspirone, a non-BZP anxiolytic, is helpful for agitation in dementia, there is little evidence to support its use in this population as an antianxiety agent.

There are no approved treatments for apathy, but stimulants (e.g., methylphenidate and dextroamphetamine) and related compounds (e.g., modafinil) are commonly used in clinical practice. In addition, there is an interest in using dopamine agonists (e.g., ropinirole and pramipexole) and norepinephrine reuptake inhibitors (e.g., atomoxetine), as there is speculation that they improve frontal lobe performance. There are small trials demonstrating the efficacy of antidepressants for affective lability, and mood stabilizers (e.g., valproic acid) are also used clinically for this condition. Finally, newer antipsychotics (e.g., risperidone and olanzapine) have been shown to decrease irritability in trials that were designed to assess the efficacy of these agents for psychosis and behavioral disturbances.

Psychosis and Behavioral Disturbances

Psychosocial interventions need to focus on the environment, the patient, and caregivers. Eliminating environmental stimulation sometimes reduces behavioral dyscontrol. Important environmental triggers include the following: unfamiliar people, places, and sounds; sensory overload; changes in routine; and isolation. Patient-related interventions often focus on unmet needs. Many individuals with late-moderate or advanced dementia have communication problems, which translate into difficulties conveying basic needs such as hunger, thirst, or a need for toileting. A need for autonomy or independence may be expressed as agitation. Caregiver interventions emphasize education about the disease and its effects; realistic expectations of the patient; enhancing communications; and support around caregiver stress.

Because there is little empirical evidence to guide decision making in selecting a medication, we begin by formulating a working hypothesis that places the patient's psychopathology in a context. For example, if "agitation" is associated with delusions of theft or harm, we might select an antipsychotic. If it is associated with tearfulness, social withdrawal, or preoccupation with themes of loss or death, we might consider an antidepressant first. If it is associated with impulsivity, aggression, lability of mood, or excessive motor activity, we might consider an antipsychotic or a mood stabilizer first.

Although clinical studies have not validated this approach to treatment, two major practice guidelines for the treatment of agitation rest on the assumption that matching target symptoms to drug class is appropriate. One was based strictly on published data *(22)*, whereas the other was based on expert clinical consensus *(23)*. After selecting a class of medication, a specific agent is chosen based both on evidence of efficacy and a favorable safety and tolerability profile. In general, optimal dosing is one or two times daily. A reduction in the frequency or severity of symptoms, rather than a full resolution, is a reasonable goal. A general principle is "start low, go slow," meaning that medication is generally started at a low dosage and gradually increased until there is evidence of either clear benefit or toxicity.

When a treatment trial is positive it is reasonable to continue treatment for a period of weeks or months, at some point considering medication reduction or discontinuation, with close monitoring for re-emergence of signs and symptoms. Where a medication appears ineffective, it is reasonable to perform an empiric trial in reverse, tapering the medication and monitoring for problems during withdrawal. This strategy may reveal behavioral problems that actually were better with treatment.

Concerning antipsychotics, two meta-analytical studies examined the use of conventional agents for behavioral disturbances and found modest treatment effects, no differences between specific medications, and troublesome side effects. Common side effects include extrapyramidal symptoms (EPS), tardive dyskinesia, sedation, peripheral and central anticholinergic effects, postural hypotension, cardiac conduction defects, and falls. As rates of tardive dyskinesia are at least fivefold greater in elderly than younger populations *(24)*, the use of conventional antipsychotics in this patient population requires careful monitoring for movement disorders.

Examining atypical antipsychotics, positive results were reported in two of three large multicenter trials of risperidone that were completed in nursing home patients with moderate-severe dementia and psychosis and/or agitation. The first positive study compared risperidone (0.5, 1, and 2 mg per day) with placebo in 625 institutionalized subjects *(25)*. EPS and somnolence emerged in roughly 25% of subjects at the 2 mg per day dose, with good tolerability and safety otherwise. The highest response rates were seen at the 1 and 2 mg per day dosages, and benefits were noted on measures of both psychosis and aggression.

More recently, a 12-week study compared placebo to a flexible dose of risperidone, up to a maximum of 2 mg per day (mean dosage 0.95 mg per day) *(26)*. At endpoint, risperidone was superior to placebo on aggression and global measures. Cerebrovascular adverse events (CVAEs) were reported in 3 patients (1.8%) treated with placebo and 15 patients (9%) treated with risperidone, 5 of whom suffered a stroke and 1 a transient ischemic attack. Of these 6 patients, 5 had either VaD or mixed dementia, and all 6 had significant predisposing factors for CVAEs. Subsequently, a pooled analysis of four placebo-controlled trials in patients with dementia ($N = 1230$) found that the incidence of CVAEs was statistically significantly greater in risperidone-treated than placebo-treated patients (3.8 vs 1.5%). Once again, the majority of patients reporting CVAEs had significant predisposing factors.

Two studies have examined the use of olanzapine in patients with dementia. One was underdosed and was not associated with either toxicity or efficacy. The other was a randomized, placebo-controlled, multicenter study for agitation and/or psychosis in 206 nursing home residents treated and used olanzapine at dosages of 5, 10, and 15 mg per day *(27)*. Measures of agitation and psychosis improved significantly at 5mg per day compared with placebo, an effect less evident at 10 mg per day and not evident at 15 mg per day. Common dose-related side effects were sedation (25–36%) and gait disturbance (20%). These results suggest an efficacious and well-tolerated target dose of 5 mg per day.

In a pooled analysis of five placebo-controlled trials in patients with dementia ($N = 1852$), the incidence of CVAEs was statistically significantly greater in olanzapine-treated than placebo-treated patients (1.3 vs 0.4%, respectively). In two active comparator trials, the risk for olanzapine was comparable to risperidone and conventional antipsychotics. The incidence of death was statistically significantly higher among olanzapine-treated than placebo-treated patients (3.5 vs 1.5%, respectively). All olanzapine-treated patients who suffered CVAEs had risk factors for cerebral ischemic events.

Quetiapine has not been as extensively studied in this population, with just one placebo-controlled comparison trial vs haloperidol for psychosis in dementia, the results of which have been presented in abstract form only. The mean doses were 120 mg per day (quetiapine) and 2 mg per day (haloperidol). Neither antipsychotic was superior to placebo, but both improved agitation. Quetiapine treatment was associated with better daily functioning than treatment with either placebo or haloperidol, and it demonstrated better tolerability than haloperidol with respect to EPS and anticholinergic side effects.

Ziprasidone has no published data on use in this patient population. Aripiprazole, a novel dopamine mixed agonist/antagonist, has been used in three large phase III studies in patients with AD and psychosis. Results published so far suggest a benefit for agitation and mood disturbance, variable impact on psychosis, and overall good tolerability at doses of 5–15 mg per day.

The atypical antipsychotics as a class are very likely better tolerated than conventional antipsychotics, and at least as efficacious. Both conventional (particularly high-potency agents) and atypical antipsychotics (particularly risperidone and olanzapine at higher dosages) are capable of producing EPS, especially parkinsonism. However, Jeste et al. *(28)* recently reported a cumulative tardive dyskinesia incidence rate of 2.6% in 330 dementia patients treated openly with risperidone (mean dose approx 1 mg per day) for a median of 273 days. This figure is considerably less than that reported in older subjects treated with conventional agents. However, we believe the risk of worsened gait, with increased dependence and increased risk of falls, mandates that special attention be paid to gait changes after initiation of any antipsychotic medication.

Most studies with BZPs have reported a reduction in agitation with short-term therapy, although few have been placebo-controlled. High rates of side effects are reported, including ataxia, falls, confusion, anterograde amnesia, sedation, and light-headedness. Thus, BZPs are reserved for agitation associated with procedures or on an as-needed basis for acute agitation. Drugs with simple hepatic metabolism and relatively short half-lives, such as lorazepam 0.5 mg one to three times daily, are selected most often.

There are mixed results from clinical trials using SSRIs for agitation in patients with dementia, although in a recent placebo-controlled comparison (citalopram vs perphenazine) study in hospitalized patients with agitation and/or psychosis, only citalopram was superior to placebo for agitation and aggression *(29)*. There are a number of case series and open trials suggesting benefit for trazodone at dosages of 50–400 mg per day. Symptoms of irritability, anxiety, restlessness, and depressed affect have been reported to improve in some cases, along with disturbed sleep. The main side effects included sedation and orthostatic hypotension. Current recommendations reserve trazodone use for insomnia. A typical starting dose is 25 mg at bedtime, with maximum doses of 100–250 mg per night.

The term *mood stabilizer* was first applied to the lithium salts but more recently has been extended to include several anticonvulsants that may have antimanic effects. Carbamazepine and valproate are the best-studied agents in the anticonvulsant class. The bulk of available evidence suggests that they have antiagitation effects more or less equivalent to other "effective" psychotropics. A placebo-controlled, parallel group study of carbamazepine in 51 patients found a significant reduction in agitation at a mean dosage of 300 mg per day *(30)*. Tolerability in carbamazepine studies was generally good, with evidence of sedation and ataxia, but there is potential for more serious side effects and drug–drug interactions.

Valproic acid, also available as a better-tolerated enteric-coated derivative (divalproex sodium), has also been widely studied. Two randomized, placebo-controlled clinical trials suggest an antiagitation effect with generally good tolerability. Side effects occurring more often in the drug group were sedation, mild gastrointestinal distress, mild ataxia, and an expected mild (but not clinically significant) thrombocytopenia *(31)*. The available evidence suggests a starting dosage of 125 mg twice daily, increasing by 125–250 mg increments every 5–7 days. The maximal dose is determined by clinical response, or in the event of clinical uncertainty a serum level of approx 60–90 µg/mL.

There is considerable evidence suggesting that cholinesterase inhibitors have psychotropic effects in patients with dementia. A placebo-controlled study of rivastigmine in patients with Lewy body dementia showed that patients on drug had fewer delusions and hallucinations than controls. Almost twice as many patients on rivastigmine were deemed responders, defined as at least 30% improvement from baseline on the sum of scores for the delusions, hallucinations, apathy, and depression subscales of the NPI *(32)*. In the only prospective study of cholinesterase inhibitors in AD with behavioral symptoms, a 6-month trial found donepezil to be superior to placebo on the apathy, depression, and anxiety subscales of the NPI.

Antipsychotics, antidepressants (particularly SSRIs), and mood stabilizers have all been used clinically for the treatment of inappropriate sexual behavior in dementia, although there have been few controlled studies of psychotropic medication for this problem. Results of preliminary research suggest benefit from the use of antiandrogen agents (e.g., medroxyprogesterone acetate, cyproterone acetate, and conjugated estrogens) and cimetidine (an H_2-receptor antagonist purported to be a nonhormonal antiandrogen) for this problem. Although beyond the scope of this chapter, recommendations exist for specific psychosocial interventions to help manage this behavior. Regardless the setting and the specific treatment that is utilized, it is important that patients with dementia and inappropriate sexual behavior be closely monitored to ensure the safety of others in the environment.

SUMMARY

Psychiatric complications are common in most types of dementia, and can roughly be grouped into disturbances in affect, behavior, and thinking. Psychiatric co-morbidity and a fluctuating course are common, which can complicate diagnosis and treatment. Psychiatric disturbances warrant clinical attention and treatment, as they are associated with poorer outcomes, decreased quality of life, increased institutionalization, and caregiver distress.

Psychotropic medication should be used only after simpler nonpharmacological interventions have been attempted. When possible, drug selection should be based on matching target symptoms to drug class. Most of the available clinical trials indicate that newer antidepressants and atypical antipsychotics are the medication classes most likely to be beneficial for the psychiatric complications commonly seen in dementia. Although combination therapy is widely used, there is little empiric evidence in support of this strategy. Given our limited knowledge, further research is clearly needed to better characterize and improve treatment for psychiatric complications in dementia.

REFERENCES

1. Alexopoulos GS, Meyers BS, Young RC, Mattis S, Kakuma T. The course of geriatric depression with "reversible dementia": a controlled study. Am J Psychiatry 1993;150:1693–1699.
2. Steffens DC, Taylor WD, Krishnan KR. Progression of subcortical ischemic disease from vascular depression to vascular dementia. Am J Psychiatry 2003;160:1751–1756.
3. Cummings JL. The Neuropsychiatry of Alzheimer's Disease and Related Dementias. London: Martin Duntz Ltd, Taylor and Francis Group; 2003.
4. Lee HB, Lyketsos CG. Depression in Alzheimer's disease: heterogeneity and related issues. Biol Psychiatry 2003;54:353–362.
5. Olin JT, Katz IR, Meyers BS, Schneider LS, Lebowitz BD. Provisional diagnostic criteria for depression of Alzheimer disease: rationale and background. Am J Geriatr Psychiatry 2002;10:264.
6. Olin JT, Schneider LS, Katz IR, et al. Provisional diagnostic criteria for depression of Alzheimer disease. Am J Geriatr Psychiatry 2002;10:125–128.
7. Ballard C, Neill D, O'Brien J, McKeith IG, Ince P, Perry R. Anxiety, depression and psychosis in vascular dementia: prevalence and associations. J Affect Disord 2000;59:97–106.
8. Groves WC, Brandt J, Steinberg M, et al. Vascular dementia and Alzheimer's disease: is there a difference? A comparison of symptoms by disease duration. J Neuropsychiatry Clin Neurosci 2000;12:305–315.
9. Lyketsos CG, Steinberg M, Tschanz JT, Norton MC, Steffens DC, Breitner JC. Mental and behavioral disturbances in dementia: findings from the Cache County Study on Memory in Aging. Am J Psychiatry 2000;157:708–714.
10. Mendez MF, Perryman KM. Neuropsychiatric features of frontotemporal dementia: evaluation of consensus criteria and review. J Neuropsychiatry Clin Neurosci 2002;14:424–429.

11. Levy ML, Miller BL, Cummings JL, Fairbanks LA, Craig A. Alzheimer disease and frontotemporal dementias: behavioral distinctions. Arch Neurol 1996;53:687–690.

12. Lyketsos CG, Sheppard JM, Steinberg M, et al. Neuropsychiatric disturbance in Alzheimer disease clusters into three groups: the Cache County study. Int J Geriatr Psychiatry 2001;16:1043–1053.

13. Frisoni GB, Rozzini L, Binetti G, et al. Behavioral syndromes in Alzheimer's disease: description and correlates. Dement Geriatr Cogn Disord 1999;10:130–138.

14. Jeste DV, Finkel SI. Psychosis of Alzheimer's disease and related dementias: diagnostic criteria for a distinct syndrome. Am J Geriatr Psychiatry 2000;8:29–34.

15. Devanand DP, Jacobs DM, Tang MX, et al. The course of psychopathological features in mild to moderate Alzheimer disease. Arch Gen Psychiatry 1997;54:257–263.

16. Hope T, Keene J, Fairburn CG, Jacoby R, McShane R. Natural history of behavioral changes and psychiatric symptoms in Alzheimer's disease: a longitudinal study. Br J Psychiatry 1999;174:39–44.

17. Snowden JS, Neary D, Mann DM. Frontotemporal dementia. Br J Psychiatry 2002;180:140–143.

18. American Geriatrics Society and American Association for Geriatric Psychiatry. Consensus statement on improving the quality of mental health care in U.S. nursing homes: management of depression and behavioral symptoms associated with dementia. J Am Geriatr Soc 2003;51:1287–1298.

19. Alexopoulous GS, Katz IR, Reynolds CF III, et al. The expert consensus guideline series: pharmacotherapy of depressive disorders in older patients. Postgraduate Medicine Special Report 2001;1–86.

20. Lyketsos CG, DelCampo L, Steinberg M, et al. Treating depression in Alzheimer disease: efficacy and safety of sertraline therapy, and the benefits of depression reduction: the DIADS. Arch Gen Psychiatry 2003;60:737–746.

21. Swartz JR, Miller BL, Lesser IM, Darby AL. Frontotemporal dementia: treatment response to serotonin selective reuptake inhibitors. J Clin Psychiatry 1997;58:212–216.

22. American Psychiatric Association Work Group on Alzheimer's Disease and Related Dementias. Practice guidelines for the treatment of patients with Alzheimer's disease and other dementias of late life. Am J Psychiatry 1997;154:1–39.

23. Alexopoulous GS, Silver JM, Kahn DA, et al. Treatment of agitation in older persons with dementia. Postgrad Med 1998; 1–88.

24. Jeste DV, Caligiuri MP, Paulsen JS, et al. Risk of tardive dyskinesia in older patients: a prospective longitudinal study of 266 outpatients. Arch Gen Psychiatry 1995;52:756–765.

25. Katz IR, Jeste DV, Mintzer JE, Clyde C, Napolitano J, Brecher M. Comparison of risperidone and placebo for psychosis and behavioral disturbances associated with dementia: a randomized, double-blind trial. J Clin Psychiatry 1999;60:107–115.

26. Brodaty H, Ames D, Snowdon JS, et al. A randomized placebo-controlled trial of risperidone for the treatment of aggression, agitation, and psychosis of dementia. J Clin Psychiatry 2003;64:134–143.

27. Street JS, Clark WS, Gannon KS, et al. Olanzapine treatment of psychotic and behavioral symptoms in patients with Alzheimer disease in nursing care facilities: a double-blind, randomized, placebo-controlled trial. Arch Gen Psychiatry 2000;57:968–976.

28. Jeste DV, Okamoto A, Napolitano J, Kane JM, Martinez RA. Low incidence of persistent tardive dyskinesia in elderly patients with dementia treated with risperidone. Am J Psychiatry 2000;157:1150–1155.

29. Pollock BG, Mulsant BH, Rosen J, et al. Comparison of citalopram, perphenazine, and placebo for the acute treatment of psychosis and behavioral disturbances in hospitalized, demented patients. Am J Psychiatry 2002;159:460–465.

30. Tariot PN, Erb R, Podgorski CA, et al. Efficacy and tolerability of carbamazepine for agitation and aggression in dementia. Am J Psychiatry 1998;155:54–61.

31. Porsteinsson AP, Tariot PN, Erb R, et al. Placebo-controlled study of divalproex sodium for agitation in dementia. Am J Geriatr Psychiatry 2001;9:58–66.

32. McKeith I, Del Ser T, Spano PF, et al. Efficacy of rivastigmine in dementia with Lewy bodies: a randomised, double-blind, placebo-controlled international study. Lancet 2000;356:2031–2036.

12

Psychiatric Complications of Strokes

Sergio E. Starkstein and Robert G. Robinson

INTRODUCTION

Depression is the most frequent psychiatric complication of stroke lesions, and is present in about 40–50% of patients with acute strokes. Depression usually lasts for about 3–12 months, and is associated with more severe physical and cognitive impairments, poor quality of life, and relatively higher mortality. Depression after stroke is readily treated with selective serotonergic reuptake inhibitors (SSRIs) and tricylcic antidepressants (TCAs). Pharmacological treatment may not only improve mood, but may also result in a relatively greater recovery from physical and cognitive deficits, and reduced mortality.

Mood and behavioral changes are rarely absent among patients with cerebrovascular lesions. Mood and anxiety disorders are the most frequent psychiatric conditions after stroke, but psychotic symptoms such as hallucinations, delusions, and manic symptoms may also occur. Other behavioral problems not included in main psychiatric nosological systems—such as apathy, pathological affective display, anosognosia, and the so-called catastrophic reaction—are frequently found among stroke patients.

Given the high frequency and great functional impact of post-stroke depression, we mostly focus on this condition, but the prevalence and clinical characteristics of other behavioral problems in stroke are discussed as well.

EPIDEMIOLOGY

The prevalence of depression during the acute and subacute stroke period is about 40–50%, but this figure is strongly related to the method and criteria for diagnosing depression in stroke, as well as the patient population being investigated. During the acute hospitalization period, the frequency of depression is about 40%, with half of these depressions meeting the Diagnostic Statistical Manual, Fourth Edition (DSM-IV) criteria for a major depression (Table 1) and the remaining half meeting the criteria for a minor (dysthymic) depression (1). The number of patients with subsyndromal depression (i.e., those admitting to depressive symptoms but not meeting criteria for major or minor depression) may be high as well. The prevalence of post-stroke depression in rehabilitation centers has been reported to range between 49 and 54% (1). The prevalence of post-stroke depression in community-based studies (i.e., all patients in a specified area who can be identified by a primary care physician as having had a stroke within a defined period) was reported to be 14% for major depression and 9% for minor depression in an Australian sample (2). In a rural Chinese community, as many as 62% of stroke survivors were reported to meet the criteria for depression (3). In 436 consecutive admissions

From: *Current Clinical Neurology: Psychiatry for Neurologists*
Edited by: D.V. Jeste and J.H. Friedman © Humana Press Inc., Totowa, NJ

Table 1
Criteria for Major Depressive Episode

Depressed mood most of the day, nearly every day, as indicated either by subjective report (e.g., feels sad or empty) or observation.

Markedly diminished interest or pleasure in all, or almost all, activities most of the day, nearly every day (as indicated either by subjective account or observation made by others).

Significant weight loss when not dieting or weight gain (e.g., a change of more than 5% of body weight in a month), or decrease or increase in appetite nearly every day.

Insomnia or hypersomnia nearly every day.

Psychomotor agitation or retardation nearly every day (observable by others, not merely subjective feelings of restlessness or being slowed down).

Fatigue or loss of energy nearly every day.

Feelings of worthlessness or excessive or inappropriate guilt (these may be delusional) nearly every day (not merely self-reproach or guilt about being sick).

Diminished ability to think or concentrate, or indecisiveness, nearly every day (either by subjective account or as observed by others).

Recurrent thoughts of death (not just fear of dying), recurrent suicidal ideation without a specific plan, or a suicide attempt or a specific plan for committing suicide.

Adapted from ref. *8*.

to a stroke regional center in Germany, Herrmann and colleagues found marked depressive symptoms in 22% at 3 months, and 21% at 1 year after stroke *(4)*. In a stroke register of patients recruited over 2 years in four different Finnish districts, Kotila and associates *(5)* found depression in more than 40% of the patients at both 3 months and 1 year after stroke.

Women were reported to have a higher prevalence of post-stroke major depression as compared with men *(4,6)* and a significant association with depression was reported between female sex, long-lasting disability, living alone after stroke, and age older than 70 years *(7)*.

In conclusion, depression is present in about 40–50% of stroke patients both in the acute stage and during the subacute rehabilitation period. Epidemiological studies reported a lower frequency of depression after stroke, which may be related to the inclusion of patients with milder strokes as compared with patients admitted to acute hospital settings.

SIGNS AND SYMPTOMS

The diagnosis of psychiatric and behavioral disorders in neurological disease should be made after a thorough mental status examination, with a specific evaluation of signs and symptoms of psychiatric disorders. Major and minor (dysthymic) depression are the affective syndromes most frequently studied in patients with stroke lesions. The DSM-IV defines post-stroke major depression as "a mood disorder due to stroke with major depressive-like episode" *(8)*. The DSM-IV includes the category of "Mood Disorder Due to a General Medical Condition" (Table 2), which consists of two subtypes: one with depressive features, whenever the predominant mood is depressed but the full criteria for a major depression are not met; and a second with major depressive-like episodes, whenever the full criteria for a major depression are met. Depression includes both physical symptoms (autonomic anxiety, morning depression, weight loss, delayed sleep, subjective anergia, early awakening, and loss of libido) and psychological symptoms (worrying, brooding, loss of interest, hopelessness, suicidal fears, social withdrawal, self-depreciation, lack of self-confidence, simple ideas of reference, guilty ideas of reference, pathological guilt, and irritability).

A lesser form of depression included in the DSM-IV, is minor depression. The "research criteria" for minor depression require depression or anhedonia with at least one, but fewer than four, additional symptoms of major depression or alternatively, a diagnosis of mood disorder resulting from stroke

Table 2
Criteria for Mood Disorder Due to a General Medical Condition

A. A prospective and persistent disturbance in mood predominates in the clinical picture and is characterized by either (or both) of the following:
   1. depressed mood or markedly diminished interest or pleasure in all, or almost all, activities.
   2. elevated, expansive, or irritable mood.
B. There is evidence from the history, physical examination, or laboratory findings that the disturbance is the direct physiological consequence of a general medical condition.
C. The disturbance is not better accounted for by another mental disorder.
D. The disturbance does not occur exclusively during the course of a delirium.
E. The symptoms cause clinically significant distress or impairment in social, occupational, or other important areas of functioning.

Types:
   With Depressive Features: if the predominant mood is depressed but the full criteria are not met for a Major Depressive Episode.
   With Major Depressive-Like Episode: if the full criteria are met for a Major Depressive Episode.
   With Manic Features: if the symptoms of both mania and depression are present but neither predominates.

Adapted from ref. *8.*

with depressive features. Another diagnostic category offered by the DSM-IV is dysthymia. One limitation of this diagnosis is that it requires that the syndromic cluster of depressive symptoms be present most of the time for more than 2 years. Because waiting for 2 years to diagnose a post-stroke dysthymic disorder is not clinically useful, many studies have used the symptom criteria for dysthymic disorder excluding the 2-year criterion.

The main diagnostic dilemma is how to diagnose depression among patients with stroke when symptoms of the putative psychiatric disorder may be produced by the neurological condition itself. Paradiso and colleagues examined this issue in a 2-year follow-up study that included 142 patients with an acute stroke *(9)*. Their main finding was that throughout the follow-up period, those patients reporting a depressed mood during the acute stroke hospitalization showed a significantly higher frequency of all autonomic and psychological symptoms of depression (Table 2) as compared to the group without in-hospital depressed mood, except for the symptoms of early morning awakening, loss of libido and weight, suicide plans, and pathological guilt. Another important finding was that three autonomic symptoms (autonomic anxiety, morning depression, and subjective anergia) were significantly more frequent in stroke patients with depressed mood as compared with patients without a depressed mood at all times throughout the 2-year follow-up period.

Fedoroff and colleagues *(10)* assessed the frequency of depressive symptoms in 205 patients with acute stroke, who were divided into those who reported a depressed mood and those who reported no depressed mood. The main finding was that patients with depressed mood had a significantly higher frequency of every autonomic and psychological symptom of depression, except for early morning awakening, as compared with patients without depressed mood. Patients with depressed mood had an average of four autonomic and four psychological symptoms of depression as compared with an average of one autonomic and one psychological symptom of depression in patients without a depressed mood. Fedoroff and colleagues estimated that the use of standardized diagnostic criteria such as the DSM-IV might falsely elevate the frequency of depression by 1–2%, and concluded that both autonomic and psychological symptoms of depression were significantly related to the presence of a depressed mood among patients with an acute stroke *(10)*.

The mental status examination in patients with neurological illness should be assessed using a semistructured interview, such as the Schedules for Clinical Assessment in Neuropsychiatry *(11)* or the Structured Clinical Interview for DSM-IV *(12)*. Depression rating scales are useful to rate the severity but not the presence of depressive disorders and may also be used as screening instruments to determine the likelihood of the presence or absence of a given psychiatric diagnosis. The most widely used depression scales include the Hamilton Depression Scale, an interviewer-rated scale *(13)*; the Beck Depression Inventory, a self-rated questionnaire *(14)*; the Zung Depression Scale, a self-rated scale *(15)*; the Montgomery-Asberg Depression Rating Scale, an interviewer-rated scale *(16)*; the General Health Questionnaire, a self-rated scale that involves several areas of assessment besides depression *(17)*; and the Center for Epidemiological Scales for Depression, another self-rated scale *(18)*.

A psychiatric assessment requires a verbal report from the patient, which may be an important limitation in those with moderate or severe language or cognitive deficits. Ross and Rush made the important suggestion that depression in aphasic patients should be diagnosed based on the presence of specific behavioral signs, such as decreased sleep or decreased food intake *(19)*. Gainotti and co-workers developed a depression rating scale designed to be used with stroke patients *(20)*. This scale rates the domains of depressed mood, guilt feelings, thoughts of death or suicide, vegetative symptoms, apathy and loss of interest, anxiety, the catastrophic reaction, hyperemotionalism, anhedonia, and diurnal mood variations. This instrument may be a useful addition to the psychiatrist assessment of stroke patients, but two major limitations should be noted. First, some of the domains purportedly rated by this scale (e.g., catastrophic reaction, hyperemotionalism) lack clear operational definitions, and their syndromical validity has not been demonstrated. Second, this instrument may not be suitable for use among patients with moderate or severe aphasia; a limitation shared with all the other diagnostic instruments. Robinson and colleagues required stroke patients to score within 10 points following re-administration of the Zung Depression Scale before a full psychiatric interview could be attempted. In later studies, these investigators required their patients to perform part 1 of the Token Test—which assesses verbal comprehension—without error *(1)*. This strategy usually excluded patients with moderate or severe fluent aphasia, and alternative strategies should be designed for those patients in whom verbal interviews were not feasible.

In conclusion, the DSM-IV criteria for major and minor depression are both valid and reliable to diagnose depression in stroke patients. Depression should be diagnosed after a thorough mental state exam. Structured interviews are useful and reliable diagnostic instruments, and depression scales should be used to rate the severity of depression and monitor response to treatment. Several strategies have been proposed to diagnose depression in aphasic patients, but no specific instrument or set of criteria has been validated.

MECHANISM

Major post-stroke depression is associated with lesions involving left cortical (mainly frontal) and subcortical (mainly basal ganglia) regions *(1)*. Moreover, there is a correlation between the distance of the lesion from the frontal pole and depression scores: the closer the lesion is to the frontal pole, the more severe the depression *(1)*. On the other hand, minor (dysthymic) depression is associated with both right and left posterior (mainly parietal) lesions *(1)*. A meta-analysis by Carson et al. *(21)* and a subsequent study by Gainotti et al. *(22)* both failed to find a significant association between post-stroke depression and lesions location. On the other hand, a recent meta-analytic study corroborated the association between depression and left anterior lesions when the analysis was restricted to patients within the first 2 months after the stroke lesion *(23)*. The anatomical correlates of post-stroke depression were reported to change over time and may explain interstudy differences in the association of lesion location with post-stroke depression *(23,24)*. Subcortical atrophy that may precede the stroke lesion and a family or personal history of psychiatric disorder were identified as relevant risk factors for post-stroke depression *(1)*. A combination of microinfarction, diffuse white matter disease, and perivascular changes was reported to be significantly related to major depression in patients with cerebrovascular disease *(25)*.

A positron emission tomography study using the serotonergic ligand N-methyl-spiperone demonstrated that stroke lesions in the right hemisphere produce a significantly higher ratio of ipsilateralto-contralateral spiperone binding in uninjured temporal and parietal cortex, as compared to comparable left hemisphere strokes *(26)*. Patients with left hemispheric strokes showed a significant inverse correlation between the amount of spiperone binding in the left temporal cortex and depression scores. Thus, a greater depletion of biogenic amines in patients with right hemispheric lesions could result in a compensatory upregulation of serotonin receptors, whereas the loss of upregulation after left hemispheric lesions could lead to left temporal dysfunction and ultimately result in depression. Supporting the role of serotonergic dysfunction in post-stroke depression, Ramasubbu and colleagues *(27)* and Morris and colleagues *(28)* both demonstrated an attenuated prolactine response after treatment with D-fenfluramine (a marker of serotonergic function) in patients with post-stroke depression as compared with nondepressed stroke individuals *(27)*.

DIFFERENTIAL DIAGNOSES

Anxiety

About 11% of patients with acute stroke may show generalized anxiety disorder, whereas in community-based samples the rate of post-stroke anxiety is of about 3% *(1)*. Anxiety disorders specifically refer to pathological states in which the intensity and duration of anxiety produces impairment in social, occupational, and other areas of functioning. The DSM-IV category of "Generalized Anxiety Disorder" is characterized by at least 6 months of persistent and excessive anxiety and worry, and three or more of the symptoms listed in Table 3. In several stroke studies, the time constraint was reduced to 1 month. The DSM-IV also includes the category of "Anxiety Disorder Due to a General Medical Condition," which is defined as a clinically significant anxiety that is considered to be the result of the direct physiological effects of a general medical condition. The International Classification of Diseases-10 includes a similar construct under the category of Organic Anxiety Disorder.

Apathy

Apathy is defined as the absence or lack of feeling, emotion, interest, or concern (Table 4). In the psychiatric literature, apathy was subsumed under different terms such as the *amotivational syndrome, emotional blunting, retardation*, or *avolition*. Starkstein and colleagues found that 11% of 80 patients with acute stroke lesions showed apathy as their only psychiatric disorder, and another 11% had both apathy and depression *(29)*. Patients with apathy (without depression) showed a significantly higher frequency of lesions involving the posterior limb of the internal capsule as compared with patients with no apathy.

Catastrophic Reaction

The catastrophic reaction is characterized by anxiety, tears, aggressive behavior, swearing, displacement, refusal, renouncement, and compensatory boasting. Starkstein and colleagues *(30)* designed a scale to specifically diagnose this syndrome (Table 5). They found the catastrophic reaction in 19% of patients with acute stroke lesions, and 66% of patients with the catastrophic reaction also had major depression *(30)*. Thus, the catastrophic reaction may characterize a specific type of post-stroke major depression.

Pathological Affective Display

Patients with stroke frequently present with sudden episodes of crying or laughing that are generically termed pathologic affective display. This entity may be subdivided into the categories of emotional lability and pathological laughing and/or crying. The former is defined as sudden laughing and/or crying that the patient is unable to suppress, which generally occurs in appropriate situations and is accompanied by a congruent alteration of mood. Pathological laughing or crying is defined as sudden laughing or crying episodes that do not correspond to an underlying emotional change. Robinson and colleagues developed the Pathological Laughing and Crying Scale to quantify aspects of pathological affective display, such as the duration of the episodes, their relation to external events, degree of

Table 3
Generalized Anxiety Disorder

A. There must be a period of at least 6 months with prominent tension, worry, and feelings of apprehension about everyday events and problems.
B. At least four of the symptoms listed below must be present, at least one of which must be from items 1–4:
   1. Autonomic arousal symptoms
      a. Palpitations or pounding heart, or accelerated heart rate;
      b. Sweating;
      c. Trembling or shaking;
      d. Dry mouth (not because of medication or dehydration);
   2. Symptoms involving chest and abdomen
      e. difficulty in breathing;
      f. feeling of choking;
      g. chest pain or discomfort;
      h. nausea or abdominal distress
   3. Symptoms involving mental state
      i. feeling dizzy, unsteady, faint, or light-headed;
      j. feelings that objects are unreal (derealization), or that the self is distant or "not really here" (depersonalization);
      k. fear of losing control, "going crazy", or passing out;
      l. fear of dying;
   4. General symptoms
      m. hot flashes or cold chills;
      n. numbness or tingling sensations;
   5. Symptoms of tension
      o. muscle tension or aches and pains;
      p. restlessness and inability to relax;
      q. feeling keyed up, on edge, or mentally tense;
      r. a sensation of a lump in the throat, or difficulty in swallowing;
   6. Other nonspecific symptoms
      s. exaggerated response to minor surprises or being startled;
      t. difficulty in concentrating, or mind "going blank", because of worrying or anxiety;
      u. persistent irritability;
      v. difficulty in getting to sleep because of worrying.

Adapted from ref. *8.*

voluntary control, inappropriateness in relation to emotions, and degree of resultant distress *(31)*. Robinson and colleagues found no significant correlations between scores of emotional lability and scores of depression, social functioning, activities of daily living (ADLs), and cognitive level, suggesting that post-stroke depression and pathological emotions may be independent phenomena *(31)*. Kim and colleagues prospectively studied 148 patients with single unilateral stroke at 2–4 months poststroke, and correlated lesion location with depression and emotional lability *(32)* They found depression in 18% of the patients and emotional lability in 34%. Anterior cortical lesion location was significantly associated with depression, whereas lenticulocapsular strokes were significantly associated with emotional lability *(32)*.

Anosognosia

Anosognosia is defined as the lack of awareness of physical, cognitive, or behavioral changes produced by stroke. Starkstein and colleagues developed the Anosognosia Questionnaire to diagnose the presence of anosognosia (i.e., full denial of illness), or anosodiaphoria (i.e., the emotional indifference to the deficit) *(33)*. About 30% of stroke patients may show anosognosia or anosodiaphoria

Table 4
Apathy Scale

Rate the patient's behavior over the *PAST MONTH* Questions	Not at all	Slightly	Some	A lot
Are you interested in learning new things?				
Does anything interest you?				
Are you concerned about your condition?				
Do you put much effort into things?				
Are you always looking for something to do?				
Do you have plans and goals for the future?				
Do you have motivation?				
Do you have the energy for daily activities?				
Does someone have to tell you what to do each day?				
Are you indifferent to things?				
Are you unconcerned with many things?				
Do you need a push to get started on things?				
Are you neither happy nor sad, just in between?				
Would you consider yourself apathetic?				

Note: For questions 1–8, the scoring system is the following: not at all = 3 points; slightly = 2 points; some = 1 point; a lot = 0 points. For questions 9–14, the scoring system is the following: not at all = 0 points; slightly = 1 point; some = 2 points; a lot = 3 points.

during the acute stage after the stroke. Anosognosia is significantly associated with poor quality of life for both patients and caregivers, and is the main clinical indicator of poor physical and functional recovery *(1)*.

COURSE

Although major post-stroke depression was reported to last about 1 year, minor (dysthymic) post-stroke depression was found to have a more variable duration, lasting from 3 months to more than 2 years *(1)*. Morris and colleagues *(34)* and House and colleagues *(35)* reported that most patients with minor depression were not depressed 3 to 6 months after the acute event. Differences in case ascertainment (acute stroke patients vs community-dwelling patients) or differences in premorbid personality characteristics may explain these discrepancies. Kauhanen and colleagues *(36)* examined the longitudinal evolution of depression in 106 post-stroke patients and found an increasing frequency of major depression during the first year following stroke. Lesion location may also influence the duration of post-stroke depression. Starkstein and colleagues demonstrated that patients with subcortical (primarily basal ganglia) or cerebellar and brainstem lesions recovered significantly faster from post-stroke depression than patients with cortical lesions *(1)*.

Depression is an important negative factor in the recovery from impairments in ADLs and is associated with a higher mortality among stroke patients. Clark and Smith *(37)* reported a significant association between post-stroke depression and worse social functioning, and Lafgren and colleagues *(38)* demonstrated a significant negative correlation between depression and psychological well-being after stroke *(39)*. Carod-Artal and colleagues examined quality of life in a series of 90 stroke survivors, 1 year after the acute event. They found that depression was among the main predictors of poor quality of life among stroke patients *(39)*.

Several investigators demonstrated a significant correlation between depression and physical impairment. Bosworth and colleagues *(40)* examined long-term patient health status in a series of 1073 individuals with an acute stroke lesion. Twelve months after the acute event the authors found that living alone, being institutionalized, decreased physical function, and depression were independently

Table 5
Catastrophic Reaction Scale

Key:
    0 = None
    1 = Slight (once during the interview)
    2 = Moderate (several times during the interview)
    3 = Extreme (most of the interview).

1. Patient appeared to be anxious (i.e., patient showed an apprehensive attitude or expressed fears).
2. Patient complained of feeling anxious or afraid (i.e., patient referred to feeling tense or having psychological concomitants of anxiety).
3. Patient became tearful (i.e., patient cried at some point during the evaluation).
4. Patient complained of feeling sad or depressed (i.e., patient spontaneously reported sad feelings during the evaluation).
5. Patient behaved in angry manner (i.e., patient shouted, contradicted the examiner, performed tasks in careless way).
6. Patient complained of feeling angry (patient reported being upset with the evaluation and/or the examiner).
7. Patient swore (patient at some point during the evaluation).
8. Patient expressed displaced anger (patient complained about the hospital, doctors, and fellow patients).
9. Patient refused to do something (patient stopped doing a task or refused to answer some questions).
10. Patient described a feeling of suddenly becoming depressed or hopeless (patient reported feeling worthless, sad, and lacking in confidence).
11. Patient boasted about self (patient reported being able to perform the tasks flawlessly and explained failures as due to lack of concentration and tiredness).

associated with lower levels of patient health status. After adjusting for physical functioning, stroke patients with significant depressive symptoms reported lower health status, which persisted over time. Singh and colleagues *(41)* found that more severe deficits in ADLs predicted a more severe depression 3 months later. Parikh and colleagues *(42)* examined the severity of functional impairments in 63 stroke patients with or without depression during a 2-year follow-up period. Although both groups were comparable in terms of physical disability while in the hospital, depressed patients showed significantly less recovery after 2 years as compared to nondepressed patients. Another study found a significant correlation between depressive symptoms and both functional outcome and handicap at 3 months and 1-year following stroke *(43)*. Morris and colleagues *(44)* examined the association between depression and deficits in ADLs in a 15-month follow-up study that included 49 patients with an acute stroke lesion. They found significantly less recovery in overall functioning and physical disability, among stroke patients with in-hospital depression as compared with those without depression. Astrom and colleagues *(45)* suggested that the failure to recover from deficits in ADLs in the early period after stroke might lead to depression, which then inhibits progress in physical recovery. In support, Robinson and colleagues found that the severity of in-hospital depression predicted the severity of deficits in ADLs 6 months later, and similarly, the severity of ADL impairment in the acute in-hospital period predicted the severity of depression 6 months later *(1)*. Thus, the relationship between depression and ADLs appears to be both time-dependent (i.e., the correlation becomes stronger from the in-hospital acute stage to 6 months later) and reciprocal (i.e., depression predicts more severe deficits in ADLs, and vice-versa). To examine whether the *persistence* of depression over time may impair the recovery in ADLs among stroke patients, Chemerinski and colleagues *(46)* examined differences on recovery of ADLs between post-stroke depressed patients with remission of their depression ($N = 21$), as compared with post-stroke depressed patients without mood recovery over the first 3 to 6 months after stroke. Whereas there were no significant between-group differences in demographic variables, lesion characteristics, and neurological symptoms, those patients who had a remission of their depression at follow-up had significantly greater recovery in ADLs at follow-up than patients without mood

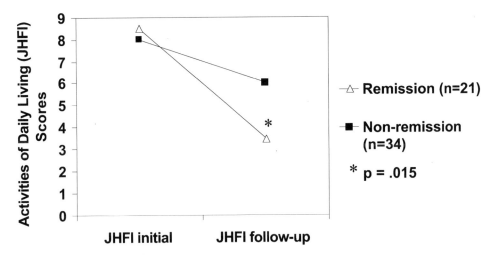

Fig. 1. Post-stroke patients with remission of depression showed significantly greater recovery in activities of daily living than non-remitted patients at the 3- or 6-month follow-up [$F = 6.37$; $df = 1$; 53, $p = 0.015$].

improvement (Fig. 1). Based on this finding the authors suggested that the poor recovery of ADLs in post-stroke depressed patients could be related to less motivation to engage in rehabilitation treatments, leading to slow recovery *(46)*.

Patients with major depression after left hemispheric lesions demonstrated significantly more severe cognitive impairments as compared to nondepressed stroke patients, and post-stroke depression may also have a negative influence on the recovery of cognitive impairment *(1)*. Given that lesion variables may account for a significant proportion of cognitive deficits, Starkstein and colleagues matched stroke patients with or without major depression for lesion size and location *(47)*. They found that patients with major post-stroke depression had significantly lower Mini-Mental State Exam (MMSE) scores than patients without depression *(47)*. Because the MMSE is a rather crude measure of cognitive functions, Bolla-Wilson and colleagues *(48)* examined depressed and nondepressed stroke patients with a comprehensive neuropsychological battery. Patients with major depression and left hemispheric lesions showed significantly more severe deficits on tasks of verbal memory, language, visuoconstructional ability, executive motor functions, and frontal lobe-related tasks than nondepressed patients with left hemispheric strokes. On the other hand, there were no significant differences on these cognitive tests between depressed and nondepressed patients with right hemispheric lesions. Downhill and Robinson *(49)* examined the longitudinal evolution of cognitive deficits in 309 patients with acute stroke lesions. At the in-hospital assessment patients with major depression after a left hemisphere stroke had significantly lower MMSE scores than nondepressed patients, and this association persisted for up to 1 year after stroke.

Post-stroke depression is associated with a relatively high mortality. Morris and colleagues *(50)* found that patients with acute in-hospital depression had a 10-year mortality of 70% as compared with a mortality of 31% for stroke patients without depression. A difference on the probability of survival between the depressed and nondepressed patients was evident as early as the first year after stroke, and continued during the first 5 years before the curves began to parallel each other (Fig. 2). A logistic regression analysis to assess the contribution of depression, social function, co-morbid medical illness, age, gender, social class, physical and cognitive impairment, and size and location of stroke demonstrated that depression remained an independent factor for mortality, with an odds ratio of 3.7. Lesion volume was the computed tomography variable most strongly associated with increased mortality: patients who died after the 10-year follow-up period had more than twice the lesion volume as

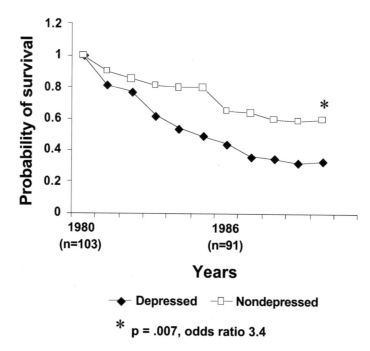

Fig. 2. Probability of survival following stroke for depressed and nondepressed patients. (From ref. *69*.)

compared with patients who survived. However, the association between depression and a higher mortality remained significant after lesion volume was ruled-out. Finally, in a series of 448 patients assessed 1 month after stroke, House and colleagues *(51)* found that the depression subscale of the General Health Questionnaire was the only significant predictor of mortality using a logistic regression to control for other variables. The only negative study reported was a 3-year follow-up study by Astrom and colleagues *(45)* that included 21 patients. These researchers reported that older age, disorientation, impairments in ADLs, and more severe cortical atrophy were significantly related to a higher mortality during the follow-up period. On the other hand, no significant association was found between post-stroke depression and a higher mortality.

In conclusion, depression has a strong negative impact on the recovery process of stroke patients. More severe depression predicts more severe functional and cognitive deficits, a relatively worse social functioning, poorer quality of life, and higher mortality.

TREATMENT

Post-stroke depression may be adequately treated with antidepressant drugs. In the first randomized, double-blind, placebo-controlled study, Lipsey and colleagues *(52)* examined the efficacy of nortriptyline in a randomized, double-blind, placebo-controlled study that included 11 patients treated with active drug and 15 patients given placebo. After 6 weeks of treatment, patients taking nortriptyline showed significantly lower Hamilton Depression scores than the placebo group. Important side effects such as delirium, confusion, drowsiness, and agitation, were found in three patients. In the second study, Andersen and colleagues *(53)* examined the efficacy of the specific serotonin reuptake inhibitor citalopram in the treatment of post-stroke depression. They found that at both 3 and 6 weeks of treatment the active group had significantly lower Hamilton Depression scores than the placebo group. Nortriptyline, fluoxetine, and placebo were compared in the treatment of depression after acute stroke *(54)*. Patients received either nortriptyline up to 100 mg per day, fluoxetine up to 40 mg per day, or placebo during a 12-week period. Nortriptyline produced a significantly higher response rate

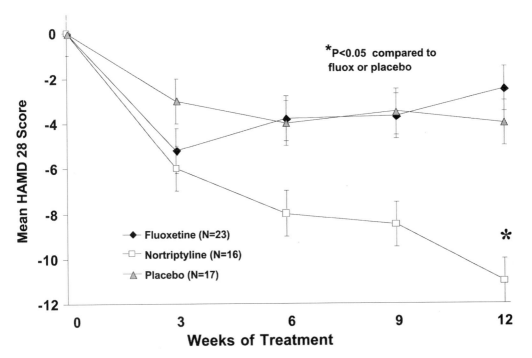

Fig. 3. Change in Hamilton Depression score (28 items) over 12 weeks of treatment for all patients who were entered in the study. Using intention-to-treat analysis there was a significant group by time interaction ($F = 3.45$, $df = 8$, 212, $p = 0.0035$) and *post-hoc* analysis showed significantly greater change in patients treated with nortriptyline compared with fluoxetine or placebo at 12 weeks. (From ref. *70*.)

than fluoxetine or placebo in the treatment of post-stroke depression, anxiety, and impairments in ADLs (Fig. 3). There was no significant difference in depression outcome between fluoxetine and placebo *(54)*. In a multicenter double-blind, placebo-controlled study for the treatment of acute hemiplegic patients with post-stroke major depression, Wiart and colleagues *(55)* found fluoxetine to produce no major side effects and to be significantly more effective than placebo. Fruehwald and colleagues *(56)* carried-out a 3-month double-blind, randomized, placebo-controlled trial of fluoxetine (20 mg per day) in 50 moderate to severe post-stroke depressed patients. The study included an 18-month open-label extension. There were no significant differences between placebo-and fluoxetine-treated patients during the initial 3-month period, but between-group differences became significant at the 18-month follow-up. Although no significant differences could be observed between both groups at 4 weeks, depression increased in the placebo group at 12 weeks; the difference was evident at 18 months, when patients treated with fluoxetine showed less depression *(56)*.

Treatment of Depression and Functional Recovery

Several studies examined whether treating depression after stroke with antidepressant medication has a positive impact on recovery from functional impairments. Reding and colleagues *(57)* demonstrated that stroke patients treated with the antidepressant trazodone showed greater improvement in ADLs as compared with patients treated with placebo. Gonzalez-Torrecillas and colleagues *(58)* compared 11 post-stroke depressed patients treated with nortriptyline, 26 depressed patients treated with fluoxetine, and 11 post-stroke depressed patients treated with placebo. After a 6-week treatment period, patients on either nortriptyline or fluoxetine had a significantly greater improvement on ADLs as compared to patients on placebo. Gainotti and colleagues *(59)* examined the influence of post-stroke depression and antidepressant therapy on the improvement of motor scores and disability. A group of

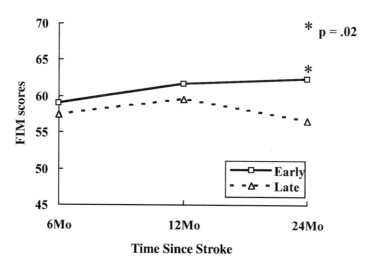

Fig. 4. Change in functional independence measure (FIM) scores over 2 years in patients who started receiving nortriptyline or fluoxetine within the first month after stroke (Early) compared to those who started after the first month post-stroke (Late). FIM scores were measured at the same times following stroke to control for group differences in time since stroke when the 12-week course of treatment was given. Note the significant deterioration in FIM scores in late treatment group. Repeated measures ANOVA between months 12 and 24 showed a significant group-by-time interaction (efficacy analysis; $F = 6.87$, $df = 1,30$, $p = 0.01$; intention-to-treat analysis; $F = 5.70$, $df = 1,53$, $p = 0.02$). (From ref. *71*.)

49 patients who suffered from depression after stroke and received either antidepressant treatment ($n = 24$) or no treatment ($n = 25$) were compared with 15 nondepressed stroke patients. Twenty-three of the 24 patients received fluoxetine monotherapy with dosages ranging from 20 to 40 mg per day. The main finding was that the physical recovery of nontreated depressed patients was significantly less than in nondepressed and depressed but treated stroke patients.

Narushima and Robinson compared early vs late treatment of depression after stroke on ADL outcomes over 2 years after treatment *(60)*. They found that patients who began antidepressants (nortriptyline or fluoxetine) within the first month after stroke had better outcome by 2 years post-stroke than patients who started antidepressant therapy more than 1 month after stroke (Fig. 4). This finding suggests that there may be a time-related therapeutic window for instituting antidepressant treatment. Based on a merged analysis of prior treatment studies, Kimura and colleagues *(61)* found that patients with post-stroke depression who responded to the antidepressant (defined as a greater than 50% reduction in HAM-D scores) had a significant improvement on MMSE scores as compared to nonresponders. Finally, preliminary evidence suggests that antidepressant treatment may decrease mortality after stroke. In a recent study, Jorge et al. examined the 9-year mortality of 104 stroke patients who were randomly assigned to receive a 12-week double-blind course of nortriptyline, fluoxetine, or placebo early in the recovery period after a stroke *(62)*. Of 53 patients who were given full-dose antidepressants, 36 (69%) were alive at follow-up, as compared with only 10 (36%) of 28 placebo-treated patients (Fig. 5). These differences remained significant after other factors associated with mortality were controlled for.

Prevention of Post-Stroke Depression

A number of recent studies examined whether treatment with antidepressant medication could prevent post-stroke depression during the acute post-stroke period. The antidepressant mianserin was evaluated in an 18-month, randomized, double-blind, placebo-controlled study that included 100 patients with acute stroke during a 1 year using a double-blind design *(63)*. There was no signif-

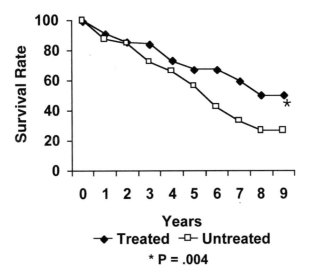

Fig. 5. Survival rates over 9-year follow-up of acute stroke patients who were entered in a 12-week double blind course of antidepressants or placebo. Data shows intention to treat analysis. (From ref. 72.)

icant difference in the frequency of major depression between mianserin- and placebo-treated patients, thus failing to demonstrate a significant efficacy for mianserin to prevent post-stroke depression.

A double-blind study by Narashima and colleagues *(60)* compared nortriptyline, fluoxetine, and placebo to prevent post-stroke depression. During the 3-month treatment period nortriptyline and fluoxetine appeared to be better than placebo in preventing depression. However, when nortriptyline was discontinued, patients were more likely to develop depression during the following 6 months. Rasmussen and colleagues, *(64)* in a double-blind trial, treated a series of patients who were less than 1 month post-stroke with sertraline or placebo for 1 year. The main finding was that 22% of the 67 patients given placebo developed depression (either major or minor) compared with only 8% for the 70 patients treated with sertraline.

Psychotherapy

Kneebone and Dunmore *(65)* reviewed the psychological management of post-stroke depression and identified cognitive behavior therapy as a potentially useful treatment modality. However, a recent randomized controlled study by Lincoln and Flannaghan *(66)* found no significant benefit of cognitive-behavioral psychotherapy for post-stroke depression. Mant and colleagues *(67)* carried out a randomized controlled trial of family support vs normal care in a series of 323 stroke patients and 26 caregivers. The main finding was that family support significantly increased social activities and improved quality of life of caregivers, with no significant effects on patients.

CONCLUSION

In conclusion, recent studies demonstrated that both TCAs and SSRIs have a significant antidepressant effect among stroke victims. Moreover, preliminary findings suggest that antidepressant treatment may also improve both physical and cognitive deficits among patients with post-stroke depression. Recent findings also suggest that treatment with antidepressant medication in the acute stage after stroke prevents the onset of depression in a significant proportion of stroke victims. Antidepressants do not seem to produce more frequent or severe side effects than placebo, but future studies will have to confirm whether the cessation of antidepressants results in a rebound of depression.

REFERENCES

1. Robinson RG. The Clinical Neuropsychiatry of Stroke. Cambridge: Cambridge University Press; 1998.
2. Burvill PW, Johnson GA, Jamrozik KD, Anderson CS, Stewart-Wynne EG, Chakera TM. Prevalence of depression after stroke: the Perth Community Stroke Study. Br J Psychiatry 1995;166:320–327.
3. Fuh JL, Liu HC, Wang SJ, Liu CY, Wang PN. Poststroke depression among the Chinese elderly in a rural community. Stroke 1997;28:1126–1129.
4. Herrmann M, Bartels C, Wallesch CW. Depression in acute and chronic aphasia: symptoms, pathoanatomical-clinical correlations and functional implications. J Neurol Neurosurg Psychiatry 1993;56:672–678.
5. Kotila M, Numminen H, Waltimo O, Kaste M. Depression after stroke: results of the FINNSTROKE Study. Stroke 1998; 29:368–372.
6. Paradiso S, Robinson RG. Gender differences in poststroke depression. J Neuropsychiatry Clin Neurosci 1998;10:41–47.
7. Hayee MA, Akhtar N, Haque A, Rabbani MG. Depression after stroke-analysis of 297 stroke patients. Bangladesh Med Res Counc Bull 2001;27:96–102.
8. American Psychiatric Association. Diagnostic and Statistical Manual of Mental Disorders, Fourth edition. Washington, DC: Amer Psychiatric Pub; 1994.
9. Paradiso S, Ohkubo T, Robinson RG. Vegetative and psychological symptoms associated with depressed mood over the first two years after stroke. Int J Psychiatry Med 1997;27:137–157.
10. Fedoroff JP, Starkstein SE, Parikh RM, Price TR, Robinson RG. Are depressive symptoms nonspecific in patients with acute stroke? Am J Psychiatry 1991;148:1172–1176.
11. World Health Organization. Schedules for Clinical Assessment in Neuropsychiatry. Version 2.0. Geneva: World Health Organization;1994.
12. Spitzer RL, Williams JB, Gibbon M, First MB. The Structured Clinical Interview for DSM-III-R (SCID). I: History, rationale, and description. Arch Gen Psychiatry 1992;49:624–629.
13. Hamilton M. A rating scale for depression. J Neurol Neurosurg Psychiatry 1960;23:56–62.
14. Beck AT, Ward CH, Mendelson M, Mock J, Erbaugh J. An inventory for measuring depression. Arch Gen Psychiatry 1961; 4:551–571.
15. Zung WW, Richards CB, Short MJ. Self-rating depression scale in an outpatient clinic. Further validation of the SDS. Arch Gen Psychiatry 1965;13:508–515.
16. Montgomery SA, Asberg M. A new depression scale designed to be sensitive to change. Br J Psychiatry 1979;134:382–389.
17. Goldberg DP, Hillier VF. A scaled version of the General Health Questionnaire. Psychol Med 1979;9:139–145.
18. Radloff LA. The CES-D Scale, a self-report depression scale for research in the general population. Applied Psychological Measurement 1977;1:385–401.
19. Ross ED, Rush AJ. Diagnosis and neuroanatomical correlates of depression in brain damaged patients. Arch Gen Psychiatry 1981;38:1344–1354.
20. Gainotti G, Azzoni A, Razzano C, Lanzillotta M, Marra C, Gasparini F. The Post-Stroke Depression Rating Scale: a test specifically devised to investigate affective disorders of stroke patients. J Clin Exp Neuropsychol 1997;19:340–356.
21. Carson AJ, MacHale S, Allen K, et al. Depression after stroke and lesion location: a systematic review. Lancet 2000;356: 122–126.
22. Gainotti G, Azzoni A, Marra C. Frequency, phenomenology and anatomoclinical correlates of major post-stroke depression. Br J Psychiatry 1999;175:163–167.
23. Narushima K, Kosier JT, Robinson RG. A reappraisal of poststroke depression, intra- and inter-hemispheric lesion location using meta-analysis. J Neuropsychiatry Clin Neurosci 2003;15:422–430.
24. Shimoda K, Robinson RG. The relationship between poststroke depression and lesion location in long-term follow-up. Biol Psychiatry 1999;45:187–192.
25. Ballard C, McKeith I, O'Brien J, et al. Neuropathological substrates of dementia and depression in vascular dementia, with a particular focus on cases with small infarct volumes. Dement Geriatr Cogn Disord 2000;11:59–65.
26. Mayberg HS, Robinson RG, Wong DF, et al. PET imaging of cortical S2 serotonin receptors after stroke: lateralized changes and relationship to depression. Am J Psychiatry 1988;145:937–943.
27. Ramasubbu R, Flint A, Brown G, Awad G, Kennedy S. Diminished serotonin-mediated prolactin responses in nondepressed stroke patients compared with healthy normal subjects. Stroke 1998;29:1293–1298.
28. Morris P, Hopwood M, Maguire K, Norman T, Schweitzer I. Blunted prolactin response to D-fenfluramine in post-stroke major depression. J Affect Disord 2003;76:273–278.
29. Starkstein SE, Fedoroff JP, Price TR, Leiguarda R, Robinson RG. Apathy following cerebrovascular lesions. Stroke 1993; 24:1625–1630.
30. Starkstein SE, Fedoroff JP, Price TR, Leiguarda R, Robinson RG. Catastrophic reaction after cerebrovascular lesions: frequency, correlates, and validation of a scale. J Neuropsychiatry Clin Neurosci 1993;5:189–194.
31. Robinson RG, Parikh RM, Lipsey JR, Starkstein SE, Price TR. Pathological laughing and crying following stroke: validation of a measurement scale and a double-blind treatment study. Am J Psychiatry 1993;150:286–293.
32. Kim JS, Choi-Kwon S. Poststroke depression and emotional incontinence. Neurology 2000;54:1805–1810.

33. Starkstein SE, Fedoroff JP, Price TR, Leiguarda R, Robinson RG. Anosognosia in patients with cerebrovascular lesions. A study of causative factors. Stroke 1992;23:1446–1453.
34. Morris PL, Shields RB, Hopwood MJ, Robinson RG, Raphael B. Are there two depressive syndromes after stroke? J Nerv Ment Dis 1994;182:230–234.
35. House A, Dennis M, Mogridge L, Warlow C, Hawton K, Jones L. Mood disorders in the year after first stroke. Br J Psychiatry 1991;158:83–92.
36. Kauhanen M, Korpelainen JT, Hiltunen P, et al. Poststroke depression correlates with cognitive impairment and neurological deficits. Stroke 1999;30:1875–1880.
37. Clark MS, Smith DS. Changes in family functioning for stroke rehabilitation patients and their families. Int J Rehabil Res 1999;22:171–179.
38. Lafgren B, Gustafson Y, Nyberg L. Psychological well-being 3 years after severe stroke. Stroke 1999;30:567–572.
39. Carod-Artal J, Egido JA, Gonzalez JL, Varela de Seijas E. Quality of life among stroke survivors evaluated 1 year after stroke: experience of a stroke unit. Stroke 2000;31:2995–3000.
40. Bosworth HB, Horner RD, Edwards LJ, Matchar DB. Depression and other determinants of values placed on current health state by stroke patients: evidence from the VA Acute Stroke (VASt) study. Stroke 2000;31:2603–2609.
41. Singh A, Black SE, Herrmann N, et al. Functional and neuroanatomic correlations in poststroke depression: the Sunnybrook Stroke Study. Stroke 2000;31:637–644.
42. Parikh RM, Lipsey JR, Robinson RG, Price TR. Two-year longitudinal study of post-stroke mood disorders: dynamic changes in correlates of depression at one and two years. Stroke 1987;18:579–584.
43. Herrmann N, Black SE, Lawrence J, Szekely C, Szalai JP. The Sunnybrook Stroke Study: a prospective study of depressive symptoms and functional outcome. Stroke 1998;29:618–624.
44. Morris PL, Raphael B, Robinson RG. Clinical depression is associated with impaired recovery from stroke. Med J Aust 1992;157:239–242.
45. Astrom M, Adolfsson R, Asplund K. Major depression in stroke patients. A 3-year longitudinal study. Stroke 1993;24:976–982.
46. Chemerinski E, Robinson RG, Arndt S, Kosier JT. The effect of remission of poststroke depression on activities of daily living in a double-blind randomized treatment study. J Nerv Ment Dis 2001;189:421–425.
47. Starkstein SE, Robinson RG, Price TR. Comparison of patients with and without poststroke major depression matched for size and location of lesion. Arch Gen Psychiatry 1988;45:247–252.
48. Bolla-Wilson K, Robinson RG, Starkstein SE, Boston J, Price TR. Lateralization of dementia of depression in stroke patients. Am J Psychiatry 1989;146:627–634.
49. Downhill JE Jr, Robinson RG. Longitudinal assessment of depression and cognitive impairment following stroke. J Nerv Ment Dis 1994;182:425–431.
50. Morris PL, Robinson RG, Andrzejewski P, Samuels J, Price TR. Association of depression with 10-year post-stroke mortality. Stroke 1993;150:124–129.
51. House A, Knapp P, Bamford J, Vail A. Mortality at 12 and 24 months after stroke may be associated with depressive symptoms at 1 month. Stroke 2001;32:696–701.
52. Lipsey JR, Robinson RG, Pearlson GD, Rao K, Price TR. Nortriptyline treatment of post-stroke depression: a double-blind study. Lancet 1984;1:297–300.
53. Andersen PS, Oster A, Johansen LK, et al. Citalopram for post-stroke pathological crying. Nucleic Acids Res 1993;21:4491–4498.
54. Robinson RG, Schultz SK, Castillo CS, et al. Nortriptyline versus fluoxetine in the treatment of depression and in short-term recovery after stroke: a placebo-controlled, double-blind study. Am J Psychiatry 2000;157:351–359.
55. Wiart L, Petit H, Joseph PA, Mazaux JM, Barat M. Fluoxetine in early poststroke depression: a double-blind placebo-controlled study. Stroke 2000;31:1829–1832.
56. Fruehwald S, Gatterbauer E, Rehak P, Baumhackl U. Early fluoxetine treatment of post-stroke depression—a three-month double-blind placebo-controlled study with an open-label long-term follow up. J Neurol 2003;250:347–351.
57. Reding MJ, Orto LA, Winter SW, Fortuna IM, Di Ponte P, McDowell FH. Antidepressant therapy after stroke. A double-blind trial. Arch Neurol 1986;43:763–765.
58. Gonzalez-Torrecillas JL, Mendlewicz J, Lobo A. Effects of early treatment of poststroke depression on neuropsychological rehabilitation. Int Psychogeriatr 1995;7:547–560.
59. Gainotti G, Antonucci G, Marra C, Paolucci S. Relation between depression after stroke, antidepressant therapy, and functional recovery. J Neurol Neurosurg Psychiatry 2001;71:258–261.
60. Narushima K, Kosier JT, Robinson RG. Preventing poststroke depression: a 12-week double-blind randomized treatment trial and 21-month follow-up. J Nerv Men Dis 2002;190:296–303.
61. Kimura M, Robinson RG, Kosier JT. Treatment of cognitive impairment after poststroke depression : a double-blind treatment trial. Stroke 2000;31:1482–1486.
62. Jorge RE, Robinson RG, Arndt S, Starkstein S. Mortality and poststroke depression: a placebo-controlled trial of antidepressants. Am J Psychiatry 2003;160:1823–1829.
63. Palomaki H, Kaste M, Berg A, et al. Prevention of poststroke depression: 1 year randomised placebo controlled double blind trial of mianserin with 6 month follow up after therapy. J Neurol Neurosurg Psychiatry 1999;66:490–494.

64. Rasmussen A, Lunde M, Poulsen DL, Sorensen K, Qvitzau S, Bech P. A double-blind, placebo-controlled study of ser-traline in the prevention of depression in stroke patients. Psychosomatics 2003;44:216–221.

65. Kneebone II, Dunmore E. Psychological management of post-stroke depression. Br J Clin Psycol 2000;39(Pt 1):53–65.

66. Lincoln NB, Flannaghan T. Cognitive behavioral psychotherapy for depression following stroke: a randomized controlled trial. Stroke 2003;34:111–115.

67. Mant J, Carter J, Wade DT, Winner S. Family support for stroke: a randomised controlled trial. Lancet 2000;356:808–813.

68. Chemerinski E, Robinson RG, Kosier JT. Improved recovery in activities of daily living associated with remission of post-stroke depression. Stroke 2001;32:113–117.

69. Morris PL, Robinson RG, Andrzejewski P, Samuels J, Price TR. Association of depression with 10-year post-stroke mortality. Am J Psychiatry 1993;150:124–129.

70. Robinson RG, Schultz SK, Castillo C, et al. Nortriptyline versus fluoxetine in the treatment of depression and in short term recovery after stroke: a placebo controlled, double-blind study. Am J Psychiatry 2000;157:351–359.

71. Narushima K, Robinson RG. The effect of early versus late antidepressant treatment on physical impairment associated with poststroke depression. Is there a time-related therapeutic window? J Nerv Ment Dis 2003;191:645–652.

72. Jorge RE, Robinson RG, Arndt S, Starkstein S. Mortality and post-stroke depression: a placebo controlled trial of anti-depressants. Am J Psychiatry 2003;160:1823–1829.

13

Neuromuscular Disorders

Jeffrey Allen Cohen and Renee Marie Vebell

INTRODUCTION

For purposes of this chapter, neuromuscular disorders can be broken into three groups. The first group is *neuropathies*, including disorders of the anterior horn cells (AHCs), for example, amyotrophic lateral sclerosis (ALS) and diabetic neuropathy. The next group is *myopathies*, for example, myotonic dystrophy. Finally, there is the *neuromuscular junction* group, for example, myasthenia gravis (MG). One usually does not consider neuromuscular disorders to have significant symptoms of psychological dysfunction, but, in the diseases that are discussed, psychiatric manifestations can be of great importance to both the patient and practitioner. The literature is in this area is sparse, with the exception of ALS and Duchenne's muscular dystrophy. The psychological manifestations of neuromuscular disorders can occur either as a direct result of the disease, for example, pseudobulbar manifestations in ALS, cognitive impairment in myotonic dystrophy, or as a secondary reaction to the illness such as depression in ALS or anxiety in MG. In this chapter, we review the major categories of neuromuscular diseases and those disorders in which the practitioner should be aware of neuropsychological factors both primary and secondary.

NEUROPATHIES

In this group, we discuss the most common form of motor neuron disease, ALS, as well as polyneuropathies such as diabetic neuropathy.

Amyotophic Lateral Sclerosis

In ALS, there are both direct effects of the illness causing psychiatric symptoms as well as secondary effects of the disease. First, we discuss the primary manifestations. ALS is a disorder of the lower motor neuron (LMN)—the AHCs and cranial nerve motor nuclei—and the upper motor neuron (UMN)—corticospinal and coticobulbar tracts). There is a progressive degeneration of these cells that results in UMN signs of spasticity weakness and pathological reflexes, and LMN signs of atrophy weakness and fasiculations. There are no significant sensory or bowel and bladder deficits. ALS can be predominately bulbar onset or limb onset. In bulbar ALS, the deficits predominately involve cranial nerve function, for example, dysarthria, dysphagia, weakness of chewing, and weakness of the facial musculature. As noted earlier there can be UMN or LMN findings in combination or a predominance of one. Pseudobulbar ALS is an example of weakness associated with only UMN signs of the cranial nerve innervated musculature (corticobulbr tracts).

From: *Current Clinical Neurology: Psychiatry for Neurologists*
Edited by: D.V. Jeste and J.H. Friedman © Humana Press Inc., Totowa, NJ

Cognition in Amyotophic Lateral Sclerosis

Cognition was thought to be preserved in ALS. Over the last decade, a number of researchers have documented cognitive impairment (CI) in ALS patients *(1,2)* using neuropsychological testing, neurophysiological recordings, and imaging studies. It should be stressed that other factors such as depression may contribute or masquerade as CI in ALS patients. The techniques used to document cognitive function may vary and interpretation of test results may not be unanimous. Despite these caveats, there are a number of investigators who feel CI is a common finding in ALS patients.

The reports of CI in ALS differ in the characterization and clinical course of CI. The onset of CI usually follows motor involvement but there is a case series where CI preceded overt motor deficits. The CI usually takes the form of a frontotemporal dementia (FTD *(3)*. ALS and FTD rarely may overlap both in familial ALS and sporadic ALS *(3)*. This frontal deficit is characterized as mild. In one study *(4)*, the CI did not significantly worsen over a 12-month observation period. In another study *(5)*, bulbar ALS patients showed greater impairment in a number of neuropsychological subtests and their CI was progressive over time. Magnetic resonance imaging (MRI) spectroscopy demonstrated a reduction of the *N*-acetylaspatate /creatine (NAA/Cr) ratio in the nondominant precentral motor strip at 6 months, having been normal at baseline. In contrast the NAA/Cr ratio obtained from the anterior cingulate at baseline was already significantly reduced in bulbar ALS patients, but not limb-onset patients. The authors concluded that bulbar-onset ALS patients with cognitive deficits and cingulate gyrus neuronal loss develop more profound neuropsychological deficits. Speech and language capabilities remained relatively preserved.

A functional MRI (fMRI) study of ALS patients was performed to better understand the pathways of CI in ALS patients *(6)* In ALS patients as compared with controls, the fMRI on a letter-fluency task and a confrontation naming task revealed impaired activation in prefrontal regions. The authors felt this study provided evidence of cerebral abnormalities in ALS patients of language and executive function networks. In addition, they stressed that both the fMRI and CI changes can be varied in ALS. A positron emission tracer scan study showed that the ALS patients with CI demonstrated impaired activation in cortical and subcortical areas *(6)*.

Event-related potentials (ERPs) have been performed in ALS patients. ALS patients with CI had abnormalities of these ERPs suggesting frontal network dysfunction *(7)*. In addition to these studies involving neuropsychological, imaging, and neurophysiological testing pathological and biochemical studies have been undertaken to ascertain the cause of CI in ALS patients.

Yang et al. *(8)* studied τ-protein metabolism in the brain tissue of ALS patents. They found that τ immunoreactive astrocytic and dense neuronal inclusions were found in CI and non-CI groups but they were found to a greater extent in the CI group. Superficial linear spongiosis and aggregates immunoreactive with specific markers (τ-1 and AT-8) were unique to CI ALS. These investigators feel that CI in ALS may be related to abnormal τ metabolism. Wilson et al. *(9)* examined the brains of ALS CI patients vs non-CI patients for the presence of ubiquittin-immunoereactive intraneuronal (Ub+) inclusions as a marker for CI. The Ub+ inclusions were found both in CI and non CI ALS patients but the presence of CI was associated with a greater distribution and load of neuropathological features both Ub+ inclusions and dystrophic neurites. In addition, CI was associated with superficial linear spongiosis suggesting that cognitive impairment in ALS patients shares a pathological feature common in FTD. Finally, it should be stressed that the cognitive changes noted in ALS may also be the result of hypoxemia, medication, and nutritional effects. Depression may also contribute to the perception of dementia. There are no good data examining the role of medications used in Alzheimer's disease to reverse or stabilize the CI in ALS patients.

Pseudobulbar

Pseudobular ALS is a specific condition that occurs in ALS when corticobulbar tract involvement is present. The patient usually has some degree of facial weakness, difficultly swallowing, dysarthric speech, exaggerated jaw jerk, and pathological crying and laughing (PLC). It is believed that PLC is related to abnormalities in the frontal-subcortical circuits, but the etiology of this disorder is unclear. McCullagh *(10)* performed a number of psychometric tests on ALS patients with and without PLC. He felt that testing abnormalities, particularly the Wisconsin Card Sorting test, suggested functional impairment of the prefrontal cortex. PLC has been associated with affective emotions by some, others feel it is devoid of such feelings. In clinical practice, we have heard ALS patients describe both situations. PLC can be successfully treated with various antidepressants including tricyclics (TCAs) and selective serotonin reuptake inhibitors (SSRIs). There are case reports of PLC being transformed to only pathological laughing, suggesting that there may be an underlying depression that is helped by treatment *(10)*. An added benefit of TCA therapy is decreasing salivary secretions and improving the silarrhea.

Depression

Depression is a common accompaniment of ALS, although some investigators doubt an increase in the frequency and severity of depression, as compared with either control groups or other patients with chronic illnesses. There are a number of studies examining the relationship among psychosocial factors, motor impairment, and depression in ALS patients.

These data are conflicting, but a number of generalizations can be made. Patients with more impaired physical function are more likely to suffer significant depression. Religiosity or spirituality may help to mitigate depression in ALS *(11)*. A rapid course of physical loss of function is related to worsening depression in ALS *(12–14)*. In our ALS clinic we have collected pilot data that confirms significant depression is common in ALS. We, like others, have found that sleep disturbances are also common in ALS. Depression in ALS can be treated using any of a number of medications; usually we use antidepressants with anti-cholinergic effects.

Sleep

ALS can be associated with significant disturbances of sleep. This may be as a result of muscle cramps, immobility, depression, and actual obstructive sleep apnea (OSA *[15]*). OSA can be caused by weakness of the palatal muscles, tongue, and neck musculature. Obviously, weakness of the diaphragm and other respiratory muscles may add to this problem. The sleep disturbances can further exacerbate the motor weakness, CI, and depression. We feel it is important to consider overnight sleep studies in ALS patients when sleep abnormalities or incipient respiratory insufficiency is suspected. A change in alertness, daytime sleepiness, or subtle CI may be a clue. It is important to realize that nocturnal respiratory insufficiency may occur with no symptoms during the day. Nocturnal hypoventilation may be very insidious treatment with either bilevel positive airway pressure or continuous positive airway pressure (CPAP) can greatly improve the patient's functional status.

Palliative Care in Amyotophic Lateral Sclerosis

With no curative treatment, palliative care is an essential issue in the care of patients with ALS. As most studies demonstrate, death is usually 2–5 years after the onset of symptoms, with 50% of patients dying within 3 years *(16)*. Providing patients and their family members with palliative assistance that includes physical, psychological, social, and spiritual needs at the time of diagnosis will help to support quality of life. Using a multidisciplinary team approach with patient care to assist in the management and anticipation of problems and symptoms can improve patient coping skills and allow the patient to die peacefully.

The multidisciplinary team includes the neurologist, physiatrist, pulmonary therapist, support groups, home health service/hospice, nurse, occupational and physical therapists, speech and respiratory therapists, psychiatrist/psychologist, social worker, and dietitian. This comprehensive approach can meet the challenging needs of the ALS patient and family, without omitting or duplicating the issues that need addressing.

Physical therapy provides exercise education and adaptive equipment to promote the patient's independence and safety. Early education can work to improve endurance, decrease fatigue, and improve muscle tone. This may also impact feelings of depression. As the disease progresses, range of motion and stretching exercises may help to prevent contractures. Suggestions on needed equipment (e.g., a wheelchair) may take time to accept when taking into consideration the psychological readiness of the patient and the family.

As the muscle weakness and fatigue progresses, occupational therapy assists with recommending devices that promote independence in activities of daily living. Built-up eating utensils or the use of a shower chair can maximize a patient's independence and self-worth. The patient may need resting hand splints to be made. Teaching about energy conservation may minimize the feelings of fatigue and helplessness.

Dysphagia and dysarthria problems can be addressed by a speech therapist. Speech therapists educate patients and families about proper positioning when eating and breathing techniques to help vocal volume and articulation. As the disease progresses, assistance with communication devices such as communication boards, writing pads, and voice amplifiers can help the patient and the family with this important need. Adjusting to these changes can be very stressful on the family and caregivers and emotional support is often indicated.

As respiratory complications are the most common cause of death, a respiratory therapist can help to monitor the forced vital capacity. A discussion of assistive breathing devices may be indicated as the forced vital capacity decreases or symptoms develop of nocturnal hypercarbia. The earlier these discussions begin, the more time the patient and family have to explore their options.

A dietitian can intervene with the problems associated with dysphagia and the potential for weight loss. Modifying the diet initially to five to six smaller meals per day and avoiding thin fluids that swallow rapidly, may be of help. Other foods that are difficult to swallow such as tough meat, lettuce, and thick-crust breads may need to be avoided. As the disease progresses, it becomes challenging to avoid dehydration and malnutrition. Sauces and liquid thickeners may be indicated. The dietitian can educate the family about meal preparations that may appeal to the patient's challenging needs.

The mental health team meets the needs of both the patient and the family members. Many different emotions are experienced at different stages of the illness. The support and guidance must be individualized for each person involved. The rate of the disease progression also impacts coping skills. Fears of the increasing disabilities often need to be addressed. The frustrations with the loss of independence, dependency on others, loneliness, isolation from the loss of employment, and fear of dying are all very real concerns that need time and support to grieve and explore these feelings.

The nurse will assess ailments and educate about issues associated with constipation, skin integrity problems, pain from immobility, coping skills, nutritional issues, and need for home health care. Educating the family on medication management, emergency measures such as suctioning and performing a Heimlich maneuver, or care of a percutaneous endoscopic gastrostomy tube may be indicated.

Home health services or a hospice team can integrate the ongoing efforts by the outpatient ALS team. They can facilitate the equipment modifications in the home. They can anticipate the patient's changing needs with diet, communication, pain issues, loss of independence, and safety challenges. Additional support may be indicated for the issues of depression, loneliness, fear, and hopelessness. Working with the family in the comfort and safety of their home may promote positive coping skills.

Terminal Care in Amyotophic Lateral Sclerosis

As the disease progresses, most patients experience a gradual decline, followed by a period of rapid change, often after a respiratory tract infection or a silent aspiration. With the support from the palliative care team of the home health services or from the hospice team, the patient can pass away peacefully with symptom management. It may be important for the family to hear that choking to death is very rare. In addition, patients not on a ventilator often progress into a drowsy then sleep state, then slip into a coma *(17)*.

Symptom management is critical for the patient and family to be able to have the time and energy to grieve the impending death. Most patients with ALS want to remain at home. The hospice team can educate the family and caregivers on the physical aspects of the care, including safe and proper use of analgesics for pain, morphine for dyspnea, anticholinergic medications for drooling and excessive chest secretions, antianxiety medications, skin care, bowel and bladder care, and moving the immobile patient.

In order to support the patient and family on the psychosocial aspects of the dying process, a trusting relationship is needed—one that has ideally developed over time. Increased emotional support and guidance, especially during the periods of rapid decline, may be necessary. Considering the multiple losses the patients face, death may come as a relief. The guilt the families may experience can be supported with bereavement services from hospice programs.

As noted, this is a very difficult topic without a clear strategy for each individual. Caution should be exercised in making blanket assumptions about individual patients. We have seen patients continue to change their decisions throughout the course of their illness.

Quality of Life Scales

A number of scales have been used in ALS as well as other neuromuscular disorders these scales can be used to monitor treatment intervention in ALS as well as to better understand the clinical course of illness *(18,19)*.

Post Polio Syndrome

This syndrome can be defined according to criteria proposed by Dalakas *(20)* and others. Post polio syndrome (PPS) is the development of new neuromuscular symptoms in patients who have suffered an acute attack of paralytic poliomyelitis. PPS is a clinical diagnosis. The following are considered in the diagnosis: (a) history of an acute febrile illness in childhood or adolescence during a polio epidemic and functional stability or recovery for at least 15 years, (b) residual muscle atrophy weakness and areflexia in at last one limb, (c) development of new neuromuscular symptoms or musculoskeletal complaints, and (d) exclusion of other causes that could explain the symptoms. Neuropsychological testing gives mixed results, but a subgroup of PPS may demonstrate stress and anxiety *(20)*. Most PPS patients report no psychopathological symptoms. There is no apparent relationship between psychopathological symptoms and the degree of motor disability *(21)*. There are very few studies that have examined cognition in PPS patients. A patient survey suggested widespread complaints in concentration *(20)*. Objective studies have not clearly confirmed these complaints. Investigators have tried to link recticular activating system and hypothalmaic pathology as the result of prior polio infection to decreased arousal and fatigue *(21)*. Despite the lack of confirming studies, we feel depression may be an accompaniment of PPS. This can be difficult because there is an overlap of the symptoms of both depression and PPS, such as sleep disturbances, fatigue, and weakness. Sleep disturbances resulting from nocturnal weakness of the palate, tongue and neck musculature can occur similar to ALS. This may cause an OSA *(21)*. Sleep studies and the use of CPAP may be helpful. Treatment of depression can be rewarding for both the patient and physician.

Guillian Barré Syndrome

Guillian Barré syndrome (GBS) is an autoimmune disorder that causes demyelination of the roots and peripheral nerves. As a result of this demyelination, patients suffer acute predominately motor weakness that may result in quadraparesis and respiratory problems. Patients may be ventilator-dependent for a prolonged period of time. Chewing and swallowing might also be impaired. Significant depression can occur as a result of these disabilities. It is important to realize that a relatively complete recovery may occur despite significant initial disability. Severe depression can occur because of the rapid onset of severe weakness and respiratory failure. The recovery may be quite prolonged and there may be months of skilled nursing care. Support, reassurance, and the use of antidepressant medications may be necessary (22). The recovery of GBS is usually maximally achieved at 2 years.

Mercury Intoxication

Mercury poisoning by accidental or deliberate means can cause a central nervous effects. CI, severe tremor, and behavioral problems can occur; the term "mad as hatter" is taken from the poisoning of workers in the felt hat-making industry. This was a result of inorganic mercury in the form of mercury salts *(23)*.

Porphyria

Porphyria is a disorder caused by the defective synthesis of heme. Neuropathy is associated with only abnormalities of liver heme metabolism—acute intermittent porphyria, hereditary coproporphhyria, and variegate porphyria. The neuropsychiatric manifestations may include restlessness, agitation, and nightmares. This may progress to psychosis with delirium, hallucinations, coma, and seizures. The disorder is usually triggered by the ingestion of certain medications as well as stress. The behavioral disturbances in porphyria are usually not specifically addressed; treatment is directed toward the avoidance of provoking medications and stress (starvation and dehydration) *(24)*.

Diabetic Neuropathy

There are a number of studies examining the association of depression and painful diabetic neuropathy *(25–27)*. The range of depression in diabetic patients is 8–27%. In some studies there is a higher rate of depression in patients with painful diabetic neuropathy; others have dismissed this link. There appears not to be a clear relationship between the pain of diabetic neuropathy and depression. Despite the clear link between diabetic neuropathy and depression, antidepressants appear to be helpful for improving pain *(26,27)*. The TCAs had success in double-blind studies. In one study, imipramine had an 81% response rate in decreasing pain (26). There are also studies pointing to the efficacy of paroxetine, citlopram, seratline, and duloxetine.

NEUROMUSCULAR JUNCTION

Myasthenia Gravis

MG is an autoimmune disorder that is usually bimodal in age distribution among young women and older men. The disorder is associated with antibodies directed against the acetylcholine (Ach) receptors on the striated muscle endplate region. MG is characterized by weakness that usually worsens as the day goes on—fatigable weakness. As in most autoimmune disorders, the disease process can improve or worsen independent of any specific factors, but it is clear that psychological stressors may be related to exacerbations of MG. There are a number of studies that relate stress to exacerbations of MG *(28)*. As the result of the judicious use of newer immunological treatments over last 10 years, severe exacerbations of MG are much less common.

Despite reports of a specific personality type in individuals with MG, there are no data to support this. There are a number of reports that suggest a stressful life event occurring just prior to the appearance of MG *(28,29)*. A common factor appears to be the association of anger and clinical worsening of MG. Men seem to be most concerned with the dysarthria associated with MG, whereas women are most concerned about facial weakness and expression *(28)*. A reported association of left-handedness and MG has been posed but not proven.

In addition, some researchers have stressed MG patients can have CI caused by abnormalities of Ach transmission within the central nervous system. Researchers have critiqued the studies reporting CI in MG and found them lacking in rigor because of confounding factors such as medications, depression, anxiety, and measurement tools. In more highly controlled studies of cognition in MG, significant deficits have not been found. The younger MG patient may find the stress of unpredictable weakness very difficult to accept *(30,31)*. As a result pervasive anxiety, a lack of regular medical follow-up, and the lack of medication adherence, these patients may be difficult to manage. The older myasthenic patient is usually less problematic. We rarely see psychotic behavior in MG patients.

Many in the field have had the experience of dealing a pseudomyasthenia syndrome. These patients are usually 30- to 40-year-old women and most commonly present with fatigue as the primary MG symptom. Other symptoms such as dysarthria, dysphagia, extremity weakness, visual blurring, and diplopia may be common. These patients have negative serology and negative repetitive stimulation and normal single electromyelogram fiber studies. Care should be taken when performing the tensilon test to use an unequivocal objective deficit. These could include ptosis, eye-movement weakness, and dysarthria. It should be cautioned that even these symptoms may not be objective and can be faked. One should never use a tensilon test when the only change being monitored is an increase in strength or an improvement in fatigue. These pseudomyasthenia patients may "respond" to therapy including intravenous immunoglobulin, plasma exchange, immunosuppression, steroids, and mestinon.

Steroid use in MG may also have side effects such as mania, depression, sleep disturbance, and depression. It is important, therefore, to use the lowest possible dosage. Alternate-day therapy may decrease these side effects. The use of immunosuppressant therapy in order to lessen the need of long-term steroid usage is common.

MYOPATHY

Duchenne Muscular Dystrophy

CI occurs in conjunction with muscular dystrophy, as recognized and described by Duchene, and was subsequently categorized as Duchene Muscular Dystrophy (DMD) *(31)*. Standardized measures of intelligence, such as the Wechsler Intelligence Scale and the Stanford Binet report full-scale IQs of approx 83, with ranges from the 40s to greater than 120. On average, the IQ among persons with DMD is approx 1 standard deviation (15 points) below the normative mean of 100 *(32)*. Recent studies have reported similar results.

In examining specific patterns of CI in DMD, results suggest that verbal IQ is more impaired than performance IQ. Significant decrement of performance IQ occurs later in the course of DMD. Studies to understand the cause of CI have yielded conflicting results. Factors that seem to affect CI most likely include socioeconomic level, as well as genetic factors based on affected siblings; there is no relationship between physical functioning and CI. In addition, there are no specific neuropathological abnormalities underlying the CI. Computed tomography, MRI, positron emission tomography, and magnetic resonance spectroscopy have yielded no consistent results. The actual time course and progression of CI is unknown *(32)*.

Myotonic Dystrophy

Like DMD, myotonic dystrophy (MD) is associated with CI. Congenital MD results in a more significant IQ decrement *(32)*. These individuals are more likely to be in the mentally retarded range. Psychometric studies report mean full-scale IQs in the range of 86.8 for congenital MD and 92.1 for noncongenital MD. Maternal inheritance results in lower full-scale IQ than paternal inherited MD. The IQ differences in various series may be greater than a 20-point decrement for maternally inherited MD *(32)*.

Studies that have attempted to characterize the specific cognitive changes in MD have yielded conflicting results. Studies that have assessed CI impairment over time have not documented progressive deterioration. Researchers have not found a clear correlation between motor function and CI. Earlier age of onset (excluding congenital MD) may be linked to greater instance of CI. Some investigators have suggested females are more cognitively impaired than males, but this is also unclear *(32)*.

Imaging studies demonstrate white matter lesions in MD patients and these may be associated with CI. The actual brain volume studies are conflicting. There is data suggesting that both studies of cognitive potentials and cerebral blood flow measures may be related to CI *(32)*.

Palliative Care in Muscular Dystrophy

Helping the patient with MD and their family to consider the difficult transition to palliative care services may be challenging. As DMD is the most common of the muscular dystrophies, it is addressed here. Several factors contribute to the challenging nature of this transition.

To start, a death that usually occurs late in adolescence is painful for both the family and the health professionals. During the course of the disease, many families develop encouraging attitudes to cope with physical dysfunction, in order to work toward living as long as possible. It is common for the child, the family, and the caregivers to be optimistic and avoid pessimistic thinking. With this in mind, when increased assistance is needed with mobilization, ventilation, and/or equipment, the physical and emotional burden of this care may become evident. As a result, early referrals to palliative care services may not be productive. On average, these services provide support for only 3–4 months *(33)*. If the family resists a palliative care referral, they may be minimally prepared when death is imminent.

The positive attitude and subsequent denial of the reality of the eventual death of the child with DMD is a common coping mechanism. Health professionals need to educate families so that they are knowledgeable of available services. The goal is to have these services in place, with the support staff already in the home setting, so that when terminal care is needed, coping skills are in place.

Another challenge is to help the family develop positive coping skills with regard to allowing the child to die at home. One study found that families have a healthier grief response when the patient with DMD died in the home environment *(32)*. Families need to learn how to access medical care for exacerbations of respiratory infections and not depend on emergency hospital care. Developing confidence in these skills will help the family to provide terminal care at home.

Utilizing palliative care services from a home care service will foster a relationship with a nurse manager. This nurse will coordinate services needed in the home, such as equipment to promote home safety, referrals for counseling services, and education of the skills needed to keep the patient in the home setting. The family can develop a trusting relationship with the nurse and learn to develop the skills to manage through successive respiratory crises.

Early referrals to palliative care services offer support not only to the family members who provide the care, but rather to the whole family. The stress of the gradually increasing physical and emotional burden of care also affects the siblings. Providing support to all members of the family will ultimately help the family unit cope with the dying process.

Terminal Care in Muscular Dystrophy

Managing the terminal stages of a patient with DMD may be problematic in meeting the psychosocial needs of the patient and the family members. Transitioning the family from helping the patient survive this debilitating and progressive illness to facing the end-of-life decisions is challenging. Ideally, the family can use skills developed from palliative care services to cope with the end-of-life issues and grieving process.

As discussed earlier, the setting of the terminal care is very important. The stress and dehumanization of a hospital setting may make it very difficult for the patient and the family to cope with the dying process. If the patient is in a home setting, maximizing the support systems, both the palliative care services and family/friend supports can promote healthy coping skills. Often times, the palliative care services can transition into hospice services, without a change in personnel.

Patient and family discussions need to address the issue of assisted ventilation. Survival levels have not been found to prolong life expectancy with preventative ventilation *(33)*. It is strongly suggested to begin these sensitive discussions early, before hypoxia and dyspnea affect level of consciousness. The patient and the family need reassurances that professional support is available, and decisions may change. Families need to know that hospice services focus on care, not cure. A natural and comfortable death is possible, often assisted with small doses of opioids to ease respiratory distress.

The bereavement support that the family receives from palliative care services will help the family grieve the child's death. There may be a large void in the family's life after the full-time physical and emotional responsibilities have ceased. This grief needs professional support over time, so that each family member may cope with this significant loss.

CONCLUSION

Neuromuscular disorders can exhibit significant symptoms of psychological dysfunction. Disorders of the peripheral nerves, muscles, and neuromuscular junction may all have significant psychological aspects. This may be the result of primary or secondary effects of the illness. Despite the lack of familiarity and paucity of literature in this area, the practitioner must anticipate and recognize these psychological symptoms that can often worsen the course of illness. This recognition can greatly help both the patient and the practitioner.

REFERENCES

1. Cavalleri F, De Renzi E. Amyotrophic lateral sclerosis with dementia. Acta Neurol Scand 1994;89:391–394.
2. Iwasaki Y, Kinoshita M, Ikeda K, Takamiya K, Shiojima T. Cognitive impairment in amyotrophic lateral sclerosis and its relation to motor disabilities. Acta Neurol Scand 1990;81:141–143.
3. Lomen-Hoerth C. Characterization of amyotrophic lateral sclerosis and frontotemporal dementia. Dement Geriatr Cogn Disord 2004;17:337–341.
4. Kilani M, Micallef J, Soubrouillard C, et al. A longitudinal study of the evolution of cognitive function and affective state in patients with amyotrophic lateral sclerosis. Amyotroph Lateral Scler Other Motor Neuron Disord 2004;5:46–54.
5. Strong MJ, Grace GM, Orange JB, Leeper HA, Menon RS, Aere C. A prospective study of cognitive impairment in ALS. Neurology 1999;53:1665–1670.
6. Abrahams S, Goldstein LH, Simmons A, et al. Word retrieval in amyotrophic lateral sclerosis: a functional magnetic resonance imaging study. Brain 2004;127:1507–1517.7.
7. Hanagasi HA, Gurvit IH, Ermutlu N, et al. Cognitive impairment in amyotrophic lateral sclerosis: evidence from neuropsychological investigation and event-related potentials Brain Res Cogn Brain Res 2002;14:234–244.
8. Yang W, Sopper MM, Leystra-Lantz C, Strong MJ. Microtubule-associated tau protein positive neuronal and glial inclusions in ALS. Neurology 2003;61:1766–1773.
9. Wilson CM, Grace GM, Munoz DG, He BP, Strong MJ. Cognitive impairment in sporadic ALS: a pathologic continuum underlying a multisystem disorder. Neurology 2001;57:651–657.
10. McCullagh S, Moore M, Gawel M, Feinstein A. Pathological laughing and crying in amyotrophic lateral sclerosis: an association with prefrontal cognitive dysfunction. J Neurol Sci 1999;169:43–48.
11. Walsh SM, Bremer BA, Felgoise SH, Simmons Z. Religiousness is related to quality of life in patients with ALS. Neurology 2003;60:1527–1529.
12. Trial M, Nelson ND, Van JN, Appel SH, Lai EC. A study comparing patients with amyotrophic lateral sclerosis and their caregivers on measures of quality of life, depression, and their attitudes toward treatment options. J Neurol Sci 2003;209:79–85.
13. Lou JS, Reeves A, Benice T, Sexton G. Fatigue and depression are associated with poor quality of life in ALS. Neurology 2003;60:122–123.
14. Simmons Z, Bremer BA, Robbins RA, Walsh SM, Fischer S. Quality of life in ALS depends on factors other than strength and physical function. Neurology 2000;55:388–392.
15. Hetta J, Jansson I. Sleep in patients with amyotrophic lateral sclerosis. J Neurol 1997;244:S7–S9.
16. Jackson CE, Bryan WW. Amyotrophic lateral sclerosis. Semin Neurol 1998;18:27–39.
17. Oliver D, Borasio GD. Diseases of the motor nerves. In: Voltz R, Bernat JL, Borasio GD, Maddocks I, Oliver D, Portenoy RK, eds. Palliative Care in Neurology. New York: Oxford University Press; 2004, 79–89.
18. Bromberg MB, Forshew DA. Comparison of instruments addressing quality of life in patients with ALS and their caregivers. Neurology 2002;58:320–322.
19. Swash M. Health outcome and quality of life measurements in amyotrophic lateral sclerosis. J Neurol 1997;244:S26–S29.
20. Grafman J, Clark K, Richardson D, Dinsmore S, Stein D, Dalakas M. Neuropsychology of post-polio syndrome. Ann NY Acad Sci 1995;753:103–110.
21. Modlin JF, Coffey DJ. Poliomyelitis, polio vaccines, and the postpoliomyelitis syndrome. In: Scheld WM, Whitley RJ, Marra C, eds. Infections of the Central Nervous System, Third Edition. Philadelphia: Lippincott Williams and Wilkins; 2004:101–104.
22. Gregory RJ. Recovery from depression associated with Guillain Barre syndrome. Issues Ment Health Nurs 2003;24:129–135.
23. Windebank AJ. Metal neuropathy. In: Dyck PJ, Thomas PK, eds. Peripheral Neuropathy, Third Edition. Philadelphia: WB Saunders; 1993:150–156.

24. Windebank AJ, Bonkovsky HL. Porphyric neuropathy. In: Dyck PJ, Thomas PK, eds. Peripheral Neuropathy, Third Edition. Philadephia: WB Saunders; 1993:1161–1168.
25. de Groot M, Anderson R, Freedland KE, Clouse RE, Lustman PJ. Association of depression and diabetes complications: a meta-analysis. Psychosom Med 2001;63:619–630.
26. Goodnick PJ. Use of antidepressants in treatment of comorbid diabetes mellitus and depression as well as in diabetic neuropathy. Ann Clin Psychiatry 2001;13:31–41.
27. Max MB, Lynch SA, Muir J, Shoaf SE, Smoller B, Dubner R. Effects of desipramine, amitriptyline, and fluoxetine on pain in diabetic neuropathy. N Engl J Med 1992;329:1250–1256.
28. Sneddon J. Myasthenia gravis: a study of social, medical, and emotional problems in 26 patients. Lancet 1980;1:526–528.
29. Doering S, Henze T, Schussler G. Coping with myasthenia gravis and implications for psychotherapy. Arch Neurol 1993; 50:617–620.
30. Paul RH, Cohen RA, Zawacki T, Gilchrist JM, Aloia MS. What have we learned about cognition in myasthenia gravis?: A review of methods and results. Neurosci Biobehav Rew 2001;25:75–81.
31. Paul RH, Cohen RA, Gilchrist JM. Ratings of subjective mental fatigue relate to cognitive performance in patients with myasthenia gravis. J Clin Neurosci 2002;9:243–246.
32. Sigford BJ, Lanham RA. Cognitive, psychosocial, and educational issues in neuromuscular disease. Phys Med Rehabil Clin N Am 1998;9:249–270.
33. Maddocks I, Stern L. Muscular dystrophy and related myopathies. In: Voltz R, Bernat JL, Borasio GD, Maddocks I, Oliver D, Portenoy RK, eds. Palliative Care in Neurology. New York: Oxford University Press; 2004:90–96.

14

Psychiatric Aspects of Parkinson's Disease

Laura Marsh and Joseph H. Friedman

INTRODUCTION

Parkinson's disease (PD) has a special place in neuropsychiatry. Along with progressive supranuclear palsy (PSP), it has been a paradigm for "subcortical" cognitive dysfunction, including dementia, as well as a model for affective disturbances occurring as an intrinsic part of the degenerative process. Although defined clinically by its motor features, PD is clearly a neurobehavioral syndrome, with 90% of patients affected by neuropsychiatric disturbances at some point during the course of the disease (1). Furthermore, psychopathology in PD constitutes a greater stress for caregivers than motor dysfunction, with dementia and psychosis the most devastating and important precipitants of nursing home placement.

GENERAL APPROACH TO THE PATIENT

Management of psychiatric disturbances in PD patients requires familiarity with the overlap and interplay of the motor, cognitive, and psychiatric aspects of PD, especially the effects of medications on mental state (2). An etiological classification scheme (Table 1) categorizes the described phenomena as either primary and inherent to the disease process or secondary to some primary aspect of the disease or its treatment. For example, dementia is a primary process, whereas excessive daytime somnolence may result from nocturia related to PD-induced bladder spasticity, hence a secondary problem; psychosis and disinhibited behaviors are iatrogenically related to anti-parkinsonian medications. The specificity of PD-related pathology as primary or secondary can be debated. However, an advantage of this approach is that it focuses on identification and interrelations of potential causes of specific psychiatric phenomena and determining which are most salient and modifiable.

DEPRESSION

Epidemiology and Phenomenology

Depressive disorders are common in PD, but reported rates vary according to the population sampled and how cases are defined (3). On average, prevalence rates for syndromic depression are 40–50%. In most studies, up to half of cases have major depressive disorders, but the majority of patients have non-major depressive syndromes that include minor depression, dysthymia, and subsyndromal depression.

From: *Current Clinical Neurology: Psychiatry for Neurologists*
Edited by: D.V. Jeste and J.H. Friedman © Humana Press Inc., Totowa, NJ

Table 1
Neuropsychiatric Disturbances in Parkinson's Disease:
Etiological Classification

Primary	Secondary
Selective cognitive deficits	Psychosis
Executive dysfunction	Hallucinations
Dementia	Delusions
Delirium	Vivid dreams
Depression[a]	Depression[a]
Apathy	Mania/depression[b]
Anxiety	
Fatigue	Fatigue
Akathisia	Hypersexuality
Sleep disorders	L-dopa abuse
REM sleep behavior disorder	Impulsive–compulsive behaviors[a]
Fragmented sleep	
Excessive daytime somnolence	
Sleep apnea (obstructive)	
Impulsive and compulsive behaviors[a]	

[a]Some disturbances may be intrinsic to the pathology, secondary to effects of treatments and/or the impact of the disease, or a combination of these factors.

[b]Mania or depression may occur in the context of "on–off" motor fluctuations (i.e., non-motor fluctuations or following deep brain stimulation, particularly in the region of the subthalamic nucleus). REM, rapid eye movement.

Signs and Symptoms

The core features of depressive disorders are the presence of a persistent and pervasive depressed or low mood and/or a decreased ability to enjoy activities that would ordinarily be enjoyed (anhedonia) and/or a decline in interest level from their usual baseline. Motor symptoms may limit pursuit of previous interests, but the depressed patient fails to find alternatives or respond to pleasurable events when they do occur. Anxiety symptoms and co-morbid anxiety syndromes, such as panic disorder, are especially common in PD-related depression. Other symptoms include indecisiveness, fatigue, poor concentration, morbid thoughts including thoughts of one's own death, emotional lability, and feelings of worthless or guilt. Some studies suggest that self-blame, a negative self-attitude, delusions, self-destructive thoughts, and anhedonia are less evident. Nonetheless, they can be present, but suicide is rare. Other psychological, vegetative, and autonomic symptoms of depression are common. Early morning awakening, anergia, and mental slowing occur at comparable rates in nondepressed PD samples.

Etiopathological Factors

A relationship between depression and structural pathology is supported by the occurrence of depressive disorders early in the disease course, even pre-dating motor symptoms. Furthermore, degenerative changes of the serotonin, norepinephrine, and dopamine neurotransmitter systems are associated with depression and effective medications influence these neurotransmitters. Functional imaging studies suggest hypometabolism of basal ganglia-frontal circuits. In general, family history of depression is not associated with development of depressive disturbances in PD. Psychological reactions can also influence the development of a persistent and pervasive depressive disorder, especially later in the disease.

Diagnosis

Direct and careful inquiry is critical for recognizing depressive disorders. Depressive disorders should be suspected when self-reported disability exceeds evidence on the examination. Patients or clinicians may resist exploration of the potential diagnosis of depression because of fears about the implications of a psychiatric diagnosis, but an unacknowledged and untreated psychiatric disturbance is ultimately more problematic.

The core symptoms of depression (low or depressed mood, anhedonia, and diminished interests) and the other nonsomatic features of depression (e.g., excessive pessimism and negative ruminations, tearfulness, hopelessness, and guilt) are important for distinguishing depressed from nondepressed PD patients. Most somatic symptoms, except for late insomnia and reduced appetite, have little sensitivity for depressive disorders *(4)*.

Many people think that mood disorders result from a lack of coping skills but the opposite actually occurs. With PD (or any chronic illness), successful coping and adaptation is virtually impossible in the face of an untreated mood disorder. Once the depressive disorder is treated, the person is better able to compensate and face the challenges associated with PD. In fact, such changes may be signs that the mood disorder is responding to treatment.

Differential Diagnosis

The differential diagnosis of depressive disorders includes normal states of grief or demoralization, interpersonal difficulties, major mood disorders (major depression, dysthymia, or bipolar disorder), adjustment disorders, anxiety syndromes, drug-induced or fluctuating mood states that correspond to "on-off" anti-parkinsonian medication effects, pathological tearfulness (also called emotionalism), dementia, apathetic states, psychosis, delirium, and thyroid disease. It is critical to distinguish whether a patient has more than one disturbance (e.g., major depression, cognitive impairment, and drug-induced mood changes).

Depressed mood states may represent a normal psychological reaction rather than a pervasive mood disorder. There is a risk for over diagnosis of depressive disorders because the term *depression* is used commonly to refer to a variety of mood states, including anger, apathy, low mood, grief, demoralization, disgust, fatigue, frustration, embarrassment, anxiety, and fearfulness.

Shared clinical features between depression and PD also increase the risk of over diagnosis of depressive disorders. Overlapping features include slowness (psychomotor retardation), hypomimia (restricted affect), hunched posture, cognitive impairment, sleep, appetite, fatigue, and impaired initiation (apathy) *(5)*. Conversely, underdiagnosis is also a problem because motor symptoms can mask depressive phenomena, clinicians may be inattentive to psychiatric disturbances, or the advanced age or the presence of PD leads individuals to "explain away" depressive disorders as "understandable" reactions.

Course and Prognosis of Depression

Little definitive information is known on the course of depressive disorders in PD *(3)*. If left untreated, depression in PD is associated with excess cognitive and motor dysfunction, accelerated disability, greater caregiver distress, economic strain, and worse quality of life. Nonmajor forms of depression often progress to major depression if untreated. There are no consistent relationships between depression onset and severity to age onset or duration of PD, motor severity, or disease stage or subtype. Patients with very mild symptoms of PD can have profound and disabling depressive disorders that have greater impact than their motor dysfunction.

Treatment

Promotion of self-management is one important component of treating patients with chronic diseases *(2)*. Accordingly, education, exercise, healthy emotional activities, pacing daily activities, avoiding sleep deprivation, and maintaining a positive attitude are very important ways to reduce stress and ward off development of more persistent depressed moods. Psychotherapy may help gain perspectives and maintain behaviors that promote well-being. "Watchful waiting" with follow-up in 2–3 weeks and encouragement of problem-solving strategies is appropriate if life stressors appear to be the prevailing problem. Occupational, physical, and speech therapies, home care programs, and social workers can be helpful in this regard. Psychiatric referral is indicated when there is diagnostic uncertainty, if the patient does not respond to initially prescribed treatments, if more time is needed to provide care than is feasible in an outpatient neurology practice, or when there are concerns about suicidality or other self-destructive behaviors.

Antidepressant medications are indicated when depressive disorders persist and contribute to significant distress and dysfunction *(2)*. The selective serotonin reuptake inhibitors (SSRIs; e.g., sertraline, escitalopram) and serotonin-norepinephrine reuptake inhibitors (SNRIs; e.g., nortriptyline, venlafaxine) are most commonly used, but there is no evidence that one compound is more effective when the patient undergoes a full course of therapy. Thus, antidepressant choices are based on drug side-effect profiles. The goal of treatment should be remission of depressive phenomena. Careful follow-up of the antidepressant response is critical because many patients are undertreated. Side effects such as weight gain and sexual dysfunction are common with the SSRIs and affect compliance. Low-dose trazodone (25–50 mg starting dose) often helps insomnia and can be tapered as the depressive disturbance resolves.

Electroconvulsive therapy (ECT) is effective for PD-depression and indicated for severe depressive disorders, especially when there is a need for a rapid response. Usually, this is when patients have depression-related psychosis or severe vegetative symptoms. Inability to tolerate standard antidepressants and failure to respond to antidepressants are also indications. ECT often improves motor function for periods lasting from hours to several weeks.

ANXIETY DISORDERS

Epidemiology

Pathological anxiety is a common and important problem in PD, but has received less attention compared with depression *(6)*. Anxiety syndromes appear in up to 40% of patients, affecting men and women equally. Particularly common are generalized anxiety disorder (GAD), social phobia, and panic disorder, which have prevalence rates of 25% in some series. Anxiety disorders and heightened anxiety can be features of depressive disorders, but they also tend to be chronic, whereas depressive disorders are more often episodic. Anxiety can be associated with fluctuations in levodopa levels, although there is not always a strict temporal relationship between anxiety and motor "off" states. Some patients have disabling mood fluctuations characterized by severe and intractable anxiety and panic.

Signs and Symptoms

Akinesia and bradykinesia may provoke anxious reactions in the course of living with PD, but anxiety disorders are distinguished by the stereotyped and persistent nature of the anxiety phenomena. In general, anxiety disorders in PD resemble those of idiopathic anxiety disorders. Affected patients who fail to meet discrete Diagnostic and Statistical Manual of Mental Disorders, Fourth Edition (DSM-IV) syndromic criteria are regarded as having anxiety disorder, not otherwise specified. Panic attacks involve the sudden onset of unprovoked apprehension accompanied by various somatic symptoms, including shortness of breath, gastrointestinal distress, palpitations, and flushing as well as fears of losing control or dying. Some patients report episodic panic attack-like states that occur at the same time daily and are associated with motor deficits. Claustrophobia, social phobia, and other phobias are states of excessive apprehension precipitated by a given circumstance. The heightened anxiety can be associated with panic features. Patients with GAD have chronic and excessive anxiety and worry over many aspects of their life. It is often associated with muscle tension, concentration problems, and fatigue. Sleep disturbances are common in most anxiety disorders. Co-morbid depressive disorders are common, but not exclusively present. An important symptom of anxiety is "inner tremor," a feeling of tremor when nothing is shaking. This can be felt in the limbs or trunk, where tremor is impossible.

Etiopathological Factors

Whereas depressed feelings in PD may be related to a sense of loss, most syndromic anxiety in PD patients is recognized as foreign and excessive. To that end, anxiety syndromes in PD appear related to the underlying disease pathology. Anxiety disorders often occur during the 3- to 8-year prodromal period before the onset of motor symptoms, as well as more remotely, and may represent a risk factor or a nonmotor symptom for the disease *(6)*. Several studies implicate noradrenergic dysfunction or an imbalance in noradrenergic/dopaminergic tone. Reports of reduced anxiety after neurosurgical treatment of PD suggests frontostriatal involvement.

Diagnosis

The key diagnostic feature is the report or observation of unwarranted or discrete anxiety that is generalized or related to a provoking circumstance.

Differential Diagnosis

Anxiety disorders include panic disorder, agoraphobia, social phobia, specific phobias, GAD, post-traumatic stress disorder, and unspecified anxiety disorder. The combination of depression and anxiety and the overlap of somatic features of anxiety with those of PD or other medical conditions can confound diagnosis. Thus, it is important to exclude medical conditions such as hypothyroidism, hypoglycemia, and cardiac disease. Anxiety associated with motor fluctuations can be associated with a more persistent anxiety disorder condition, but initial treatment should focus on minimizing "on–off" fluctuations *(7)*.

Course and Prognosis

There are no studies on the course and prognosis of anxiety disorders in PD. Some anxious patients relay worries about their motor status even when they are doing relatively well. If the anxiety disturbance is unrecognized, this can lead to overmedication with anti-parkinsonian medications and earlier onset of complications of therapy, such as "on–off" phenomena, dyskinesias, and psychosis.

Treatment

There are no formal studies on treatment of anxiety in PD. Many SSRI and SNRI antidepressant agents are indicated for treatment of idiopathic anxiety disorders (e.g., panic disorder, social phobia, GAD) and they also tend to benefit PD patients with similar conditions. Despite the putative role of noradrenergic dysfunction, there is no evidence that SNRIs will work better than SSRIs for treatment of anxiety in PD. Nortriptyline at low doses (e.g., beginning at 10 mg at bedtime) can be helpful in promoting nocturnal sleep and reducing daytime generalized anxiety. The low dose limits the side effects of nortriptyline, which is also relatively inexpensive compared to most other antidepressants. Benzodiazepines can be cautiously prescribed in very low starting doses (e.g., lorazepam 0.25 mg) for short-term or intermittent use with heightened symptoms; over the long term, their regular use often leads to drug tolerance, dependence, and interdose withdrawal phenomena with heightened anxiety and adverse cognitive effects. However, a few individuals with chronic anxiety disorders actually do best on chronic low doses of benzodiazepines. Atypical antipsychotics such as quetiapine at low doses (e.g., 6.25 mg starting dose) can also be tried. Co-morbid depressive disorders, which are common, should be treated to remission.

APATHY

Epidemiology

Previous studies show that apathy, defined as a state of diminished motivation, occurs in PD as an independent syndrome in about 12% of patients and co-exists with depressive disorders in at least 25% of patients. There are no clear predictors of apathy. The data are contradictory as to whether patients with independent apathetic syndromes have greater cognitive impairment. Certainly, apathy is a common component of dementia, delirium, or demoralization.

Signs and Symptoms

Apathy is manifest as a lack of motivation or initiative along with indifference about the degree of inactivity *(8)*. There is usually diminished perseverance, interest in new things, and concerns over one's health. Such patients generally enjoy themselves at arranged or structured activities, but they return to their usual inert state once the event is over. Patients fail to take an active interest in others and may be less conversational. They do not exhibit negativism, active social withdrawal, or anhedonia as seen with depressive disorders. Apathy is usually not distressing to the patient, but their inactivity and lack of spontaneous effort are frustrating to family members and caregivers, who tend to initiate complaints and wonder if the patient has a depressive disorder.

Etiopathological Factors

Goal-directed activity is associated with intact dopaminergic and prefrontal cortical activity, but apathetic syndromes commonly involve basal ganglia pathology. Evidence for neuronal loss in the locus coeruleus implicates a role for noradrenergic dysfunction. A role for abnormalities in frontal-subcortical circuitry is thus suggested. Parallels between features of apathy and those of PD, especially bradyphrenia and bradykinesia, suggest shared pathophysiological processes among these cognitive, behavioral, and motor aspects of the disease. One study showed strong associations between apathy, executive dysfunction, impairments in instrumental activities of daily living, and higher levodopa doses. No clear demographic or historic features distinguish apathetic syndromes from PD in general or compared with PD with depression.

Diagnosis

DSM-IV Text Revision(TR) uses the term "personality change with apathy secondary to a general medical condition (PD)" when there is an apathetic syndrome. There are no established criteria for diagnosing apathetic syndromes. Persistent and pervasive apathetic phenomena are often overlooked or misdiagnosed as a primary depressive disorder. Recognition of the symptoms or syndrome is important in order to guide treatment *(8)*.

Differential Diagnosis

Neurological signs and symptoms such as akinesia, hypomimia, hypophonia, cognitive dysfunction, and bradyphrenia can confound recognition of apathy. It is critical to exclude other explanations, such as a depressive disorder or delirium. SSRI antidepressants, which are most frequently prescribed for depression in PD, can also cause apathy, but this has not been demonstrated specifically in PD.

Course and Prognosis

There are no specific studies on the course of apathy in PD or its impact on the long-term course of the disease. Physical inactivity contributes to physical deconditioning, which can aggravate motor disability and compound caregiver burdens.

Treatment

There are no studies on the treatment of apathy. Caregivers should be educated about apathy, executive dysfunction, and their manifestations. Families need to learn how to respond appropriately to the patient's lack of motivation and encourage health-promoting behaviors, including medication compliance, which the patient is unlikely to initiate. Treatment of co-morbid depression is an obvious first step pharmacologically. There are reports of improved function with dopaminergic or noradrenergic medications, such as amphetamines, levodopa, dopamine receptor agonists, selegeline, amantadine. Anecdotally, the cognitive-enhancing agents that are cholinesterase inhibitors or N-methyl-D-aspartate antagonists have been helpful.

SELECTIVE COGNITIVE IMPAIRMENTS AND DEMENTIA

Epidemiology and Phenomenology

Nearly all patients with PD demonstrate some degree of cognitive impairment that ranges from mild selective deficits to dementia *(9)*. Commonly, cognitive decline is not obvious clinically and scores on dementia screening tests, such as the Mini-Mental State Exam (MMSE), are often in the "normal range," even for individuals with dementia. Early in the disease course, the impairments are more selective and generally affect the domains of executive and visuospatial functions, memory, and attention. Cross-sectionally, about 25–40% of patients have dementia *(10)*.

Signs and Symptoms

Executive dysfunction, which is especially common, involves impairments in the ability to process new information and anticipate, plan, initiate, maintain, and change behaviors. Patients with executive dysfunction complain of disorganization and distractibility that prevents them from completing tasks. Other affected cognitive domains include information-processing speed (bradyphrenia), explicit recall (with relative sparing of recognition memory), spatial planning, verbal fluency, and attention. The impact of these types of such deficits depends on individual circumstances, but they may contribute to disability that affects employment or independent living.

Patients with more global impairments fall into three general subgroups. The first consists of an intensification of the selective deficits, especially in memory and information-processing speed. A second group shows wider involvement of cortical functions, including aphasia, apraxia, and memory deficits, but the clinical presentation remains distinct from Alzheimer's disease (AD). A third group has clinical features consistent with both PD and AD, and the language deficits are especially pronounced relative to the two other subgroups.

Etiopathological Factors

Postmortem and imaging studies suggest that dementia in PD is associated with neuronal loss of the cholinergic cells of the basal forebrain. In addition to the typical findings of PD (Lewy bodies and neuronal loss in the substantia nigra *pars compacta*), there are often Alzheimer-type neuropathological changes (senile plaques and neurofibrillary tangles) in the limbic system and/or the cortex. However, most cases of PD-dementia do not meet neuropathological criteria for definite AD. Cortical Lewy bodies are observed in PD patients with and without dementia. Some PD patients will meet neuropathological criteria for dementia with Lewy bodies at more advanced stages. The selective cognitive impairments may involve dysfunction of nonmotor neural circuits, including mesolimbic and mesocortical dopaminergic projections. Bradyphrenia may be associated with noradrenergic cell loss. Dementia is also associated with increasing age, family history of dementia, depression, and more severe motor dysfunction. Anticholinergic medications, medication interactions, disturbed sleep, and co-morbid medical illnesses are extrinsic factors that contribute to cognitive impairment.

Diagnosis

There are no operational criteria for the diagnosis of cognitive impairments or dementia in PD. Patients and families should be asked specifically about acquired changes in thinking abilities, memory, language, and executive functions and how these changes affect function at work and home.

Differential Diagnosis

Because dementia is not inevitable in PD, it is important to exclude other conditions. As for all patients with dementia, there should be a metabolic work-up. Brain imaging, although justifiable, is rarely of value. Cognitive impairments can lead to reduced social interactions, and this may be interpreted as a sign of depression. However, depressive disorders are also associated with increased cognitive impairment, and can either aggravate or cause a dementia syndrome. Anti-parkinsonian and other medications with psychoactive effects can also have deleterious cognitive effects. As frank dementia develops later in the course of PD, early-onset dementia (i.e., coinciding with onset of PD motor signs or within the first few years), suggests dementia with Lewy bodies.

Course and Prognosis

The course and prognosis of selective cognitive deficits and dementia in PD is unclear, in part because of the lack of operational definitions. At end stages of the disease, about 70% of the patients have a severe dementia syndrome. Dementia is associated with an increased likelihood of co-morbid depression and/or psychosis, which increases caregiver burden and not uncommonly leads to nursing home admission.

Treatment

There are no standard treatments of cognitive deficits in PD. Factors, such as anticholinergic medications, that contribute to cognitive impairment and dementia should be addressed. Education about cognitive deficits, their impact, and potential compensatory strategies is helpful to patients and their families. Formal neuropsychological testing can help clarify areas of relative strengths versus vulnerabilities and serial testing can assess individual change. Cholinesterase inhibitors were shown to improve cognition in three double-blind placebo-controlled studies *(11–13)*. Effects of other potential cognitive-enhancing agents (e.g., memantine, and neuroprotective agents) await further assessment.

PSYCHOSIS

Epidemiology and Phenomenology

The term *psychosis* refers to the specific phenomena of hallucinations (sensory perceptions without a stimulus), delusions (fixed false beliefs despite evidence to the contrary), and thought disorder (a disturbance in the form of speech). The development of psychosis in PD is invariably associated with dopaminergic therapy. When hallucinations, particularly visual hallucinations, occur in the absence of dopaminergic treatment, the diagnosis of dementia with Lewy bodies should be considered. Hallucinatory experiences are considered "benign" when the patient has insight into their non-real nature and is not disturbed by them, but the ability to discriminate can vary, especially in the setting of dementia. "Illusions," sensory distortions of real objects, are not strictly hallucinations, but are grouped with that category. A lamp is seen as a person, a fire hydrant as a dog, or a shadow as a lurking animal. Many PD patients seem to develop illusions before hallucinations, but the prognostic significance of this is uncertain. Often, patients have insight into the non-real nature of these experiences, but may not reveal them to clinicians or family unless asked specifically.

Hallucinations involve any sensory modality and occur in nearly 50% of patients over the course of the disease. Cross-sectionally, about 25–40% of patients experience hallucinations *(14)*. The hallucinations are predominantly visual, and usually take the form of nonthreatening people—sometimes strangers, sometimes family or friends—who look real. They are often outside the house, people fixing the road, children climbing trees, and so on. Some people experience "presence hallucinations," defined as the compelling feeling that someone is in the room behind the patient, forcing him or her to turn. "Passage" hallucinations consist of brief sightings of someone or something passing in the peripheral visual field. The patient typically sees the same hallucination each time. They may occur in the light or the dark, and tend to occur when the patient is alone, relaxing, watching TV, or reading. They usually ignore the patient although they may interact among themselves. Patients with insight into the non-real nature of their hallucinatory experiences may find them amusing. Patients who lack insight can become distressed and may have associated paranoia. Some patients feel a responsibility for their "house guests" and attempt to feed or tend to their presumed needs.

Less than half the patients with visual hallucinations suffer from other types of hallucinations. About 10% of patients have auditory hallucinations; olfactory, tactile, and visceral hallucinations are less common *(15)*. These forms of hallucinations almost invariably occur in people who also have visual hallucinations. In general, they are indistinct phenomena that do not involve the visual hallucination. That is, the patient may hallucinate people who are silent, and, at other times hear party noises or muffled speech outside the room.

Reported prevalence rates for delusions are 3–30%. Delusions are generally of a paranoid nature. A common delusion is of spousal infidelity. Other delusional themes include concerns about abandonment, or people living in the house, planning harm, stealing money, purposefully misplacing items, spying, and so on. In nondemented patients the sensorium is clear and scores on tests of cognitive function, including the MMSE are normal. Frequently complicating the psychosis are both anxiety and depression.

Other Etiopathological Factors

Cognitive impairment, especially dementia, is the major risk factor for the development of psychosis *(14)*. Aside from dementia, systemic disorders, particularly infections, contribute to development of psychotic symptoms, usually in the context of a delirium. Medication toxicity is also common. Renal failure, even if partial, will increase the risk of amantadine toxicity because it is excreted via the kidneys. Each of the anti-PD medications can induce delirium or psychosis with a normal sensorium, so drug toxicity from excess dosing should always be considered, as a patient may accidentally overdose. Other psychoactive medications (e.g., benzodiazepines, non-PD anticholinergic medications, antihistamines, opiates, steroids) can result in psychosis. In the absence of other contributing factors, such as a delirium, it should be kept in mind that the development of psychotic symptoms is "state-dependent." Thus, the psychotic symptoms are dependent on several factors, including degree of sleep deprivation and stress, and not on the brain drug level alone. Goetz et al. demonstrated this by hospitalizing a cohort of patients who had visual hallucinosis on L-dopa in their homes. None developed any psychotic symptoms with intravenous infusions of L-dopa in the hospital.

Diagnosis

The diagnosis of psychosis rests on the presence of hallucinations or delusions, irrespective of whether the patient has insight. A key diagnostic issue is whether the patient has psychotic symptoms in the context of a normal sensorium or if there is evidence for an encephalopathy, with fluctuating levels of awareness, alertness, and attention. It is common for the psychotic symptoms to be context-dependent. Thus, hallucinations are rarely experienced in the office setting and reports of delusions are more common than the actual experience of them in the presence of the doctor. It is critical to obtain information about the presence of psychotic symptoms from an informant because patients may not have adequate insight to report their abnormal beliefs or experiences, or simply forget about them when they are not present.

Differential Diagnosis

The differential diagnosis of PD-related psychosis includes encephalopathy (delirium), during which a global change in mentation with fluctuating levels of alertness and attention is frequently accompanied by confusion, disorientation, and psychotic symptoms. In patients with a dementia, there will be greater confusion over their baseline level. The distinction between drug-induced visual hallucinations from Bonnet's syndrome, in which elderly people, particularly those with visual impairment, develop benign complex visual hallucinations, may be impossible. If the hallucinations are drug-induced they should resolve with reductions in the medications. Parasomnias can also be difficult to distinguish from psychosis. Patients may act out a dream, as in rapid eye movement (REM) sleep behavior disorder, or awaken from a dream to experience its continuation while awake, or suffer a "REM intrusion" while awake but in a near sleep state. "REM intrusions" are brief dreams in twilight state. Vivid dreams will be reported the next morning as if the events had truly occurred. This can mimic hallucinatory experiences or delusional thinking.

Course and Prognosis

The enhanced use of safe and effective drugs to treat psychosis in PD has improved outcomes but the presence of psychosis carries a poor prognosis *(16)*. Despite demonstrated improvements in psychotic symptoms in each of the two randomized controlled trials with low-dose clozapine, there was a 10% mortality rate during the 3-month trial, with deaths split evenly between the placebo- and drug-treated subjects. In a follow-up of the cohort from one clozapine trial, mortality was 25% at 22 months and nursing home placement occurred in 42%. There were, in addition, multiple hospitalizations, often for nonpsychiatric problems. Despite the use of clozapine in the first follow-up report, 69% of treated patients remained psychotic, albeit to a milder extent. Nondemented psychotic patients often developed dementia during the 22-month follow-up. This contrasted with a follow-up study on such patients before clozapine was used and there was 100% mortality by 16 months.

Treatment

When patients have insight, the first approach to treatment is to exclude a contributing medical condition such as pneumonia or urosepsis. Once this is done, medications must be reduced or economized as far as possible. Sometimes, non-PD medications such as anticholinergics, used for bladder hyperactivity, or anxiolytics can be discontinued. PD medications should be reduced or stopped depending on the effect on motor function. Although it has not been studied, we recommend tapering and discontinuing one drug at a time rather than tapering all the drugs simultaneously. Cholinesterase inhibitors have been shown in open-label studies to reduce psychosis in PD and improve cognition, which may reduce the risk for psychosis. Thus, their use can be considered although definitive studies have not been conducted. Addition of an atypical antipsychotic should be considered when the psychotic symptoms are bothersome or if there is associated agitation, oppositional, or aggressive behavior that affects caregiving *(17)*. Strong data supports the use of clozapine. Doses as low as 6.25 mg at bedtime are often effective, but the mean dose required in most studies is 25 mg per day. A large number of PD patients have been successfully treated with quetiapine. Because quetiapine does not require any blood monitoring and clozapine does, quetiapine has become the initial antipsychotic of choice for most American PD experts. Several randomized controlled trials have demonstrated that olanzapine worsens motor function in PD patients so it should be avoided. The limited published data on risperidone also indicates that it worsens motor function. As of this writing, a single report, an open-label retrospective study suggests that aripiprazole is neither helpful nor well tolerated, however, further study will be needed to draw conclusions.

BRAIN SURGERY FOR PD

After a lengthy hiatus in which surgery for PD was extremely rare, limited primarily to thalamotomies for the treatment of refractory tremor, functional neurosurgery was resurrected to treat several motor problems in PD *(18)*. It became apparent that ablative lesioning could be improved on by electrical stimulation to reduce the actual damage to the brain while simultaneously allowing a variety of stimulation parameters to be altered to better cope with individual variation and plasticity over time.

Signs and Symptoms

Deep brain stimulation (DBS) in PD has been associated with a variety of psychiatric outcomes *(19)*. Most of these are direct physiological effects, whereas others occur because of profound changes in function that often alter family psychodynamics. The direct physiological consequences of DBS on mood have been reported, with some cases in detail *(20,21)*. Observed effects include acute depression, delayed-onset depression, immediate relief of depression, apathy, euphoria, disinhibition, hallucinations, and a 10% incidence of acute mania in some series *(22)*. A sub-clinical effect described in one report is a decline in the ability of patient who had received bilateral subthalamic nucleus (STN) DBS to assess facial emotions in other people. This type of effect could have a significant but hard to detect impact on patients' quality of life *(23)*. We note this only to illustrate that there may be subtle changes associated with DBS.

Pallidotomy can cause affective and cognitive changes, but these appear to be less marked or common.

Neurobiology

The mechanisms for the various responses to STN DBS are unknown. The medial STN is believed to be connected to the limbic portion of the globus pallidus, the striatum, the prefrontal and cingulate cortices. There is a rich connection between portions of the frontal lobes and the STN.

Other Etiopathological Factors

Most of the factors inducing behavioral changes in the DBS patients remain unknown. Electrode location is a critical factor; too low a placement has induced depression, and relatively small changes in stimulator settings have been associated with dramatic alterations of mood. The presence of significant cognitive impairment puts the patient at risk for further cognitive declines after surgery.

Diagnosis

Identification of postoperative behavioral changes is not difficult, although it may be difficult to distinguish a primary effect of the stimulation from a secondary effect. A patient who has a poor response to surgery may develop a pervasive depressive disturbance, which presumably is different from a depressive disturbance induced physiologically by the stimulator settings.

Differential Diagnosis

Some behavioral effects may mimic drug-related effects, particularly psychosis. In general, anti-PD medications can be reduced with STN surgery, hence behavioral changes that are possibly medication-related may be handled by drug reduction.

Course and Prognosis

Whether the course of the behavioral abnormalities associated with DBS is the same or different than those that evolve naturally is unknown. The discrete stimulation-induced syndromes are recognized by either their appearance or resolution following DBS adjustment, and their resolution within seconds, which is atypical for sustained depressive or manic syndromes.

Treatment

DBS adjustments need to be made when a behavioral change is thought to be associated with the DBS itself.

FATIGUE

Fatigue is a symptom complex that has multiple meanings. Whereas PD patients suffer from objectively measurable muscle fatigue with repeated muscle contractions, the fatigue discussed here is a "sense of tiredness, lack of energy or total body give out" *(25)*. It is a subjective perception that is one of the most common symptoms in all of medicine. There are few disorders, physical or mental, not associated with an increase in fatigue.

Epidemiology

Hoehn and Yahr noted in 1967 that fatigue alone was a rare presenting feature of PD. In surveys of PD patients, however, fatigue was common, affecting half, and was typically long lasting. In addition, half the patients who suffer from fatigue consider it to be as bad as their other symptoms.

Neurobiology

The underlying physiology of fatigue is unknown. Evoked potentials have demonstrated differences in responses in fatigued versus nonfatigued PD populations but how these relate to the perception of fatigue is unknown. Objectively demonstrable muscle fatigue, and physiological measures of exercise efficiency such as oxygen utilization for exercise tasks do not correlate with perceptions of fatigue *(26)*. The overlap between mood and fatigue is so large that it is likely multiple factors are involved in the development of fatigue, which often predates the diagnosis of PD.

Etiopathological Factors

The "causes" of fatigue are unknown. There is an association between fatigue and depressed mood, but nondepressed patients often suffer from fatigue *(27)*. Fatigue may be associated with sleep disturbances but successful treatment of excessive daytime sleepiness may not improve true fatigue. Fatigue does not correlate with motor dysfunction, duration of disease, or age. It does correlate with the self-perception of poor health.

Diagnosis

The diagnosis of fatigue rests on the patient's report, or response to questioning *(28)*. It cannot be demonstrated on examination as it does not correlate with muscular fatigue.

Differential Diagnosis

The overlap between fatigue and depression is large enough that fatigued patients should be evaluated for depression. They may have both. Other explanations for the fatigue should be considered, particularly other medical illnesses such as heart failure, anemia, hypothyroidism, and the like. Low blood pressure is another consideration, although not documented in published series. The overlap between sleepiness and fatigue is another area where interventions may be helpful. Patients should be evaluated for excessive daytime sleepiness, which may be perceived as fatigue and which may be treatable.

Course and Prognosis

Only one study has been published looking at long-term outcome. Those results were discouraging. Patients who were fatigued when the first prevalence survey was taken remained fatigued when assessed 9 years later, despite treatment attempts. On the other hand, patients who were not suffering with depression initially were very unlikely to develop it. Overall, the fatigue worsened over time.

Treatment

There is no treatment known for fatigue in PD. Whereas amantadine improves fatigue in multiple sclerosis , there is no data to suggest it helps in PD *(28)*. Dopamine agonists have been implicated in worsened fatigue but this may be a confound resulting from their sedating side effect. Modafinil has been shown to improve excessive daytime sleepiness but not fatigue. Antidepressants have not been adequately studied but appear to improve mood without resolving the fatigue. Endurance training has been shown to improve fatigue in patient with other medical conditions including chemotherapy and cancer. It has not been tested in PD. Patients often reject this intervention, describing themselves as desirous but too fatigued to begin an exercise program. A role for stimulants such as amphetamines has been advocated but no data supports their use.

IMPULSE CONTROL AND COMPULSIVE BEHAVIORS

Although rare, there are behavioral abnormalities that appear to be drug-related that have attracted much attention and can be especially problematic *(29)*. The first is hypersexuality. When L-dopa was first introduced, it was considered by some to be an aphrodisiac. In recent times, the anti-PD medications have been recognized as causing hypersexuality as well as abnormal sexual behaviors such as cross-dressing, exhibitionism, and even zoophilia *(30)*. These activities are rare but can be very disruptive or distressing. The treatment approach is uncertain. Reducing dopaminergic medications, especially dopamine agonists, behavioral counseling, and antipsychotic and medications are the usual treatment routes. Medications that help with impulsivity, such as SSRIs, or mood stabilizers are also tried. The patient's day should be structured so opportunities for the behavior are limited, especially if it carries a risk of harm to others or the patient. Psychiatric hospitalization may be necessary to gain behavioral control.

Pathological gambling resulting from anti-PD medications is relatively rare, but devastating *(29, 31)*. Patients and families should be specifically warned about the potential for pathological gambling as most patients are not aware that this behavioral change is related to medication changes. Even those who have never gambled may attribute their behavior to changes in circumstances and, until it becomes problematic, finding a new source of enjoyment. As with hypersexual behavior, the treatment is uncertain, but the same medication approaches are used. In addition, families or others often need to take complete control of the finances and limit the patient's access to money and gambling opportunities.

"Punding," a syndrome first described in amphetamine addicts, refers to an obsessive-compulsive-like fascination *(29)* with handling objects and taking them apart, usually with less success at putting them together again. Patients may catalog their jewelry or enter sums on a calculator, as in balancing a checkbook, endlessly. Although patients may recognize their behaviors as abnormal, they do not find them disquieting and thus do not ask for help. These behaviors, however, may lead to inattention to other more vital matters, which can cause others to raise concerns.

Less problematic are other perseverant behaviors that also are drug-related, such as producing soft "sucking" sounds, humming single tunes, or making stereotyped gestures. In some cases, these behaviors are compulsive (i.e., repetitive acts that the patient feels driven to perform and leads to a relief in anxiety). Unlike the punding and gambling, these syndromes may bother patients so that they complain about them. Treatment involves lowering or altering the anti-PD medications or possibly adding an SSRI.

ACKNOWLEDGMENTS

Support for manuscript preparation by Dr. Marsh provided by the Johns Hopkins Medical Institutions Morris K. Udall Parkinson's Disease Research Center of Excellence (NIH, P50-NS-58377).

REFERENCES

1. Aarsland D, Larsen JP, Lim NG et al. Range of neuropsychiatric disturbances in patients with Parkinson's disease. J Neurol Neurosurg Psychiatry 1999; 67:492–496.
2. Menza M, Marsh L. Psychiatric issues in Parkinson's disease: a practical guide. London: Taylor and Francis. In press.
3. McDonald WM, Richard I, DeLong MR. Prevalence, etiology, and treatment of depression in Parkinson's disease. Biol Psychiatry 2003;54:1363–1375.
4. Leentjens AFG, Marinus J, Van Hilten JJ, Lousberg R, Verhey FRJ. The contribution of somatic symptoms to the diagnosis of depressive disorder in Parkinson's disease: a discriminant analytic approach. J Neuropsychiatry Clin Neurosci 2003:15:74–77.
5. Shulman LM, Taback RL, Rabinstein AA, Weiner WJ. Non-recognition of depression and other non-motor symptoms in Parkinson's disease. Parkinsonism Rel Disord 2002;8:193–197.
6. Marsh L. Anxiety disorders in Parkinson's Disease. Intl Rev Psychiatry 2000;12:307–318.
7. Richard IH, Justus AW, Kurlan R. Relationship between mood and motor fluctuations in Parkinson's disease. J Neuropsychiatry Clin Neurosci 2001;13:35–41.
8. Pluck GC, Brown RG. Apathy in Parkinson's disease. J Neurol Neurosurg Psychiatry 2002;73:636–642.
9. Dubois B, Pillon B. Cognitive deficits in Parkinson's disease. J Neurol 1997; 244:2–8.

10. Dubois B, Pillon B. Dementia in Parkinson's disease. In: Wolters EC, Sheltens Ph, Berendse HW, eds. Mental dysfunction in Parkinson's disease II. Utrecht: Academic Pharmaceutical Productions; 1999:165–176.

11. Aarsland D, Laake K, Larsen JP, Janvin C. Donepezil for cognitive impairment in Parkinson's disease: a randomized controlled study. J Neurol Neurosurg Psychiatry 2002;72:708–712.

12. Leroi I, Brandt J, Reich SG, et al. Randomized placebo-controlled trial of donepezil for cognitive impairment in Parkinson's disease. Intl J Ger Psychiatry 2004;19:1–8.

13. Emre M, Aarsland D, Albanese A, et al. Rivastigmine for dementia associated with Parkinson's disease. N Engl J Med 2004;351(24):2509–2518.

14. Aarsland D, Larsen JP, Cummings JL, Laake K. Prevalence and clinical correlates of psychotic symptoms in Parkinson Disease. A community-based study. Arch Neurol 1999;56:595–601.

15. Poewe W. Psychosis in Parkinson's disease. Mov Disord 2003;18:S80–S87.

16. Factor SA, Feustel PJ, Friedman JH, et al. Long term outcome of Parkinson's disease patients with psychosis. Neurology 2003;60:1756–1761.

17. Fernandez HH, Trieschmann ME, Friedman JH. Treatment of psychosis in Parkinson's disease: Safety considerations. Drug Saf 2003;26:643–659.

18. Baron MS, Vitek JL, Bakay RA, et al. Treatment of advanced Parkinson's disease by unilateral posterior GPi pallidotomy: 4-year results of a pilot study. Mov Disord 2000; 5:230–237.

19. Anderson KE, Mullins J. Behavioral changes associated with deep brain stimulation surgery for Parkinson's disease. Curr Neurol Neurosci Rep 2003;3:306–313.

20. Berney A, Vingerhoets F, Perrin A, et al. Effect on mood of subthalamic deep brain stimulation for Parkinson's disease: a consecutive series of 24 patients. Neurology 2002;59:1427–1429.

21. Funkiewiez A, Ardouin C, Caputo E, et al. Long term effects of bilateral subthalamic nucleus stimulation on cognitive function, mood and behavior in Parkinson's disease. J Neurol Neurosurg Psychiatry 2004;75:834–839.

22. Kulisevsky J, Berthier ML, Gironell A, Pascual-Sedano B, Molet J Parés P. Mania following deep brain stimulation for Parkinson's disease. Neurology 2002;59:1421–1424.

23. Dujardin K, Blairy S, Debfevre L, et al. Subthalamic nucleus stimulation induces deficits in decoding emotional facial expressions in Parkinson's disease. J Neurol Neurosurg and Psychiatry 2004;75:202–208.

24. Saint-Cyr JA, Trepanier LL, Kumar R, Lozano AM, Lang AE. Neuropsychological consequences of chronic bilateral stimulation of the subthalamic nucleus in Parkinson's disease. Brain 2000;123:2091–2108.

25. Friedman JH, Chou KL. Sleep and fatigue in Parkinson's disease. Parkinsonism Relat Disord 2004;10(Suppl 1):S27–S35.

26. Garber CE, Friedman JH. Effects of fatigue on physical activity in patients with Parkinson's disease. Neurology 2003;60:1119–1124.

27. Herlofson K, Larsen JP. The influence of fatigue on health-related quality of life in patients with Parkinson's disease. Acta Neurol Scand 2003;107:1–6.

28. Krupp LB, LaRocca NG, Muir-Nash J, Steinberg AD. The fatigue severity scale. Application to patients with multiple sclerosis and systemic lupus erythematosis. Arch Neurol. 1989;46:1121–1123.

29. Kurlan R. Disabling repetitive behaviors in Parkinson's disease. Mov Disord 2004;19:433–437.

30. Uitti R, Tanner CM, Rajput AH, Goetz CG, Klawans HL, Thiessen B. Hypersexuality with antiparkinsonian therapy. Clin Neuropharmacol 1989;12:375–383.

31. Voon V. Repetition, repetition, and repetition: compulsive and punding behaviors in Parkinson's disease. Mov Disord 2004;19:367–370.

15

Neuropsychiatric Disorders in Multiple Sclerosis

David C. Mohr and Darcy Cox

INTRODUCTION

In this chapter, we review the empirical literature on the epidemiology, etiology, consequences, and treatment of neuropsychiatric disturbance associated with multiple sclerosis (MS). We focus primarily on depression and neuropsychological impairment, as most of the empirical literature examined these two areas. However, we briefly describe other areas including pathological laughing and crying (PLC), anxiety, anger, and bipolar disorder.

EPIDEMIOLOGY AND ETIOLOGY

Depression

It is widely agreed that depression is one of the more common symptoms in MS (1–3). Twelve-month prevalence of major depressive disorder (MDD) is 15–26%, with younger patients being more likely to be depressed (4). However, nearly half of all MS patients experience significant levels of depressive symptoms at any given point in time (5), and the lifetime prevalence of MDD following an MS diagnosis is approx 50% (6). These rates of depression are higher in MS than in other chronic illnesses (7,8) and other neurological disorders (9,10). Whereas the natural history of depression in MS has not been adequately studied, examination of control conditions in intervention studies suggest that depression in MS, left untreated, is not self-limiting (11).

Depression in MS likely has multiple etiologies. It clearly has psychosocial origins. Loss of function in MS is unpredictable, and for many patients, unrelenting. Although absolute level of cognitive and physical impairment is not necessarily related to adjustment or depression (9,12–14), patient's perceptions of the uncertainty (15), variability in disease (16), and the perceived intrusiveness of disease on daily activities (17–19) are all related to depression and adjustment. Loss of social support and social role functioning, which are associated with the disease, have also been shown to be associated with depression (20–23).

Although the psychological sequelae of MS are associated with depression, this alone does not account for the higher rates of depression in MS compared to rates found in patients with other progressive diseases. We have, therefore, proposed an etiological model that includes increased risk from both MS pathological and MS pathogenic factors. MS brain lesion volume, particularly in the frontal and temporal regions, have consistently been associated with increased risk of MDD and greater severity of depressive symptoms (24–26). It is increasingly accepted that some proinflammatory cytokines can induce and/or aggravate symptoms of depression in the general population (27). Consistent with this literature, there is evidence in MS that depression is strongly associated with disease exacerbation,

From: *Current Clinical Neurology: Psychiatry for Neurologists*
Edited by: D.V. Jeste and J.H. Friedman © Humana Press Inc., Totowa, NJ

measured both clinically and by gadolinium-enhancing magnetic resonance imaging (MRI) *(28,29)*. Thus, depression may be a product of specific MS-related autoimmune disease processes, as well as the neurological damage caused by these processes. This would indicate that depression could be both a complication associated with MS, as well as a symptom of MS.

In rare cases, depression may be an iatrogenic effect of medications. The oral or intravenous gluco-corticoids used to treat exacerbations can produce changes in mood and cognition *(30)*. There has also been some speculation that new-onset or increased depression may be an iatrogenic effect associated with some of the disease modifying medications (DMMs) commonly used to treat MS. Specifically, early uncontrolled studies suggested that the interferon (IFN)-β may be associated with increased risk of depression *(31–33)*. However, more recently studies have consistently and clearly shown that IFN-β does not cause increases in depressive symptoms *(34,35)*. Some patients may show an increase in depressive symptoms following initiation of DMMs, however, this is likely an artifact resulting from a pre-initiation drop in depression associated with increased optimism immediately prior to initiation *(36)*. Thus, an observed increase in depression represents a return to baseline depression rather than an effect of the medication.

Anxiety and Anger

Compared to depression, little has been written on anxiety in MS. Given the degree of uncertainty and the perceived potential threat of the disease *(15,37,38)* it is not surprising that the rates of anxiety are higher in MS than those found in the normal population *(39)*. The point prevalence of problems with anxiety has been estimated at between 19 and 34% *(40–42)*. One study has suggested that anxiety is more common than depression *(43)*.

Anxiety can have several sequelae. Anxiety can aggravate depression in MS and is associated with increased rates of suicidal ideation, compared to depressed MS patients with little or no anxiety *(43)*. Anxiety is also related to decreased adherence to DMMs, which are all administered by injection. Anticipatory injection anxiety is related whether or not the patient is able to self-inject, and self-injection is associated with adherence *(44)*. Experienced injection anxiety is also directly related to adherence.

Clinicians have frequently noted anger in MS patients *(45,46)*. However, there is little empirical literature in this area. Anger is an appropriate response to the frustrations of having a chronic illness and encountering new physical limitations. It becomes problematic when the intensity of the anger causes distress, and/or when the anger is displaced onto others in the environment. This is an important area that deserves greater research efforts.

Pathological Laughing and Crying (PLC) and Euphoria

PLC has been used synonymously with pseudobulbar affect. PLC is defined as bouts of uncontrollable laughing, crying, or both in response to nonspecific stimuli in the absence of a matching mood state *(47)*. It is estimated that PLC occurs in approx 5–10% of MS patients *(48)*. It is generally associated with greater physical and cognitive disability. PLC is generally responsive to fluoxetine *(49)* and fluvoxamine *(50)*. Euphoria is a similar condition in which the patient's mood is consistently cheerful and he or she is seemingly unaware or unconcerned with his or her condition. Estimates of the prevalence of euphoria vary from 5 to 48%, although in our experience the lower number is likely more accurate. Euphoria is a symptom of MS because it is associated with greater lesion load in the brain *(9,51)*. Extreme caution should be used in ascribing symptoms such as PLC or euphoria to psychological causes such as repression or denial, particularly in patients with substantial cognitive impairment.

Cognitive Impairment

Cognitive impairment is very common in MS, with an estimated point prevalence of 40–75% and a lifetime prevalence closer to 75%. Whereas prevalence is higher in patients with advanced disease, significant cognitive impairment symptoms can also present at onset or early in the disease course, and in patients with very low levels of physical disability *(52,53)*.

Cognitive disorders produce a decline in cognitive functioning that leads to impairment in the patient's ability to fulfill his or her responsibilities in daily life. The Diagnostic and Statistical Manual of Psychiatric Disorders, Fourth Edition (DSM-IV) lists two cognitive disorders caused directly by MS: "Dementia due to Multiple Sclerosis" and "Cognitive Disorder Not Otherwise Specified (NOS) due to Multiple Sclerosis" *(54)*. Patients can also experience cognitive dysfunction as a result of severe depression, severe fatigue, or medication side effects.

Cognitive disorder NOS due to MS, the most common form of cognitive impairment, is a much milder condition than dementia due to MS. Patients with cognitive disorder NOS due to MS may complain of a number of subtle cognitive problems, including difficulty with memory, attention, multitasking, word-finding, visuospatial learning, memory, and organization, and problems with organization and scheduling *(55–59)*. The presentation of cognitive problems across patients is heterogeneous. It is also important to recognize that patients can have significant cognitive problems, but can have memory function preserved.

Dementia due to MS is characterized by severe memory impairment and severe impairment in at least one other cognitive domain, which may manifest as aphasia, apraxia, agnosia, or disturbed executive functioning. This impairment must be of sufficient severity to produce a readily apparent functional decline in most areas of the patient's life, regardless of the patient's level of physical functioning. Fortunately, dementia due to MS is relatively uncommon. It typically occurs either very late in the disease course or in the course of unusually aggressive disease.

A number of neuropathological findings have been associated with cognitive dysfunction in MS patients. Lesion volumes derived from conventional T2 and T1 MRI have generally shown moderate correlations with cognitive dysfunction *(60–64)*. More recently, atrophy has been found to play significant role in the development of cognitive difficulties in MS, perhaps particularly in patients with frontal syndromes and more severe behavioral difficulties. Atrophy also can begin very early in the disease course *(65)*. Frontal atrophy, supratentorial atrophy, increased third ventricle volume, and atrophy of the corpus callosum have been shown to correlate with a number of cognitive problems, including problems with learning and memory, behavioral disturbance, impaired reasoning, and poor attention, as well measures of global cognitive impairment and dementia *(65–69)*. Current research is examining the relationships between newer imaging techniques, such as magnetization transfer ratio, proton magnetic resonance spectroscopy, and functional imaging, which also appear to be more strongly correlated with cognitive impairment than conventional imaging *(70)*.

Other Psychiatric Disorders

There has been some suggestion that bipolar affective disorder may occur more frequently among patients with MS than in normal controls *(71,72)*. However, in the more than 15 years since publication of these findings, there have been no reported replications of these findings. Psychotic symptoms are also sometimes mentioned as being associated with MS, but there is no convincing evidence that psychotic symptoms occur at greater rates among MS patients compared with the general population generally.

DIAGNOSIS

As noted above, although patients with MS can show a variety of psychiatric symptoms, depression and cognitive impairment have received the greatest attention. Therefore, the remainder of this chapter focuses on these two prevalent neuropsychiatric conditions.

Depression

To diagnose MDD, a patient must have had either depressed mood or decreased interest or pleasure in activities (anhedonia) for at least 2 weeks, plus at least four additional symptoms including among the following: change in appetite, change in sleep, psychomotor retardation or agitation, fatigue, sense of worthlessness, problems in concentration, and thoughts of suicide (*see* Chapter 4). Other depressive diagnoses such as dysthymia or subthreshold depressions may include subsets of these symptoms. It is important to note that the cardinal symptoms are depressed mood *or* anhedonia. Many depressed MS patients may not feel sad, but may have lost motivation or interest in engaging in activities.

There have been some suggestions that some symptoms of depression are confounded with symptoms of MS *(73)*. For example, fatigue, cognitive impairment, insomnia, and change in weight could all potentially be symptoms of either MDD or MS. However, more recent evidence suggests that these symptoms may not caused by only one source, but may be multiply determined. Indeed, a recent study has shown that all symptoms of depression improve with treatment for depression, including those that might be confounded with MS *(74)*. Thus, in diagnosing depression, we do not recommend excluding symptoms of depression for a diagnosis of MDD just because they may also be related to MS. We recommend that any symptom of depression be considered a symptom of depression if it occurs in the presence of either depressed mood or anhedonia.

Depression is under diagnosed in MS *(7)*. Estimates are that 67% of MS patients with MDD receive no treatment for their depression *(75)*. This is likely a result of the "don't ask, don't tell" rules around depression—most patients do not tell their physicians and most physicians do not routinely ask. A number of screening questionnaires have been shown to effectively identify MS patients who likely have MDD *(76)*. However, the use of screening questionnaires for depression has not been widely adopted, in part because they require some level of organization within a clinic to have them scored and the information presented to the provider before the visit ends.

Many health care organizations, including the Veterans Affairs Administration, have adopted the use of two questions asked by the provider annually: "have you been consistently depressed or down, most of the day, nearly every day, for the past 2 weeks?" and "in the past 2 weeks, have you been much less interested in most things or much less able to enjoy the things you used to enjoy most of the time?" Consistent with findings from primary care *(77)*, these two questions very reliably identify MS patients with depression, with high rates of "hits" and low rates of false-positives *(75)*. It is important to note that MDD requires depressed mood *or* anhedonia (loss of interest). We strongly urge that MS patients be screened for depression at each visit.

Cognitive Impairment

Patients are not always accurate in reporting their cognitive symptoms. It is not uncommon for patients with little or no impairment to report significant symptoms, and those with severe symptoms to minimize the severity *(78)*. Level of cognitive impairment cannot be inferred from physical impairment as the two are not well correlated. As such, formal neuropsychological assessment performed by a neuropsychologist is usually required for a clear and objective evaluation of level of impairment and areas of function that are impacted. If the patient is disabled because of cognitive symptoms, a neuropsychologist's assessment may prove useful as the patient attempts to obtain appropriate disability benefits. Unfortunately, there are a number of potential problems associated with neuropsychological assessment. A full battery can often take several hours to administer. This can lead to a number of difficulties, including problems related to the patient's fatigue, issues with cost and reimbursement, and issues of accessibility.

Brief screening tools generally used by neurologists, such as the Mini-Mental State Exam, do not have adequate sensitivity and specificity to identify probable Cognitive Disorder NOS in MS patients. In addition, this measure may misdiagnose patients who have psuedodementia resulting from severe depression, rather than cognitive dysfunction resulting from MS. The most simple and accurate screen is the report of a spouse, partner, or other family member. Reports of family members have shown much stronger correlations with objective assessment than have reports of patients *(79)*.

CONSEQUENCES OF NEUROPSYCHIATRIC PROBLEMS

Depression has been shown to have the largest impact on quality of life in MS, exceeding the effects of physical impairments and mobility problems *(80)*. Depression can significantly increase disability by reducing a person's ability to work effectively or fulfill other social roles in the family and elsewhere. In addition to reducing quality of life and engagement in significant roles, depression increases the risk of suicide in MS *(81)*. Patients with MS have been shown to be more than seven times more likely to commit suicide than the general population *(82)*.

Cognitive impairment can also significantly reduce a patient's ability to work or engage in daily activities. Some research has found that cognitive impairments are the largest cause for disability, exceeding the impact of physical impairments *(83)*. Given the importance of cognition in the modern workplace, this is perhaps not surprising. Cognitive impairments can also impact the patient's relationships with others. People may attribute the patient's symptoms or forgetfulness or inattention to willful behavior, rather than acknowledging the presence of cognitive difficulty. Patients themselves may misattribute cognitive symptoms to depression, stress, aging, or "losing their minds."

Mild and moderate cognitive impairment often can require occupational accommodations, short-term or permanent disability benefits, or unemployment *(83,84)*, and may require additional assistance with scheduling, organization, and other tasks. More severe dementia can impair many important daily activities, including employment, driving, food preparation, care of small children, shopping, or management of finances. Patients with dementia resulting from MS may make unsafe or unwise decisions, and may be sufficiently functionally impaired to require legal conservatorship.

TREATMENT

Depression

Evidence suggests that depression in MS, left untreated, will not improve *(11)*. Although the etiology of depression in MS may include disease-specific factors such as brain lesions or inflammation, the treatment literature has found that, as a group, patients with MS respond to treatment for depression about as well as patients without MS.

Antidepressant Medications

Open-label studies have suggested that treatment with serotonin-specific reuptake inhibitors, tricyclics (TCAs), and other classes of antidepressant medications are effective at reducing depression *(85,86)*. To date there has been only one small placebo-controlled trial of the TCA, desimipramine, which showed mixed outcomes *(87)*. Whereas 5 weeks of treatment showed significant improvements the Hamilton Rating Scale for Depression *(88)*, an interviewer-rated measure, there was no significant improvement, compared to placebo, on self-reported severity of symptoms using the Beck Depression Inventory *(89)*. Upon conclusion of the trial, most patients were receiving the either the minimal clinical dosage of 150 mg per day or less. A more recent study compared a 16-week treatment of sertraline to two forms of psychotherapy for MDD among MS patients *(90)*. Sertraline produced significant reductions in depressive symptoms on both objective and subjective measures of depression. But it should be noted that physicians met every 4 weeks with patients and the median daily dosage by the end of treatment was 150 mg, or three times the minimum clinical dosage. To the best of our knowledge, there is no indication in the literature that there is any difference in efficacy between sertraline and desimipramine. Thus, the difference between the two trials is likely that patients in the sertraline trial received more potent dosing, compared to those in the desimipramine trial.

Physician Care for Depression

Most guidelines for the treatment of depression with pharmacotherapy, such as the Agency for Health Care Policy and Research guidelines, require follow-up approximately every 4 weeks after the initiation of antidepressant medication because most medications require 4–6 weeks to achieve their full effect *(91–94)*. The prescribing physician should monitor for response to treatment, side effects, and adherence. If the patient has not achieved full symptom relief, the dose should be adjusted upwards or treatment should be augmented with another medication. Adjustments in dose and medication should be made to manage significant side effects. Adherence, a significant problem in the treatment of depression, should be monitored closely. Most patients require several times the minimal dosage to achieve full symptom relief *(95)*.

A recent study examining the care of 260 patients with MS cared for by neurologists in a large health maintenance organization, found that 26% of these met MDD criteria. Of those patients meeting MDD criteria, 67% received no antidepressant, 30% received antidepressant treatment that was at threshold or below threshold, and only 3% received doses that exceeded minimal clinical dosages *(75)*. Data suggests that most MS patients treated for MDD require doses greater than the minimal clinical dosages to achieve full symptom relief. These findings are highly consistent with the literature from primary care, which shows that physicians tend not to assess depression adequately and generally do not provide adequate treatment *(91)*.

There are many reasons why physicians who are not mental health specialists do not provide pharmacotherapy that is adequate to produce full symptom relief. We believe one principal reason is that the care models for depression do not fit with the care models in outpatient medical clinics. Most neurologists who treat MS do not see their patients every 4 weeks, making it difficult to follow up. Thus, for most clinics, alternative methods of supporting treatment for depression must be developed. A number of studies have examined alternative methods of following depressed patients in primary care and other non-mental health specialty care clinics. Most of these have used nurse telephone follow-up to monitor symptoms of depression, side effects, adherence and management of life stressors *(96,97)*. Although such programs have not yet been developed or tested for MS, findings from other settings suggest that depression outcomes can be significantly enhanced through such programs.

Psychotherapy

There have been several studies examining the efficacy of psychotherapy for the treatment of depression in patients with MS *(11,90)*. The literature suggests that psychotherapies focused on improving the coping skills of patients are just as effective as antidepressant medications. Psychotherapies that focus solely on provision of social support are less effective for patients with MS. Data from the general psychiatric literature suggest that psychotherapy and antidepressant medications results in significantly greater rates of improvement than providing either treatment alone *(98)*. There is no reason to believe this finding would not be true for patients with MS as well. Thus, particularly for patients with more severe depression or depression that is refractory to a single treatment approach, combined psychotherapy and pharmacotherapy may be indicated.

Predictions of Response and Relapse

In general, research has not found any disease-related predictors of outcome. Patients with physical and cognitive impairment appear to show initial responses to pharmaco- and psychotherapies that are similar to those who do not have these impairments. However, patients with greater lesion load and greater levels of cognitive impairment are significantly less likely to maintain the treatment gains at 6-month follow-up *(99)*. This suggests that MS patients with cognitive impairment and high lesion load who are treated for depression should be followed closely to ensure maintenance of treatment gains.

Although psychotherapy and antidepressant medications produce similar results in populations of depressed patients, there may be some instances when one is preferable to the other. Studies for the general psychiatric literature indicate that antidepressant medications are more likely to be effective than psychotherapy in patients with severe depression *(100)*. There is also an emerging literature suggesting that antidepressant medications may be less effective than psychotherapy in patients with one class of neuropsychological deficits, executive dysfunction (e.g., deficits in planning, organizing, sequencing, and problem solving), associated with frontal and fronto-subcortical brain lesions. This effect was first seen in the treatment of depression in the elderly *(101–103)*. Our group has recent shown similar findings among patients with MS *(104)*.

Cognitive Impairment

The DMMs appear to have a small to moderate impact on progression of cognitive symptoms. Intramuscular IFN-β 1-a and IFN-β 1-b have been shown to help preserve cognitive functioning, whereas no effect on cognition has been seen for glatiramer acetate *(105–107)*. IFN-β 1-b has been shown to have a positive impact on visual memory in a small group of relapsing-remitting MS (RRMS) patients *(106)* and intramuscular IFN-β 1-a has been shown reduce decline across a broader number of areas of cognitive functioning in RRMS, including processing speed, visuospatial learning and memory, and executive functioning *(108)*. No data on the effects of subcutaneous IFN-β 1-a on cognitive functioning are currently available, and the impact of chemotherapy agents frequently used as adjuncts to the DMMs are unknown.

There is little data on cognitive-enhancing drugs. A small open-label trial of donepezil HCl suggested a limited benefit on cognition in MS *(109)*. A small functional MRI study finds differences in activation in left medial prefrontal areas and the right basal ganglia between cognitively intact MS patients and controls performing a reading task following administration of rivastigmine *(110)*. Further research on the potential of this class of medications to slow progression of cognitive dysfunction in MS is required before recommendations can be made.

At present, the most common strategies for managing cognitive difficulties encourage the patient to develop compensatory and accommodation strategies. Neuropsychology, speech therapy, and occupational therapy can be very useful in designing individualized compensation plans. External memory aids (lists and reminders), reducing distractions, and structuring tasks tend to be the most useful strategies, as well as pacing activity and rest periods to manage physical and cognitive fatigue. Compensating for these kinds of difficulties frequently involves significant assistance and cooperation from others in the patient's life.

EFFECTS OF PSYCHOLOGICAL VARIABLES ON MULTIPLE SCLEROSIS

Whereas it is generally accepted that MS can have profound effects on psychological functioning in patients, the notion that depression and/or stressful life events might affect MS is more controversial.

The Effects of Stress on Multiple Sclerosis

Many patients report that stress results in disease exacerbation. This notion was first considered by Charcot, one of the earliest investigators of MS, who speculated that grief, vexation, and adverse changes in social circumstance were related to the onset of MS *(111)*. A recent meta-analysis of 14 empirical studies supported the hypothesis that stressful life events significantly increase the risk of exacerbation *(112)*. Consistent with this meta-analysis, stressors associated with the family and work have been associated with the subsequent development of new gadolinium-enhancing MRI brain lesions, an objective marker of inflammation *(113)*. However, these data also suggested that different types of stress may have differential effects. Whereas most of the studies examined the effects of common, often more chronic stressors, such as family or work problems, one study examined the effects of a traumatic stressor: being an Israeli civilian under actual or threatened missile attack during the first Persian Gulf War *(114)*. Contrary to all other studies, these investigators found a decreased risk of exacerbation associated with traumatic stress. Given that such trauma causes a marked rise in the release of endogenous glucocorticoids, this finding is perhaps not surprising. However, it does suggest that if stress effects MS exacerbation then these effects may be variable depending on a number of factors, including severity and chronicity.

To date, there is considerable support for the hypothesis that stress is associated with increased risk of exacerbation. However, this literature is very underdeveloped and there is much that is unknown. The mechanisms that underlie this association are unclear and there is no conclusive evidence of a causal relationship. For example, it is certainly possible that the patient's subjective experience of stress is an early sign of exacerbation. Furthermore, we cannot link exacerbations to stressful life events in

Table 1
Recommendations for the Treatment of Depression by Neurologists

Identify depression: Screen for depression at each visit by verbal assessment of mood and anhedonia using the following two questions:
- "Over the past 2 weeks, have you felt down, depressed, or hopeless, more days that not?"
- "Over the past 2 weeks, have you found that you have had little interest or pleasure in doing things, more days than not?"

Explain treatment options: If a patient is depressed, explain options including antidepressant medications, psychotherapy, or both.

If the patient selects psychotherapy: Follow-up to ensure the patient makes the appointment.

If patient agrees to initiate pharmacotherapy: Initiate treatment with a standard antidepressant medication and follow-up at least every 4 weeks until full response is achieved.
- At each follow-up visit assess adherence and problem solve around adherence lapses.
- At each follow-up visit, adjust dose upwards or augment with additional medications if symptoms remain.
- At each follow-up visit, check for side effects. Problem-solve around management of side effects. Change medication or reduce dosage when management strategies fail.

Maintenance of Gains: Continue follow-up at increasingly greater intervals. If patient shows significant signs of cognitive impairment, follow the patient frequently to prevent relapse of depression.

any given individual patient. Finally, it is important to acknowledge that the evidence an association between stressful life events and MS exacerbation should not be interpreted as evidence that patients are in any way responsible for exacerbations or disease progression.

Effects of Depression on Multiple Sclerosis

There are at least three potential pathways by which depression might affect MS disease:

1. Depression can affect MS indirectly by affecting behaviors such as adherence to DMMs that affect MS exacerbation or progression.
2. Depression can affect patient's perceptions of the severity of symptoms.
3. Depression might affect MS directly via effects on the immune system.

There is some support for the indirect hypothesis. A longitudinal study of patients initiating an IFN medication found that depression was associated with decreased adherence to medications used to treat MS *(31)*. However, successful treatment for depression with either psychotherapy or antidepressant medications significantly reduces risk of discontinuation of DMMs *(115,116)*.

There is also some support for the idea that depression may increase symptom severity. For example, cross-sectional and longitudinal studies have reported that depression is associated with fatigue *(117,118)*. Treatment of depression results in significant improvements in fatigue *(119)*. In addition, depression has direct negative impact on performance of measures of cognitive function involving frontal executive systems, frontally mediated executive functions, such as working memory, timed tasks of reasoning and problem-solving, speeded attentional processing, and planning ability. It is likely that this relationship is reciprocal in real-world scenarios, with depressed MS patients demonstrating slowed processing and making poorer choices, which leads to unwanted outcomes that further worsen depression. It is currently unknown whether effective treatment for depression in MS might reduce the impact of some of these difficulties.

Finally, there is also some evidence that depression may affect MS pathogenic factors. IFN-γ, a cytokine produced by T-cells, been shown both to precede and to cause MS exacerbation *(120,121)*. Successful treatment for depression has been shown to result in significant decreases in T-cell production of IFN-γ *(122)*.

Table 2
Recommendations for Managing Cognitive Impairment in Multiple Sclerosis

Include family members in as many patient visits as possible. At each patient contact ask family member about problems with:

- W   Word-finding
- A   Attention
- M   Memory
- M   Multi-tasking

If the patient and family express no concerns:

- Monitor at future visits

If the patient expresses mild concern but family members are not concerned about.

- Consider possible mild cognitive impairment.
- Probable depression—evaluate for depression and treat.
- Consider referral for neuropsychological assessment or screening.

If the patient and family both express concern:

- This suggests probable moderate cognitive impairment and possible co-morbid depression.
- Evaluate for depression and treat.
- Initiate referral for neuropsychological evaluation.

If the family expresses concern, but patient denies concern:

- Screen for PLC, euphoria.
- Probable severe cognitive impairment and possible co-morbid depression.
- Consider possibility of dementia, initiate dementia screens.
- Initiate referral for neuropsychological evaluation if indicated.

SUMMARY

In this chapter we have reviewed the essential empirical literature on the epidemiology, assessment, treatment, and consequences of neuropsychiatric disturbance in MS, principally depression and cognitive impairment. Based on this literature we have made recommendations for the care of these disorders. Table 1 displays a recommended algorithm for the treatment of depressive disorders. An algorithm for assessment and management of cognitive dysfunction is offered in Table 2.

ACKNOWLEDGMENTS

Manuscript preparation was supported by NIH grants R01 MH59708 and R01 HD043323-01 to Dr. Mohr.

REFERENCES

1. Andersson P-B, Goodkin DE. Current pharmacologic treatment of multiple sclerosis symptoms. West J Med1996;165: 313–317.
2. Schapiro RT. Symptom management in multiple sclerosis. Ann Neurol 1994;36(Suppl):S123–S129.
3. Thompson AJ. Multiple sclerosis: symptomatic treatment. J Neurol 1996;243:559–565.
4. Patten SB, Beck CA, Williams JV, Barbui C, Metz LM. Major depression in multiple sclerosis: a population-based perspective. Neurology 2003;61:1524–1527.
5. Chwastiak L, Ehde DM, Gibbons LE, Sullivan M, Bowen JD, Kraft GH. Depressive symptoms and severity of illness in multiple sclerosis: epidemiologic study of a large community sample. Am J Psychiatry 2002;159:1862–1868.
6. Sadovnick AD, Remick RA, Allen J, et al. Depression and multiple sclerosis. Neurology 1996;46:628–632.
7. Minden SL, Orav J, Reich P. Depression in multiple sclerosis. Gen Hosp Psychiatry 1987;9:426–434.
8. Surridge D. An investigation into some psychiatric aspects of multiple sclerosis. Br J Psychiatry 1969;115:749–764.
9. Rabins PV, Brooks BR, O'Donnell P, et al. Structural brain correlates of emotional disorder in multiple sclerosis. Brain 1986;109:585–597.
10. Whitlock FA, Siskind MM. Depression as a major symptom of multiple sclerosis. J Neurol Neurosurg Psychiatry 1980;43:861–865.

11. Mohr DC, Goodkin DE. Treatment of depression in multiple sclerosis: review and meta-analysis. Clin Psychol Sci Prac 1999;6:1–9.

12. McIvor GP, Riklan M, Reznikoff M. Depression in multiple sclerosis as a function of length and severity of illness, age, remissions, and perceived social support. J Clinical Psychol 1984;40:1028–1033.

13. Millefiorini E, Padovani A, Pozzilli C, et al. Depression in the early phase of MS: influence of functional disability, cognitive impairment and brain abnormalities. Acta Neurol Scand 1992;86:354–358.

14. Rao SM, Leo GJ, Bernardin L, Unverzagt F. Cognitive dysfunction in multiple sclerosis. I. Frequency, patterns, and prediction. Neurology 1991;41:685–691.

15. Wineman NM, Schwetz KM, Goodkin DE, Rudick RA. Relationships among illness uncertainty, stress, coping, and emotional well-being at entry into a clinical drug trial. Appl Nurs Res 1996;9:53–60.

16. Schiaffino KM, Shawaryn MA, Blum D. Examining the impact of illness representations on psychological adjustment to chronic illness. Health Psychol 1998;17:262–268.

17. Devins GM, Edworthy SM, Paul LC, et al. Restless sleep, illness intrusiveness, and depressive symptoms in three chronic illness conditions: rheumatoid arthritis, end-stage renal disease, and multiple sclerosis. J Psychosom Res 1993;37:163–170.

18. Devins GM, Edworthy SM, Seland TP, Klein GM, Paul LC, Mandin H. Differences in illness intrusiveness across rheumatoid arthritis, end-stage renal disease, and multiple sclerosis. J Nerv Ment Dis 1993;181:377–381.

19. Devins GM, Styra R, O'Connor P, et al. Psychosocial impact of illness intrusiveness moderated by age in multiple sclerosis. Psychology, Health, and Medicine 1996;1:179–191.

20. Barnwell AM, Kavanagh DJ. Prediction of psychological adjustment to multiple sclerosis. Soc Sci Med 1997;45:411–418.

21. Gilchrist AC, Creed FH. Depression, cognitive impairment and social stress in multiple sclerosis. J Psychosom Res 1994; 38:193–201.

22. Gulick EE. Correlates of quality of life among persons with multiple sclerosis. Nurs Res 1997;46:305–311.

23. Pakenham KI. Adjustment to multiple sclerosis: application of a stress and coping model. Health Psychol 1999;18:383–392.

24. Feinstein A, Roy P, Lobaugh N, Feinstein K, O'Connor P, Black S. Structural brain abnormalities in multiple sclerosis patients with major depression. Neurology 2004;62:586–590.

25. Zorzon M, Zivadinov R, Nasuelli D, et al. Depressive symptoms and MRI changes in multiple sclerosis. Eur J Neurol 2002;9:491–496.

26. Bakshi R, Czarnecki D, Shaikh ZA, et al. Brain MRI lesions and atrophy are related to depression in multiple sclerosis. Neuroreport 2000;11:1153–1158.

27. Capuron L, Dantzer R. Cytokines and depression: the need for a new paradigm. Brain Behav Immun 2003;17(Suppl 1): S119–S124.

28. Dalos NP, Rabins PV, Brooks BR, O'Donnell P. Disease activity and emotional state in multiple sclerosis. Ann Neurol 1983;13:573–577.

29. Fassbender K, Schmidt R, Mossner R, et al. Mood disorders and dysfunction of the hypothalamic-pituitary-adrenal axis in multiple sclerosis: association with cerebral inflammation. Arch Neurol 1998;55:66–72.

30. Medical Economics. Physicians' Desk Reference, Fifty Second Edition. Montvale, NJ: Medical Economics Data Production Company; 1998.

31. Mohr DC, Goodkin DE, Likosky W, et al. Therapeutic expectations of patients with multiple sclerosis upon initiating interferon beta–1b: relationship to adherence to treatment. Mult Scler 1996;2:222–226.

32. Mohr DC, Likosky W, Boudewyn AC, et al. Side effect profile and adherence to in the treatment of multiple sclerosis with interferon beta-1a. Mult Scler 1998;4:487–489.

33. Neilley LK, Goodin DS, Goodkin DE, Hauser SL. Side effect profile of interferon beta-1b in MS: results of an open label trial. Neurology 1996;46:552–554.

34. Borràs C, Río J, Porcel J, Barrios M, Tintoré M, Montalbon X. Emotional state of patients with relapsing-remitting MS treated with interferon beta-1b. Neurology 1999;52:1636–1639.

35. Feinstein A, O'Connor P, Feinstein K. Multiple sclerosis, interferon beta-1b and depression: a prospective investigation. J Neurol 2002;249:815–820.

36. Mohr DC, Likosky W, Dwyer P, Van Der Wende J, Boudewyn AC, Goodkin DE. Course of depression during the initiation of interferon beta-1a treatment for multiple sclerosis. Arch Neurol 1999;56:1263–1265.

37. Wineman NM. Adaptation to multiple sclerosis: the role of social support, functional disability, and perceived uncertainty. Nurs Res 1990;39:294–299.

38. Wineman NM, Durand EJ, McCulloch BJ. Examination of the factor structure of the Ways of Coping Questionnaire with clinical populations. Nurs Res 1994;43:268–273.

39. Maurelli M, Marchioni E, Cerretano R, et al. Neuropsychological assessment in MS: clinical neuropsychological and neuro-readiological relationships. Acta Neurol Scand 1992;86:124–128.

40. Minden SL, Schiffer RB. Mood disorders in multiple sclerosis. Neuropsychiatry Neuropsychol Behav Neuro 1991;4:62–77.

41. Pepper CM, Krupp LB, Friedberg F, Doscher C, Coyle PK. A comparison of neuropsychiatric characteristics in chronic fatigue syndrome, multiple sclerosis, and major depression. J Neuropsychiatry Clin Neurosci 1993;5:200–205.

42. Stenager E, Knudsen L, Jensen K. Multiple sclerosis: correlation of anxiety, physical impairment and cognitive dysfunction.

Ital J Neurol Sci 1994;15:97–101.

43. Feinstein A, O'Connor P, Gray T, Feinstein K. The effects of anxiety on psychiatric morbidity in patients with multiple sclerosis. Mult Scler 1999;5:323–326.

44. Mohr DC, Cox D. Managing difficulties with adherence to injectable medications due to blood, injection, and injury phobia and self-injection anxiety. Am J Drug Deliv 2003;1:215–221.

45. Minden SL. Psychotherapy for people with multiple sclerosis. Neuropsychiatry 1992;4:198–213.

46. Mohr DC, Cox D. Multiple Sclerosis. Clinical Handbook of Health Psychology: A Practical Guide to Effective Interventions, Second Edition. USA: Hogrefe and Huber; 2004.

47. Poeck K. Pathophysiology of emotional disorders associated with brain damage. In: Vinken PJ, Bruyn GW, eds. Handbook of Clinical Neurology. Amsterdam: North Holland Publishing; 1969:343–367.

48. Feinstein A, Feinstein K, Gray T, O'Connor P. Prevalence of neurobehavioral correlates of pathological laughing and crying in multiple sclerosis. Arch Neurol 1997;54:1116–1121.

49. Seliger GM, Hornstein A, Flax J, Herbert J, Schroeder K. Fluoxetine improved emotional incontinence. Brain Inj 1992;6: 267–270.

50. Iannaccone S, Ferini-Strambi L. Pharmacologic treatment of emotional lability. Clin Neuropharmacol 1996;19:532–535.

51. Kahana E, Leibowitz U, Alter M. Cerebral multiple sclerosis. Neurology 1971;21:1179–1185.

52. Achiron A, Barak Y. Cognitive impairment in probable multiple sclerosis. J Neurol Neurosurg Psychiatry 2003;74:443–446.

53. Ruggieri RM, Palermo R, Vitello G, Gennuso M, Settipani N, Piccoli F. Cognitive impairment in patients suffering from relapsing-remitting multiple sclerosis with EDSS < or = 3.5. Acta Neurol Scand 2003;108:323–326.

54. American Psychiatric Association. Diagnostic and statistical manual of mental disorders, Fourth Edition. Washington DC: Amer Psychiatric Pub; 1994.

55. Thornton AE, Raz N. Memory impairment in multiple sclerosis: a quantitative review. Neuropsychology 1997;11:357–366.

56. Zakzanis K. Distinct neurocognitive profiles in multiple sclerosis subtypes. Arch Clin Neuropsychol 2000;15:115–136.

57. Kujala P, Portin R, Ruutianen J. Memory deficits and early cognitive deterioration in MS. Acta Neurol Scand 1996;93: 329–335.

58. Brassington JC, Marsh NV. Neuropsychological aspects of multiple sclerosis. Neuropsychol Rev 1998;8:43–77.

59. DeLuca J, Barbieri-Berger S, Johnson SK. The nature of memory impairments in multiple sclerosis: acquisition versus retrieval. Journal of clinical and experimental Neuropsychology 1994;16:183–189.

60. Rovaris M, Filippi M, Falautano M, et al. Relation between MR abnormalities and patterns of cognitive impairment in multiple sclerosis. Neurology 1998;50:1601–1608.

61. Camp S, Stevenson V, Thompson A, et al. Cognitive function in primary progressive and transitional progressive multiple sclerosis: a controlled study with MRI correlates. Brain 1999;122:1341–1348.

62. Comi G, Filippi M, Martinelli V, et al. Brain MRI correlates of cognitive impairment in primary and secondary progressive multiple sclerosis. J Neurol Sci 1995;132:222–227.

63. Foong J, Rozewicz L, Quaghebeur G, et al. Executive function in multiple sclerosis: The role of frontal lobe pathology. Brain 1997;120:15–26.

64. Hohol MJ, Guttmann CR, Orav J, et al. Serial neuropsychological assessment and magnetic resonance imaging analysis in multiple sclerosis. Arch Neurol 1997;54:1018–1025.

65. Zivadinov R, Sepcic J, Nasuelli D, et al. A longitudinal study of brain atrophy and cognitive disturbances in the early phase of relapsing-remitting multiple sclerosis. J Neurol Neurosurg Psychiatry 2001;70:773–780.

66. Edwards S, Liu C, Blumhardt L. Cognitive correlates of supratentorial atrophy on MRI in multiple sclerosis. Acta Neurol Scand 2001;104:214–223.

67. Benedict R, Bakshi R, Simon JH, Priore R, Miller C, Munschauer F. Frontal cortex atrophy predicts cognitive impairment in multiple sclerosis. J Neuropsychiatry Clin Neurosci 2002;14:44–51.

68. Huber SJ, Rammohan KW, Bornstein RA, Christy JA. Depressive symptoms are not influenced by severity of multiple sclerosis. Neuropsychiatry Neuropsychol Behav Neuro 1993;6:177–180.

69. Benedict R, Weinstock-Guttman B, Fishman I, Sharma J, Tjoa C, Bakshi R. Prediction of neuropsychological impairment in multiple sclerosis: comparison of conventional magnetic resonance imaging measures of atrophy and lesion burden. Arch Neurol 2004;61:226–230.

70. Cox D, Pelletier D, Genain C, et al. The unique impact of changes in normal appearing brain tissue on cognitive dysfunction in secondary progressive multiple sclerosis patients. Mult Scler 2004;10:626–629.

71. Schiffer RB, Weitkamp LR, Wineman NM, Guttormsen S. Multiple sclerosis and affective disorder. Family history, sex, and HLA-DR antigens. Arch Neurol 1988;45:1345–1348.

72. Schiffer RB, Wineman NM, Weitkamp LR. Association between bipolar affective disorder and multiple sclerosis. Am J Psychiatry 1986;143:94–95.

73. Mohr DC, Goodkin DE, Likosky W, Beutler L, Gatto N, Langan MK. Identification of Beck Depression Inventory items related to multiple sclerosis. J Behav Med 1997;20:407–414.

74. Moran PJ, Mohr DC. The validity of Beck Depression Inventory and Hamilton Rating Scale for Depression items in the assessment of depression among patients with multiple sclerosis. J Behav Med 2005;35–41.

75. Mohr DC, Hart S, Merluzzi N, Fonareva I, Tasch ES. Depression in Multiple Sclerosis: Screening and Treatment. Under review.

76. Sullivan MJ, Weinshenker B, Mikail S, Bishop SR. Screening for major depression in the early stages of multiple sclerosis. Can J Neurol Sci 1995;22:228–231.

77. Whooley MA, Avins AL, Miranda J, Browner WS. Case-finding instruments for depression. Two questions are as good as many. J Gen Intern Med 1997;12:439–445.

78. Schwartz CE, Kozora E, Zeng Q. Towards patient collaboration in cognitive assessment: Specificity, sensitivity, and incremental validity of self-report. Ann Behav Med 1996;18:177–184.

79. Benedict RH, Munschauer F, Linn R, et al. Screening for multiple sclerosis cognitive impairment using a self-administered 15-item questionnaire. Mult Scler 2003;9:95–101.

80. Provinciali L, Ceravolo MG, Bartolini M, Logullo F, Danni M. A multidimensional assessment of multiple sclerosis: relationships between disability domains. Acta Neurol Scand 1999;100:156–162.

81. Feinstein A. An examination of suicidal intent in patients with multiple sclerosis. Neurology 2002;59:674–678.

82. Sadovnick AD, Eisen K, Ebers GC, Paty DW. Cause of death in patients attending multiple sclerosis clinics. Neurology 1991;41:1193–1196.

83. Rao SM, Leo GJ, Ellington L, Nauertz T, Bernardin L, Unverzagt F. Cognitive dysfunction in multiple sclerosis II. Impact on employment and social functioning. Neurology 1991;41:692–696.

84. Amato M, Ponziani G, Siracusa G, Sorbi S. Cognitive dysfunction in early-onset multiple sclerosis: a reappraisal after 10 years. Arch Neurol 2001;58:1602–1606.

85. Scott TF, Allen D, Price TR, McConnell H, Lang D. Characterization of major depression symptoms in multiple sclerosis patients. J Neuropsychiatry Clin Neurosci 1996;8:318–323.

86. Flax JW, Gray J, Herbert J. Effect of fluoxetine on patients with multiple sclerosis. Am J Psychiatry 1991;148:1603.

87. Schiffer RB, Wineman NM. Antidepressant pharmacotherapy of depression associated with multiple sclerosis. Am J Psychiatry 1990;147:1493–1497.

88. Hamilton M. A rating scale for depression. J Neurol Neurosurg Psychiatry1960;23:56–62.

89. Beck AT, Ward CH, Medelson M, Mock J, Erbaugh J. An inventory for measuring depression. Arch Gen Psychiatry 1961;4: 561–571.

90. Mohr DC, Boudewyn AC, Goodkin DE, Bostrom A, Epstein L. Comparative outcomes for individual cognitive-behavior therapy, supportive-expressive group psychotherapy, and sertraline for the treatment of depression in multiple sclerosis. J Consult Clin Psychol 2001;69:942–949.

91. Simon GE. Evidence review: efficacy and effectiveness of antidepressant treatment in primary care. Gen Hosp Psychiatry 2002;24:213–224.

92. Munoz RF, Hollon SD, McGrath E, Rehm LP, VandenBos GR. On the AHCPR depression in primary care guidelines. Further considerations for practitioners. Agency for Health Care Policy and Research. AHCPR. Am Psychol 1994;49: 42–61.

93. Schulberg HC, Block MR, Madonia MJ, et al. The 'usual care' of major depression in primary care practice. Arch Fam Med 1997;6:334–339.

94. Hirschfeld RM, Keller MB, Panico S, et al. The National Depressive and Manic-Depressive Association consensus statement on the undertreatment of depression. JAMA 1997;277:333–340.

95. Simon GE, Lin EH, Katon W, et al. Outcomes of "inadequate" antidepressant treatment. J Gen Intern Med 1995;10:663–70.

96. Hunkeler EM, Meresman JF, Hargreaves WA, et al. Efficacy of nurse telehealth care and peer support in augmenting treatment of depression in primary care. Arch Fam Med 2000;9:700–8.

97. Simon GE, VonKorff M, Rutter C, Wagner E. Randomised trial of monitoring, feedback, and management of care by telephone to improve treatment of depression in primary care. BMJ 2000;320:550–554.

98. Keller MB, McCullough JP, Klein DN, et al. A comparison of nefazodone, the cognitive behavioral-analysis system of psychotherapy, and their combination for the treatment of chronic depression. N Engl J Med 2000;342:1462–1470.

99. Mohr DC, Epstein L, Luks TL, et al. Brain lesion volume and neuropsychological function predict efficacy of treatment for depression in multiple sclerosis. J Consult Clin Psychol 2003;71:1017–1024.

100. Elkin I, Gibbons RD, Shea MT, et al. Initial severity and differential treatment outcome in the National Institute of Mental Health Treatment of Depression Collaborative Research Program. J Consult Clin Psychol 1995;63:841–847.

101. Alexopoulos GS, Kiosses DN, Choi SJ, Murphy CF, Lim KO. Frontal white matter microstructure and treatment response of late-life depression: a preliminary study. Am J Psychiatry 2002;159:1929–1932.

102. Alexopoulos GS, Meyers BS, Young RC, et al. Executive dysfunction and long-term outcomes of geriatric depression. Arch Gen Psychiatry 2000;57:285–290.

103. Kalayam B, Alexopoulos GS. Prefrontal dysfunction and treatment response in geriatric depression. Arch Gen Psychiatry 1999;56:713–718.

104. Julian L, Mohr DC. Executive functioning is a differential predictor for response to treatment for depression in multiple sclerosis. Under review.

105. Fischer JS, Priore R, Jacobs L, et al. Neuropsychological effects of interferon beta-1a in relapsing multiple sclerosis. Multiple Sclerosis Collaborative Research Group. Ann Neurol 2000;48:885–892.

106. Pliskin N, Hamer D, Goldstein D, et al. Improved delayed visual reproduction test performance in multiple sclerosis patients receiving interferon beta-1b. Neurology 1996;47:1463–1468.

107. Weinstein A, Schwid SIL, Schiffer RB, McDermott MP, Giang DW, Goodman AD. Neuropsychologic status in multiple sclerosis after treatment with glatiramer. Arch Neurol 1999;56:319–324.

108. Fischer JS, Priore RL, Jacobs LD, et al. Neuropsychological effects of interferon beta-1a in relapsing multiple sclerosis. Multiple Sclerosis Collaborative Research Group. Ann Neurol 2000;48:885–892.

109. Greene Y, Tariot P, Wishart H, et al. 12-week, open trial of donepezil hydrocholoride in patients with multiple sclerosis and associated cognitive impairments. J Clin Psychopharmacol 2000;20:350–356.

110. Allyson MMP, Scott RB, Palace J, Smith S, Matthews PM. Potentially adaptive functional changes in cognitive processing for patients with multiple sclerosis and their acute modulation by rivastigmine. Brain 2003;126:2750–2760.

111. Charcot JM. Lectures on Diseases of the Nervous System. Sigerson G, Translator. London: New Sydenham Society; 1877.

112. Mohr DC, Hart SL, Julian L, Cox D, Pelletier D. Association between stressful life events and exacerbation in multiple sclerosis: a meta-analysis. BMJ 2004;328:731.

113. Mohr DC, Goodkin DE, Bacchetti P, et al. Psychological stress and the subsequent appearance of new brain MRI lesions in MS. Neurology 2000;55:55–61.

114. Nisipeanu P, Korczyn AD. Psychological stress as risk factor for exacerbations in multiple sclerosis. Neurology 1993;43: 1311–1312.

115. Mohr DC, Goodkin DE, Likosky W, Gatto N, Baumann KA, Rudick RA. Treatment of depression improves adherence to interferon beta-1b therapy for multiple sclerosis. Arch Neurol 1997;54:531–533.

116. Mohr DC, Likosky W, Bertagnolli A, et al. Telephone-administered cognitive-behavioral therapy for the treatment of depressive symptoms in multiple sclerosis. J Consult Clin Psychol 2000;68:356–361.

117. Bakshi R, Shaikh ZA, Miletich RS, et al. Fatigue in multiple sclerosis and its relationship to depression and neurologic disability. Mult Scler 2000;6:181–185.

118. Schwartz CE, Coulthard-Morris L, Zeng Q. Psychosocial correlates of fatigue in multiple sclerosis. Arch Phys Med Rehabil 1996;77:165–170.

119. Mohr DC, Hart SL, Goldberg A. Effects of treatment for depression on fatigue in multiple sclerosis. Psychosom Med 2003;65:542–547.

120. Lu CZ, Jensen MA, Arnason BG. Interferon gamma- and interleukin-4-secreting cells in multiple sclerosis. J Neuroimmunol 1993;46:123–128.

121. Panitch HS, Hirsch RL, Schindler J, Johnson KP. Treatment of multiple sclerosis with gamma interferon: exacerbations associated with activation of the immune system. Neurology 1987;37:1097–1102.

122. Mohr DC, Goodkin DE, Islar J, Hauser SL, Genain CP. Treatment of depression is associated with suppression of nonspecific and antigen-specific T(H)1 responses in multiple sclerosis. Arch Neurol 2001;58:1081–1086.

W. Curt LaFrance, Jr. and Andres M. Kanner

INTRODUCTION

Psychiatric disorders can be identified in 25–50% of people with epilepsy (PWE), with higher prevalence among patients with poorly controlled seizures. These disturbances include depression, anxiety, psychotic disorders, cognitive and personality changes occurring in the interictal or ictal/post-ictal states. Three areas of focus in epilepsy include co-morbid primary psychiatric processes, integrated symptoms secondary to epilepsy, and nonepileptic seizures. Research in epilepsy and depression suggests a possible shared pathogenic mechanism between seizures and mood disorders.

PWE have been found to be at higher risk of suffering from mood, anxiety, psychotic, and attention deficit disorders (ADD [1–19]; *see* Table 1). The wide ranges reflect the different patient populations surveyed and the different assessment techniques.

Some General Principles

The evaluation of any type of psychopathology in PWE must be approached with the following questions in mind.

1. Is this psychiatric disturbance temporally related to the occurrence of seizures?
2. Is the onset of psychiatric symptoms associated with the remission of seizures? We consider the peri-ictal psychiatric symptoms (pre-ictal and post-ictal) as well as inter-ictal symptoms associated with the onset or remission of seizures as an expression of a para-ictal process.
3. Are the psychiatric symptoms the result of the introduction of an anti-epileptic drug (AED) with potential negative psychotropic properties, or did they appear after discontinuation of an AED with positive psychotropic properties (mood stabilizing, antidepressant, and anxiolytic properties)?
4. Do the symptoms meet diagnostic criteria of the Diagnostic and Statistical Manual of Mental Disorders (DSM-IV), or the International Classification of Diseases or do these symptoms present as an atypical disorder?
5. What is the impact of the psychiatric disorder at hand on the quality of life of patients?
6. What is the treatment for the psychiatric disorder? If pharmacotherapy is required, how do psychotropic drugs interact with AEDs and what is the impact of psychotropic drugs on the seizure threshold?

DEPRESSION IN EPILEPSY

Depression is the most frequent psychiatric disorder in PWE. It is more common in patients with partial seizure disorders of temporal or frontal lobe origin and among patients with poorly controlled seizures *(2–4,6)*. In three community-based studies, prevalence rates of depression ranged between 21 and 33% among patients with persistent seizures and 4–6% among seizure-free patients *(2–4)*. Blum

From: *Current Clinical Neurology: Psychiatry for Neurologists*
Edited by: D.V. Jeste and J.H. Friedman © Humana Press Inc., Totowa, NJ

Table 1
Prevalence-Rates of Psychiatric Disorders in Epilepsy and the General Population

	Prevalence rates	
Psychiatric disorder	Epilepsy	General population
Depression	11–80%	3.3%: Dysthymia
		4.9–17%: Major depression
Psychosis	2–9.1%	1%: Schizophrenia
		0.2%: Schizophreniform disorder
Generalized anxiety disorder	15–25%	5.1–7.2%
Panic disorder	4.9–21%	0.5–3%
Attention deficit hyperactivity disorder	12–37%	4–12%

et al. recently reported the results of a population-based survey that investigated a lifetime prevalence of depression, epilepsy, diabetes, and asthma in 185,000 households *(5)*. Among the 2900 PWE, 29% reported having experienced at least one episode of depression. This contrasted with 8.6% prevalence among healthy respondents, 13% among patients with diabetes, and 16% among people with asthma.

Recent data have suggested that the relationship between epilepsy and depression is not unidirectional, but bidirectional. Indeed, two population-based controlled studies of newly diagnosed adult-onset epilepsy, carried out in Sweden and the United States, respectively, showed that a history of depression *preceding the onset of epilepsy* was three to seven times more frequent among PWE than controls *(20,21)*.

Suicide in People With Epilepsy

The suicide rate in depressed PWE is 9 to 25 times higher in patients with partial seizures of temporal lobe origin than expected in the overall population *(22–24)*. In a recent review of the literature, Gilliam and Kanner concluded that suicide has one of the highest standardized mortality rates (SMRs) of all causes of death in PWE *(25)*. Robertson reviewed 17 studies pertaining to mortality in epilepsy and found that suicide was 10 times more frequent than in the general population *(22)*. Rafnsson et al. recently reported the results of a population-based incidence cohort study in PWE from Iceland in which suicide had the highest SMR (5.8) of all causes of death *(23)*. A Swedish study of cause-specific mortality among 9000 previously hospitalized PWE found an SMR of 3.5 *(24)*.

Depression As a Para-Ictal Phenomenon

Pre-ictal symptoms of depression and depressive episodes typically present as a dysphoric mood in which the prodromal symptoms may extend for hours or even 1–3 days prior to the onset of a seizure. In children, this dysphoric mood often takes the form of irritability, poor frustration tolerance, and aggressive behavior. Blanchet and Frommer *(26)* assessed mood changes during 56 days in 27 PWE who rated their mood on a daily basis. Mood ratings pointed to a dysphoric state 3 days prior to a seizure in 22 (81%) patients. This change in mood was greatest during the 24 hours preceding the seizure. Patients or parents of children with epilepsy often report that dysphoric symptoms completely resolve the day after the ictus.

Post-ictal symptoms of depressive and depressive episodes have been recognized for decades but have been investigated in a systematic manner in only one study *(27)*. The presence of post-ictal symptoms of depression was identified in 43 of 100 consecutive patients with refractory partial seizure disorders. These symptoms occurred after more than 50% of seizures and their duration ranged from 0.5 to 108 hours, with a median duration of 24 hours. Other studies have shown that symptoms of depression can outlast the ictus for up to 2 weeks, and, at times, have led patients to suicide *(28,29)*.

Ictal symptoms of depression or a depressive episode are the clinical expression of a simple partial seizure in which the depressive symptoms are the sole (or predominant) semiology. Ictal symptoms of depression ranked second after symptoms of anxiety/fear as the most common type of ictal affect in one study *(30)*. This presentation occurred in 21% of 100 PWE who reported auras consisting of psychiatric symptoms *(31,32)*. Yet, the actual prevalence of ictal symptoms of depression is yet to be established in larger studies. The most frequent symptoms include feelings of anhedonia, guilt, and suicidal ideation. Such mood changes were typically brief, stereotypical, occurred out of context, and wee associated with other ictal phenomena. More typically, however, ictal symptoms of depression are followed by an alteration of consciousness as the ictus evolves from a simple to a complex partial seizure.

Depression As Co-Morbid Disorder: Inter-Ictal Depressive Disorders

Inter-ictal forms of depression in epilepsy can be identical to depressive disorders described in patients without epilepsy (i.e., major depression, bipolar disorder, cyclothymia, dysthymia and minor depression). Nevertheless, a review of the literature has clearly shown an atypical clinical presentation of inter-ictal depressive episodes that fail to meet any of the DSM categories. Blumer coined the term of Interictal Dysphoric Disorder to describe this atypical presentation, found in about one third of patients with mood disorders in epilepsy *(33)*. It is characterized by a chronic "dysthymic-like" state, where symptoms tend to occur intermittently, intermixed with brief euphoric moods, explosive irritability, anxiety, paranoid feelings, and somatoform symptoms (e.g., anergia, atypical pain, and insomnia). This type of depression is often unrecognized.

Depression As an Iatrogenic Process

AED-Related Depression

AEDs can cause psychiatric symptoms *(34)*. AEDs with γ-aminobutyric acid properties, primarily phenobarbital, primidone, the benzodiazepines, tiagabine, and vigabatrin *(35–39)*, are more likely to cause depression. Other AEDs that have been linked to depression include felbamate, topiramate, levetiracetam and zonisamide *(40–42)*. The addition of AEDs with mood-stabilizing properties, such as carbamazepine, valproic acid (VA), and lamotrigine, can occasionally cause depressive episodes, albeit with a significantly lower frequency than other AEDs. More often than not, these AEDs are associated with the occurrence of depression *upon their discontinuation* in patients with a prior history of depression or panic disorder, which had been kept in remission by these AEDs *(43)*.

Depression Following Epilepsy Surgery

There have been an increasing number of reports of depressive disorders following an anterotemporal lobectomy *(44)*. It is not unusual to see "mood lability" within the initial 6 weeks after surgery. Often, these symptoms subside, but in up to 30% of patients, overt symptoms of depression become apparent within the first 6 months. Characteristically, symptoms of depression vary in severity from mild to very severe, including suicidal attempts. In most instances, these depressive disorders respond readily to pharmacological treatment with antidepressant drugs (see later discussion). Patients with a prior history of depression are at greater risk, and this risk is independent of the postsurgical control of seizures. All patients undergoing epilepsy surgery, therefore, should be advised of this potential complication, *prior to surgery*.

Impact of Depression on Quality of Life in Epilepsy Patients

Depression has a significant negative impact on the quality of life of PWE. Lehrner et al. *(45)* found that depression was the single strongest predictor for each domain of health-related quality of life that persisted after controlling for seizure frequency, seizure severity, and other psychosocial variables. Perrine et al. *(46)* found that mood had the highest correlations with scales of the Quality of Life in Epilepsy Inventory-89 (QOLIE-89) and was the strongest predictor of poor quality of life in regression analyses. In a study of patients with pharmaco-resistant temporal lobe epilepsy (TLE), Gilliam et al. found that high ratings of depression and neurotoxicity from AEDs were the only independent variables significantly associated with poor quality of life scores on the QOLIE-89 summary score. The authors *did not* find any correlation between the type and/or the frequency of seizures. Gilliam et al. also found that mood status was the strongest predictor of the patients' assessment of their own health status in a group of 125 patients more than 1 year after temporal lobe surgery *(47,48)*.

Treatment of Depression in Epilepsy

Before starting a patient on an antidepressant drug (AD), it is important to determine if the seizures may be related to starting or stopping an AED. In all cases inquiry into suicidality is mandatory.

Do ADs worsen seizures? The variables associated with an increased risk of seizure occurrence with ADs in patients without epilepsy include (a) high plasma serum concentrations, (b) rapid dose increments, (c) the presence of other drugs with proconvulsant properties, and (d) the presence of central nervous system (CNS) pathology, abnormal electroechocardiogram (EEG), and personal and family history of epilepsy *(49–52)*. Thus, patients should be started at low doses with small increments until the desired clinical response is reached. This will minimize the risk of causing or exacerbating seizures.

In general, the selective serotonin reuptake inhibitor (SSRI) class is safe in patients with epilepsy. In one study, sertraline was found to definitely worsen seizures in only 1 out of 100 patients with refractory epilepsy *(53)*. Blumer has also reported using tricyclic antidepressants (TCAs) alone and in combination with SSRIs in epileptic patients without seizure exacerbation *(54)*. Monoamine oxidase inhibitors have not been known to cause seizures in patients without epilepsy. The ADs that should be avoided in PWE include maprotiline, bupropion, amoxapine, and clormipramine *(34,52)*. There is little anecdotal data on the safety of the newer ADs of the serotonin and norepinephrine reuptake inhibitor family (SNRI), venlafaxine and mirtazapine.

Pharmacokinetic Interactions Between ADs and AEDs

Most ADs are metabolized in the liver, and their metabolism is accelerated in the presence of AEDs with enzyme-inducing properties, which include phenytoin, carbamazepine, phenobarbital, primidone at regular doses, and oxcarbazepine and topiramate at higher doses. This pharmacokinetic effect is not observed with the new AEDs (i.e., gabapentin, lamotrigine, tiagabine, levetiracetam, and zonisamide). Conversely, some of the SSRIs are inhibitors of one or more isoenzymes of the cytochrome P450 (CYP 450) system. These include fluoxetine, paroxetine, fluvoxamine and, to a lesser degree, sertraline *(55–57)*. Citalopram, on the other hand, does not have pharmacokinetic interactions with AEDs *(34)*. Sertraline has been shown rarely to increase phenytoin levels, and this is thought to be associated with displacement by tight protein binding, or by inhibition of the CYP 450 system *(58,59)*.

Choice of Antidepressant

The SSRI class should be considered as the first line treatment in depressed PWE. They are safe with respect to seizure propensity, are less likely to result in fatalities after an overdose, and generally have a favorable adverse effects profile. Furthermore, their efficacy in dysthymic disorders and in symptoms of irritability and poor frustration tolerance makes this class of ADs more attractive among PWE who have atypical forms of depression. SSRIs with no or minimal effects on CYP 450 isoenzymes, such as citalopram and sertraline, should be considered in patients taking hepatically metabolized AEDs to avoid pharmacokinetic interactions.

In open, uncontrolled trials, TCAs have also been reported to yield a good clinical response, but the cardiotoxic effects and severe complications seen in overdose make these drugs a second-line AD choice. Blumer has anecdotal reports of the utility of low-dose TCA in PWE and Interictal Dysphoric Disorder *(54)*.

A cautionary note is in order. Before starting an AD, clinicians must rule out a history of a manic or hypomanic episode that may be suggestive of a bipolar disorder, as ADs can potentially trigger a manic or hypomanic episode in the short term, and it may worsen the course of the bipolar disorder in the long term, particularly in the case of rapid-cycling bipolar disease. In such cases, an AED with mood-stabilizing and antidepressant properties such as lamotrigine must be considered. Carbamazepine and valproate may be added in case of persistent symptoms. Lithium should be considered if these AEDs are unable to yield a euthymic state.

Other Types of Psychiatric Treatments

Lithium was the first "mood-stabilizing drug" used for the treatment of patients with bipolar disorder. Its use in epileptic patients with affective disorders, however, has been fraught with several problems, including changes in EEG recordings and proconvulsant effects at therapeutic serum concentrations in patients without epilepsy *(34,60)*. Lithium's neurotoxicity and related increase in seizure risk increases with the concurrent use of neuroleptic drugs, in the presence of EEG abnormalities, and with a history of CNS disorder.

Electroconvulsive therapy is not contraindicated in depressed PWE *(61–63)*. It is a well-tolerated treatment and is worth considering in PWE with very severe depression that fails to respond to ADs. Furthermore, there is no evidence that ECT increases the risk of epilepsy *(64)*.

In addition to pharmacological intervention, the value of psychotherapy for the treatment of depression in PWE should not be overlooked. Surveys reveal that fear of the next seizure is rated as the greatest concern in PWE *(65)*. Counseling and psychotherapy can be very useful in helping the patient deal with the stressors and limitations of living with epilepsy.

ANXIETY DISORDERS IN EPILEPSY

Anxiety is the second most common psychiatric co-morbidity in PWE, with an estimated prevalence between 15 and 25% *(2–4,66,67)*. In 174 consecutive PWE from five epilepsy centers, a current DSM-IV diagnosis of anxiety disorder was found in 30% of patients *(66)*.

The various forms of anxiety disorders (generalized anxiety disorder, panic disorder, phobias, obsessive-compulsive disorder, and posttraumatic stress disorder) can present *interictally* with the same clinical manifestations as anxiety disorders in the general population. The peri-ictal presentations of anxiety symptoms often differ from their inter-ictal manifestations, however.

Anxiety Episodes as Para-Ictal Processes

Ictal fear or panic is the most frequent ictal psychiatric symptom. It is the sole or predominant clinical expression of a simple partial seizure (aura) or the initial symptom of a complex partial seizure and usually has a mesial temporal lobe origin.

A careful history can help distinguish inter-ictal from ictal panic. Ictal panic is typically less than 30 seconds in duration, is stereotypical, occurs out of context to concurrent events, and is associated with other ictal phenomena such as periods of confusion of variable duration and subtle or overt automatisms. The intensity of the sensation of fear is mild to moderate and rarely reaches the intensity of a panic attack. On the other hand, inter-ictal panic attacks consist of episodes of 5–20 minutes duration, which at times may persist for several hours. The feeling of fear or panic is very intense ("feeling of impending doom") and is associated with a variety of autonomic symptoms, including tachycardia, diffuse diaphoresis, and dyspnea. Patients may become so completely absorbed by the panic that they may not be able to report what is going on around them; however, there is no confusion or loss of consciousness, as seen in complex partial seizures. It is not infrequent for patients to develop agoraphobia resulting from the fear of experiencing a panic attack. EEG recordings with sphenoidal electrodes placed under fluoroscopic guidance may be necessary to demonstrate the mesial temporal lobe epileptiform activity that generates ictal panic *(68)*.

Patients with ictal panic may also suffer from inter-ictal panic attacks, which have been identified in up to 25% of PWE *(67)*.

Post-ictal symptoms of anxiety can be relatively frequent among patients with refractory partial epilepsy. In a recently published study of 100 consecutive patients with pharmaco-resistant partial epilepsy, we identified a mean of 2±1 post-ictal symptoms of anxiety (range: 1 to 5; median = 2) in 45 patients *(27)*. These symptoms occurred after more than 50% of their seizures and had a median duration of 24 hours (range: 0.5 to 148 hours). Thirty-two patients reported symptoms of generalized anxiety and/or panic; an additional 10 patients also reported symptoms of compulsions and 29 patients experienced post-ictal symptoms of agoraphobia. In 44 of these 45 patients, post-ictal symptoms of depression were also reported, which included anhedonia, feelings of helplessness, crying bouts, suicidal ideation, and feelings of guilt.

Treatment of Anxiety Disorders in Epilepsy

Antidepressants belonging to the SSRI class can prevent the occurrence of inter-ictal panic attacks as well as treat generalized anxiety disorder. On the other hand, there is as of yet no evidence that these drugs have any impact on post-ictal psychiatric symptoms. ADs of the SNRI family have been also been used with success, but no controlled studies exist in PWE. Benzodiazepines have been used for years in the management of anxiety disorders. We do not recommend their chronic use because of the development of tolerance and sedating adverse events. However, short trials with clonazepam can be quite effective.

PSYCHOSIS OF EPILEPSY

Psychotic disorders can present as a schizophreniform disorder, indistinguishable from those of patients without epilepsy. However, the term psychosis of epilepsy implies the presence of certain characteristics that distinguish these disorders from those of patients without epilepsy.

Psychosis As an Expression of a Para-Ictal Process

Post-Ictal Psychotic Symptoms and Psychotic Episodes

Post-ictal psychotic phenomena can present in the form of isolated symptoms or as psychotic episodes defined as a cluster of symptoms of at least 24 hours duration. The prevalence of post-ictal psychotic disorders in PWE is yet to be established, but has been estimated to range between 6 and 10% *(69,70)*. Habitual post-ictal psychotic symptoms have been found in 7% of 100 consecutive patients with refractory partial epilepsy *(27)*. Common findings include the following:

1. A delay between the onset of psychiatric symptoms and the time of the last seizure.
2. A relatively short duration.
3. An affect-laden symptomatology.
4. Clustering of symptoms into delusional and affective-like psychosis.
5. An increase in the frequency of secondarily generalized tonic-clonic seizures preceding the onset of post-ictal psychosis (PIP).
6. Onset of PIP after having seizures for a mean period of more than 10 years.
7. Prompt response to low-dose neuroleptic medication or benzodiazepines *(70–74)*.

In a study with 8 years of follow-up on patients with PIP, 3 developed chronic psychosis and 4 of 14 patients died *(73)*.

In most cases, insomnia is the initial presenting symptom. In patients with recurrent PIP episodes, families need to learn to recognize these symptoms so that a timely administration of 1 to 2 mg of risperidone may avert the episode. Risperidone should be given for 2–5 days and then discontinued.

The occurrence of PIP episodes also has important localizing implications. PIP suggests the presence of bilateral independent *ictal foci (72–74)* so that patients undergoing surgical evaluation may require longer video-EEG (VEEG) monitoring studies and possibly the use of intracranial electrodes. If recordings with depth or subdural electrodes are used, prophylactic treatment with low-dose risperidone or haloperidol can avert the occurrence of such episodes during the invasive VEEG monitoring studies *(70)*.

Ictal psychotic symptoms or episodes should always be considered in the differential diagnosis of PIP and psychosis of epilepsy (POE), as a whole. It is typically a result of nonconvulsive status epilepticus. The presence of unresponsiveness and automatisms should increase the suspicion. Yet, confirmation with EEG recordings is of the essence as certain psychotic processes, such as catatonic states, can be associated with unresponsiveness and mannerisms that mimic automatisms.

Alternative Psychosis or "Forced Normalization"

The concept of alternative psychosis, developed from observations by Landoldt in 1953, *(26)* is an inverse relation between seizure control and psychotic symptom occurrence. He described a "normalization" of EEG recordings with the appearance of psychiatric symptoms and coined the term "forced normalization." Forced normalization has been reported in patients with TLE and generalized epilepsies. Dongier reported the disappearance of a focal discharge during a psychotic episode in 15% of 318 patients with peri-ictal psychoses *(69)*. Prevalence rates of alternative psychosis are reported to be 11–25% *(75)*. As with other forms of POE, the psychotic manifestations were identified after a 15.2-year history of epilepsy in 23 patients reported by Wolf *(76)*. The dopamine (DA) system has been implicated in forced normalization. DA antagonists provoke seizures, and DA agonists have anticonvulsant properties but may precipitate psychosis. Both Landoldt and Wolf reported a pleomorphic clinical presentation with a paranoid psychosis without clouding of consciousness being the most frequent manifestation. A premonitory phase involving insomnia, anxiety, a feeling of oppression, and social withdrawal may occur in a prodomal phase. Forced normalization may then manifest as psychosis, conversion symptoms, hypochondriasis, depression or mania.

INTER-ICTAL PSYCHOSIS OF EPILEPSY

Inter-ictal psychotic disorders can present with delusions, hallucinations, referential thinking, and thought disorders, as in patients without epilepsy. Slater coined the term of inter-ictal POE to describe certain clinical characteristics, particularly, psychotic episodes seen inter-ictally in patients with chronic epilepsy *(77)*. The description of these cases is remarkable for *the absence* of negative symptoms, better pre-morbid history, and less common deterioration of the patients' personality. The psychosis is less severe and more responsive to therapy.

Iatrogenic Psychotic Disorders

AED-Related Psychosis

Psychotic disorder as an expression of a drug toxicity has been reported with several AEDs, most prominently ethosuximide, phenobarbital, and primidone as well as the newer AEDs topiramate and levetiracetam *(34)*. Psychotic disorders can occasionally follow the discontinuation of AEDs, particularly those with mood-stabilizing properties. Ketter et al. reported the development of some cases who experienced psychosis among 32 inpatients who were withdrawn from carbamazepine, phenytoin, and valproic acid *(43)*. Acute withdrawal from benzodiazepines is well known to result in an acute psychotic episode *(78)*.

Psychosis Following Temporal Lobectomy

Temporal lobectomy has been associated with postoperative psychosis. In a series of 100 of Falconer's patients, Taylor reported 7 with *de novo* postoperative psychosis *(79)*. Jensen and Vaernet reported *de novo* psychotic disorders in 9 of 74 patients *(80)*. Trimble calculated postoperative *de novo* psychoses to range between 3.8 and 35.7% (mean, 7.6%) of patients and suggested that in at least some cases a causal relation by way of forced normalization was possible *(81)*.

Many epilepsy centers currently do not consider patients with a preoperative history of psychosis as candidates for epilepsy surgery. Thus, more recent reports of postsurgical psychosis in patients are primarily *de novo* psychoses, which would be expected to be of lower incidence than postoperative exacerbations of pre-existing psychosis.

Yet, a history of psychosis should not be considered an absolute contraindication to epilepsy surgery, provided that the patient can cooperate during the presurgical evaluation, has a clear understanding of the nature of the surgical procedure, and can provide a fully informed consent.

Drug Treatment of Psychosis in Epilepsy Patients

Antipsychotic drugs (APDs) are necessary in the management of psychotic disorders in epilepsy patients despite their proconvulsant properties. Although it is essential that the risk of seizure occurrence be always carefully considered when starting APDs in these patients, it should never be a reason not to treat a patient in need of APD.

The seizure rate associated with the use of APDs has ranged between 0.5 and 1.2% among patients without epilepsy *(82)*. The risk is higher with certain drugs, and in the presence of the following factors: a history of epilepsy, abnormal EEG recordings, history of CNS disorder, rapid titration of the APD dose, high doses of APD, and the presence of other drugs that lower the seizure threshold *(34)*. For example, when chlorpromazine is used at doses above 1000 mg per day, the incidence of seizures was reported to increase to 9%, in contrast to a 0.5% incidence when lower doses are taken *(83)*. Clozapine has been reported to cause seizures in 4.4% when used at doses above 600 mg per day, whereas at a doses lower than 300 mg, the incidence of seizures is less than 1% *(84)*. Although these two drugs have been associated with the higher frequencies of seizures, most APDs have been associated with seizure occurrence in the presence of the risk factors just cited.

Unfortunately, the impact of APD on seizure occurrence among PWE has not been properly studied. Pacia and Devinsky reviewed the incidence of seizures among 5629 patients treated with clozapine *(85)*. Sixteen of these patients had epilepsy before the start of this APD and all patients experienced worsening of seizures while on the drug: 8 patients at doses lower than 300 mg per day, 3 patients at doses between 300 and 600 mg per day, and 5 at doses higher than 600 mg per day. Higher doses of clozapine were associated with greater risk of seizures than lower dose therapy *(85)*. It goes without saying that clozapine should be avoided or used in exceptional circumstances with extreme caution in PWE.

Most APD can cause EEG changes consisting of slowing of the background activity particularly when used at high doses. In addition, some APDs, particularly clozapine, can cause paroxysmal electrographic changes in the form of inter-ictal sharp waves and spikes. This type of epileptiform activity, however, is not predictive of seizure occurrence. Data from studies by Tiihonen et al. suggest that a severe disorganization of the EEG recordings is a better predictor of seizure occurrence *(86)*.

Clozapine followed by chlorpromazine and loxapine are the three APD with the highest risk of seizure occurrence. Those with a lower seizure risk include haloperidol, molindone, fluphenazine, perphenazine, trifluoperazine, and the atypical, risperidone. The PDR data available on the atypicals report seizures during clinical trials occurring with olanzapine (0.9%), quetiapine (0.8%), risperidone (0.3%) and ziprasidone (0.4%) *(59)*. Whether the presence of AEDs at adequate levels protects patients with epilepsy from breakthrough seizures upon the introduction of APD with proconvulsant properties, is yet to be established. AEDs are sometimes started when clozapine is used at greater than 600 mg per day.

In addition to the proconvulsant properties of APD, clinicians must also consider the pharmacokinetic and pharmacodynamic interactions between APD and AEDs. Induction of hepatic enzymes on the introduction of enzyme-inducing AEDs may result in an increase of the clearance of most APD. By the same token, discontinuation of an AED with enzyme-inducing properties may result in a decrease in the clearance of APD, which in turn can lead to extrapyramidal side effects caused by an increase of their serum concentrations. Finally, certain AEDs, like VA , can inhibit the glucuronidation metabolism of APD like clozapine.

ATTENTION DEFICIT DISORDERS AND BEHAVIOR DISTURBANCES

In a population-based study carried out in the Isle of White in Great Britain, Rutter and colleagues found behavioral disorders in 28.6% of children with uncomplicated seizures, and 58.3% of children with both seizures and additional CNS pathology *(16)*. In a separate population-based study of children with seizures, cardiac disorders, and controls, McDermott and colleagues found that children with epilepsy had more behavioral problems than either the children with cardiac disease or the controls. The children with epilepsy presented with higher rates of hyperactive behavior (28.1 vs 12.6% in cardiac children and 4.9% in controls), headstrong or oppositional behavior (28.1 vs 18.3% of cardiac children and 8.6% of controls), and antisocial behavior (18.2 vs 11.6% of cardiac children and 8.8% of controls) *(17)*.

Symptoms of ADD and Behavior Disorders As an Expression of Para-Ictal Phenomena

Pre-Ictal Symptoms and Episodes

Pre-ictal irritability, impulsive behavior, and poor frustration-tolerance have all been reported by parents of epileptic without attention deficit hyperactivity disorder (ADHD). Their actual prevalence rates are yet to be established, however. Blanchet and Frommer identified pre-ictal irritability as a prominent symptom, associated with symptoms of depression *(26)*. These changes were more accentuated during the 24 hours preceding the seizure.

Post-Ictal Symptoms of ADD and Behavioral Disturbances

In the study on clinical characteristics and prevalence of post-ictal psychiatric symptoms cited previously *(27)*, post-ictal irritability was seen in 30 patients and poor frustration tolerance in 36, with a median duration of 24 hours for each symptom (range: 0.5 to 108 hours).

ADD and Behavioral Disturbances As an Expression of Other Para-Ictal Processes

Behavior disturbances and ADD are frequent expressions of para-ictal processes, remitting or improving significantly upon reaching seizure control. Examples include "epileptic encephalopathies" such as the acquired epileptic aphasia of childhood (also known as Landau-Kleffner Syndrome) *(87)*.

Aggressive behavior and ADD can be seen in children with gelastic seizures associated with hypothalamic hamartomas. These psychiatric symptoms remit with cessation of epileptic seizures *(88)*.

ADD and Behavioral Disturbances As a Co-Morbid Disorder:
Inter-Ictal ADD and Behavioral Disturbances

The prevalence of ADHD in PWE is reported to range from 10 to 40% *(16–18)*. Many of the AEDs can cause symptoms of behavioral disturbances. The most frequent offenders include GABAergic drugs such as the barbiturates, benzodiazepines, and vigabatrin. Among the newer AEDs, topiramate and levetiracetam have been implicated. Valproic acid can cause behavioral disturbances at higher doses and encephalopathy even with therapeutic doses.

Treatment of Attention Deficit Hyperactivity Disorder in Patients With Epilepsy

The pharmacologic treatment of ADHD in PWE is the same as that of patients without seizures. In general, there is no pharmacokinetic interaction between CNS stimulants and AEDs, though there have been two reports that methylphenidate can increase blood levels of phenytoin and phenobarbital *(34)*.

NONEPILEPTIC SEIZURES

Nonepileptic events are either physiologic or psychological in origin. Psychological nonepileptic seizures (NES) resemble epileptic seizures (ES) presenting as a sudden, involuntary, time-limited alteration in behavior, motor activity, autonomic function, consciousness, or sensation. However, unlike epilepsy, NES do not result from epileptogenic pathology and are not accompanied by an epileptiform electrographic ictal pattern. Patients with NES are often disabled and difficult to treat.

Epidemiology

Of the 1% of the US population with epilepsy, between 5 and 20% have NES *(89)*. They are usually women (approx 80%) and are between 15 to 35 years old (approx 80%) *(90)*, although young children and the elderly can also develop NES. The patients, their family, and society bear an enormous cost if psychiatric care is not provided or if inappropriate neurological therapy is instituted. NES are not directly treated by AEDs, and yet most patients with NES receive unnecessary AEDs *(91)*. Extensive observational data suggest that AEDs are ineffective or may worsen NES *(92)*. In some cases, potentially dangerous invasive diagnostic studies, toxic parenteral medications, or emergent intubation are administered. Diagnostic and therapeutic challenges are complicated by the 10–30% rate of co-morbid NES and ES. Misdiagnosis and mistreatment of NES as ES costs an estimated $110–920 million annually on diagnostic evaluations, inappropriate administration of AEDs, and emergency department utilization *(93)*.

Pathology

Although we do not have a specific "lesion" that explains NES, we do have an understanding of the co-morbid psychopathology in patients with NES. The phenomenology of NES, also referred to as pseudoseizures, is well defined, with systematic assessments of diagnostic co-morbidities and psychological testing *(94,95)*. Studies have informed us of risk factors for NES (e.g., sexual or physical abuse, head injury) *(96,97)*, and good prognostic features for NES resolution (e.g., female, independent lifestyle, short duration of NES) *(98–101)*. Negative prognostic factors include longer duration of NES, co-morbid neurological and/or psychiatric disease, and pending litigation, among others. Interestingly, CNS pathology and abnormal EEG did not predict outcome in two studies *(102,103)*.

No single psychopathogenic process causes NES. NES are clinically classified under different DSM-IV diagnoses, including conversion, somatization, and dissociation disorders and a much smaller percentage as factitious disorder and malingering. A psychosocial stressor (e.g., sexual or physical abuse, loss of a relationship, work stress, parental divorce) *(104)* is often identified but may take months to uncover. Many patients with NES also suffer from mood (12–100%), anxiety (11–80%), personality (33–66%), nonseizure conversion/somatoform (20–100%), and nonseizure dissociative disorders (up to 90%) co-occurring with their primary NES diagnosis of conversion, somatoform, or dissociative disorder *(99)*.

Diagnosis of Nonepileptic Seizures

Obtaining an accurate diagnosis of NES is the essential first step for instituting proper therapy and avoiding unnecessary and potentially dangerous therapies. Clinical features of ES and NES overlap, however, and there is no one clinical feature that reliably distinguishes ES from NES. Subjective visceral, sensory or psychic phenomena, alterations in responsiveness, and convulsive motor activity can be present in both disorders. Ictal presentations range from uncoordinated disorganized motor activity to unresponsiveness without motor signs in NES. Clinical differentiation between NES and ES has also been based on other identifiers such as the presence of pre-ictal pseudosleep (where patients report being asleep but EEG shows them to be awake), and geotropic eye movements (forced downward deviation of the eyes toward the floor with head turning) with NES, and the presence of post-ictal headache and post-ictal nose rubbing with epilepsy. The use of suggestion in order to both provoke and stop NES is documented. With the issue of disclosure and informed consent, activation procedures have drawn fire recently as a potentially unethical intervention *(105)*. However, when properly employed, seizure induction can act as a "stepping stone" to treatment if the patient develops insight into the events *(106)*. The distinction between epilepsy physiologic nonepileptic events and psychological NES is based on the combination of thorough history, physical exam in the peri-ictal period, and neurophysiologic monitoring.

VEEG monitoring led to an explosion of NES knowledge beginning in the 1980s *(107–110)*. A recent article reviewing the diagnostic tests, including EEG, neuroimaging, prolactin levels, and personality testing provides the sensitivities and specificities for each of these tests *(111)*. It was once thought that absence of physical injury sustained during a seizure was a diagnostic indicator differentiating NES from ES; however, more than half of all patients with NES actually do have physical injury associated with their NES *(112)*. Other injuries occur as a result of iatrogenic issues that are also prevalent in NES, and death has resulted in medically aggressive treatment of NES *(113)*. Up to one half of NES patients have had "pseudostatus epilepticus" and 27.8% of patients with NES are admitted to intensive care units inappropriately for treatment *(114)*.

Nonepileptic seizures are not associated with epileptiform discharges on VEEG recordings, the gold standard for NES diagnosis *(115)*. Humility in diagnosing NES without VEEG—and sometimes with VEEG—is critical. In one study, prediction of the nature of unusual seizures by the admitting neurologist was accurate in only 67% of cases. When observing these events without accompanying EEG, determination from observations of unit personnel and neurologists was correct in less than 80% of episodes *(116)*. Lancman et al. strongly assert "no matter how suggestive the clinical manifestation of a paroxysmal event may be of pseudoseizures, such diagnosis should never be made without electrographic confirmation" *(117)*. The co-occurrence of ES and NES in a patient further complicates diagnosis and therapy. The diagnosis of mixed ES/NES comes through careful history and thorough review of medical records that can identify different episode types and assessment of the supportive data.

Electroencephalographic abnormalities in patients with NES do not necessarily confirm the diagnosis of ES. For example, EEGs showing "sharpish waves" or paroxysmal slowing provide little support of ES. A positive neurological history was present in one-fourth of patients with NES and a positive family history of epilepsy was present in 37.6% of NES patients *(118)*. Although neurological signs/symptoms and history are important to note in seizure patients, they are in no way pathognomic in distinguishing NES from ES. A recent paper described three criteria in NES patients admitted for VEEG, yielding a positive predictive value of 85% *(119)*. The criteria were: (a) at least two NES per week, (b) refractory to at least two AEDs, and (c) at least two EEGs without epileptiform activity. Using "the rule of two's" documenting seizure frequency, EEG abnormalities, and drug treatment response prior to VEEG may help with definitive diagnosis of NES.

Treatment Literature

Despite diagnostic advances, there is no standardized, effective treatment for NES. Even as our knowledge of NES phenomenology continues to grow, there are no published randomized placebo-controlled trials for treatment of NES. The literature provides widely divergent views on natural history and outcome, as well as the value of psychotherapy, psychotropic medication, and other interventions for NES *(100,120–122)*. We still lack controlled studies on treatment of this costly and disabling disorder, despite our knowledge of it for three centuries.

A systematic review of all of the NES treatment literature has been published *(123)*. There are only four references to a prospective series in the NES treatment literature published. Ataoglu et al. *(124)*, randomized 30 patients with NES, half to paradoxical intention (PI) inpatient psychotherapy, and the other half to oral benzodiazepine therapy. PI consists of the therapist suggesting that the patient engage in the undesired activity intentionally. The authors found greater improvements in anxiety scores and mildly better seizure control in the PI group than in the diazepam group. An uncontrolled individualized psychological therapeutic program for 16 patients with NES for an average of 12 weeks resulted in complete cessation of NES in half of the patients *(125)*. More recently, two prospective, open trials of cognitive-behavioral therapy and group psychotherapy showed reduction in NES frequency and posttraumatic symptoms, respectively *(126,127)*.

In a follow-up cohort study, 11 of 14 (79%) inpatients with NES experienced cessation or significant improvement after receiving a combination of hypnosis, group therapy, family therapy, and individual therapy *(128)*. A follow-up study at a comprehensive epilepsy center (CEP) *(121)* suggested that CEP psychotherapists and CEP neurologists have a similar favorable treatment outcome, underscoring the beneficial impact of continuity of care and explanation of the nature of the seizures. The study also showed that the absence of communication with a NES patient about the diagnosis yields no improvement or worsening in their seizures. Rusch et al. *(129)* found that matching specific psychotherapies to the patient's co-morbid diagnoses produced greater seizure-free rates, with 21 of 33 patients (63%) reaching event-free status at the end of treatment.

TREATMENT OF NES

Despite our preliminary understanding of risk factors, treatment for patients with NES is poorly understood. One of the main reasons for this is the lack systematic intervention studies. The void of generalizable, effective treatments for NES leaves only consensus recommendations *(120)*. Although psychotherapy is the mainstay of treatment recommendations, *(120,121)* its efficacy remains unproven. Further, no medications have been proven effective in the treatment of NES. Clinicians do, however, use psychotropic medications to treat co-morbid mood, anxiety, and elements of personality disorders, which often occur in patients with NES.

Treatment Theories

Etiological approaches for NES include biomedical, psychodynamic, cognitive-behavioral, and family theory models *(130–132)*. The diagnosis of NES is often seen as a unitary disorder or syndrome. Just as the behavioral manifestations of NES vary tremendously, the underlying etiologies are also varied. Precursors to psychogenic NES include childhood sexual abuse, physical abuse, co-morbid psychiatric conditions, minor head trauma, disability claims, and reinforced behavioral patterns, among others. In identifying signs, symptoms, and situations that are associated with NES in a patient, we can then provide interventions to promote the mental, physical, and social health of the patient *(133)*.

Biomedical approaches highlight the absence of epileptiform activity during NES, demonstrating a functional-neuroanatomic dissociation model for NES *(134,135)*. AEDs do not treat NES and in some patients can worsen NES *(136)*. Antidepressant, antianxiety, and antipsychotic therapies (e.g., medication, relaxation techniques) can treat symptomatic co-morbid disorders and are currently being studied to evaluate if medications may indirectly improve NES frequency or severity.

NES are currently treated as a neuropsychiatric illness with psychological underpinnings. Both psychotherapeutic and psychopharmacological interventions are used to treat psychological conflicts and to treat the psychiatric co-morbid diagnoses. These approaches fall under the headings of psychodynamic psychotherapy, cognitive-behavioral therapies, family systems therapies, behavioral modification (mainly for mentally handicapped individuals), and biological psychiatric treatments.

Conceptualization for Treatment Recommendations

Bowman recommends the "four Es" for interventions by neurologists: explanation, exploration, exportation (for treatment), and do not exile. The circumspect neurologist will exercise caution when deciding whether or not to "explore" a patient's trauma history. The "exile" issue is of greatest importance. Once the VEEG diagnosis of NES is confirmed, the difficult work of collaboratively treating the patient with colleagues in psychiatry is just begun.

Treatment and outcome vary considerably with the underlying psychopathology. Patients with NES generally have poor to fair treatment outcomes, but children and adolescents tend to do better than adults. In one study, outcome was significantly better for the younger patients at 1, 2, and 3 years after diagnosis (seizure free percentages: children 73, 75, 81%, and adults 25, 25, 40%, respectively). The authors proposed that different psychological mechanisms at different ages of onset and greater effectiveness with earlier intervention may be factors leading to better outcome for children and adolescents *(139)*.

Higher success rates are noted in the treatment articles and chapters describing longer inpatient admissions where patients were managed by a multidisciplinary team familiar with NES *(140)*. More recent reviews, however, reveal that roughly one-third of the patients have NES cessation, and another one-third have reduction in their NES *(141)*. In one NES outcome study, 71% of patients reported persistence of their seizures, despite 41% of the patients having had inpatient psychiatric treatment *(114)*. Of the patients with lone NES, 40% continued to receive AEDs inappropriately, impacting quality of life. Quigg et al. found that quality-of-life measures improve, however, when patients reach NES freedom, and not when their NES are merely reduced *(142)*. Even with NES improvement, up to half of the patients remain on government or family support and are unemployed *(132)*, and patients with NES generally do not expect to return to work *(143)*. One study found that patients with NES scored higher on hypochondriasis and somatic-complaint scales of the Minnesota Multiphasic Personality Inventory when compared with PWE, reflective of a focus on bodily function and neurological complaints *(144)*. Poor quality of life in patients with NES may partly result from their somatic focus. A factor analysis of predictors of health-related quality of life revealed that patients with NES had more bodily concern than those with epilepsy *(145)*, and that somatic focus may influence health-related quality of life.

Noting the good prognosis if NES has a recent onset, Gates suggested that psychiatric treatment be based on NES chronicity: short-term psychotherapy for those with NES less than 6 months, and more intensive inpatient therapy for longstanding NES *(146)*. Although patients who receive feedback about their diagnosis and psychotherapy have better outcomes than those who do not *(121)*, the difference may reflect baseline characteristics of the groups, rather than the effects of intervention.

Based on the clinical and research reports to date, we suggest the following assessment and treatment approach by a multispecialty neuropsychiatric team:

1. Proper diagnosis: VEEG for each patient with suspected NES, refractory, or pharmacoresistant seizures.
2. Presentation: explain the NES diagnosis in a clear, positive, nonpejorative manner. The patient may make the diagnosis presentation to the family members if cognitively and emotionally capable. This process helps reveal the level of understanding and initial acceptance of the diagnosis by the patient. Clarifications can be made by the physician who is present. Communicate the diagnosis unambiguously to the referring physician and explain the need to eliminate unnecessary medications in lone NES, or modification in mixed ES/NES.
3. Psychiatric treatment: conduct a thorough psychiatric assessment to identify predisposing factors (including co-morbid psychiatric disorders), seizure precipitants, and perpetuating factors. As diagnosis informs treatment, a dual-armed approach ensues with pharmacotherapy and/or psychotherapy, as indicated by the individual needs of the patient with NES.

Psychopharmacology begins with tapering and discontinuing ineffective AEDs for patients with lone NES, unless a specific AED has a documented beneficial psychopharmacological effect in the patient. In patients with mixed ES/NES, reduce high-dose or multiple AED therapy if possible. Use psychopharmacological agents to treat mood, anxiety, or psychotic disorders.

CONCLUSIONS

Psychological NES are likely the result of a complex interaction between psychiatric disorders, psychosocial stressors, dysfunctional coping styles, and CNS vulnerability *(147)*. Identifying the underlying stressors and providing supportive psychotherapy can help some patients but is often insufficient or ineffective. Studies consistently identify three main co-morbid diagnoses in patients with NES: major depressive disorder, posttraumatic stress disorder, and cluster B personality traits characterized by impulsivity/hostility *(148,149)*. Three additional critical areas of dysfunction in the NES population are: emotion regulation, family dynamics, and unemployment/disability *(122,150,151)*. Poorer outcomes to treatment may be associated with the high number of co-morbid psychiatric disorders and psychosocial stressors *(152)*. Therefore, treatment for patients with NES may require coordination between neurologists and psychiatrists/psychologists with combined psychological education, psychotherapy, and pharmacotherapy, while simultaneously eliminating ineffective AEDs. There is a great need for these interventions to be studied in randomized, controlled trials.

In conclusion, a significant number of PWE have psychiatric disorders that accompany their seizures, and/or integrated mood/anxiety/psychotic and personality integrated symptoms secondary to their epilepsy. Management of epilepsy is also complicated by the presence of NES. Further research in these three areas is needed to inform diagnosis, pathophysiology, and treatment of these neuropsychiatric aspects of epilepsy.

REFERENCES

1. Kogeorgos J, Fonagy P, Scott DF. Psychiatric symptom patterns of chronic epileptics attending a neurological clinic: a controlled investigation. Br J Psychiatry 1982;140:236–243.
2. Jacoby A, Baker GA, Steen N, Potts P, Chadwick DW. The clinical course of epilepsy and its psychosocial correlates: findings from a U.K. Community study. Epilepsia 1996;37:148–161.
3. O'Donoghue MF, Goodridge DM, Redhead K, Sander JW, Duncan JS. Assessing the psychosocial consequences of epilepsy: a community-based study. Br J Gen Pract 1999;49:211–214.
4. Edeh J, Toone B. Relationship between interictal psychopathology and the type of epilepsy. Results of a survey in general practice. Br J Psychiatry 1987;151:95–101.
5. Blum D, Reed M, Metz A. Prevalence of major affective disorders and manic/hypomanic symptoms in persons with epilepsy: a community survey. Neurology 2002;58(Suppl2):A174.
6. Mendez MF, Cummings JL, Benson DF. Depression in epilepsy. Significance and phenomenology. Arch Neurol 1986;43: 766–770.
7. Regier DA, Farmer ME, Rae DS, et al. One-month prevalence of mental disorders in the United States and sociodemographic characteristics: the Epidemiologic Catchment Area study. Acta Psychiatr Scand 1993;88:35–47.
8. Kessler RC, McGonagle KA, Zhao S, et al. Lifetime and 12-month prevalence of DSM-III-R psychiatric disorders in the United States. Results from the National Comorbidity Survey. Arch Gen Psychiatry 1994;51:8–19.
9. Schmitz B, Wolf P. Psychosis in epilepsy: frequency and risk factors. J Epilepsy 1995;8:295–305.
10. Onuma T, Adachi N, Ishida S, Katou M, Uesugi S. Prevalence and annual incidence of psychosis in patients with epilepsy. Psychiatry Clin Neurosci 1995;49:S267–S268.
11. Bredkjaer SR, Mortensen PB, Parnas J. Epilepsy and non-organic non-affective psychosis. National epidemiologic study. Br J Psychiatry 1998;172:235–238.
12. Currie S, Heathfield KW, Henson RA, Scott DF. Clinical course and prognosis of temporal lobe epilepsy. A survey of 666 patients. Brain 1971;94:173–190.
13. Perini GI, Tosin C, Carraro C, et al. Interictal mood and personality disorders in temporal lobe epilepsy and juvenile myoclonic epilepsy. J Neurol Neurosurg Psychiatry 1996;61:601–605.
14. Pariente PD, Lepine JP, Lellouch J. Lifetime history of panic attacks and epilepsy: an association from a general population survey. J Clin Psychiatry 1991;52:88–89.
15. Roy-Byrne PP, Stein MB, Russo J, et al. Panic disorder in the primary care setting: comorbidity, disability, service utilization, and treatment. J Clin Psychiatry 1999;60:492–499.
16. Rutter M, Graham P, Yule W. A Neuropsychiatric Study in Childhood. Philadelphia: JB Lippincott; 1970.
17. McDermott S, Mani S, Krishnaswami S. A population-based analysis of specific behavior problems associated with childhood seizures. J Epilepsy 1995;8:100–110.
18. Semrud-Clikeman M, Wical B. Components of attention in children with complex partial seizures with and without ADHD. Epilepsia 1999;40:211–215.
19. Brown RT, Freeman WS, Perrin JM, et al. Prevalence and assessment of attention-deficit/hyperactivity disorder in primary care settings. Pediatrics 2001;107:E43.
20. Forsgren L, Nystrom L. An incident case-referent study of epileptic seizures in adults. Epilepsy Res 1990;6:66–81.
21. Hesdorffer DC, Hauser WA, Annegers JF, Cascino G. Major depression is a risk factor for seizures in older adults. Ann Neurol 2000;47:246–249.
22. Robertson MM. Suicide, parasuicide, and epilepsy. In: Pedley T, Engel J, eds. Epilepsy: A Comprehensive Textbook. Philadelphia: Lippincott-Raven; 1997.
23. Rafnsson V, Olafsson E, Hauser WA, Gudmundsson G. Cause-specific mortality in adults with unprovoked seizures. A population-based incidence cohort study. Neuroepidemiology 2001;20:232–236.
24. Nilsson L, Tomson T, Farahmand BY, Diwan V, Persson PG. Cause-specific mortality in epilepsy: a cohort study of more than 9,000 patients once hospitalized for epilepsy. Epilepsia 1997;38:1062–1068.
25. Gilliam F, Kanner AM. Treatment of depressive disorders in epilepsy patients. Epilepsy Behav 2002;3:2–9.
26. Blanchet P, Frommer GP. Mood change preceding epileptic seizures. J Nerv Ment Dis 1986;174:471–476.
27. Kanner AM, Soto A, Gross-Kanner H. Prevalence and clinical characteristics of postictal psychiatric symptoms in partial epilepsy. Neurology 2004;62:708–713.
28. Hancock JC, Bevilacqua AR. Temporal lobe dysrhythmia and impulsive or suicidal behavior: preliminary report. South Med J 1971;64:1189–1193.
29. Anatassopoulos G, Kokkini D. Suicidal attempts in psychomotor epilepsy. Behav Neuropsychiatry 1969;1:11–16.
30. Williams D. The structure of emotions reflected in epileptic experiences. Brain 1956;79:29–67.
31. Weil AA. Depressive reactions associated with temporal lobe-uncinate seizure. J Nerv Ment Dis 1955;121:505–510.

32. Daly D. Ictal affect. Am J Psychiatry 1958;115:97–108.

33. Blumer D, Altshuler, LL. Affective disorders. In: Engel J, Pedley TA, eds. Epilepsy: A Comprehensive Textbook, Version II. Philadelphia: Lippincott-Raven; 1998:2083–2099.

34. McConnell H, Duncan, D. Treatment of psychiatric comorbidity in epilepsy. In: McConnell H, Snyder P, eds. Psychiatric Comorbidity in Epilepsy.Washington, DC: American Psychiatric Press;1998:245.

35. Brent DA, Crumrine PK, Varma RR, Allan M, Allman C. Phenobarbital treatment and major depressive disorder in children with epilepsy. Pediatrics 1987;80:909–917.

36. Ferrari M, Barabas G, Matthews WS. Psychologic and behavioral disturbance among epileptic children treated with barbiturate anticonvulsants. Am J Psychiatry 1983;140:112–113.

37. Smith DB, Mattson RH, Cramer JA, Collins JF, Novelly RA, Craft B. Results of a nationwide Veterans Administration Cooperative Study comparing the efficacy and toxicity of carbamazepine, phenobarbital, phenytoin, and primidone. Epilepsia 1987;28(Suppl 3):S50–S58.

38. Barabas G, Matthews WS. Barbiturate anticonvulsants as a cause of severe depression. Pediatrics 1988;82:284–285.

39. Ring HA, Reynolds EH. Vigabatrin and behaviour disturbance. Lancet 1990;335:970.

40. McConnell H, Duffy J, Cress K. Behavioral effects of felbamate. J Neuropsychiatry Clin Neurosci 1994;6:323.

41. Kanner AM, Faught E, French J, et al. Psychiatric adverse events caused by topiramate and lamotrigine: a postmarketing prevalence and risk factor study. Epilepsia 2000;41:169.

42. Mula M, Trimble MR. The importance of being seizure free: topiramate and psychopathology in epilepsy. Epilepsy Behav 2003;4:430–434.

43. Ketter TA, Malow BA, Flamini R, White SR, Post RM, Theodore WH. Anticonvulsant withdrawal-emergent psychopathology. Neurology 1994;44:55–61.

44. Savard G, Andermann LF, Reutens D, Andermann F. Epilepsy, surgical treatment and postoperative psychiatric complications: a re-evaluation of the evidence. In: Trimble M, Schmitz B, eds. Forced Normalization and Alternative Psychosis of Epilepsy. Petersfield: Writson Biomedical Publishing Ltd; 1998:179–192.

45. Lehrner J, Kalchmayr R, Serles W, et al. Health-related quality of life (HRQOL), activity of daily living (ADL) and depressive mood disorder in temporal lobe epilepsy patients. Seizure 1999;8:88–92.

46. Perrine K, Hermann BP, Meador KJ, et al. The relationship of neuropsychological functioning to quality of life in epilepsy. Arch Neurol 1995;52:997–1003.

47. Gilliam F, Kuzniecky R, Faught E, Black L, Carpenter G, Schrodt R. Patient-validated content of epilepsy-specific quality-of-life measurement. Epilepsia 1997;38:233–236.

48. Gilliam F. Optimizing health outcomes in active epilepsy. Neurology 2002;58(Suppl 5):S9–S20.

49. Rosenstein DL, Nelson JC, Jacobs SC. Seizures associated with antidepressants: a review. J Clin Psychiatry 1993;54:289–299.

50. Preskorn SH, Fast GA. Tricyclic antidepressant-induced seizures and plasma drug concentration. J Clin Psychiatry 1992;53:160–162.

51. Curran S, de Pauw K. Selecting an antidepressant for use in a patient with epilepsy. Safety considerations. Drug Saf 1998; 18:125–133.

52. Swinkels J, Jonghe F. Safety of antidepressants. Int Clin Psychopharmacol 1995;9:19–25.

53. Kanner AM, Kozak AM, Frey M. The use of sertraline in patients with epilepsy: Is It Safe? Epilepsy Behav 2000;1:100–105.

54. Blumer D, Zielinksi J. Pharmacologic treatment of psychiatric disorders associated with epilepsy. J Epilepsy 1988;1: 135–150.

55. Grimsley SR, Jann MW, Carter JG, D'Mello AP, D'Souza MJ. Increased carbamazepine plasma concentrations after fluoxetine coadmistration. Clin Pharmacol Ther 1991;50:10–15.

56. Pearson HJ. Interaction of fluoxetine with carbamazepine. J Clin Psychiatry 1990;51:126.

57. Fritze J, Unsorg B, Lanczik M. Interaction between carbamazepine and fluvoxamine. Acta Psychiatr Scand 1991;84: 583–584.

58. Haselberger MB, Freedman LS, Tolbert S. Elevated serum phenytoin concentrations associated with coadmistration of sertraline. J Clin Psychopharmacol 1997;17:107–109.

59. Physicians' Desk Reference, Fifty-Sixth Edition. Montvale, NJ: Medical Economics; 2002.

60. Bell AJ, Cole A, Eccleston D, Ferrier IN. Lithium neurotoxicity at normal therapeutic levels. Br J Psychiatry 1993;162: 689–692.

61. Sackeim HA, Decina P, Prohovnik I, Malitz S, Resor SR. Anticonvulsant and antidepressant properties of electroconvulsive therapy: a proposed mechanism of action. Biol Psychiatry 1983;18:1301–1310.

62. Regenold WT, Weintraub D, Taller A. Electroconvulsive therapy for epilepsy and major depression. Am J Geriatr Psychiatry 1998;6:180–183.

63. Fink M, Kellner CH, Sackeim HA. Intractable seizures, status epilepticus, and ECT. J ECT 1999;15:282–284.

64. Blackwood DH, Cull RE, Freeman CP, Evans JI, Mawdsley C. A study of the incidence of epilepsy following ECT. J Neurol Neurosurg Psychiatry 1980;43:1098–1102.

65. Fisher RS, Vickrey BG, Gibson P, et al. The impact of epilepsy from the patient's perspective I. Descriptions and subjective perceptions. Epilepsy Res 2000;41:39–51.

66. Jones JE, Hermann BP, Barry JJ, Gilliam FG, Kanner AM, Meador KJ. Rates and risk factors for suicide, suicidal ideation, and suicide attempts in chronic epilepsy. Epilepsy Behav 2003;4:31–38.

67. Vazquez B, Devinsky O. Epilepsy and anxiety. Epilepsy Behav 2003;4:S20–S25.

68. Kanner AM, Ramirez L, Jones JC. The utility of placing sphenoidal electrodes under the foramen ovale with fluoroscopic guidance. J Clin Neurophysiol 1995;12:72–81.

69. Dongier S. Statistical study of clinical and electroencephalographic manifestations of 536 psychotic episodes occurring in 516 epileptics between clinical seizures. Epilepsia 1959;1:117–142.

70. Kanner AM, Stagno S, Kotagal P, Morris HH. Postictal psychiatric events during prolonged video-electroencephalographic monitoring studies. Arch Neurol 1996;53:258–263.

71. Lancman ME, Craven WJ, Asconape JJ, Penry JK. Clinical management of recurrent postictal psychosis. J Epilepsy 1994;7: 47–51.

72. Devinsky O, Abramson H, Alper K, et al. Postictal psychosis: a case control series of 20 patients and 150 controls. Epilepsy Res 1995;20:247–253.

73. Logsdail SJ, Toone BK. Post-ictal psychoses. A clinical and phenomenological description. Br J Psychiatry 1988;152: 246–252.

74. Umbricht D, Degreef G, Barr WB, Lieberman JA, Pollack S, Schaul N. Postictal and chronic psychoses in patients with temporal lobe epilepsy. Am J Psychiatry 1995;152:224–231.

75. Trimble MR, Schmitz B. The Neuropsychiatry of Epilepsy. Cambridge, UK & New York: Cambridge University Press; 2002.

76. Wolf P, Trimble MR. Biological antagonism and epileptic psychosis. Br J Psychiatry 1985;146:272–276.

77. Slater E, Beard AW, Glithero E. The schizophrenialike psychoses of epilepsy. Br J Psychiatry 1963;109:95–150.

78. Sironi VA, Franzini A, Ravagnati L, Marossero F. Interictal acute psychoses in temporal lobe epilepsy during withdrawal of anticonvulsant therapy. J Neurol Neurosurg Psychiatry 1979;42:724–730.

79. Taylor DC. Mental state and temporal lobe epilepsy. A correlative account of 100 patients treated surgically. Epilepsia 1972;13:727–765.

80. Jensen I, Vaernet K. Temporal lobe epilepsy. Follow-up investigation of 74 temporal lobe resected patients. Acta Neurochir (Wien) 1977;37:173–200.

81. Trimble MR. Behaviour changes following temporal lobectomy, with special reference to psychosis. J Neurol Neurosurg Psychiatry 1992;55:89–91.

82. Whitworth AB, Fleischhacker WW. Adverse effects of antipsychotic drugs. Int Clin Psychopharmacol 1995;(Suppl 5): 21–27.

83. Logothetis J. Spontaneous epileptic seizures and electroencephalographic changes in the course of phenothiazine therapy. Neurology 1967;17:869–877.

84. Toth P, Frankenburg FR. Clozapine and seizures: a review. Can J Psychiatry 1994;39:236–238.

85. Pacia SV, Devinsky O. Clozapine-related seizures: experience with 5,629 patients. Neurology 1994;44:2247–2249.

86. Tiihonen J, Nousiainen U, Hakola P, et al. EEG abnormalities associated with clozapine treatment. Am J Psychiatry 1991; 148:1406.

87. Morrell F, Whisler WW, Smith MC, et al. Landau-Kleffner syndrome. Treatment with subpial intracortical transection. Brain 1995;118(Pt 6):1529–1546.

88. Fohlen M, Lellouch A, Delalande O. Hypothalamic hamartoma with refractory epilepsy: surgical procedures and results in 18 patients. Epileptic Disord 2003;5:267–273.

89. Gates JR, Luciano D, Devinsky O. The classification and treatment of nonepileptic events. In: Devinsky O, Theodore WH, eds. Epilepsy and Behavior. New York: Wiley-Liss; 1991:251–263.

90. Shen W, Bowman ES, Markand ON. Presenting the diagnosis of pseudoseizure. Neurology 1990;40:756–759.

91. de Timary P, Fouchet P, Sylin M, et al. Non-epileptic seizures: delayed diagnosis in patients presenting with electro-encephalographic (EEG) or clinical signs of epileptic seizures. Seizure 2002;11:193–197.

92. Krumholz A, Niedermeyer E, Alkaitis D, Morel R. Psychogenic seizures: a 5-year follow-up study. Neurology 1980;30:392.

93. Martin RC, Gilliam FG, Kilgore M, Faught E, Kuzniecky R. Improved health care resource utilization following video-EEG-confirmed diagnosis of nonepileptic psychogenic seizures. Seizure 1998;7:385–390.

94. Gram L, Johannessen SI, Oterman PO, Sillanpaa M. Pseudo-Epileptic Seizures, First Edition. Petersfield, UK: Wrightson Biomedical Publishing; 1993.

95. Gates JR, Rowan AJ. Non-Epileptic Seizures, Second Edition. Boston, MA: Butterworth-Heinemann; 2000.

96. Alper K, Devinsky O, Perrine K, Vazquez B, Luciano D. Nonepileptic seizures and childhood sexual and physical abuse. Neurology 1993;43:1950–1953.

97. Westbrook LE, Devinsky O, Geocadin R. Nonepileptic seizures after head injury. Epilepsia 1998;39:978–982.

98. Chabolla DR, Krahn LE, So EL, Rummans TA. Psychogenic nonepileptic seizures. Mayo Clin Proc 1996;71:493–500.

99. Bowman ES. Nonepileptic seizures: psychiatric framework, treatment, and outcome. Neurology 1999;53(Suppl 2):S84–S88.

100. Barry JJ. Nonepileptic seizures: an overview. CNS Spectr 2001;6:956–962.

101. Ettinger AB, Dhoon A, Weisbrot DM, Devinsky O. Predictive factors for outcome of nonepileptic seizures after diagnosis. J Neuropsychiatry Clin Neurosci 1999;11:458–463.

102. Lelliott PT, Fenwick P. Cerebral pathology in pseudoseizures. Acta Neurol Scand 1991;83:129–132.
103. Kanner AM, Parra J, Frey M, Stebbins G, Pierre-Louis S, Iriarte J. Psychiatric and neurologic predictors of psychogenic pseudoseizure outcome. Neurology 1999;53:933–938.
104. Wyllie E, Glazer JP, Benbadis S, Kotagal P, Wolgamuth B. Psychiatric features of children and adolescents with pseudoseizures. Arch Pediatr Adolesc Med 1999;153:244–248.
105. Smith ML, Stagno SJ, Dolske M, et al. Induction procedures for psychogenic seizures: ethical and clinical considerations. J Clin Ethics 1997;8:217–229.
106. Devinsky O, Fisher R. Ethical use of placebos and provocative testing in diagnosing nonepileptic seizures. Neurology 1996;47:866–870.
107. Penin H. Elektonische Patientenuberwachung in der Nervenklinik Bonn [Electronic patient monitoring in the neurologic hospital of Bonn]. Umsschau in Wissenschaft und Technik 1968;7:211–212.
108. Desai BT, Porter RJ, Penry JK. The psychogenic seizure by videotape analysis: a study of 42 attacks in 6 patients. Neurology (Minneap.) 1979;29:602.
109. Boon PA, Williamson PD. The diagnosis of pseudoseizures. Clin Neurol Neurosurg 1993;95:1–8.
110. Jedrzejczak J, Owczarek K, Majkowski J. Psychogenic pseudoepileptic seizures: clinical and electroencephalogram (EEG) video-tape recordings. Eur J Neurol 1999;6:473–479.
111. Cragar DE, Berry DT, Fakhoury TA, Cibula JE, Schmitt FA. A review of diagnostic techniques in the differential diagnosis of epileptic and nonepileptic seizures. Neuropsychol Rev 2002;12:31–64.
112. Kanner AM. Psychogenic nonepileptic seizures are bad for your health. Epilepsy Curr 2003;3:181–182.
113. Reuber M, Baker GA, Gill R, Smith DF, Chadwick DW. Failure to recognize psychogenic nonepileptic seizures may cause death. Neurology 2004;62:834–835.
114. Reuber M, Pukrop R, Bauer J, Helmstaedter C, Tessendorf N, Elger CE. Outcome in psychogenic nonepileptic seizures: 1 to 10-year follow-up in 164 patients. Ann Neurol 2003;53:305–311.
115. Ghougassian DF, d'Souza W, Cook MJ, O'Brien TJ. Evaluating the Utility of Inpatient Video-EEG Monitoring. Epilepsia 2004;45:928–932.
116. King DW, Gallagher BB, Murvin AJ, et al. Pseudoseizures: diagnostic evaluation. Neurology 1982;32:18–23.
117. Lancman ME, Lambrakis CC, Steinhardt MI. Psychogenic pseudoseizures: a general overview. In: Ettinger AB, Kanner AM, eds. Psychiatry Issues in Epilepsy: A Practical Guide to Diagnosis and Treatment, First Edition. Philadelphia, PA: Lippincott, Williams & Wilkins; 2001:341–354.
118. Lancman ME, Brotherton TA, Asconape JJ, Penry JK. Psychogenic seizures in adults: a longitudinal analysis. Seizure 1993;2:281–286.
119. Davis BJ. Predicting nonepileptic seizures utilizing seizure frequency, EEG, and response to medication. Eur Neurol 2004; 51:153–156.
120. Ramani V. Treatment of the adult patient with non-epileptic seizures. In: Gates JR, Rowan AJ, eds. Non-Epileptic Seizures, Second Edition. Boston, MA: Butterworth-Heinemann; 2000:300–316.
121. Aboukasm A, Mahr G, Gahry BR, Thomas A, Barkley GL. Retrospective analysis of the effects of psychotherapeutic interventions on outcomes of psychogenic nonepileptic seizures. Epilepsia 1998;39:470–473.
122. Walczak TS, Papacostas S, Williams DT, Scheuer ML, Lebowitz N, Notarfrancesco A. Outcome after diagnosis of psychogenic nonepileptic seizures. Epilepsia 1995;36:1131–1137.
123. LaFrance WC Jr, Devinsky O. The treatment of nonepileptic seizures: historical perspectives and future directions. Epilepsia 2004;45(Suppl 2):1–7.
124. Ataoglu A, Ozcetin A, Icmeli C, Ozbulut O. Paradoxical therapy in conversion reaction. J Korean Med Sci 2003;18: 581–584.
125. McDade G, Brown SW. Non-epileptic seizures: management and predictive factors of outcome. Seizure 1992;1:7–10.
126. Goldstein LH, Deale AC, Mitchell-O'Malley SJ, Toone BK, Mellers JD. An evaluation of cognitive behavioral therapy as a treatment for dissociative seizures: a pilot study. Cogn Behav Neurol 2004;17:41–49.
127. Zaroff CM, Myers L, B. Barr W, Luciano D, Devinsky O. Group psychoeducation as treatment for psychological nonepileptic seizures. Epilepsy Behav 2004;5:587–592.
128. Kim CM, Barry JJ, Zeifert PA. The use of inpatient medical psychiatric treatment for nonepileptic events. Epilepsia 1998;39 (Suppl 6):242–243.
129. Rusch MD, Morris GL, Allen L, Lathrop L. Psychological treatment of nonepileptic events. Epilepsy Behav 2001;2: 277–283.
130. Ziegler FJ, Imboden JB. Contemporary conversion reactions. II. A conceptual model. Arch Gen Psychiatry 1962;6: 279–287.
131. Swingle PG. Neurofeedback treatment of pseudoseizure disorder. Biol Psychiatry 1998;44:1196–1199.
132. Krawetz P, Fleisher W, Pillay N, Staley D, Arnett J, Maher J. Family functioning in subjects with pseudoseizures and epilepsy. J Nerv Ment Dis 2001;189:38–43.
133. LaFrance WC, Jr., Devinsky O. Treatment of nonepileptic seizures. Epilepsy Behav 2002;3(Suppl 1):S19–S23.
134. Brown RJ, Trimble MR. Dissociative psychopathology, non-epileptic seizures, and neurology. J Neurol Neurosurg Psychiatry 2000;69:285–288.

135. Blumer D. On the psychobiology of non-epileptic seizures. In: Gates JR, Rowan AJ, eds. Non-Epileptic Seizures, Second Edition. Boston, MA: Butterworth-Heinemann; 2000:305–310.
136. Niedermeyer E, Blumer D, Holscher E, Walker BA. Classical hysterical seizures facilitated by anticonvulsant toxicity. Psychiatr Clin (Basel) 1970;3:71–84.
137. Chand SP, al Khalili K. Pseudoseizures associated with doll phobia. Int J Psychiatry Med 2000;30:93–96.
138. Shulman KI, Silver IL. Hysterical seizures as a manifestation of "depression" in old age. Can J Psychiatry 1985;30: 278–280.
139. Wyllie E, Friedman D, Luders H, Morris H, Rothner D, Turnbull J. Outcome of psychogenic seizures in children and adolescents compared with adults. Neurology 1991;41:742–744.
140. Ramani V, Gumnit RJ. Management of hysterical seizures in epileptic patients. Arch Neurol 1982;39:78–81.
141. Reuber M, Elger CE. Psychogenic nonepileptic seizures: review and update. Epilepsy Behav 2003;4:205–216.
142. Quigg M, Armstrong RF, Farace E, Fountain NB. Quality of life outcome is associated with cessation rather than reduction of psychogenic nonepileptic seizures. Epilepsy Behav 2002;3:455–459.
143. Pestana EM, Foldvary-Shaefer N, Marsillio D, Morris HH III. Quality of Life in Patients With Psychogenic Seizures. Neurology 2003;60:A355.
144. Owczarek K. Somatisation indexes as differential factors in psychogenic pseudoepileptic and epileptic seizures. Seizure 2003;12:178–181.
145. Testa SM, Szaflarski JP, Fargo JD, Dulay MF, Schefft BK. Psychological correlates of health-related qality of life (HRQOL) in epileptic and nonepileptic seizures. Neurology 2003;60:A383.
146. Gates JR. Diagnosis and treatment of nonepileptic seizures. In: McConnell HW, Snyder PJ, eds. Psychiatric Comorbidity in Epilepsy. Basic mechanisms, diagnosis, and treatment, First Edition.Washington, DC: American Psychiatric Press; 1998:187–204.
147. Mokleby K, Blomhoff S, Malt UF, Dahlstrom A, Tauboll E, Gjerstad L. Psychiatric comorbidity and hostility in patients with psychogenic nonepileptic seizures compared with somatoform disorders and healthy controls. Epilepsia 2002;43: 193–198.
148. Bowman ES, Markand ON. Psychodynamics and psychiatric diagnoses of pseudoseizure subjects. Am J Psychiatry 1996; 153:57–63.
149. Rechlin T, Loew TH, Joraschky P. Pseudoseizure "status." J Psychosom Res 1997;42:495–498.
150. Holmes MD, Dodrill CB, Bachtler S, Wilensky AJ, Ojemann LM, Miller JW. Evidence that emotional maladjustment is worse in men than in women with psychogenic nonepileptic seizures. Epilepsy Behav 2001;2:568–573.
151. Griffith JL, Polles A, Griffith ME. Pseudoseizures, families, and unspeakable dilemmas. Psychosomatics 1998;39:144–153.
152. Carson AJ, Ringbauer B, MacKenzie L, Warlow C, Sharpe M. Neurological disease, emotional disorder, and disability: they are related: a study of 300 consecutive new referrals to a neurology outpatient department. J Neurol Neurosurg Psychiatry 2000;68:202–206.

17

Tourette's Syndrome

Cathy Budman and Roger Kurlan

INTRODUCTION

The text revision Diagnostic and Statistical Manual of Psychiatry, Fourth Edition (DSM-IV-TR) lists the following diagnostic criteria for Tourette's syndrome (TS) *(1)*:

1. Both multiple motor and one or more vocal tics have been present at some time during the illness, although not necessarily concurrently.
2. The tics occur many times a day (usually in bouts) nearly every day or intermittently throughout a period of more than 1 year, and during this period there was never a tic-free period of more than 3 consecutive months.
3. The onset is before age 18 years.
4. The disturbance is not the result of the direct physiological effects of a substance (e.g., stimulants) or a general medical condition (e.g., Huntington's disease or post-viral encephalitis).

Whereas these categorical criteria encompass the essential diagnostic features of TS, its clinical manifestations are most commonly encountered in association with a spectrum of behavioral symptoms (Table 1).

PHENOMENOLOGY

Tics are recurrent, nonrhythmic, stereotyped movements (motor tics) or sounds produced by moving air through the nose, mouth, or throat (vocal tics) *(2)*. Simple motor tics are sudden, brief, isolated movements of a single muscle group such as an eye blink, a facial grimace, or a head jerk. Although most simple motor tics are fast and abrupt, some may appear as slower, sustained, tonic movements (e.g., neck twisting, abdominal or buttock tightening) that resemble dystonia and are therefore termed *dystonic tics (3)*. Complex motor tics consist of more coordinated and complicated movements engaging several muscle groups. Some manifest as touching, tapping, smelling, copropraxia (obscene gestures), and echopraxia (mimicking movements performed by others).

Simple vocal tics include a variety of inarticulate noises and sounds, such as throat clearing, sniffing, and humming. Complex vocal tics have linguistic meaning and consist of full or truncated words, such as echolalia (repeating the words of others), palilalia (repeating the individual's own words), and coprolalia (obscene words). Coprolalia, given its colorful, dramatic presentation, is perhaps responsible for the public notoriety of TS, yet this symptom occurs in only a minority of patients and certainly is not required for the diagnosis.

The patient often experiences an irresistible urge to tic. This urge can usually be suppressed temporarily, but at the expense of a build-up of psychic tension that can be relieved only by the performance

From: *Current Clinical Neurology: Psychiatry for Neurologists*
Edited by: D.V. Jeste and J.H. Friedman © Humana Press Inc., Totowa, NJ

Table 1
Clinical Heterogenity of Tourette's Syndrome

The tic disorder

Tic types
1. Simple motor tics
2. Simple vocal tics
3. Complex motor tics
4. Complex vocal tics
5. Tic variants
    a. Dystonic tics
    b. Sensory tics
Primary tic disorder syndromes
1. Tourette's syndrome
2. Chronic tic disorder (motor or vocal)
3. Transient tic disorder
Associated psychiatric disorders
A. Obsessive-compulsive disorder (OCD)
B. Attention deficit hyperactivity disorder
C. Non-OCD anxiety disorders
D. Mood disorders
E. Other behavioral disturbances

of a tic. Recent attention has focused on sensory symptoms that may occur in TS. "Sensory tics" are patterns of uncomfortable somatic sensations, such as pressure, tickle, or warmth, that are localized to specific body regions, such as the face, shoulder, or neck *(4,5)*. Patients attempt to relieve the uncomfortable sensations with movements often interpreted as voluntary, usually tonic tightening or stretching of muscles indicative of a dystonic tic. Relief is temporary, however, and the movements are repeated. Some patients produce vocalizations that are responses to a sensory stimulus in the larynx or throat. Sensory tics, reported by about 40% of surveyed TS patients, may be the most prominent feature of illness for some patients and are often misdiagnosed.

Typically, the motor and vocal tics of TS follow a waxing and waning pattern, such that there are periods lasting days or weeks of tic exacerbation followed by other periods during which tics are quiescent or less severe. More common tics such as eye blinking or coughing may go largely unrecognized or mistakenly ascribed to "habits," nervousness, or psychopathology.

In summary, current evidence suggests that TS and related tic disorders are quite common in the general population. For the most part, they appear to represent mild, nondisabling symptoms that do not lead to medical attention or therapy.

EPIDEMIOLOGY

There is a 3:1 male predominance among patients with TS *(6)*. The disorder has been identified in all races and appears to be uniformly distributed across socioeconomic classes *(6)*. Its clinical features are consistent among different cultural groups except that coprolalia is particularly uncommon in Japanese patients *(6)*. Whereas traditionally TS was viewed as a rare disorder, recent evidence suggests that milder forms are more common than generally appreciated. An accurate lifetime prevalence rate for TS has not been established. Past estimates, ranging from 0.03 to 1.6% *(7)*, have been based largely on case series of patients referred for medical evaluation or on data obtained from questionnaires without direct clinical examinations *(8–10)*. Several lines of evidence suggest that these approaches are likely to be inaccurate and lead to gross underestimates of disease prevalence.

Systematic analysis of large TS kindreds using a family study method in which all available members are directly interviewed and examined indicates that most cases of TS do not come to medical attention and that the disorder is unrecognized and misdiagnosed by physicians *(7,11)*.

More recent studies that employed modern diagnostic criteria have identified TS fairly commonly in studied school populations. Mason et al. studied all ninth-grade pupils in a single school and found that 2.9% met criteria for TS (excluding the impairment criterion) *(12)*. A school-based study in Sweden assessed children at age 7 who were followed for up to 4 years and found a 1% prevalence for TS *(13)*.

NEUROBIOLOGY

Although genetic factors are now recognized as those most important for the development of TS and related tic disorders, investigators continue to search for underlying neuroanatomic and neurochemical disturbances that may be manifestations of the gene defect and involved in the pathogenesis of the disorder. Several lines of evidence have supported the notion that striatal dopamine receptor supersensitivity at least partly underlies the tic disorder: (a) dopamine receptor antagonists are the most effective drugs for suppressing tics, (b) tics may be exacerbated by dopaminergic medications such as amphetamines, (c) reduced levels of the dopamine (DA) metabolite homovanillic acid have been identified in the cerebrospinal fluid of patients with TS *(14)*, and (c) the phenomenon of tardive tics following chronic DA antagonist therapy *(15)*. However, more recent observations that the DA agonist pergolide *(16)*, the dopaminergic agent levodopa *(17)*, and the psychostimulant methylphenidate *(18)* all lessen tics, have challenged this hypothesis. The reported absence of staining for dynorphin in the globus pallidus of a postmortem brain from a patient with TS *(19)* and clinical observations that drugs affecting the endogenous opioid system may influence the symptoms of TS *(20–22)* have focused attention on the role of this neurochemical system in the pathogenesis of the disorder. Another study of postmortem TS brains revealed reduced concentrations of cyclic adenosine 3, 5-monophosphate in the cerebral cortex and suggests a possible dysfunction of secondary neurochemical messengers *(23)*. Other authors have suggested that sex hormone influences on brain development and function may be important in the pathogenesis of TS *(24,25)*. Recent studies involving cerebral magnetic resonance imaging have revealed that the basal ganglia in patients with TS do not have the volumetric asymmetry (left greater than right) seen in normal controls *(26,27)*.

DIFFERENTIAL DIAGNOSIS

Distinguishing Tics From Other Movement Disorders

Tics must be distinguished from other stereotyped repetitive movement disorders, such as myoclonus, tardive dyskinesia, and dystonias (e.g., blepharospasm, torticollis) *(2)*. Movements associated with mental retardation, psychosis, autism, or congenital blindness and deafness, may be difficult to distinguish from motor tics and both tics and sterotypies often co-occur in this population. The tendency to wax and wane in severity, change in location, and present in context of other more typical tic symptoms can be helpful in differentiating these two phenomenon.

Distinguishing Tourette's From Other Tic Disorders

Primary tic disorders include chronic motor or vocal tic disorder, transient tic, and TS *(6)*. Chronic motor or vocal tic disorders differ from TS in that either motor or vocal tics, but not both, are present for greater than a 1-year period. Transient tic disorder is diagnosed when the duration or the symptoms is less than 1 year. However, many regard these presentations as clinical variants of TS *(28,29)*.

Although it is generally believed that the primary tic disorders occur on a hereditary basis *(30)*, occasional cases of acute or chronic tics may represent these phenocopies *(31)*, and examples include chronic neuroleptic exposure (tardive TS) *(11)*, viral encephalitis *(31,32)*, head trauma *(33)*, carbon monoxide intoxication, *(34)* and Sydenham's chorea *(35)*. A recently proposed and highly controversial hypothesis suggests that some cases of TS occur on the basis of an autoimmune process following streptococcal infection as part of a spectrum of neurobehavioral symptoms termed pediatric autoimmune neuropsychiatric disorders associated with streptococcal infection (PANDAS) *(36)*. Secondary tic disorders may also occur in a number of neurological disorders, including Huntington's disease, Parkinson's disease, progressive supranuclear palsy, neuroacanthocytosis, Meige's syndrome, startle disorders, and developmental basal ganglia syndrome *(31,37)*.

COURSE AND PROGNOSIS

The onset of tics occurs between the ages of 2 and 15 years in most cases, with the mean age at onset being 7 years *(38)*. The initial tics usually occur in the upper body, commonly involving the eyes (e.g., eye blinking) or other parts of the face. Vocal tics represent the initial manifestation of illness for a minority of patients.

Over the short term, tics characteristically change in type and wax and wane in severity. The longer term, lifelong course of the TS tic disorder has been investigated in several studies. Erenberg found that 73% of adult TS subjects reported that over a period of years their tics had either lessened considerably or almost disappeared *(39)*. Bruun followed 136 TS patients from 5 to 15 years and found that tic severity lessened over time, with 59% rated mild-moderate initially and 91% rated so at follow-up *(40)*. Over time, 28% came off medications and 52% reported spontaneous improvement. Shapiro and Shapiro observed that 5–8% of TS patients recover completely and permanently in adolescence; tics become less severe in 35% of cases during adolescence and less severe in "most patients" in adulthood *(38)*. Thus, many patients with TS experience an improvement or resolution of tics after adolescence.

TREATMENT OF TICS

Most patients with mild tics who have made a good adaptation in their lives can avoid the use of any medications. Educating patients, family members, peers, and school personnel regarding the nature of TS, restructuring the educational environment, and supportive counseling are measures that may be sufficient to avoid drug therapy. Pharmacotherapy should be considered once it is determined that the tics are functionally disabling and not remediable to psychosocial interventions. The goal in treating tics is generally to achieve "satisfactory" suppression or control rather than to attempt to make the patient completely "tic free." For the patient with mild or moderate tics, treatment is usually initiated with an α-agonist *(41)*. Clonidine (Catapres®) is initiated at 0.05 mg at bedtime, and the dosage is increased by 0.05 mg every few days until satisfactory control of tics is achieved or unacceptable side effects are encountered. Most patients respond to one tablet (0.1 mg) three times a day (before and after school and at bedtime for children), but the maintenance dose should be the lowest one that gives satisfactory suppression of tics. Because of a short duration of action, particularly in children, four times daily dosing may be required. When necessary, higher doses of clonidine (generally up to 0.6 mg per day) can be used, although adverse effects (usually sedation) can be the dose-limiting factor. Transdermal clonidine (Catapres TTS®) is an alternative dosing form, particularly for children who cannot swallow pills, but this formulation may often cause skin irritation and is impractical during summer months. Guanfacine (Tenex®) is a newer α-agonist that has the advantages of single or twice daily dosage and causes less sedation than clonidine. It is initiated at 0.5–1 mg at bedtime and gradually titrated as needed to a maximum dosage of 4 mg.

If an α-agonist alone is insufficient, an antipsychotic drug can be added (if partial relief with an α-agonist was observed) or the α-agonist can be replaced with an antipsychotic (if no benefit was perceived). When clonidine or guanfacine are to be discontinued, the drug should be tapered over 7–10 days in order to avoid potential withdrawal phenomena, such as tachycardia or rebound hypertension.

The newer atypical antipsychotics have generally supplanted the conventional antiypsychotics as second-line tic suppressants because of better side-effect profiles. The atypical agents can generally be given in a single bedtime dose. Those atypical antipsychotics with reported tic-suppressing actions include risperidone (Risperidal®; 0.25 mg–16 mg per day), olanzapine (Zyprexa®; 2.5–15 mg per day), and ziprasidone (Geodon®; 20–200 mg per day). When the atypical antipsychotics are ineffective or not tolerated, a trial of a classical neuroleptic antipsychotic may be indicated. Haloperidol (Haldol®) remains one of the most commonly used classical antipsychotics neuroleptics for treating tics. The drug is initiated at 0.25 mg at bedtime, increasing as necessary; most patients have a favorable response to 2 mg per day or less, given at bedtime. If haloperidol is unsuccessful or produces unacceptable side effects, one can then switch to pimozide (Orap®), fluphenazine (Prolixin®) or another neuroleptic. For patients with very severe tics that are extremely problematic, one can initiate therapy with an antipsychotic, rather than an α-agonist. Local intramuscular injections of botulinum toxin have been used to treat patients with painful dystonic tics *(42)*.

Other medications that have been reported to improve tics include tetrabenazine, clonazepam, and topiramate.

ASSOCIATED PSYCHIATRIC DISORDERS

In his 1825 paper, Jean Itard first described the ticking and cursing symptoms of the 26-year-old Marquise de Dampierre, noting the peculiar contrasts between her disinhibited behaviors and her otherwise distinguished manners and intellect *(43)*. Sixty years later, a subsequent report on this unfortunate woman and similar cases by Gilles de la Tourette, student of the famous neurologist Charcot, further emphasized an association of behavioral and emotional symptoms such as obsessions, compulsions, phobias, and mood lability with the involuntary movements and vocalizations *(44)*.

Co-morbid psychiatric disorders such as obsessive-compulsive disorder (OCD), attention deficit hyperactivity disorder (ADHD), affective disorders (including depression, bipolar spectrum disorders, and non-OCD anxiety disorders), and impulse control disorders are commonly encountered when treating TS in the clinical setting *(45)*. Recent studies have demonstrated that up to 50% of outpatients with TS suffer from behavioral and emotional symptoms that would meet threshold criteria for a co-morbid psychiatric disorder *(46)*. Because distress and impairment caused by psychiatric co-morbidities often surpasses that by tics, active screening and specific treatment of associated emotional and behavioral symptoms in TS is essential. The two psychiatric conditions most commonly associated with TS—OCD and ADHD—are further highlighted in this chapter.

OBSESSIVE-COMPULSIVE DISORDER

Obsessions are defined as intrusive, recurrent thoughts, impulses, or images that are experienced as unwanted, inappropriate, and distressing. Obsessive symptoms cause marked anxiety or distress and are not simply excessive worries about real-life problems.

Obsessive thoughts may include contamination fears, aggressive thoughts, or images of harming others or of harm befalling oneself, an unreasonable need to know or remember, or fears of saying certain things or of not saying the "right" thing. Typically, the person attempts to suppress or ignore his or her obsessive thoughts, impulses, or images, or to neutralize them with some other thought or action. In contrast to true delusional thinking, the person with obsessive symptoms is aware that these phenomena are generated by his or her own mind and views these symptoms as unreasonable and excessive *(47)*.

Compulsions represent repetitive behaviors or mental acts that a person feels driven to perform in response to an obsession or according to rules that must be rigidly obeyed. Such behaviors, which typically include repetitive hand-washing, ordering, counting, or checking rituals, are directed at averting or reducing distress at preventing some dreaded event from occurring. The repetitious, excessive and seemingly uncontrollable, anxiety-driven features of compulsions distinguish these symptoms from usual goal-directed behaviors *(47)*.

A formal diagnosis of OCD is made when the disturbance cannot be attributed to the direct physiological effect of a substance such as an illegal drug or medication or to a general medical condition or other axis I psychiatric disorder, and when obsessive-compulsive symptoms (OCS) cause marked distress, consume more than 1 hour per day, or significantly interfere with the person's normal functioning *(47)*.

TIC-ASSOCIATED OBSESSIVE-COMPULSIVE SYMPTOMS

Phenomenology and Epidemiology

Studies have shown rates of OCS in TS ranging from 11 to 80% *(48)*. Although OCS are fairly common, the prevalence of symptoms sufficiently severe to warrant a formal diagnosis of OCD in most clinical studies of TS is considerably less, probably closer to 30% *(49)*. Although most specialists now view OCS as an integral part of TS, it is apparent that the majority of individuals with primary OCD do not suffer from a tic disorder *(50)*.

Increasing evidence from neurobiological and clinical studies suggest that tic-related obsessive-compulsive symptomatology may constitute a distinct phenotype of OCD. Tic-related OCS are associated with an earlier age of onset, a greater proportion of male gender, and a family history of tic disorder *(51)*.

Signs and Symptoms

Tic-associated OCD or OCS are characterized by a predominance of obsessions with aggressive or sexual themes, preoccupation with symmetry and exactness, feelings of incompleteness, "just-right" phenomenon (e.g., repeating an action until it "feels just right"), ordering, arranging counting, touching, and doing/re-doing compulsions. Classic contamination obsessions or cleaning compulsions common in OCD alone, occur with less frequency in OCD with tics *(52)*.

Neurobiology of Obsessive-Compulsive Disorder

In addition to TS, a number of other movement disorders such as Parkinson's, Huntington's, and Wilson's diseases, are also associated with OCS *(53)*. Recent neuroimaging studies have implicated abnormalities of the orbitofrontal cortex and basal ganglia metabolism (i.e., elevated glucose metabolic rates) that normalize with successful treatment *(54–56)*.

Other Potential Etiological Factors

It has been proposed that some forms of tics and/or OCD may be the sequelae of infectious processes. In such cases, the explosive onset or exacerbation of tics and/or OCS appears to occur with a temporal relationship to recent streptococcal or viral infection *(57,58)*. The PANDAS hypothesis suggests that a spectrum of pediatric neurobehavioral conditions may arise as the consequence of postinfectious autoimmune mechanisms *(59)*. Although this hypothesis is intriguing, further research is still needed before any causal relationship can be assumed.

Other potential environmental risk factors for OCD include perinatal insults and cocaine abuse *(60–62)*.

Differential Diagnosis of Obsessive-Compulsive Disorder

Compulsions in TS can be difficult to distinguish from complex motor tics because both manifest repetitive, unwanted behaviors. Whereas tic symptoms are often preceded by premonitory urges or performed to achieve a "just-right" somatosensory experience, they are not typically associated with or executed in response to a specific fear or cognitive phenomenon *(63)*. Unlike tics, compulsions are often associated with specific rules (i.e., are ritualistic), such as needing to be repeated a certain number of times or in a particular order.

The differentiation between compulsions and perseverative behaviors or stereotypies can also be challenging, particularly in individuals with mental retardation, psychosis, or developmental disabilities such as autism who may not easily communicate their associated obsessional thinking.

A variety of primary psychiatric disorders including anorexia nervosa, body dysmorphic disorder, delusional disorders, schizotypal personality, schizophrenia, somatization disorder, phobias, posttraumatic stress disorder, generalized anxiety disorder, and mood disorders may include OCS. Obsessive-compulsive personality disorder (OCPD)—which is characterized by a lifelong preoccupation with orderliness, control, efficiency, and perfectionism that interferes with task completion and/or interpersonal relationships—can also be confused with OCD. However, in the case of OCPD, symptoms are more disruptive and disturbing to others who experience such individuals as rigid, stubborn, and aloof. In contrast, in OCD, obsessions and compulsions are primarily a source of distress and anxiety to the individual who suffers from these ego-dystonic symptoms. The individual with OCPD experiences his or her symptoms as enhancing his or her control over others and the environment, whereas the individual with OCD longs for self-control and freedom from the intrusive demands of his or her symptoms.

Course and Prognosis of Obsessive-Compulsive Disorder Associated With Tics and Tourette's Syndrome

Little data is available concerning the long-term course of OCS in TS. There is evidence that OCS wax and wane in severity over time, similar to tics. Symptoms are typically worsened during periods of emotional or physical stress. Clinical experience suggests that although remission or considerable improvement of tic symptoms may occur by early adulthood, OCS often persist throughout the lifetime and can be a source of considerable morbidity.

Treatment of Obsessive-Compulsive Disorder Associated With Tics and Tourette's Syndrome

It is important to screen for OCS/OCD as part of the routine examination of patients with tics/TS. Types of symptoms, frequency, intensity, and impairment of both current and past symptoms should be documented. Inquiries about other members of the family (such as a parent or spouse) are recruited to either participate in the compulsive rituals or assist in the avoidance of known stimuli that regularly precipitate OCS are very informative and may also serve to educate family members about this behavioral comorbidity.

The tricyclic antidepressant (TCA) clomipramine (Anafranil®) was the first drug to demonstrate efficacy for treatment of OCD but is associated with a number of troublesome side effects, including prolongation of the QT-interval, tachycardia, orthostasis, sedation, dry mouth, sweating, tremor, lowered seizure threshold, constipation, urinary retention, and weight gain. Like other TCAs, clomipramine has a narrow therapeutic index and is highly toxic in overdose. Age-related and genetically determined metabolic profiles influence the dosing of clomipramine but most individuals should be started on low doses (i.e., 25 mg daily at bedtime) and increased approximately every 3–5 days to a maximum of 3 mg/kg per day up to 250 mg daily *(64,65)*. Improvement should not be expected before 3 weeks and can take up to 12 weeks.

Treatment of OCD has been advanced by the availability of selective serotonin reuptake inhibitors (SSRIs) although recent evidence indicates that approx 30–40% of patients with OCD will show little or no response after adequate trials with these agents *(66)*. The response to pharmacotherapy of tic-associated OCD is even less robust than that of OCD alone and may require augmentation with a conventional or atypical antipsychotic *(67–70)*. Of the six SSRIs currently on the market, which include fluoxetine, fluvoxamine, sertraline, paroxetine, citalopram, and escitalopram, all but escitalopram have demonstrated efficacy in the treatment of OCD in adults *(71–73)*. Fluoxetine, fluvoxamine, sertaline and paroxetine have been demonstrated to be effective treatments for OCD in children *(74–76)*. Whereas their comparative safety profiles render the SSRIs easier to use than the conventional TCAs, headaches, nausea, vomiting, diarrhea, anorexia, weight change, insomnia, sedation, akathisia, sexual dysfunction, and agitation can be common side effects. More recently, there has been increased concern about the risk for increased suicidal ideation and behavior in children treated with SSRIs based on data from several pediatric depression studies in Great Britain. Although treatment with paroxetine specifically was associated with a higher frequency of self-injurious behaviors and ideation in depressed children, the Food and Drug Administration (FDA) has suggested caution when using all SSRIs in the pediatric population until further data becomes available from controlled studies *(77)*.

The SSRIs differ in their chemical structure, potency in blocking serotonin at the presynaptic nerve terminal, and in their active metabolites and inhibition of various cytochrome P450 hepatic isoenzymes; the latter characteristics have important clinical implications particularly in patients who are receiving other medications concurrently because blood levels can be dangerously increased, particularly when using fluoxetine, fluvoxamine, or paroxetine *(78)*. The usual starting dose for fluoxetine is 5–20 mg with increases approximately every 5–7 days to approx 10–80 mg daily. Sertraline can be started at 25–50 mg daily and increased similarly every 5–7 days to approx 50–200 mg daily. Fluvoxamine can be started at 25–50 mg daily and increased every 5 days to approx 50–300 mg daily. Paroxetine is started at 5–10 mg daily and increased to approx 10–60 mg daily. Citalopram can be started at 5–10 mg daily and increased to approx 20–40 mg daily. Similarly to clomipramine, the SSRIs can take 8–12 weeks, often at higher doses, before a clinical effect will be noted. Most authorities recommend switching to a second SSRI when an adequate trial of the first does not produce the desired clinical response *(79)*. Unfortunately, relapse of OCD symptoms occurs in up to 90% of patients within a few weeks of withdrawal from medication *(80,81)*.

Nonpharmacological interventions are also important in the treatment of OCD, particularly cognitive-behavioral therapy (CBT) using exposure and response prevention. The utility of CBT has been demonstrated in both children and adults with OCD *(82–84)*. The combination of CBT and medication for the treatment of OCD often leads to greater and more sustained therapeutic responses than either intervention alone *(85)*. However, although preliminary studies are encouraging, it remains unclear whether CBT is equally effective, either alone or in combination with medication management, for the treatment of tic-associated OCD *(86,87)*.

Psychosurgical approaches including anterior cingulotomy, limbic leucotomy, subcaudate tactotomy, and anterior capsulotomy have been used for patients with severe, treatment-refractory OCD with variable success *(88–92)*. Deep brain stimulation may offer another treatment option for treatment-refractory individuals *(93)*.

ATTENTION DEFICIT HYPERACTIVITY DISORDER

Problems with concentration, distractability, impulsivity, and motoric hyperactivity may accompany a variety of medical and behavioral disorders. The core constellation of symptoms comprising the disorder currently known as attention deficit hyperactivity disorder (ADHD) was described in young boys by Still in 1902 *(94)*. Similar symptoms were observed in children during the early 1920s following the worldwide encephalitis lethargica epidemic *(95)*. However, since that time, the nosology of ADHD has undergone several permutations.

Current classification using the DSM-IV-TR *(5)* divides ADHD into three subcategories: predominantly inattentive type, predominantly hyperactive-impulsive type, and combined type. By current DSM-IV-TR diagnostic criteria, symptoms must have been present before age 7 years, have persisted for at least 6 months to a degree that is maladaptive and inconsistent with developmental level, and result in impairment of function in two or more settings (e.g., at home and in school). Accurate diagnosis and assessment of ADHD requires information from multiple informants including parents, other relative, and teachers as well as careful clinical evaluation of core symptoms.

Phenomenology of Attention Deficit Hyperactivity Disorder and Tics

The cardinal symptoms of ADHD include persistent problems since early childhood with inattention, impulsivity, and hyperkinesis. ADHD is highly associated with psychiatric comorbidities, including learning disabilities, mood disorders, and TS *(96,97)*. When TS and ADHD co-occur, ADHD symptoms typically emerge during early childhood, precede the onset of tics by a few years, and often persist well into adulthood, in contrast to tic symptoms, which often improve or remit by late adolescence *(98)*.

Many children with ADHD and tics/TS are described by their parents as extremely active during infancy, often not napping during the daytime or showing difficulties falling asleep at night, and demanding constant parental attention. Peer problems may become more evident once the child enters nursery school where such children are typically described as accident-prone, aggressive, impulsive, lacking social boundaries, and requiring frequent redirection. In many cases, particularly when tic symptoms are rather mild or subtle, it is the presence of ADHD symptoms that prompts medical evaluation, usually as a result of the child's academic and/or social problems upon entering school; in the classroom such children show difficulties remaining seated, talking out of turn, intruding on others, or performing consistently academically. However, intellectually gifted children with ADHD, particularly if they have good social skills, may go unrecognized until the later years of elementary school or even upon entry into middle school or high school, at which time the demands for organization, transitioning, and focused attention exceed their capacities to compensate.

Although there are few studies of ADHD and tics in adults, clinical experience suggests that persistent ADHD symptoms are far more disruptive in most cases than persistent tics. Adult ADHD is frequently accompanied by other psychiatric co-morbidities such as mood disorders, anxiety disorders, and substance abuse, and often leads to significant impairments of occupational and social functioning *(99)*.

ADHD is believed to have an inherited basis. Parents of children with ADHD are more likely to have ADHD than are parents of non-ADHD children and increased rates of motoric hyperactivity occur in the biological relatives of hyperactive children when compared with controls *(100)*. Based on earlier genetic studies, it has been proposed that there are two different types of ADHD in TS: an earlier onset, "classic ADHD" that presents before tic symptoms occur and represents a true co-morbidity, and a later onset, "tic-related ADHD" *(101)*. However, tic-related ADHD appears to run a distinct course from the underlying tic diathesis. Whereas the presence of tic symptoms has little impact clinically on ADHD, the presence of comorbid ADHD with tics accounts for considerable morbidity in TS. There is growing evidence that the presence of multiple psychiatric co-morbidities, peer problems, neuropsychological deficits, and disruptive behaviors in TS are primarily a function of comorbid ADHD and not specific to TS *(102–105)*.

Epidemiology

ADHD is the most common childhood psychiatric disorder, affecting approx 2–10% of school-age children *(106–108)*. Like TS, ADHD appears more frequently in male children than in females with a range from 4:1 to 9:1. However, because children with disruptive behaviors are more likely to referred for treatment, and disruptive behaviors are reported in approximately twice as many boys as girls, this excess may reflect referral bias. It is estimated that about 4.5% of adults suffer from ADHD, although until fairly recently few adults with residual ADHD symptoms received this diagnosis. Prevalence of ADHD in clinically diagnosed patients with TS ranges from 50 to 90% *(109)*.

Neurobiology of Attention Deficit Hyperactivity Disorder

Structural neuroimaging studies in children with ADHD implicate disturbances of circuitry involving the prefrontal cortex, cerebellum, and the corpus collosum *(110)*. Available data from adult functional imaging studies have primarily implicated frontal brain regions. Reduced global and regional glucose metabolism of the premotor cortex and superior prefrontal cortext has been shown in adults with ADHD using positron emission tomography *(111)*. Additional physiological data suggests that ADHD in adults in characterized by prefrontal dopaminergic hypoactivity *(112,113)*.

Differential Diagnosis

Many different disorders of childhood onset may present with similar and overlapping symptoms of ADHD. It is essential to first exclude any potential underlying medical conditions such as hyperthyroidism, phenylketonuria, anemia, asthma, seizure disorder, or medication side effects. Similarly, obtaining a thorough psychosocial history is important for excluding factors such as neglect, abuse, or acute stresses that may be causing or contributing to symptoms. The diagnosis of ADHD is one of exclusion and relies primarily on an accurate, detailed clinical history, physical examination, and laboratory assessment of symptoms that cannot be otherwise better accounted for. In primary ADHD, physical examination and routine laboratory studies are typically normal.

Inattention, fidgetiness, poor concentration, irritability, and low frustration tolerance are common symptoms in children with anxiety disorders like OCD, generalized anxiety disorder, separation anxiety disorder, and social anxiety disorder. Approximately 25% of children with ADHD have a co-morbid anxiety disorder *(114)*. A tendency toward catastrophic thinking, vigilant apprehension, over dependence on others, and rituals may help distinguish anxiety symptoms from ADHD. It must also be kept in mind that psychotropic medications commonly used to treat anxiety or mood disorders, such as the SSRIs, can transiently worsen anxiety symptoms, and/or cause akathisia, thereby mimicking symptoms of ADHD.

Similarly, premonitory symptoms and tics themselves can be very distracting and annoying; many children with tics will experience difficulties with concentration, motoric hyperactivity, increased irritability, and impatience during periods of tic exacerbation that can be confused with primary ADHD symptoms. Side effects from medications used for tic suppression also commonly induce akisthisia, anxiety, and cognitive blunting that may be difficult at times to distinguish from an underlying co-morbid ADHD.

Mood disorders, such as major depression and bipolar affective disorder typically manifest with inattention, poor concentration, impaired impulse control, and difficulties completing tasks that can be hard to distinguish from clinical symptoms of ADHD. Symptoms of major depression typically include a persistently dysphoric mood, physiological disturbances (e.g., changes in appetite, and/or weight, abnormal sleep patterns), social withdrawal, and anhedonia that are unusual in uncomplicated ADHD. Symptoms of extreme mood lability, irritability, severe sleep disturbances including hypersomnia or profound sleep reduction without daytime lethargy, unmodulated increased energy, and grandiosity with the pursuit of multiple goal-oriented activities are symptoms that help distinguish an underlying bipolar affective disorder from primary ADHD. However, there is considerable bidirectional symptom overlap between these two disorders with a significant co-morbidity of affective disorders and ADHD *(115)*. Results of recent systematic studies of children and adolescents with bipolar disorder indicate rates of ADHD ranging from 60 to 90% in pediatric patients with mania *(116)*. Pharmacological treatment of mood disorders is also commonly accompanied by cognitive and behavioral medication side effects that may resemble primary ADHD symptoms.

Substance and alcohol use disorders are also frequently co-morbid with ADHD and may present with considerable overlapping symptoms. Both acute intoxication and withdrawal states may be accompanied by motoric restlessness, distractibility, irritability, easy frustration, and inattentiveness. Approximately 50% of untreated adults with ADHD will have a substance use disorder at some point in their lives; the ultimate risk of substance use disorders can be reduced however by effective pharmacotherapy of ADHD *(117)*.

Finally, a variety of learning disorders (LDs) may present with academic underachievement, inattention, impatience, disorganization, and low frustration tolerance and have been reported in approx 22% of school-age children with TS *(118,119)*. However, recent studies of TS that controlled for the presence of co-morbidities indicate that LDs are highly correlated with an underlying ADHD and not necessarily related to TS itself. Neuropsychological testing can be extremely valuable for detecting subtle LDs that may require school modifications and interventions, although such problems are less apt to respond to medication interventions.

Course and Prognosis

As previously stated, ADHD is a condition associated with considerable morbidity. When untreated, it renders greater risk for accidents, academic failure or underperformance, impaired social relationships, marital and occupational disruption. Co-morbid ADHD accounts for a significant proportion of the morbidity associated with TS both during childhood and adulthood, and may be responsible for the multiple psychiatric disorders often encountered in complex TS patients. ADHD also appears more likely to persist into adulthood in contrast to tic symptoms that more typically will diminish in severity over time.

Treatment

There is substantial data from numerous controlled clinical trials documenting the clinical efficacy of the psychostimulants (such as methylphenidate®, dextoamphetamine®, pemoline®, and mixed amphetamine salts) for the treatment of ADHD in children and adolescents, and approx 70–80% of ADHD patients will experience a satisfactory response to psychostimulant therapy *(120,121)*.

Immediate-release stimulant preparations include methylphenidate (Ritalin®, Methyllin®, a dye-free preparation) onset of action within 20–60 minutes and duration of action from 3 to 6 hours, D-amphetamine (Dexedrine®) onset of action within 20–60 minutes and 4–6 hours duration of action and D,L-amphetamine (Adderall®) onset of action around 30–60 minutes and duration of action from 4 to 6 hours. Short acting stimulants must be dosed at least—two to three times daily.

First-generation sustained-release preparations of methylphenidate (Ritalin-SR®) with onset of action within 60–90 minutes and lasting for 5–8 hours or D-amphetamine (Dexedrine Spansule®) with an onset of action within 60–90 minutes and duration of action from 6 to 8 hours were developed to circumvent some of the practical limitations of the shorter acting stimulants, but have shown overall less clinical efficacy.

The currently available second-generation extended-release formulations of methyphenidate including Ritalin LA®, Metadate CD®, or Concerta®, and amphetamine compounds such as Adderall XR® have demonstrated excellent efficacy in well-controlled clinical trials. These agents have shown a rapid onset of action and longer duration of therapeutic effect, making possible once daily dosing for most patients *(122)*. Some of these preparations (e.g., Ritalin-LA, Metadate CD, Adderall XR) can be sprinkled on food while retaining clinical efficacy and enabling a wider range of dosing options.

The first released of these medications was Concerta, which has an osmotically mediated, timed drug-delivery system, and a duration of effect of approx 12 hours. The pharmacokinetic profile of Concerta was designed to replace immediate-release methylphenidate that requires three times a day dosing 18 mg of Concerta compares roughly with 5 mg three times a day immediate-release methylphenidate. Recent evidence from clinical studies in adolescents suggests that higher doses of Concerta (i.e., 54 mg to 72 mg) yield improved responses when compared with 18 mg to 36 mg daily *(123)*. Metadate CD was the second approved extended-release methlyphenidate preparation approved by the US FDA and contains a mixture of immediate-release and extended-release methylphenidate in a 30:70 ratio that provides an 8-hour duration of action. Because higher plasma concentrations are achieved within the first 6 hours, it is most helpful during the usual school day but effects will wane by later afternoon. Ritalin-LA is the most recent addition to this group of long-acting methylphenidate preparations and has a mixture of immediate-release and delayed-release in a 50:50 ratio, designed to replace immediate-release methylphenidate twice a day. Similar to Metadate CD, improvement of ADHD symptoms can be expected during the usual school or work day but not into evening hours. A shorter acting but more specific methylphenidate isomer, D-threo-methylphenidate (Focalin™) is also now available and has shown clinical efficacy *(124)*.

Short-acting amphetamines such as Dexedrine tablets and short-acting Adderall have been available for a number of years but suffer from similar practical limitations to short-acting methylphenidate. Dexedrine spansule provides longer duration of action (i.e., approx 6 hours) but tends to be less effective in the morning when compared with the two short-acting preparations. Adderall XR contains a mixture of neutral sulfate salts of D-amphetamine, the D-isomer of Amphetamine saccharate and D, L-amphetamine aspartate monohydrate, with a 50:50 ratio of immediate and delayed-release drug-containing beads. This once-daily preparation was designed to replace twice-daily short-acting

Adderall and has a duration of action of 10–12 hours. Dose-dependent responses also occur with Adderall XR, where 30 mg daily showed superior efficacy to 10 mg daily in a well-controlled clinical trial (125).

There is an approx 2:1 difference in potency between D, L-amphetamine and methylphenidate. Therefore, suggested dosing for D, L-amphetamine is 0.5–1 mg/kg per day and for methylphenidate 1–2 mg/kg per day. Medication titration can occur every 3–7 days as indicated up to a dose that either demonstrate clinical efficacy or intolerable side effects. Clinical response is usually robust and relatively prompt.

The most common side effects with psychostimulant medications are sleep disturbances (i.e., delayed sleep onset), reduced appetite with weight loss, stomach aches, headaches, tics, increased nervousness, and irritability. Children with underlying anxiety and/or mood disorders appear particularly susceptible to the latter behavioral side effects. Shorter acting preparations may be associated with a symptomatic rebound as drug action wanes.

Because of concerns that psychostimulants may precipitate or exacerbate tics, for a number of years these medications were not regularly used in children with tics/TS and ADHD. However, a body of data from prospective trials and well-controlled studies has demonstrated that the vast majority of children with co-morbid tics/TS and ADHD tolerate psychostimulant treatment very well with clinically insignificant and/or transient effects on tics and substantial improvement of ADHD symptoms (126–28). Results from the Treatment of Attention Deficit Disorder in Children with Tics study suggest that the combination of the α-agonist clonidine and methylphenidate appears to be an optimal strategy for treating ADHD symptoms in children with tics/TS (128).

Nonetheless, there is a minority of patients with both tics/TS and ADHD who do experience transient but disruptive exacerbations of tics when exposed to psychostimulant medication and in such cases alternative treatment strategies must be devised (129).

Although the TCA desipramine (Norpramin®) has been demonstrated to be an effective treatment of ADHD in children with comorbid tics/TS at a mean dose of 3.4 mg/kg per day, concerns about its potential cardiotoxicity and narrow therapeutic index have limited the usage of this agent (130). Additional anticholinergic side effects such as dry mouth, blurred vision, weight gain, postural hypotension and sedation can also be problematic when using TCAs.

Therefore, a further advance for the treatment of comorbid ADHD and tics/TS became possible with the introduction of the specific noradrenergic reuptake inhibitor atomoxetine (Strattera®), which shows no effect on the QTc or other cardiac conduction problems (131). Atomoxetine is well-tolerated by children with ADHD and co-morbid tic disorders, is efficacious for treating core ADHD symptoms, and has showed a trend toward decreasing tic severity in preliminary clinical trials (132). Atomoxetine is generally dosed between 1.0 and 1.4 mg/kg daily and can be administered in either a single or divided doses. Adverse side effect may include sedation, nausea, vomiting, headache, and dizziness, and can sometimes be attenuated or eliminated by using a divided dosing regimen and/or administering with a high-fat/high-protein meal. Unlike the psychostimulants, which show nearly immediate efficacy, atomoxetine must be first titrated to an appropriate dose range and then takes approx 2–4 weeks before clinical efficacy becomes apparent.

Although their clinical effects have not been consistently demonstrated, the α-adrenergic receptor agonists clonidine (Catapres) and guanfacine (Tenex) may be reasonable treatment options for children with co-morbid ADHD and TS/tic disorder because these agents may have some impact on both tics and core ADHD symptoms (133,134). Clonidine is available in an oral and transdermal, time-released preparation (Catapres TTS). It is typically given in divided doses—two to four times daily that are gradually titrated every 3–5 days to a maximum of 0.6 mg daily. Sedation, irritability, dizziness, headache, hypotension, and skin sensitivity in the case of the patch are common side effects.

The newer agent modafinil (Provigil®), which has been approved for the treatment of narcolepsy and for hypersomnia, has shown efficacy in a controlled trial for the treatment of ADHD in children and is potentially another option for treating ADHD with co-morbid TS/tics (135). Reported side effects include higher rates of insomnia, abdominal pain, and anorexia. It is usually prescribed between 100 and 300 mg daily, either in a single morning dose or divided dose.

A variety of secondary agents including buprorion (Wellbutrin®), venlafaxine (Effexor®), and even SSRIs have been employed to treat ADHD when first-line agents either fail or have intolerable side effects. The aminoketone-class antidepressant buproprion has shown efficacy for the treatment of ADHD in double-blind, placebo-controlled trials at doses ranging from 50 mg to 250 mg daily, but reports of tic exacerbation in ADHD patients with co-morbid TS have tempered enthusiasm for using this agent in this population *(136)*.

CONCLUSION

The treatment of TS and its co-morbidities poses great challenges for the clinician, particularly because medications that may improve one condition may inadvertently exacerbate others. Appropriate assessment and accurate diagnosis is an essential first step in the management of TS and its associated disorders, after which a hierarchy of symptoms, morbidities must be established so as to prioritize treatment goals. Although OCD and ADHD are among the most common psychiatric co-morbidities in TS, careful evaluation of underlying mood and anxiety disorders, developmental, and learning difficulty is also necessary. It is rarely true that tics in TS are the main cause of dysfunction; identification and appropriate treatment of psychiatric co-morbidities and/or medication side effects plays a paramount role in improving qualify of life in TS for both patient and his or her family.

REFERENCES

1. American Psychiatric Association. Diagnostic and Statistical Manual of Psychiatry, Fourth Edition, revised. Washington, DC: Amer Psychiatric Pub; 2000.
2. The Tourette Syndrome Classification Study Group. Definitions and classification of tic disorders. Arch Neurol 1993;50: 1013–1016.
3. Jankovic J, Stone L. Dystonic tics in patients with Tourette's syndrome. Mov Disord 1991;6:248–252.
4. Kurlan R, Lichter D, Hewitt D. Sensory tics in Tourette's syndrome. Neurology 1989;39:731–734.
5. Scahill LD, Leckman JF, Marek KL. Sensory phenomena in Tourette's syndrome. Adv Neurol 1995;65:273–280.
6. Tanner CM. Epidemiology. In: Kurlan R, ed. Handbook of Tourette's Syndrome and Associated Tic and Behavioral Disorders. New York: Marcel Dekker; 1993.
7. Kurlan R, Behr J, Medved L, Shoulson I, Pauls D, Kidd KK. Severity of Tourette's syndrome in one large kindred: implication for determination of disease prevalence rate. Arch Neurol 1987;44:268–269.
8. Burd L, Kerbeshian J, Wikenheiser M, Fisher W. Prevalence of Gilles de la Tourette's syndrome in North Dakota adults. Am J Psychiatry 1986;143:787–788.
9. Burd L, Kerbeshian J, Wikenheiser M, Fisher W. A prevalence study of Gilles de la Tourette syndrome in North Dakota school-age children. J Am Acad Child Psychiatry 1986;4:552–555.
10. Caine ED, McBride MC, Chiverton P, Bamford KA, Redress S, Shiao J. Tourette's syndrome in Monroe County school children. Neurology 1988;38:472–475.
11. McMahon WM, Leppert M, Filloux F, van de Wetering BJ, Hasstedt S. Tourette symptoms in 161 related family members. Adv Neurol 1992;58:159–165.
12. Mason A, Banerjee S, Eapen V, Zeitlin H, Robertson MM. The prevalence of Tourette syndrome in a mainstream school population. Dev Med Child Neurol 1998;40:292–296.
13. Kadesjoe B, Gilbert C. Tourette's syndrome: epidemiology and comorbidity in primary school children. J Am Acad Child Adolesc Psychiatry 2000;39:548–555.
14. Singer HS, Butler IJ, Tune LE, Seifert WE Jr, Coyle JT. Dopaminergic dysfunction in Tourette's syndrome. Ann Neurol 1982;12:361–366.
15. Klawans HL, Falk DK, Nausieda PA, Weiner WJ. Gilles de la Tourette's syndrome after long-term chlorpromazine therapy. Neurology 1978;28:1064–1068.
16. Gilbert DL, Sethuraman G, Sine L, Peters S, Sallee FR. Tourette's syndrome improvement with pergolide in a randomized, double-blind, crossover trial. Neurology 2000;54:1310–1315.
17. Black KJ, Mink JW. Response to levodopa challenge in Tourette syndrome. Mov Disord 2000;15:1194–1198.
18. Kurlan R, The Tourette Syndrome Study Group. Treatment of attention-deficit hyperactivity disorder in children with Tourette's syndrome (TACT Trial). Ann Neurol 2000;48:953.
19. Haber SN, Kowall NW, Vonsattel JP, Bird ED, Richardson EP Jr. Gilles de la Tourette's syndrome: a postmortem neuropathological and immunohistochemical study. J Neurol Sci 1986;75:225–241.

20. Gilman MA, Sandyk R. The endogenous opioid system in Gilles de la Tourette syndrome: a postmortem neuropathological and immunohistochemical study. Med Hypotheses 1986;19:371–378.

21. Lichter D, Majumdar L, Kurlan R. Opiate withdrawal unmasks Tourette's syndrome. Clin Neuropharmacology 1988;11: 559–564.

22. Kurlan R, Majumdar L, Deeley C, Mudholkar GS, Plumb S, Como PG. A controlled trial of propoxyphene and naltrexone in Tourette's syndrome. Ann Neurol 1991;30:19–23.

23. Singer HS, Hahn IH, Krowiak E, Nelson E, Moran T. Tourette's syndrome: a neurochemical analysis of postmortem cortical brain tissue. Ann Neurol 1990;27:443–446.

24. Kurlan R. The pathogenesis of Tourette's syndrome: a possible role for hormonal and excitatory neurotransmitter influences in brain development. Arch Neurol 1992;49:874–876.

25. Peterson BS, Leckman JF, Scahill L, et al. Steroid hormones and CNS sexual dimorphisms modulate symptom expression in Tourette's syndrome. Psychoneuroendocrinolgoy 1993;17:553–563.

26. Peterson B, Riddle MA, Cohen DJ, et al. Reduced basal ganglia volume in Tourette's syndrome using three-dimensional reconstruction techniques from magnetic resonance images. Neurology 1993;43:941–949.

27. Singer HS, Reiss AL, Brown JE, et al. Volumetric MRI changes in basal granglia of children with Tourette's syndrome. Neurology 1993;43:950–956.

28. Kurlan R, Behr J, Medved L, Como PG. Transient tic disorder and the clinical spectrum of Tourette's syndrome. Arch Neurol 1988;45:1200–1201.

29. Kurlan R. What is the spectrum of Tourette's syndrome? Curr Opinion Neurol Neurosurg 1988;1:294–298.

30. Pauls DL. The inheritance pattern. In: Kurlan R, ed. Handbook of Tourette's Syndrome and Related Tic and Behavioral Disorders. New York: Marcel Dekker; 1993:307–315.

31. Jankovic J. Tics in other neurologic disorders. In: Kurlan R, ed. Handbook of Tourette's Syndrome and Related Tic and Behavioral Disorders. New York: Marcel Dekker; 1993:167–182.

32. Sacks OW. Acquired tourettism in adult life. In: Friedhoff AJ, Chase TN, eds. Gilles de la Tourette's Syndrome. New York: Raven Press; 1982:89–92.

33. Fahn S. A case of post-traumatic tic syndrome. In: Friedhoff AJ, Chase TN, eds. Gilles de la Tourette's Syndrome. New York: Raven Press; 1982:349–350.

34. Pulst SM, Walshe TM, Romero JA. Carbon monoxide poisoning with features of Gilles de la Tourette syndrome. Arch Neurol 1983;40:443–444.

35. Cardoso F, Eduardo C, Silva AP, Mota CC. Chorea in fifty consecutive patients with rheumatic fever. Mov Disord 1997; 12:701–703.

36. Swedo SE, Leonard HL, Garvey M, et al. Pediatric autoimmune neuropsychiatric disorders associated with streptococcal infections: clinical description of the first 50 cases. Am J Psychiatry 1998;155:264–271.

37. Palumbo D, Maughan A, Kurlan R. Hypothesis III: Tourette's syndrome is only one of several causes of a developmental basal ganglia syndrome. Arch Neurology 1997;54:475–483.

38. Shapiro AK, Shapiro ES, Young JG, Feinberg TE. Gilles de la Tourette Syndrome, Second Edition. New York: Raven Press; 1988.

39. Erenberg G, Cruse RP, Rothner AD. The natural history of Tourette syndrome. A follow-up study. Ann Neurol 1987;22: 383–385.

40. Bruun RD. The natural history of Tourette's syndrome. In: Cohen DJ, Bruun RD, Leckman J, eds. Tourette's Syndrome and Tic Disorders: Clinical Understanding and Treatment. New York: John Wiley; 1988:21–39.

41. Chappell PB, Riddle MA, Scahill L, et al. Guanfacine treatment of comorbid attention-deficit hyperactivity disorder in Tourette's syndrome: preliminary clinical experience. J Am Acad Child Adolesc Psychiatry 1995;34:1140–1146.

42. Jankovic J. Botulinum toxin in the treatment of tics associated with Tourette's syndrome. Neurology 1993;43 (Suppl 2): A310.

43. Itard, Jean MG. Memoire sur Quelques Fonctions Involontaires des Appareils de la Locomotion, de la Prehension et de la Vox. Arch Generales de Medicine 1825;8:385–407.

44. Gilles de la Tourette G. Etude sur une Affecton Nereuse Caracterisee par de I'Incoordination Motrice Accompagnee d'Echolalie et de Coprolalie. Archives de Neurologic 1885;9:19–42.

45. Robertson M. Tourette syndrome, associated conditions and the complexities of treatment. Brain 2000;42:436–447.

46. Coffey B, Park K. Behavioral and emotional aspects of Tourette syndrome. Neurol Clin 1997;15:277–289.

47. American Psychiatric Association. Diagnostic and Statistical Manual of Mental Disorder, Fourth Edition, revision. Washington, DC: Amer Psychiatric Pub; 2000.

48. Robertson M, Yakley J. Obsessive compulsive disorder and self-injurious behavior. In: Kurlan R, ed. Handbook of Tourette's Syndrome and Related Tic and Behavioral Disorders. New York: Marcel Dekker; 1993:45–87.

49. King R, Leckman J, Scahill L, Cohen D. Obsessive-compulsive disorder, anxiety, and depression. In: Leckman J, Cohen D, eds. Tourette's Sydnrome: Tics, Obsessions, Compulsions Developmental Psychopathology and Clinical Care. New York: Wiley; 1999:44.

50. Rappoport J. The neurology of obsessive-compulsive disorder. J Am Med Assoc 1988;260:2888–2890.

51. Leckman J, Grice D, Barr L, et al. Tic-related vs. non-tic related obsessive-compulsive disorder. Anxiety 1995;1:208–215.

52. Cath D, Spinhoven P, van de Wetering B, et al. The relationship between types and severity of repetitive behaviors in Gilles de la Tourette's disorder and obsessive-compulsive disorder. J Clin Psychiatry 2000;61:505–513.

53. Rosenblatt A, Leroi I. Neuropsychiatry of Huntington's disease and other basal ganglia disorders. Psychosomatics 2000; 41:24–30.

54. Schwartz J, Stoessel P, Baxter L, Martin K, Phelps M. Systemic changes in cerebral glucose metabolic rate after successful behavior modification treatment of obsessive-compulsive disorder. Arch Gen Psychiatry 1996;53:109–113.

55. Fitzgerald K, MacMaster F, Paulson L, Rosenberg D. Neurobiology of childhood obsessive-compulsive disorder. Child Adolesc Psychiatry Clin N Am 1999;8:533–575.

56. Stein D. Neurobiology of obsessive-compulsive spectrum disorders. Biol Psychiatry 2000;47:296–304.

57. Allen A, Leonard H, Swedo S. Case study: a new infection-triggered, autoimmune subtype of pediatric OCD and Tourette's syndrome. J Am Acad Child Adolesc Psychiatry 1995;65:1428–1436.

58. Kiessling L, Marotte A, Benson M, Kuhn C, Wrenn D. Relationship between GABHS and childhood movement disorders. Pediatr Res 1993;33:12A.

59. Swedo S, Leonard H, Garvey M, et al. Pediatric autoimmune neuropsychiatric disorders associated with streptococcal infections: clinical description of the first 50 cases. Am J Psychiatry 1998;155:264–271.

60. Maina G, Albert U, Bogetto F, Vaschetto P, Ravizza L. Recent life events and obsessive-compulsive disorder (OCD): the role of pregnancy/delivery. Psychiatry Res 1999;89:49–58.

61. Capstick N, Seldrug J. Obsessional states: a study in the relationship between abnormalities occurring at the time of birth and the subsequent development of obsessional symptoms. Acta Psych Scan 1977;56:427–431.

62. Crum R, Anthony J. Cocaine use and other suspected risk factors for obsessive compulsive disorder: a prospective study with data from the epidemiologic catchment area surveys. Drug Alcohol Depend 1993;31:281–295.

63. Miguel E, Baer L, Rauch S, et al. Repetitive motor behaviors in obsessive-compulsive disorder and Tourette's syndrome: phenomenological differences. Br J Psychiatry 1997;170:140–145.

64. DeVeaugh-Geiss J, Katz R, Landau P, Goodman W, Rasmussen S. Clinical predictors of treatment response in obsessive-compulsive disorder: exploratory analyses from multicenter trials of clomipramine. Psychopharmacol Bull 1990;26:54–59.

65. Carpenter Leckman J, Scahill L, McDougle C. Pharmacological and other somatic approaches to treatment. In: Leckman J, Cohen D, eds. Tourette's Syndrome: Tics, Obsessions, Compulsions Developmental Psychopathology and Clinical Care. New York: Wiley; 1999, pp. 383–384.

66. Greist J, Jefferson J, Kobak K, Katzelnick D, Serlin R. Efficacy and tolerability of serotonin transport inhibitors in obsessive-compulsive disorder. Arch Gen Psychiatry 1995;52:53–60.

67. Kurlan R, Como P, Deeley C, McDermott M. A pilot controlled study of fluoxetine for obsessive-compulsive symptoms in children with Tourette's syndrome. Clin Neuropharmacol 1993;16:167–172.

68. McDougle D, Fleischmann R, Epperson C, Wasylink S, Leckman J, Price L. Risperidone addition in fluvoxamine-refractory obsessive compulsive disorder: three cases. J Clin Psychiatry 1995;56:526–528.

69. McDougle C, Goodman W, Leckman J, Lee N, Heninger G, Price L. Haloperidol addition to fluvoxamine-refractory obsessive compulsive disorder: a double-blind placebo-controlled study in patients with and without tics. Arch Gen Psychiatry 1994;51:302–308.

70. McDougle C, Goodman W, Leckman J, Barr L, Heninger G, Price L. The efficacy of fluvoxamine in obsessive compulsive disorder: effects of comorbid chronic tic disorder. J Clin Psychopharmacol 1993;13;354–358.

71. Koponen H, Lepola U, Leinonen E, Jokinen R, Penttinen J, Turtonen J. Citalopram in the treatment of obsessive-compulsive disorder: an open pilot study. Acta Psychiatr Scand 1997;96:343–346.

72. Greist J, Jefferson J, Kobak K, Katzelnick D, Serlin R. Efficacy and tolerability of serotonin transport inhibitors in obsessive compulsive disorder. Arch Gen Psychiatry 1995;52:53–60.

73. Jenike M. Clinical practice obsessive compulsive disorder. New Eng J Med 2004;350:259–265.

74. Geller D, Hoog S, Heiligenstein J, et al. Fluoxetine Pediatric OCD Study Team. Fluoxetine treatment for obsessive-compulsive disorder in children and adolescents: a placebo-controlled clinical trial. J Amer Acad Child Adolesc Psychiatry 2001;40:773–770.

75. March J, Biederman J, Wolkow R, et al. Sertraline in children and adolescents with obsessive-compulsive disorder: a multicenter randomized controlled trial. JAMA 1998;280:1752–1756.

76. Geller D, Biederman J, Stewart S, et al. Which SSRI? A metanalysis of pharmacotherapy trials in pediatric obsessive compulsive disorder. Am J Psychiatry 2003;160:1919–1928.

77. Food and Drug Administration Center for Drug Evaluation and Research. Summary Minutes of the Psychopharmacologic Drugs Advisory Committee Meeting February 2, 2004. Available at www.fda.gov.ohrms.docket/ac/04/minutes/4006MI/finalpdf.

78. Erenshefsky L, Riesenman C, Lam Y. Serotonin selective reuptake inhibitor drug interactions and the cytochrome P450 system. J Clin Psychiatry 1996;57:17–24.

79. Denys D, van Megen H, van der Wee N, Westenberg H. A double-blind switch study of paroxetine and venlafaxine in obsessive compulsive disorder. J Clin Psychiatry 2004;65:37–43.

80. Pato M, Murphy D, DeVane C. Sustained plasma concentrations of fluoxetine and/or norfluoxetine four and eight weeks after fluoxetine discontinutation. J Clin Psychopharmacol 1991;11:224–225.

81. Pato M, Zohar-Kadouch R, Zohar J, Murphy D. Return of symptoms after discontinuation of clomipramine in patients with obsessive-compulsive disorder. Amer J Psychology 1988;145:1521–1525.
82. Scahill L, Vitulano L, Brenner E, Lynch K, King R. Behavioral therapy in children and adolescents with obsessive com-pulsive disorder: a pilot study. J Child Adolesc Psychopharmacol 1996;6:191–202.
83. March J. Cognitive-behavioral psychotherapy for children and adolescents with OCD: a review and recommendations for treatment. J Amer Acad Child Adolesc Psychiatry 1995;34:7–18.
84. Foa E, Steketee G, Grayson J, Turner R, Latimer P. Deliberate exposure and blocking of obsessive-compulsive rituals: immediate long-term effects. Behav Ther 1984;15:450–472.
85. Cottraux J, Mollard E, Bouvard M, Marks I. Exposure therapy, fluvoxamine, or combination treatment in obsessive-compulsive disorder: one year follow-up. Psychiatry Res 1993;49:63–75.
86. Himle J, Fischer D, Van Etten M, Janeck A, Hanna G. Group behavioral therapy for adolescents with tic-related and non-tic related obsessive-compulsive disorder. Depress Anxiety 2003;17:73–77.
87. Piacentini J, Chang S. Behavioral treatments for Tourette syndrome and tic disorders: state of the art. Adv Neurol 2001;85:319–331.
88. Greenberg B, Price L, Rauch S, et al. Neurosurgery for intractable obsessive-compulsive disorder and depression: criti-cal issues. Neurosurg Clin N Am 2003;14:199–212.
89. Cosgrove G, Rausch S. Sterotacti cingulatomy. Neurosurg Clin N Am 2003;14:225–235.
90. Baer L, Rauch S, Ballantine H, et al. Cingulotomy for intractable obsessive-compulsive disorder. Arch Gen Psychiatry 1995;52:384–392.
91. Mindus P, Jenike M. Neurousurgical treatments of malignant obsessive-compulsive disorder. Psychiatr Clin North Am 1992;15:921–938.
92. Kurlan R, Kersun J, Ballantine H, Caine E. Neurosurgical treatment of severe obsessive-compulsive disorder associated with Tourette's syndrome. Mov Disord 1990;5:152–155.
93. Greenberg B. Update on deep brain stimulation. J ECT 2002;18:193–199.
94. Still G. The Coulstonian lectures on some abnormal physical conditions in children. Lecture 1. Lancet 1902;i:1008–1012.
95. Ebaugh F. Neuropsychiatric sequelae of acute epidemic encephalitis in children. Am J Dis Child 1923;25:89–97.
96. Barkley R. Attention-Deficit/Hyperactivity Disorder: A Handbook for Diagnosis and Treatment. New York: Guilford Press; 1998.
97. Walkup J, Khan S, Schuerholz L, Paik, Y, Leckman, J, Schultz R. Phenomenology and natural history of tic-related ADHD and learning disabilities. In: Leckman J, Cohen D, eds. Tourette's Syndrome: Tics, Obsessions, Compulsions. Develop-mental Psychopathology and Clinical Care. New York: Wiley; 1990:63.
98. Leckman J. Phenomenology of tics and natural history of tic disorders. Brain Dev 2003;25:S24–S28.
99. Biederman J, Faraone S, Spencer T, et al. Patterns of psychiatric comorbidity, cognition, and psychosocial functioning in adults with attention deficit hyperactivity disorder. Am J Psychiatry 1993;150:1792–1798.
100. Faraone S, Biederman J. Is attention deficit hyperactivity disorder familial? Harv Rev Psychiatry 1994;1:271–287.
101. Pauls D, Leckman J, Cohen D. Familial relationship between Gilles de la Tourette syndrome, attention deficit disorder, learning disabilities, speech disorders, and stuttering. J Amer Acad Child Adolesc Psychiatry 1993;32:1044–1050.
102. Stokes A, Bawden H, Camfield P, Backman J, Dooley M. Peer problems in Tourette's disorder. Pediatrics 1991;87:936–942.
103. Yeates K, Bornstein R. Attention deficit disorder and neuropsychological functioning in children with Tourette's syndrome. Neuropsychology 1994;8:65–74.
104. Spencer T, Biederman J, Harding M, et al. Disentangling the overlap between Tourette's disorder and ADHD. J Child Psychol Psychiatry 1998;39:1037–1044.
105. Sukhodolsky D, Scahill L, Zhang H, et al. Disruptive behavior in children with Tourette's syndrome: association with ADHD comorbidityt severity, and functional impairment. J Am Acad Child Adolesc Psychiatry 2003;42:98–105.
106. Bauermeister J, Canino G, Bird H. Epidemiology of disruptive behavior disorders. Child Adolesc Psychiatr Clin N Am 1994;3:177–194.
107. Jensen P, Kettle L, Roper M, et al. Are stimulants over-prescribed? Treatment of ADHD in four US communities. J Am Acad Child Adolesc Psychiatry 1999;38:797–804.
108. Goldman L, Genel M, Bezman RJ, Slanetz PJ. Diagnosis and treatment of attention deficit hyperactivity disorder in chil-dren and adolescents. JAMA 1998;279:1100–1107.
109. Walkup et al. 1999.
110. Castellanos F. Toward a pathophysiology of attention deficit/hyperactivity disorder. Clin Pediatr 1997;36:381–393.
111. Zametkin A, Nordahl T, Gross M, et al. Cerebral glucose metabolism in adults with hyperactivity of childhood onset. N Eng J Med 1990;323:1361–1366.
112. Ernst M, Zametkin A, Matochik J, Jons P, Cohen R. DOPA decarboxylase activity in attention deficit hyperactivity dis-order adults. A (fluorine-18) fluorodopa positron emission tomographic study. J Neurosci 1998;18:5901–5907.
113. Dougherty D, Bonab A, Spender T, Rausch S, Madreas B, Fischman A. Dopamine transporter density is elevated in patients with ADHD. Lancet 1999;354:2132–2133.
114. Biederman J, Newcorn J, Sprich S. Comorbidity of attention deficit hyperactivity disorder with conduct, depressive, anxi-ety and other disorders. Am J Psychiatry 1991;148:564–577.

115. Biederman J, Faraone S, Milberger S, et al. A prospective 4-year follow-up study of attention-deficit hyperactivity and related disorders. Arch Gen Psychiatry 1996;53:437–446.

116. Geller B, Zimerman B, Williams M, et al. Diagnostic characteristics of 93 cases of a prepubertal and early adolescent bipolar disorder phenotype by gender, puberty and comorbid attention deficit hyperactivity disorder. J Child Adolesc Psychopharmacol 2000;10:157–164.

117. Wilens T, Faraone S, Biederman J, Gunawardene S. Does stimulant therapy of attention-deficit hyperactivity disorder beget later substance abuse? A meta-analytic review of the literature. Pediatrics 2003;111:179–185.

118. Abwender D, Como P, Kurlan R, et al. School problems in Tourette's syndrome. Arch Neurol 1996;53:509–511.

119. Erenberg G, Cruse R, Rothner A. Tourette syndrome: an analysis of 200 pediatric and adolescent cases. Cleve Clin Q 1986;53:127–131.

120. Spencer T, Biederman J, Wilens T, Harding M, O'Donnell D, Griffin S. Pharmacotherapy of attention deficit hyperactivity disorder across the lifecycle: a literature review. J Am Acad Child Adolesc Psychiatry 1996;35:409–432.

121. Swanson J, Kramer H, Hinshaw S, et al. Clinical relevance of the primary findings of the MTA: success rates on severity of ADHD and ODD symptoms at the end of treatment. J Am Acad Child Adolesc Psychiatry 2001;40:168–179.

122. Biederman J. Practical considerations in stimulant drug selection for the attention-deficit/hyperactivity disorder patient— efficacy, potency and titration. Today's Therapeutic Trends 2002;20:311–328.

123. Greenhill L. Efficacy and safety of OROS methylphenidate in adolescents with ADHD. resented at the 49th annual meeting of the American Academy of Child and Adolescent Psychiatry, San Francisco, October 22–27, 2002.

124. West S, Johnson D, Wigal S, Zeldis J. Withdrawal trial of dex-methylphenidate HCL Focalin in children with ADHD. NR341. Presented at the 155th annual meeting of the American Psychiatric Association, Philadelphia, May 22, 2002.

125. Biederman J, Lopez F, Boellner S, Chandler M. A randomized, double-blind, placebo-controlled parallel group study of SL1381 (Adderall XR) in children with attention-deficit/hyperactivity disorder. Pediatrics 2002;110:258–266.

126. Sverd J, Gadow K, Paolicelli L. Methylphenidate treatment of attention-deficit hyperactivity disorder in boys with Tourette's syndrone. J Am Acad Child Adolesc Psychiatry 1989;28:574–579.

127. Gadow K, Nolan E, Sverd J. Methylphenidate in hyperactive boys with comorbid tic disorder 1. Short-term behavioral effects in school setting. J Am Acad Child Adolesc Psychiatry 1992;31:462–471.

128. The Tourette's Syndrome Study Group Treatment of ADHD in children with tics. A randomized controlled trial. Neurology 2002;58:527–536.

129. Castellanos F. Stimulants and tic disorders: from dogma to data. Arch Gen Psychiatry 1999;56:337–338.

130. Spencer T, Biederman J, Coffey B, et al. A double-blind comparison of desipramine and placebo in children and adolescents with chronic tic disorder and comorbid attention-deficit/hyperactivity disorder. Arch Gen Psychiatry 2002;59:649–656.

131. Wernicke J, Kratochvil D, Milton D, et al. Long-term safety of Atomoxetine in children and adolescents with ADHD. NR338. Presented at the 155th annual meeting of the American Psychiatric Association, Philadelphia, May 22, 2002.

132. McCracken J, Sallee R, Leonard H, et al. Improvement of ADHD by Atomoxetine in Children with Tic Disorders. Paper presented at the 50th annual meeting of the American Academy of Child and Adolescent Psychiatry, Miami FL, 2003.

133. Chappell P, Riddle M, Scahill L, et al. Guanfacine treatment of comorbid attention-deficit hyperactivity disorder in Tourette's syndrome: preliminary clinical experience. J Amer Acad Child Adolesc Psychiatry 1995;34:1140–1146.

134. Hunt R, Capper L, O'Connell P. Clonidine in child and adolescent psychiatry. J Child Adolesc Psychopharmacol 1990;I:87–102.

135. Biederman R, Swanson J, Lopez F. Modafinil improves ADHD symptoms in children in a randomized, double-blind placebo-controlled study. Scientific and Clinical Report Session 12, No 36. Presentation at the 156th annual meeting of the American Psychiatric Association, San Francisco, May 17–22, 2003.

136. Spencer T, Biederman J, Steingard R, Wilens T. Buproprion exacerbates tics in children with attention-deficit hyperactivity disorder and tic disorder or Tourette Syndrome. J Amer Acad Child Adolesc Psychiatry 1993;32:211–214.

18

Huntington's Disease

Karen E. Anderson and Karen S. Marder

INTRODUCTION

Huntington's disease (HD) is an autosomal dominant, progressive, neurodegenerative disorder first described in detail by George Huntington in 1872. Symptoms of HD include an extrapyramidal motor disorder, cognitive impairment, and psychiatric syndromes. Impairments in all three domains may occur simultaneously in an individual patient, or separately over the course of the illness. Behavioral and cognitive changes may precede the onset of neurological signs. Because few psychiatrists have experience in caring for patients with HD, the neurologist often must be adept in evaluation and treatment of both neurological and behavioral abnormalities.

NEUROLOGICAL SYMPTOMS AND GENETICS

Worldwide prevalence of HD is estimated at approx 4 to 7 per 100,000 people *(1)*. The disorder is less common among those of non-European ancestry. Typically, onset is in the 30s or 40s. Onset as early as age 2 or as late as 80 has been observed.

Clinical Features

Neurological signs and symptoms seen in HD include abnormal involuntary movements (chorea and dystonia) and disorders of voluntary movement (gait impairment, impairment of saccades, smooth pursuit, speech, and swallowing). The disease worsens gradually leading, in most cases, to severe disability. Patients with juvenile-onset HD, defined as age of onset less than 20 years, sometimes called the Westphal variant, comprise less than 6% of cases. They often present with a very different clinical picture, including Parkinsonism, seizures, and myoclonus, with rapid progression of the illness. School failure is often reported, and may be the earliest sign of the disease. Chorea is often minimal, whereas bradykinesia and dystonia predominate. Individuals with onset of HD in their sixth or seventh decade generally have a more indolent course with relative sparing of cognition. These later onset patients are sometimes misdiagnosed as having a parkinsonian syndrome because they are occasionally responsive to levodopa *(2)*.

Genetics and Age of Onset

The genetic abnormality underlying HD is caused by an abnormal expansion of trinucleotide repeats coding for glutamine at the N-terminus of the "huntingtin" protein *(3)*. The increase occurs in sequences of cytosine, adenine, and guanine (CAG) in exon 1 of the HD gene on the short arm of chromosome 4. The gene, known as *IT 15*, which encodes the protein huntingtin, is expressed throughout

From: *Current Clinical Neurology: Psychiatry for Neurologists*
Edited by: D.V. Jeste and J.H. Friedman © Humana Press Inc., Totowa, NJ

the brain; however, pathologically there appears to be selective vulnerability in the striatum and to a lesser extent the globus pallidus *(4)*. The normal function of huntingtin, a predominantly cytoplasmic protein, is unknown, but may include neuroprotective effects, such as "anti-apoptotic" properties. Excitotoxic effects of glutamatergic transmission, mitochondrial dysfunction, and dysregulation of CREB-binding protein-mediated gene expression (transcriptional dysregulation) have all been proposed as possible mechanisms for neuronal damage and death in HD *(5–7)*. Several compounds have been tested in mouse models of HD (generally the R6/2 mouse) with some success including riluzole, minocyline, coenzyme Q10, creatine, ascorbate, and remacemide hydrochloride *(8)*, however, none to date have been shown to be neuroprotective in humans. Two histone deacetylase inhibitors— suberoylanilide hydroxamic acid and sodium phenylbutrate—are also under investigation, as is cystamine, a transglutaminase inhibitor *(9)*.

The discovery of the gene in 1993 led to the development of direct testing for HD in individual patients from a blood sample *(3)*. Normal individuals have between 9-26 CAG repeats, with most having approx 18 repeats on each allele. Those who develop clinically apparent symptoms of HD have a higher number of repeats, usually greater than 40, on the allele inherited from the affected parent. CAG repeat number is inversely correlated with the age of disease onset. However, clinicians must be aware that it is impossible to predict exact age of disease onset in any individual patient based on CAG repeat length, and a great deal of interindividual variability occurs, especially in the 40–50 repeat range seen in most HD cases. Those with juvenile-onset HD have a repeat size of 50 or greater. Those who have an HD gene with 36–39 repeats may or may not develop the symptoms of HD, and generally have a later disease onset. They are, however, at risk of transmitting the disorder to their children, because the CAG repeats expand in each successive generation. No individual with 35 or fewer CAG repeats has been reported to develop HD symptoms. Table 1 summarizes the clinical implications of differing repeat numbers. Although those with 26–35 repeats will not develop HD themselves, they may pass the mutation on to their progeny through CAG repeat expansion in successive generations. Paternal transmission tends to produce greater CAG expansion (as a result of meiotic instability) and earlier disease onset in successive generations than that seen with maternal transmission. The link between CAG repeat length and disease progression remains controversial. A recent review by Myers provides a comprehensive overview of genetics in HD *(9a)*. Rare cases of pedigrees that produce phenocopies of HD but derive from different CAG expansions have been reported ("Huntington's disease-like 2") *(10)*. It is of interest that other CAG repeat disorders, including several spinocerebellar ataxias, show an inverse relationship between abnormal CAG repeat expansion number and disease onset *(11)*.

Asymptomatic or "At-Risk" Testing

Genetic counseling at a certified testing program is recommended by the Huntington's Disease Society of America (HDSA) for those seeking presymptomatic testing for the HD gene *(12)*. During counseling, individuals should be urged to explore the impact of positive or negative genetic test results on decisions in many areas of their life. Career and educational choices (such as entering a more or less demanding or lucrative field based on genetic status) should be discussed. The influence of genetic test results on marriage and childbearing decisions should also be considered. It is important for those counseling someone contemplating predictive genetic testing to address whether the individual is being coerced into testing by others (such as a potential spouse) who may end the relationship if the person carries the mutation, adding yet another loss. Although few people who enter the testing process will have answers to all of these questions, it is important for the counselor to determine that they have considered the full ramifications of learning their own genetic information about a condition for which there is currently no cure.

The potential impact on other family members who may be at risk for HD but may not wish to know their own genetic status should also be addressed. For example, a daughter, whose mother is from a known HD family, requests genetic testing. The mother, who feels she does not have symptoms of

Table 1
Assessment of CAG Repeat Length in Huntington's Disease (HD)

CAG repeat number	Description	Clinical picture	Comments
Less than 26		Normal	Normal individuals typically have CAG repeat number of 20 or less.
27–35	Meiotic instability	Normal phenotype	May pass on expanded CAG repeats to offspring, little is known at this time about true phenotype of these rare cases.
36–39	Reduced penetrance	HD	May have much later disease onset, but will still pass HD gene to 50% of offspring and may pass on higher number expansion.
40 or greater	Abnormal expansion	HD	Individual will develop HD symptoms; caution should be used in attempts to predict age of disease onset for any individual patient based on CAG repeat length.

HD, states she does not want to be tested herself. Meeting with the mother and daughter to facilitate communication and explore the mother's feelings about testing is vital in this situation, because if the daughter is tested independently and is found to be gene-positive, her mother's genetic status would be revealed. Adverse outcomes, including precipitation of major psychiatric illness, and suicides, have occurred following predictive genetic testing for HD, generally in the first 6 months after test results are given *(13)*. Survivor guilt may also be seen in those who test negative if other family members are affected with HD. Patients who have clinically apparent symptoms of HD but seek genetic testing for confirmation of the diagnosis may also benefit from genetic counseling prior to testing. The HDSA recommends that minors not be tested, except in extenuating circumstances.

Neurobiology

The distinctive neuropathological change seen in HD is the reduction in the medium spiny neurons in the striatum *(14)*. Caudate changes are the most prominent, but cell death also occurs throughout the striatum, globus pallidus, thalamus, and cerebellum *(15)*. Magnetic resonance imaging studies have shown quantifiable decline in caudate volume over time, correlating with age of disease onset and with trinucleotide repeat length *(16,17)*. Basal ganglia atrophy has been found in gene positive, asymptomatic individuals up to 7 years prior to onset of motor symptoms *(18)*. Receptor studies of HD patients have found reductions in striatal dopamine receptor binding, related to duration of illness *(19,20)*. As the disease advances, widespread atrophy occurs *(14,15,21)*.

Differential Diagnosis

A number of other conditions, some of which have prominent psychiatric and cognitive signs and symptoms, should be considered in the workup of a patient with chorea or in other cases of suspected HD. These include medication-related chorea, lupus, chorea gravidarum, Sydenham's chorea, polycythemia vera, hyperthyroidism, chorea following toxin exposure, Wilson's disease, neuroacanthocytosis, dentatorubralpallidoluysian atrophy, and cerebral vascular accidents leading to acute hemi-chorea/ballismus. As noted earlier, late-onset HD may be confused with parkinsonian disorders. In patients with psychiatric disorders, exposure to neuroleptics and subsequent tardive dyskinesia may confound the clinical picture. A family history absent of HD may be misleading, especially in cases of adoption, mistaken paternity, or if one family member has taken it on him or herself to conceal presence of a movement disorder in prior generations. A careful neurological exam and history and a detailed pedigree, along with confirmatory genetic testing, if desired by the family, is sufficient to determine the diagnosis in cases with a known family history of HD. In those cases with unclear or missing family history, appropriate laboratory tests and neuroimaging can also be helpful in determination of the diagnosis.

Treatment of Neurological Symptoms

At this time, there is no proven treatment to prevent HD symptom onset or slow disease progression. Treatment of chorea is not recommended unless the chorea is extremely disabling because the agents used to suppress chorea may worsen other symptoms. If chorea is treated, tetrabenazine, a reversible dopamine depletor that is only available with an investigational new drug application, can be extremely useful, as can an irreversible depletor, reserpine. Several of the glutamate antagonists, such as amantadine, riluzole, and remacemide may reduce chorea. If psychiatric symptoms, such as aggression, irritability, or psychosis are also present in addition to chorea, a standard or atypical neuroleptic may be used to treat both. Haloperidol is usually the treatment of choice in these cases because it provides the most effective suppression of chorea in a dosing range with the fewest side effects. Pharmacotherapy for the movement disorder is outlined in Table 2.

Measures to maintain function in HD patients can be extremely useful and may lead to much improved quality of life. They include physical therapy, speech and swallowing assessments and therapy, and dietary interventions including increased calories to maintain weight and modification of food to prevent choking. As motor and behavioral symptoms progress, patients with advanced HD may become wheelchair or bedbound, incontinent of urine and feces, and have drastically decreased caloric intake resulting from dysphagia. Common causes of death in patients with advanced HD include injuries related to serious falls, poor nutrition, choking, aspiration pneumonia, and other infections. It is important for physicians and other clinicians to discuss these potential complications with patients and their families in an empathetic manner, and to assist in planning for these events in accordance with the patient's wishes while they are still able to participate in decision making for matters such as writing advanced directives. A multidisciplinary approach to care of advanced patients can greatly improve their quality of life despite significant impairment *(22)*.

Summary of Experimental Treatments Under Investigation

Research is underway to investigate agents that have shown a potential neuroprotective effect in animal models such as transgenic mice, and in in vitro studies. These agents include creatine, which has been shown to slow disease progression in transgenic mice, and minocycline, a caspase inhibitor with beneficial effects in mouse models. Coenzyme Q10, remacemide, and lamotrigene, have all been studied for their potential to reduce oxidative stress *(23)*.

COGNITIVE IMPAIRMENT AND DEMENTIA

HD patients are generally found to have deficits in the domains of visuospatial, memory, and executive task performance. Early HD patients typically show slowed thought processes, which may be manifested as significant delay in responding to questions, and impaired ability to manipulate information, which is more readily apparent in patients with more cognitively demanding vocations *(24)*. Visuospatial problems may be some of the other earliest cognitive changes seen in HD *(25)*. Memory deficits in HD include slowed rates of learning and deficits in recall. Free recall improves with cued recall and recognition in HD patients, unlike those with Alzheimer's disease *(26)*. Retention is relatively normal in HD, and is often cited as a useful differentiating factor of HD from Alzheimer's on formal neuropsychological assessments. Executive dysfunction is also reported consistently in studies of HD patients on various types of tasks, including planning and sequencing working memory

Table 2
Management of the Movement Disorder in Huntington's Disease[a]

Commonly used medications	Starting dose (Dosing ranges for total daily dose)	Dosing	Potential side effects
Haloperidol	0.5–1.0 mg QD (5–10 mg QD)	Use BID or TID dosing	TD, acute dystonic reaction, akathisia, swallowing and gait impairment, parkinsonism
Tetrabenazine	12.5 mg QD, increase by 12.5 mg every 5–7 days (100–200mg)	TID dosing	Parkinsonism, depression, drowsiness, hypotension
Reserpine	0.1 mg, increase by 0.1 mg every 5–7 days (2–3 mg)	QID or TID dosing	Same as above May cause severe depression—do not use in patients with history of mood disorders.
Risperidone	0.5 mg QHS, increase by 0.5 mg every 3–5 days as tolerated (4–6 mg)	BID dosing	Parkinsonism, drowsiness, increased, risk of developing diabetes. Atypicals are generally less efficacious for suppression of chorea than standard neuroleptics.
Olanzapine	2.5 mg, increase by 2.5 mg every 2–3 days (5–20 mg)	BID dosing	Drowsiness, weight gain, increased risk of developing diabetes. Atypicals are generally less efficacious for suppression of chorea than standard neuroleptics.
Quetiapine	25 mg, increase by 25 mg every 3–5 days as tolerated (100–300mg)	BID dosing	Transient and asymptomatic liver function test increases possible, increased risk of developing diabetes. Atypicals are generally less efficacious for suppression of chorea than standard neuroleptics.
Baclofen	10 mg, increase by 10 mg every 2–3 days (60–80 mg)	BID or TID dosing	Drowsiness, dizziness, ataxia, seizures

[a]Note that treatment of chorea is only advised in cases where chorea is socially or functionally disabling, because of the side effects associated with these medications. QD, each day; QHS, at bedtime; BID, twice a day; TID, three times a day; QID, four times a day; TD, tardive dyskinesia.

and set shifting *(27,24)*. Procedural memory is also impaired, as is seen in tests of skill and motor learning *(28)*.

Executive and attentional deficits are seen in mild to moderate HD *(29)*. Formal neuropsychological testing can be very helpful in early in the disease to delineate the extent of cognitive involvement and follow cognitive change over time. A recent cross sectional analysis of 226 gene-positive, presymptomatic, individuals suggests that cognitive impairment and striatal atrophy are present before a clinical diagnosis of HD can be made *(30)*. There is currently no treatment available to slow progression of cognitive decline in HD, and most patients become demented in later stages of the illness. However, judicious evaluation of medications, and elimination or reduction, when possible, of those known to contribute to impairment of cognition, can be helpful in many cases. Any precipitous decline in cognitive function in an HD patient should be viewed with suspicion, and evaluation for occult infection or other undiagnosed medical illness should be undertaken. Given the extensive atrophy seen in many cases, HD patients are also particularly prone to subdural hematomas, which can severely alter mental status.

There have been reports of cholinesterase inhibitor use in HD to treat both motor and cognitive decline, but open label studies have not been conducted to date *(31,32)*.

AN OVERVIEW OF PSYCHIATRIC SYMPTOMS

Psychiatric symptoms may occur at any point in the course of HD; they predate the onset of motor abnormalities in one-fourth to one-half of all patients *(33–36)*. Unlike the generally predictable progression of motor and cognitive symptoms, no clear time course for psychiatric disease has been demonstrated. CAG repeat length has not been shown to correlate positively with age of onset of psychiatric symptoms or with presence of psychiatric disorders *(37)*. There is some work suggesting that apathy may correlate with progression of cognitive and motor symptoms. Other symptoms that have received extensive study in HD, such as depression and irritability, have not been reliably shown to correlate with progression of the disease, although depression tends to occur early on in the illness but often persists. Psychiatric symptoms add greatly to the burden of caregivers, distress suffered by patients, and are one of the main factors in decisions to institutionalize HD patients. The impairment in executive function, described previously, probably contributes greatly to psychiatric morbidity in HD by resulting in decreased flexibility and problems in changing behavior to suit an evolving environment. Changes in personality are very common in HD, but have received little study. Many HD patients with psychiatric symptoms respond to standard pharmacotherapy; lower dosing ranges are generally recommended, at least at the initiation of treatment. A review by Anderson and Marder summarizes the limited research on treatment of behavioral symptoms in HD to date *(38)*. Table 3 summarizes treatment guidelines for selected psychiatric symptoms in HD patients. Treatment of selected behavioral symptoms is also discussed in the vignettes at the end of the chapter.

IRRITABILITY AND AGGRESSION

Irritability is one of the most common behavioral symptoms in HD, affecting more than 50% of all patients at some point in the illness and often accompanied by verbal or physical aggression. A study of 960 HD patients found that more than 60% of HD patients or caregivers reported aggressive behavior by the patient at their first visit to an HD clinic *(39)*. This suggests that, although the majority of the work to date studying aggression and irritability in HD has been conducted with those who are institutionalized, these symptoms can appear quite early in the illness and may precede onset of motor abnormalities. More than one-third of HD patients in nursing homes were found to be aggressive in a retrospective study *(40)*. Dewhurst and others *(41)* found that violence was the main reason for hospitalization in 25% of 102 HD psychiatric inpatients. Aggression in HD was found to occur with similar frequency in men and women in another nursing home study, which differs from the general population within which the preponderance of aggressive acts are committed by males *(33)*. In the case of these patients, mild aggression occurred in 26% and moderate aggression in 11%, but seldom resulted in serious injury to the patients or to others. This may be partly a result of nursing home staff having experience and training in dealing with aggressive patients.

Because irritability is often directed toward individuals known to the patients, educating caregivers on how to identify and avoid situations that trigger irritability and how to minimize its effects if it does occur is vitally important. Behavioral interventions may prove helpful in prevention of irritability and aggression in HD by removing precipitating factors. This includes adherence to a schedule to avoid surprising the patient and provoking an outburst *(22)*. Caregivers should be advised to stop an activity, such as assistance with dressing or grooming, if aggressive behavior begins to escalate because irritability may be precipitated by assistance with activities of daily living in many patients.

Table 3
Suggested Agents for Treatment of Psychiatric Symptoms

Target symptom(s)	Examples of psychopharmacological agents used for treatment (dosing ranges)	Potential side effects	Overall comments
Irritability and aggression	Escitalopram (10–20 mg)	Initially may cause anxiety or agitation.	Generally best to start with an SRRI, then add a neuroleptic if needed. However, in cases of extreme aggression, a neuroleptic should be started first.
	Sertraline (100–200 mg)	Initially may cause anxiety or agitation.	
	Olanzapine (10–20 mg)	Weight gain, which can be helpful in some patients, sedation, possible EPS.	Standard neuroleptics will provide the most rapid sedation in these cases. *See* Table 2 for dosing of standard neuroleptics such as haloperidol.
	Quetiapine (100–300 mg, may go higher in select cases)	Sedation, possible EPS.	
Depressed mood	Escitalopram (10–20 mg)	Initially may cause anxiety or agitation. GI side effects are common, as is sedation.	Patients and caregivers should be reminded that response to an antidepressant may take 4 weeks.
Anxiety disorders (generalized anxiety, OCD, panic attacks)	Fluoxetine (40–80 mg)	Agitation, GI symptoms, insomnia.	Higher doses than those used to treat depression may be needed in the treatment of anxiety disorders.
Sleep disorders	Clonazepam (0.5–1.0 mg) at bedtime	Sedation; may cause paradoxical disinhibition in some patients, increased fall risk, confusion.	Suppresses movements so patients can fall asleep.
Psychosis	Olanzapine (10–20 mg)	Weight gain, which can be helpful in some patients, sedation, possible EPS.	Starting with an atypical neuroleptic is preferable, but a standard neuroleptic should be used in more severe cases.
	Quetiapine (100–300 mg, may go higher in select cases.	Sedation, possible EPS.	

OCD, obsessive-compulsive disorder; EPS, extrapyramidal symptoms; SSRI, selective serotonin reuptake inhibitor.

They should also be counseled not to argue with patients if it appears that irritability is escalating. If threats of physical aggression occur, they should walk away from the patient and contact emergency medical services for assistance. Obviously, guns and other weapons should be removed from the home. The patient should be prevented from accessing alcohol and illicit drugs because use of these substances, even in small quantities, may contribute greatly to disinhibition and disruptive behavior in patients with a neurodegenerative condition. In extreme cases, law enforcement agencies may need to intervene to prevent injury to the patient or to family members. Careful evaluation by a medical professional to rule out medical illness, delirium, medication toxicity, or physical discomfort should be conducted, especially in patients who have not been disruptive previously, or in those for whom communication may be impaired *(42)*. Underlying psychiatric illness should also be considered, such as depression, anxiety, or psychosis. Akithisia may occur, with concomitant restlessness and irritability, in patients who are being treated with neuroleptics for suppression of chorea or for psychiatric symptoms. Irritability and aggression both respond to phamacotherapy in many cases, sometimes in combination with behavioral interventions.

APATHY

Apathy is present in more than 50% of all HD patients and has been shown to increase with duration of illness, although it certainly occurs early in many cases *(43)*. It may also correlate positively with progression of cognitive decline and motor impairment. This may be a result of increasing pathological changes in frontostriatal circuitry affecting cognition, especially in planning and other executive functions. Apathy is often difficult to differentiate from depression, especially as the disease progresses and communication becomes impaired. Generally, apathy is more distressing to caregivers than to patients. No treatment that has been found to be definitively effective for apathy, although, as with irritability, structuring of daily activities may be useful. Patients may engage in activities if they are encouraged to do so and are not presented with too many choices *(44)*. Education of family members to promote reasonable expectations of patient behavior is often the most beneficial intervention.

MOOD DISORDERS

Up to 50% of HD patients have an affective disorder at some point in the illness, with depression as the predominant condition. Depression may occur at any point in the illness, including prodromally or concomitantly with the onset of the movement disorder, an observation that argues against a purely reactive depression. Suicide rates in HD are increased fourfold compared with the general population *(45)*. Rates from 3 to 7% have been reported, with more than 25% of patients attempting suicide at some point in the illness; suicide risk is particularly increased among patients in their fifth or sixth decade *(46)*. This overall increase in suicidality in HD may be partly the result of the high frequency of impulsivity seen in these patients *(47)*. Risk factors for suicidal behavior in HD patients are similar to those in the general population, and include depression, living alone, childlessness, being unmarried, substance abuse, and having access to guns *(48)*. Thus, HD patients who are depressed should receive careful evaluation for suicidal ideation, and all threats of suicide should be treated with utmost seriousness. There should be a low threshold for psychiatric hospitalization for observation and treatment.

The prevalence of mania and hypomania are also increased in HD. From the limited data available, mania appears to occur in approx 5% of patients. Folstein reported episodes of mania or hypomania in 10% of HD patients *(35)*.

Affective disorders in HD respond well to standard pharmacotherapy in most cases. Little work has been done to evaluate the efficacy of selective serotonin reuptake inhibitors (SSRIs) and other newer antidepressants in patients with HD, but clinical observations suggest they are as effective as older agents, such as tricyclic antidepressants, and have fewer side effects. Mood stabilizers are also useful in patients with mania. Supportive psychotherapy may be extremely helpful to patients at various stages in the illness, and is often invaluable for those who are undergoing asymptomatic, predictive genetic testing.

ANXIETY DISORDERS

Anxiety disorders have received relatively little study in HD, but they probably occur with high frequency. Anxiety was described as a common prodromal symptom of HD in some older work *(41)*. Clinical observation suggests that anxiety occurs with depression in many HD patients. Paulsen et al. *(49)* found that anxiety was reported by more than 50% of HD patients or their caregivers in a clinic setting. Obsessions and compulsions, a particular subset of anxiety symptoms, have been found to occur with high frequency in HD patients. Of HD patients, 20–50% have been reported to have obsessions or compulsions, depending on the assessment performed *(50,39)*. Other illnesses affecting the basal ganglia, including Tourette's syndrome, basal ganglia lesions, and Sydenham's chorea, also show a high frequency of obsessions and compulsions, supporting the theory that abnormalities of frontostriatal circuitry may contribute to development of these symptoms.

PSYCHOTIC DISORDERS

Psychotic symptoms are seen in approx 4% of patients. Psychosis is generally thought to be more prevalent in patients with younger onset of disease. Delusions of persecution are probably the most common psychotic symptoms; catatonia, complex delusional systems, and other symptoms seen in schizophrenia are rare, and most HD patients with psychosis do not meet diagnostic criteria for schizophrenia. These symptoms may result from effects of dopaminergic hyperactivity, interacting with subcortical limbic pathology.

SUBSTANCE ABUSE

There has been little work describing substance abuse in patients with HD. Anecdotally, HD patients are thought to be at increased risk for substance abuse, given their impulsivity and high prevalence of mood disorders. It is also unclear whether those at risk for HD are also at higher risk for abuse of alcohol and other drugs. Berrios et al. *(51)* did not find a significantly different incidence of alcohol abuse when comparing asymptomatic gene carriers to those from HD families who were gene-negative.

SLEEP DISTURBANCES

Sleep disturbances are quite common in HD; many patients have difficulty falling asleep because their movements keep them awake. Chorea may throw bedclothes off the patient and, in extreme cases, cause them to fall out of bed. Sleep changes have been reported in HD, leading to poor overall quality of sleep. Daytime fatigue obviously contributes to decreased cognitive function and may worsen psychiatric symptoms such as irritability. Judicious nighttime use of benzodiazepines in small doses is often helpful in suppression of the movements until patients fall asleep, at which time the movements generally cease.

PERSONALITY ALTERATIONS AND OTHER BEHAVIORAL SYMPTOMS

Development of personality alterations nonspecific to any one psychiatric diagnosis have been reported for many years by those who study HD *(41)*. Personality changes are probably one of the most frequent, and least studied, of all behavioral abnormalities in HD. Reports indicate that personality changes occur in anywhere from 10 to 41% of HD patients; these figures may be artificially low because many studies exclude irritability and apathy *(52)*. Aside from apathy and irritability, which are discussed above, impulsivity, emotional lability, and lack of empathy for others are all probably quite common.

Personality changes are described in individuals who carry the HD mutation who are asymptomatic. Increased anger and hostility have been reported among family members most at risk to develop HD, and irritability has been shown to be increased in asymptomatic, gene-positive individuals *(51)*.

Several groups have concluded that personality changes are among the earliest signs of HD, preceding motor and cognitive changes *(41,53)*. However, a recent study comparing asymptomatic carriers to individuals from HD families who were gene-negative found that both groups had elevated scores on tests for personality disorders, suggesting a role for family environment *(51)*.

Both hyper- and hypoactive sexual desire is reported in HD. Hypersexual behaviors were reported in 12% of men and 7% of women in an early study *(36)*. Those family members in known HD families who are ultimately diagnosed with HD are more fecund than those who do not develop the illness *(35)*. However, male impotence is also increased in HD *(35)*. Paraphillias including exhibitionism, voyeurism, pedophilia, and sexual aggression were reported in very early HD work, but have received little recent study *(54)*. Infidelity has been reported to occur early in the illness, probably as a result of impulsivity *(54,55)*. Nonviolent crimes are committed more frequently by men with HD than their first-degree relatives, a finding that is also probably related to impulsivity *(56)*.

VIGNETTES

Case 1

Mr. L is a 30-year-old malewith a diagnosis of HD who has had symptoms of the movement disorder for 2 years. His wife is concerned that he is increasingly impatient with their children, ages 6 and 3 (e.g., throwing their toys in the trash when they do not put them away each evening). Last week, he deliberately drove his car over his son's bike because the child left it out in the rain. He also curses at his wife, and becomes extremely angry when he cannot watch specific television shows because she wants to watch a program. He has difficulty falling asleep, and his wife reports that he throws the bedclothes around and sometimes falls out of bed. He is isolated from his friends, has stopped attending church, and has become focused on the 15th anniversary of his father's death, which is in a few weeks. Mr. L's father hanged himself after losing his job as a CEO of a large corporation as a result of his HD symptoms.

Evaluation and Treatment Suggestions

This patient may be in the midst of an episode of major depression, which is contributing to irritability. A mood disorder is suggested by his social withdrawal and also his focus on his father's death. He should receive prompt and careful evaluation for depression and for suicidal ideation, which is also possible given the upcoming anniversary of his father's death. In the general population, completed suicide by a close relative increases suicide risk in an individual; this is probably also the case in HD.

Treatment could begin with standard doses of an antidepressant, such as an SSRI. This may help to quell the irritability. A neuroleptic could be added later if the antidepressant is not adequate in controlling the irritability. The patient's wife may need to modify behavior, for example taping programs she wants to see on television and walking away rather than engaging in arguments with him. If symptoms escalate and she fears physical aggression, the wife should be instructed to leave the house immediately with the children and call emergency medical services from a neighbor's house. Property destruction may be predictive of future physical violence against other people.

Sleep deprivation may be worsening his mood and increasing irritability and impulsivity in this patient. The difficulty falling asleep could be a result of his depressed mood, but may also result from movements that are keeping the patient awake. Suppression of chorea with a small dose of benzodiazepine may allow the patient to fall asleep, at which point the movements will cease on their own.

Case 2

Mrs. K is a 55-year-old woman who has had HD symptoms for more than 15 years. She is cared for by her family at home, and requires constant supervision because of frequent falls. Her family is very concerned because she spends most of her day on the couch in the family room watching a blank TV screen and smoking. When family members ask if they can turn on any shows for her, she simply shrugs and yawns. She shows little interest in her grandchildren and no longer asks to have her daughter put cosmetics on for her or to be taken to the salon. She is eating well, with occasional choking, maintaining her weight, and sleeping through the night. The family denies that she is sad or tearful, and when asked about mood she states she is "fine."

Evaluation and Treatment Suggestions

This patient could be depressed, which would explain her social withdrawal and lack of interest in things around her. However, it is more likely that she is apathetic, a common symptom in HD that may increase in frequency with disease progression. Family education may be the most important intervention in this case, if depression is ruled out on evaluation. The family should be counseled to lower their expectations for her participation in activities. They should attempt to engage her in limited, structured activities and to offer her "yes" or "no" choices rather than open-ended questions. Reassuring the family that she is not "suffering" or depressed is very important.

Case 3

Mr. G is a 45-year-old gentleman who has had motor symptoms of HD for 7 years. His wife says he was always very conscientious and very orderly. In the past few years he has become more so, to the point where he can not go to bed at night unless he has personally checked all locks and windows in his house exactly four times. He also insists on keeping all his clothes in order by color and year of purchase. He collects newspaper clippings on local history, and spends hours each day reading through the newspapers; in the last 2 years he has accumulated more and more boxes of newspapers to be read and sorted in their garage, so that they must now leave their car outside. He became furious at his wife when she threw out a box of newspapers he saved that had been destroyed by mice, but the next day did not remember where that box had gone, and spent the afternoon searching for it.

Evaluation and Treatment Suggestions

This patient probably has obsessions and compulsions and may meet criteria for obsessive-compulsive disorder. He has checking, ordering, and hoarding symptoms. As with many patients, he becomes enraged when his obsessive and compulsive activities are thwarted. He may also have cognitive impairment, which exacerbates his psychiatric symptoms. A trial of an SSRI would probably help to reduce his obsessive and compulsive symptoms. Higher doses than those used to treat depression may be needed. His other medications should be evaluated and, if possible, those with anticholinergic effects should be reduced or eliminated to help maximize cognitive function.

SUMMARY

Although HD is widely known for its distinctive neurological symptoms, cognitive impairment and psychiatric symptoms often cause the preponderance of distress and impact greatly on caregiver burden. Predictive genetic testing in asymptomatic individuals can have far reaching impact on many areas of that person's life, and may have ramifications for others in the family also; it should therefore be conducted by those with experience in genetic counseling for HD. Combinations of different behavioral changes may make diagnosis and treatment of these symptoms difficult in HD patients, especially in patients for whom communication is problematic. Cognitive impairment can also confuse the clinical picture and worsen other behavioral symptoms. Despite these challenges, successful treatment of behavioral disturbances can greatly improve quality of life for patients and family members, and offers an area of tremendous positive impact in an incurable disease.

REFERENCES

1. Harper PS. The epidemiology of Huntington's disease. Hum Genet 1992; 89:363–376.
2. Reuter I, Hu MT, Andrews TC, Brooks DJ, Clough C, Chaudhuri KR. Late onset levodopa responsive Huntington's disease with minimal chorea masquerading as Parkinson plus syndrome. J Neurol Neurosurg Psychiatry 2000;68:238–241.

3. Huntington's Disease Collaborative Research Group. A novel gene containing a trinucleotide repeat that is expanded and unstable on Huntington's disease chromosomes. Cell 1993;72:971–983.

4. Vonsattel JP, DiFiglia M. Huntington disease. J Neuropathol Exp Neurol 1998;57:369–384.

5. Difiglia M. Excitotoxic injury of the neostriatum is a model for Huntington's disease. Trends Neurosci 1990;13:286–289.

6. Beal MF. Does impairment of energy metabolism result in excitotoxic neuronal death in neurodegenerative illnesses? Ann Neurol 1992;31:119–130.

7. Nucifora FC Jr, Sasaki M, Peters MF, et al. Interference by huntingtin and atrophin-1 with cbp-mediated transcription leading to cellular toxicity. Science 2001;291:2423–2428.

8. Hersch SM, Ferrante RJ. Translating therapies for Huntington's disease from genetic animal models to clinical trials. Neurorx 2004;1:298–306.

9. Feigin A, Zgaljardic D. Recent advances in Huntington's disease: implications for experimental therapeutics. Curr Opin Neurol 2002 Aug;15:483–489.

9a. Myers RH. Huntington's disease genetics. Neurorx 2004;1:255–262.

10. Margolis RL, O'Hearn E, Rosenblatt A, et al. A disorder similar to Huntington's disease is associated with novel CAG repeat expansion. Ann Neurol 2001;50:373–380.

11. Ross CA. Polyglutamine pathogenesis: emergence of unifying mechanisms for Huntington's disease and related disorders. Neuron 2002;35:819–822.

12. Hersch S, Jones R, Koroshetz W, Quaid K. The neurogenetics genie: testing for the Huntington's disease mutation. Neurology 1994;44:1369–1373.

13. Almqvist EW, Bloch M, Brinkman R, Craufurd D, Hayden MR. A worldwide assessment of the frequency of suicide, suicide attempts or psychiatric hospitalization after predictive testing for Huntington disease. Am J Hum Genet 1999;64: 1293–1304.

14. Hedreen JC, Folstein SE. Early loss of neostriatal striosome neurons in Huntington's disease. J Neuropathol Exp Neurol 1995;54:105–120.

15. Vonsattel JP, Myers RH, Stevens TJ, Ferrante RJ, Bird ED, Richardson EP Jr. Neuropathological classification of Huntington's disease. J Neuropahtol Exp Neurol 1985;44:559–577.

16. Rosas HD, Goodman J, Chen YI, et al. Striatal volume loss in HD as measured by MRI and the influence of CAG repeat. Neurology 2001;57:1025–1028.

17. Aylward EH, Li Q, Stine OC, et al. Longitudinal change in basal ganglia volume in patients with Huntington's disease. Neurology 1997;48:394–399.

18. Aylward EH, Codori AM, Rosenblatt A, et al. Rate of caudate atrophy in presymptomatic and symptomatic stages of Huntington's disease. Mov Disord 2000;15:552–560.

19. Turjanski N, Weeks R, Dolan R, Harding AE, Brooks DJ. Striatal D1 and D2 receptor binding in patients with Huntington's disease and other choreas: a PET study. Brain 1995;118:689–696.

20. Ginovart N, Lundin A, Farde L, et al. PET study of pre and post-synaptic dopaminergic markers for the neuordegenerative process in Huntington's disease. Brain 1997;120:503–514.

21. Rosas HD, Feigin AS, Hersch SM. Using advances in neuroimaging to detect, understand, and monitor disease progression in Huntington's disease. Neurorx 2004;1:263–272.

22. Moskowitz CB, Marder K. Palliative care for people with late-stage Huntington's disease. Neurol Clin 2001;19:849–865.

23. Hersch SM. Huntington's disease: prospects for neuroprotective therapy 10 years after the discovery of the causative genetic mutation.Curr Opin Neurol 2003;16:501–506.

24. Brandt J. Cognitive impairments in Huntington's disease: insights into the neuropsychology of the striatum. In: Corkin S, Grafman J, Boller F, eds. Handbook of Neuropsychology, Vol 5. Amsterdam: Elsevier; 1991.

25. Brouwers P, Cox C, Martin A, Chase T, Fedio P. Differential perceptual-spatial impairment in Huntington's and Alzheimer's dementias. Arch Neurol 1984;41:1073–1076.

26. Hodges JR, Salmon DP, Butters N. Differential impairment of semantic and episodic memory in Alzheimer's and Huntington's diseases: a controlled prospective study. J Neurol Neurosurg Psychiatry 1990;53:1089–1095.

27. Lange KW, Sahakian BJ, Quinn NP, Marsden CD, Robbins TW. Comparison of executive and visuospatial memory function in Huntington's disease and dementia of Alzheimer type matched for degree of demetia. J Neurol Neurosurg Psychiatry 1995;58:598–606.

28. Paulsen JS, Butters N, Salmon DP, Heindel WC, Swenson MR. Prism adaptation in Alzheimer's and Huntington's disease. Neuropsychology 1993;7:73–81.

29. Ho AK, Sahakian BJ, Brown RG, et al. NEST-HD Consortium. Profile of cognitive progression in early Huntington's disease. Neurology 2003 23;61:1702–1706.

30. Ross CA, Aylward EH, Stout JC, et al. Clinical and Radiographic features among presymptomatic individuals carrying an expanded CAG repeat in the Huntington's disease gene: Analysis of baseline characteristics of the PREDICT-HD cohort. Abstract, S44.001, American Academy of Neurology 56th Annual Meeting, 2004.

31. Rot U, Kobal J, Sever A, Pirtosek Z, Mesec A. Rivastigmine in the treatment of Huntington's disease. Eur J Neurol 2002;9: 689–690.

32. Fernandez HH, Friedman JH, Grace J, Beason-Hazen S. Donepezil for Huntington's disease. Mov Disord 2000;15: 173–176.

33. Shiwach RS, Patel V. Aggressive behavior in Huntington's disease: a cross-sectional study in a nursing home population. Behav Neurol 1993;6:43–47.

34. Mendez MF. Huntington's disease: update and review of neuropsychiatric aspects. Int J Psychiatry Med 1994;24:189–208.

35. Folstein SE. Huntington Disease: A Disorder of Families, First Edition. Baltimore: The Johns Hopkins Press;1989.

36. Dewhurst K, Oliver JE, McKnight AL. Socio-psychiatric consequences of Huntington's disease. Br J Psychiatry 1970;116: 255–258.

37. Weigell-Weber M, Schmid W, Spiegel R. Psychiatric symptoms and CAG expansion in Huntington's disease. Am J Med Genet 1996;67:53–57.

38. Anderson KE, Marder KS. An overview of psychiatric symptoms in Huntington's disease. Curr Psychiatry Rep 2001;3: 379–388.

39. Marder K, Zhao H, Myers RH, et al. Rate of functional decline in Huntington's disease. Huntington Study Group. Neurology 2000;54:452–458.

40. Nance MA, Sanders G. Characteristics of individuals with Huntington disease in long-term care. Mov Disord 1996;11: 542–548.

41. Dewhurst K, Oliver J, Trick KL, McKnight AL. Neuro-psychiatric aspects of Huntington's disease. Confin Neurol 1969; 31:258–268.

42. Ranen NG, Peyser CE, Folstein SE. A Physician's Guide to the Management of Huntington's Disease: Pharmacologic and Nonpharmacoligic Interventions. New York: Huntington's Disease Society of America; 1993.

43. Paulsen JS, Butters N, Sadek JR, et al. Distinct cognitive profiles of cortical and subcortical dementia in advanced illness. Neurology 1995;45:951–956.

44. Caine ED, Shoulson I. Psychiatric syndromes in Huntington's disease. Am J Psychiatry 1983;140:728–733.

45. Di Maio L, Squitieri F, Napolitano G, Campanella G, Trofatter JA, Conneally PM. Suicide risk in Huntington's disease. J Med Genet 1993;30:293–295.

46. Schoenfeld M, Myers RH, Cupples LA, Berkman B, Sax DS, Clark E. Increased rate of suicide among patients with Huntington's disease. J Neuro Neurosurg Psychiatry 1984;47:1283–1287.

47. Leonard DP, Kidson MA, Brown JG, Shannon PJ, Taryan S. A double blind trial of lithium carbonate and haloperidol in Huntington's chorea. Aust N Z J Psychiatry 1975;9:115–118.

48. Lipe H, Schultz A, Bird TD. Risk factors for suicide in Huntingtons disease: a retrospective case controlled study. Am J Med Genet 1993;48:231–233.

49. Paulsen JS, Ready RE, Hamilton JM, Mega MS, Cummings JL. Neuropsychiatric aspects of Huntington's disease. J Neurol Neurosurg Psychiatry 2001;71:310–314.

50. Anderson KE, Louis ED, Stern Y, Marder KS. Cognitive correlates of obsessive and compulsive symptoms in Huntington's disease. Am J Psychiatry 2001;158:799–801.

51. Berrios GE, Wagle AC, Markova IS, Wagle SA, Rosser A, Hodges JR. Psychiatric symptoms in neurologically asymptomatic Huntington's disease gene carriers: a comparison with gene negative at risk subjects. Acta Psychiatr Scand 2002;105: 224–30.

52. Cummings JL. Behavioral and psychiatric symptoms associated with Huntington's disease. Adv Neurol 1995;65:179–86.

53. Lishman AW. Senile dementias, presenile dementias, and pseudodementias. In: Lishman AW, ed. Organic Psychiatry: The Psychological Consequences of Cerebral Disorder. Oxford: Blackwell Science; 1998:468–469.

54. Lion EG, Kahn E. Experiential aspects of Huntington's chorea. Am J Psychiatry 1938;95:717–727.

55. James WE, Mefferd RB Jr, Kimbell I Jr. Early signs of Huntington's chorea. Dis Nerv Syst 1969;30:556–559.

56. Jensen P, Fenger K, Bolwig TG, Sorensen SA. Crime in Huntington's disease: a study of registered offences among patients, relatives, and controls. J Neurol Neurosurg Psychiatry 1998;65: 467–471.

19

Psychiatry of the Cerebellum

Russell L. Margolis

INTRODUCTION

Since the pioneering early 19th-century studies of Luigi Rolando, the cerebellum has been recognized as a critical modulator of movement. Landmarks include the descriptions of hereditary disorders affecting the cerebellum by Friedreich in 1863 and Marie in 1893, and the pre-World War II work of Holmes, who established much of the terminology and many of the methods for assessing the motor functions of the cerebellum still in clinical use today. Every contemporary neurology text, and every neurology course for students, emphasizes the anatomy and physiology underlying the motor role of the cerebellum, and the motor signs and symptoms to be elicited in the clinical examination of cerebellar function. In contrast, the normal role of the cerebellum in cognition and emotion, and the potential impact of cerebellar damage on cognition and emotion, receives scant attention. In textbooks of neuropsychiatry, the cerebellum is hardly mentioned at all (Fig. 1).

The motor-only conception of the cerebellum is an idea of the past. Striking findings in the past 20 years, using contemporary tools of neuroanatomy, neuroimaging, neuropsychology, and psychiatric diagnosis, leave little doubt that the normal cerebellum plays an important role in cognition and emotion, and that diseases of the cerebellum may lead to cognitive impairment and psychiatric disorders. As many of these nonmotor consequences of cerebellar damage may be at least partially amenable to treatment, it is obligatory for the neurologist to vigorously search for them. This chapter outlines the causes and epidemiology of cerebellar disease, the preclinical basis for assuming a role of the cerebellum in modulating human emotion and cognition, and the direct evidence demonstrating that cerebellar damage results in cognitive and noncognitive psychopathology. Although many causes of cerebellar disease exist, much of the emphasis here is on patients with the chronic conditions in which neurologists will most often confront psychiatric disorders, primarily structural lesions such as strokes and tumors, and progressive degenerative disorders such as the spinocerebellar ataxias.

DISEASES AFFECTING THE CEREBELLUM

Epidemiology

The total prevalence of cerebellar disorders is unknown. At least 50% of patients who have alcohol-dependence syndromes may develop clinical or histological evidence of cerebellar disorder (1); alcohol is clearly the single most common cause of cerebellar damage worldwide. The cerebellum is affected in 1.5–8% of all strokes (2), so this is probably the second most common cause of cerebellar damage. In children, the annual incidence of tumors affecting the cerebellum is between 0.25 and 1 per 100,000 per year. In adults, primary tumors of the cerebellum are even less common, but metastases

From: *Current Clinical Neurology: Psychiatry for Neurologists*
Edited by: D.V. Jeste and J.H. Friedman © Humana Press Inc., Totowa, NJ

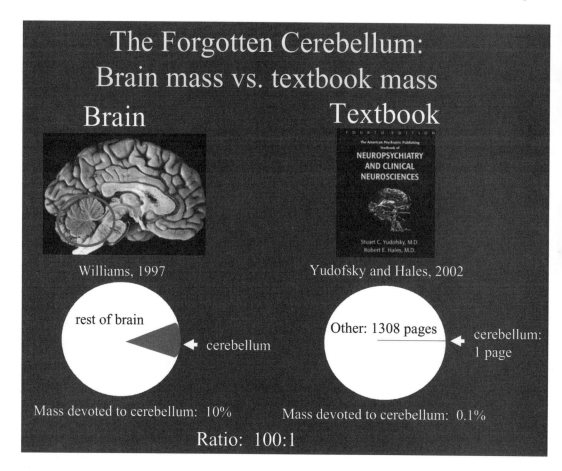

Fig. 1. The neglected cerebellum. Cover of *Textbook of Neuropsychiatry and Clinical Neurosciences* reprinted with permission from American Psychiatric Publishing, Inc., copyright 2004.

are more common. The prevalence of recessive (almost all Friedreich's ataxia), dominant, and sporadic neurodegenerative diseases that primarily affect the cerebellum is, in each case, about 2 per 100,000 *(3,4)*. Other causes of cerebellar lesions are rare.

Etiology

Table 1 lists many of the diseases that cause permanent injury to the cerebellum. With the exception of some strokes, tumors, and degenerative conditions, most of these disorders are unlikely to affect the cerebellum in isolation. This leads to a distinction between the more theoretical issue of the cognitive and emotional roles of the cerebellum itself, and the more clinical issue of the neuropsychiatric manifestations of diseases that affect the cerebellum.

PRECLINICAL EVIDENCE LINKING THE CEREBELLUM TO COGNITION AND EMOTION

Recent insights into the neuroanatomical links between the cerebellum and brain regions with known cognitive or emotional functions, coupled with a variety of animal studies in which cerebellum lesions have been shown to cause cognitive impairments and alter emotion, provide a strong basis for the role of the cerebellum in human cognition and emotion.

Neuroanatomy

The most exciting finding in cerebellar neuroanatomy over the past 20 years has been discovery of relatively closed loops that connect different regions of the cerebral cortex, including nonmotor regions, with the cerebellar cortex (Fig. 2). The pathway from the cerebral cortex to the cerebellum originates with axons in cortical layer Vb in motor, somatosensory, association, and paralimbic regions *(5,6)*. Areas of special note include posterior parietal association cortex *(7)*, portions of superior temporal sulcus and gyrus *(8)*, parastriate and parahippocampal regions *(9)*, and dorsolateral, medial, and to a lesser extent, ventral lateral prefrontal regions *(10)*. These prefrontal areas, including Brodmann regions 8A, 9, 10, 9, 32, 45B, and 46, are critical for attention, working memory, planning, motivation, decision-making, and language. After synapse in the pons, where topographical distinctions among the different sources of input is maintained, the pathway continues as projections into the cerebellar cortex. Prefrontal regions apparently project to lobes VII-VIII *(11)*, but the precise cerebellar target regions of most pontine projections is unclear.

The pathways between the cerebellum and the cerebral cortex begin with axons projecting from cerebellar Purkinje cells to the deep cerebellar nuclei, where the pathway again remains topographically defined. These nuclei then project to both "motor" and "nonspecific" nuclei of the thalamus *(12)*. Both types of thalamic nuclei project to posterior parietal, superior temporal, prefrontal association regions, and the intralaminar nuclei also project to limbic regions (cingulate, parahippocampus).

The use of retrograde tracers has established that this corticocerebellar circuit is formed of discreet and relatively closed loops *(13)*, similar to those detected in the circuitry between the basal ganglia and the cerebral cortex *(14)*. The basal ganglia and the cerebellar pathways intersect in many common regions of the cortex, including frontal and prefrontal cortex, inferotemporal cortex, and posterior parietal cortex. Not all regions of the cortex receive input from both pathways; for instance, projections to prefrontal area 12 (roughly corresponding to orbital cortex) have been detected from the basal ganglia, but not from the cerebello-thalamic system *(13)*. In general, the basal ganglia-cortical circuits are somewhat more widespread and dense then the cerebellar-cortical circuits.

Other cerebellar circuits of potential relevance for emotion and cognition include reciprocal pathways between the cerebellum and brain stem catecholaminergic (locus coeruleus) *(15)* and serotoninergic nuclei (dorsal raphe) *(16)*, between the cerebellum and the hypothalamus *(17)*, and between the cerebellum and the brainstem reticular formation, which may have a role in modulating overall alertness and activation *(18)*.

In addition to its connections with the cerebral cortex and other brain regions, the other aspect of cerebellar anatomy important to affect and cognition are the "cerebellar cortical modules" *(19)*. These modules exist as radially oriented, structurally identical units that comprise the cerebellar cortex. Each module consists of a Purkinje cell (numbering about 15–30 million in the human cerebellum), granule cells that receive input from outside of the cerebellum and innervate the Purkinje cell, and inhibitory interneurons (basket, stellate, and Golgi cells). The Purkinje cell thus serves to integrate excitatory and inhibitory input.

Animal Studies

A series of investigations have used the eye-blink conditioned response to explore the role of the cerebellum in associative learning. In this paradigm, the conditional stimulus is typically a brief tone, the unconditional stimulus is a corneal airpuff, and the eye-blink is the conditioned reflex. Purkinje cells spike patterns are altered by training, lesions of the cerebellar cortex or the interpositus nucleus prevent learning, and loss of Purkinje cells in a mutant mouse strain significantly impairs learning. *(20,21)*. Consistent with lesion studies, functional magnetic resonance imaging (fMRI) studies of eye-blink conditioning in rabbits suggests bilateral cerebellar cortex involvement *(22)*. Even this simple reflex, however, is more complex than initially thought, as it is now recognized to consist of multiple components, each at least partially mediated by different circuits *(23)*.

Table 1
Etiologies of Cerebellar Disorders

Hereditary degenerative autosomal dominant
   Spinocerebellar ataxia types 1-26
   Dentatorubro-pallidoluysian atrophy
   Huntington's disease (uncommonly)
   Hereditary prion diseases
   Episodic ataxias type 1 and 2
Hereditary autosomal recessive (metabolic)
   betalipoproteinemia
   Neiman-Pick Type C
   Hexosaminidase A deficiency (Tay-Sachs)
   Glutamic aciduria
   Hydroxyglutamic aciduria
   Cholestanolosis (cerebrotendinous xanthomatosis)
   Metachromatic leukodystrophy
   Galactocereberosidase deficiency (Krabbe disease)
   α-tocopherol deficiency (vitamin E deficiency)
   Hartnup disease
   Refsum disease (phytanic acid oxidase deficiency)
   Biotinidase deficiency
   Co-enzyme Q deficiency
Hereditary autosomal recessive, DNA repair
   Ataxia-telangenctasia
   Xeroderma pigmentosum
   Cocakyne Syndrome
Hereditary X-linked
   Pelizaeus-Merzbacher disease
   Adrenoleukodystrophy
   Rett syndrome
Mitochondrial
   Kearns-Sayre syndrome
   Myoclonic epilepsy associated with ragged-red fibers (MERRF)
   Neuropathy, ataxia, and retinitis pigmentosa (NARP)
   Leiber hereditary optic neuropathy (LHON)
Nutritional/dietary
   Vitamin E
   Thiamine (often in association with alcoholism)
   Celiac disease
Toxic
   Ethanol
   Phenytoin
   Lithium
Oncologic
   Primary tumors
   Metastases
   Paraneoplastic (small cell carcinoma of lung, breast, female genital tract, lymphomas)
Infectious/postinfectious
   Abscesses
   Whipple disease
   Subacute sclerosing panencephalitis
   Progressive rubella panencephalitis
   Infectious prion disease

Table 1 *(continued)*

Other
    Multiple sclerosis
    Sporadic late-onset cerebellar degeneration
    Multisystem atrophy
    Trauma
    Radiation
Vascular
    Embolic, hemorrhagic, or occlusive
Congenital (some autosomal-recessive or x-linked hereditary)
    Marinesco-Sjogren syndrome
    Joubert syndrome
    Dysequilibrium syndrome
    Early onset ataxia with hypogonadism, retinopathy, or deafness

AR, ; XL, .Modified and reprinted with permission from ref. *4a.*

Visuospatial learning also at least partially depends on intact input from the cerebellum. In the Morris water maze, mice or rats are required to find a platform while swimming in a tank of opaque water, using the memory of various visual cues. Testing rats with different cerebellar lesions on this task revealed dissociation between place learning (influenced by lateral regions of the cerebellum) and cued learning (influenced by midline cerebellar regions) *(24)*. Species, task details, and lesion location all influence results *(25)*.

The functional implication of the neuroanatomical link between the frontal cortex and the cerebellum has also been explored in animal studies. For instance, in primate studies, neurons in the ventral dentate, and in the prefrontal cortex to which the ventral dentate projects, had similar electrophysiological responses to tasks demanding working memory or motor planning *(26)*.

Modulation of emotion by the cerebellum has also been detected in animals. Early studies found that stimulation of the cerebellar vermis led to a state of emotional arousal *(27)* and that aggressive rhesus monkeys became much calmer after midline cerebellar lesions, but not after neocerebellar lesions *(28)*. More recently, the cerebellum has been shown to participate in the consolidation phase of fear conditioning *(29)*.

THE NEUROPSYCHOLOGY OF THE CEREBELLUM

The Cerebellum and Cognition

Evidence in humans that the cerebellum is involved in cognition and emotion has emerged from functional neuroimaging studies of normal individuals engaged in various cognitive tasks and from neuropsychological testing of individuals with cerebellar lesions. As a whole, this very large body of work makes a compelling case that the cerebellum is an active participant in multiple forms of cognition and in the generation of emotion. However, in detail, the studies must be evaluated cautiously. Were all necessary controls performed to eliminate the confounding effects of motor-based cerebellar activation? In neuroimaging studies, was the cerebellar activation a cause, consequence, or epiphenomenon of the activity under investigation? In patients with cerebellar lesions, was the lesion focal or diffuse? Where was it? Were other brain regions also involved?

One problem arises from the two different questions that have been asked: some, perhaps most, investigators have asked about the cognitive or emotional role of the cerebellum *per se*, whereas others have asked about the cognitive or emotional manifestations of diseases that affect the cerebellum, but which in many cases may also involve other brain regions. Addressing the first question requires strict attention to the location of cerebellar lesions. Strokes and tumors potentially provide the most spatial

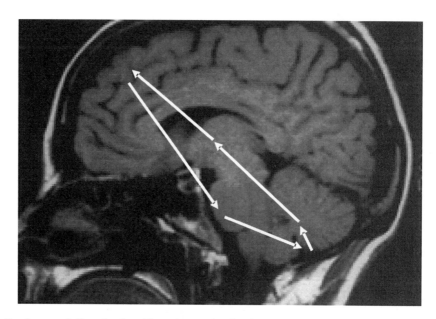

Fig. 2. Cerebro-cerebellar circuitry. The primary circuitry between the cerebral cortex and the cerebellum. Purkinje cell project to the deep cerebellar nuclei, and these neurons project to the thalmus. Thalamic nuclei project to the cerebral cortex. Cortical pyramidal cell project to the pons which then project back to the cerebellar cortex.

resolution, but spread of the lesion to other regions within or beyond the cerebellum and additional lesions (such as other cerebrovascular insults) in other brain regions in the same person may confound interpretation of data. Degenerative diseases that affect the cerebellum in most cases also affect other brain regions, although at times subtlely. These factors must be taken into account when considering neuropsychological studies of the cerebellum, as well as the age and premorbid capacities of a subject, and the duration of degenerative illness or time since a stroke or tumor resection.

The cerebellum has been shown to influence multiple cognitive spheres. Language functions mediated by the cerebellum include verb generation *(30,31)*, perception of temporal distinctions among phonemes *(32)*, verbal fluency and word generation *(33)*, and verbal working memory *(34)*. Learning with a basis in the cerebellum has been demonstrated in an eye-blink conditioning paradigm similar to that observed in rabbits and mice *(35,36)* and in a variety of procedural learning paradigms *(37)*. Sensory discrimination may also be regulated by the cerebellum *(38)*.

Executive function, which includes aspects of verbal processing, learning, and memory, may also be under the influence of the cerebellum. Tasks modulated by the cerebellum appear to include set shifting *(39)*, the performance of multiple simultaneous tasks *(40)*, and attention *(41)*. There is direct evidence that ties the cerebellum to frontal processing, especially during executive tasks. Cerebellar hypometabolism has been consistently observed after contralateral frontal lesions, a phenomenon known as crossed cerebellar diaschisis *(34)*. As predicted, the opposite phenomenon, crossed neocortical diaschisis, has been observed after cerebellar infarction *(42,43)*. Right frontal cortex activation is often accompanied by left cerebellar activation in tasks requiring episodic retrieval, whereas left frontal cortex and right cerebellar activation occurs during retrieval of semantic information, such as generating an appropriate verb when presented with a particular noun *(34)*. A comparison of working memory to rehearsal tasks, using the Sternberg verbal working memory task, revealed a correlation between superior cerebellum and frontal cortex activation in articulatory control. The extent of cerebellar involvement in executive function may depend on the motor demands, automaticity, and fluency demanded by a given task *(44)*.

Given the repetitive nature of the cerebellar microcircuit, an important general concept is that the same type of processing—an information transform—may apply to multiple cerebellar functions. Application of this theory to the consequences of cerebellar injury has led to the hypothesis of "cognitive dysmetria" *(8)*. The concept is that the cerebellum acts to dampen oscillations, and thereby smooths cognition and emotion in a manner parallel to its smoothing effect on motion. Cerebellar lesions, known to result in abnormalities of rate, force, rhythm, and accuracy of movement, would therefore be predicted to result in abnormalities of the speed, accuracy, and adaptability of cognition and emotion *(45)*. Alternative and by no means mutually exclusive theories suggest that the cerebellum serves as an error detector *(46)* or a central timing device *(47)*.

The Cerebellum and Emotion

A link between the cerebellum and emotion in humans has been established using neuroimaging protocols. For instance, the superior semilunar lobule of the cerebellum is activated in human subjects shown an unpleasant stimulus relative to the activation elicited by a pleasant stimulus *(48)*. Similarly, the cerebellum was activated when subjects were shown pictures with either positive or negative emotional valence *(49)*. In a more naturalistic experiment involving women who had lost a first-degree relative in the past year, evocation of grief activated midline and lateral cerebellar regions along with multiple other brain regions, suggested that the cerebellum is one part of an integrated pathway that modulates grief *(50)*. Pathological laughing and crying have been tentatively linked to cerebellar-mediated circuitry *(51)*. Schmahmann suggests that the posterior lobe of the cerebellum is probably most related to affect and cognition and that midline lesions of the cerebellum are particularly associated with affective changes, potentially through pathways linking the vermis, via the fastigial nucleus, with limbic cortex *(52)*.

DISEASE AND COGNITION

Cognition and Focal Cerebellar Lesions

The frequency of cognitive manifestations observed following cerebellar lesions (predominantly infarcts or hemorrhages in adults and tumors in children) is generally high. Cognitive deficits have been reported in 35–100% of patients after cerebellar strokes *(53–55)* with the lowest estimate derived from the most systematic study. As predicted by the multiple cognitive domains influenced by the cerebellum, the nature of the deficits caused by these lesions varies, and may include executive, language, praxic, memory, or visuospatial dysfunction. In many cases, the abnormalities are relatively mild *(54)*, and one study found only mild naming deficits *(42)*. Many patients improved over time. Predictably, more global lesions are associated with broader cognitive deficits, and deficits associated with infarction of the posterior inferior cerebellar artery are generally milder than those associated with superior cerebellar artery or anterior inferior cerebellar infarction.

Resection of midline posterior fossa tumors in children leads to the "posterior fossa syndrome" in 13% of cases, a condition characterized by mutism, oropharyngeal dyspraxia, impaired initiation of voluntary movements, oculomotor apraxia, incontinence, emotional liability, and personality changes that have been reported to include onset of an autistic-like syndrome *(56,57)*. Resection of tumors located elsewhere in the cerebellum may have other effects. In a series of 26 children undergoing surgery for cerebellar tumors, the 7 with resection of right hemisphere cerebellar tumors demonstrated disturbances of language processing and auditory sequential memory. The 8 children with resections of left hemisphere cerebellar tumors had disturbed spatial and visual sequential memory *(57)*.

Degenerative Cerebellar Disease and Cognition

Most but not all evidence suggests that subjects with moderate degenerative disease of the cerebellum develop a mild subcortical dementia. Kish and co-workers *(58)* studied 11 patients with standardized cognitive tests and found prominent impairments in the recall of stories, as well as deficits in verbal and nonverbal intelligence and executive functions. Because these patients were not aphasic, aphasic, apraxic, or agnosic, the authors described their mental state as a mildly disabling subcortical dementia. In a follow-up study of 43 patients with a variety of cerebellar disorders, mildly ataxic patients performed almost normally on a battery of neuropsychological tests, moderately ataxic patients displayed executive functioning deficits and mild memory deficits that could not be explained by depression, and severely ataxic patients had more pervasive deficits but were nonetheless not aphasic *(59)*. On verbal list-learning tasks, deficient immediate and delayed free recall with preservation of yes/no or forced-choice recognition is often taken as the *sine qua non* of subcortical dementia *(60)*. This finding is typical among patients with cerebellar degeneration *(61)*. Comparing matched groups of patients with degenerative disease affecting the cerebellum, Huntington's disease, and normal controls *(62)*, Brandt and colleagues found that patients with cerebellar disease were most impaired in the executive domain and least impaired in the memory domain. In contrast, the HD patients, although generally more impaired than cerebellar patients, were most impaired in visuospatial and memory domains. These findings suggest that the pattern of deficits in degenerative cerebellar disease, although consistent with a mild subcortical dementia, differs in important ways from the subcortical dementia that arises in disease most prominently affecting the basal ganglia.

A few studies have systematically examined the cognitive manifestations of one or more specific genetic diseases affecting the cerebellum, including SCA1, SCA2, SCA3, SCA6, SCA19, cerebellar ataxia with oculomotor apraxia type 1, and Friedreich's ataxia *(63–68)*. The general conclusion is that executive dysfunction is typical in these diseases. SCA1, among the more common of these disorders, produces the most global and severe deficits. The deficits in SCA6, in which pathology is largely limited to cerebellar Purkinje cells, are quite mild. Investigations of Friedreich's ataxia have yielded more variable results, with some studies finding little evidence of cognitive impairment while others have found substantial impairment in multiple cognitive modalities. An important point is that executive function may be impaired in degenerative diseases affecting the cerebellum even in the setting of overall normal intelligence and a normal bedside cognitive exam. For instance, in cerebellar ataxia with oculomotor apraxia type 1, patients with normal IQ scores showed memory deficits and executive dysfunction with impairments in initiation, conceptualization, verbal fluency. In our study of 31 patients with a variety of cerebellar degenerative diseases (average disease duration of 12 years), the rate of dementia or cognitive impairment (Diagnostic and Statistical Manual of Mental Disorders, Fourth Edition [DSM-IV] criteria) was 20%. This may well be an underestimate, as the diagnosis of cognitive impairment depended on family members attributing functional impairment to cognitive rather than motor deficits. Furthermore, the extent of cognitive impairment is certainly correlated with disease duration, and the percentage of patients with cognitive impairment would undoubtedly be higher in a group with a longer disease duration.

Noncognitive Psychopathology in Cerebellar Disease

Among cerebellar stroke patients, Robinson and colleagues *(69)* found elevated rates of mild and often short-lived depression acutely following cerebellar/brainstem strokes. Episodes of depression were generally less severe and less prolonged than after strokes in the basal ganglia or left frontal cortex. The patients in the case series of Schmahmann and Sherman *(53)*, in addition to executive dysfunction, also were described as having affective abnormalities (although formal psychiatric evaluations were not performed), leading the authors to coin the term "cognitive-affective syndrome" to describe the abnormalities in their patients. Anecdotal reports also report psychiatric syndromes related to cerebellar tumors, the resection of cerebellar tumors, and inflammatory or infectious insults of the cerebellum in adults.

Psychiatric Syndromes Accompanying Neurodegenerative Diseases of the Cerebellum

Numerous case reports have suggested the presence of psychiatric syndromes in patients with degenerative disease affecting the cerebellum. Woodward *(70)* described a family with a cerebellar

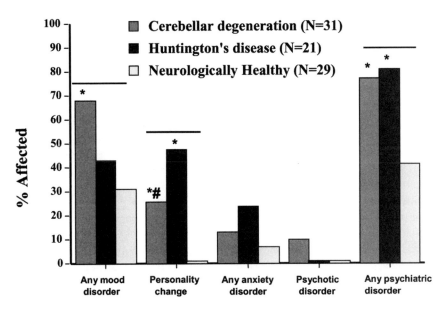

Fig. 3. Psychopathology in degenerative cerebellar disease compared to Huntington's disease. Mood disorders include major depression, brief recurrent depression, minor depressive disorder, dysthymia, and bipolar disorder, mania. Personality change diagnoses were made independent of cognitive status. Anxiety disorders included generalized anxiety disorder, panic disorder, obsessive-compulsive disorder, phobia, and post-traumatic stress disorder. Psychotic disorders included schizophrenia and psychotic disorder not otherwise specified. Results of by χ^2 analysis: lines over a given disorder indicates significant difference ($p < 0.02$) across all three groups; * indicates significant difference from neurologically healthy group ($p < .001$); and # indicates significant difference between CD and HD ($p < 0.01$). Modified and reprinted with permission from the American Journal of Psychiatry, copyright © 2002, American Psychiatric Association.

degenerative disorder in which one affected individual was "petulant and disagreeable at slight provacation," another experienced "jealous delusions, flare-ups of temper over trivia," and a third person was "withdrawn into deep despondency." Cases of "psychosis" *(71)*, and schizophrenia *(72)* have been reported. Moderate to severe levels of depression and increased apathy were noted in a small series of patients with SCA3 *(64)*. The first systematic study was performed by Skre in 1975 *(73)*. Subjects with any type of hereditary ataxia were diagnosed by undefined methods using a now obsolete psychiatric diagnostic scheme. Psychiatric disorders, including mood disorders, were found in approx 23% of subjects, 12% of their neurologically normal family members, and 3% of neurologically normal individuals from families without neurological disease. Kish (59), studying 41 subjects with cerebellar degeneration, found that 12% had clearly elevated Hamilton Depression Rating Scale (HDRS) scores. Fourteen percent were also "mildly euphoric" and 12% were "impulsive," based on "incidental observations."

To systematically determine the extent to which psychiatric disorders occur in degenerative diseases affecting the cerebellum, we examined 31 individuals with diseases affecting the cerebellum, 21 individuals with Huntington's disease (HD; which primarily affects the basal ganglia and cerebral cortex), and 29 neurologically healthy individuals *(74)*. The neurological diagnosis of the cerebellar group was based on review of all available records, including neurological history and examination, neuroimaging, and genetic testing. Diagnoses included sporadic cerebellar ataxia (35%), the cerebellar form of multisystem atrophy (16%), and familial cerebellar ataxia of various types (48%). Individuals with basal ganglia findings on exam or by neuroimaging were excluded from the study. Past and current psychiatric diagnoses were made on the basis of an interview by an experienced neuropsychiatrist using the

Structured Clinical Interview for DSM-IV axis I disorders, nonpatient version. A consensus diagnosis was made in conjunction with a second neuropsychiatrist who was blind to the neurological diagnosis. The three groups were matched on age, sex, education, and estimated premorbid IQ. The disease groups were additionally matched for extent of neurological impairment and disease duration.

The key finding was that the percentage of patients with a history of any psychiatric disorder was very similar in patients with cerebellar degeneration and HD (about 80% in each group), and twice the rate of neurologically healthy controls (Fig. 3). Most striking, the rate of mood disorders was 67% in the cerebellar group, nearly twice the rate ($p < 0.01$) observed in the neurologically healthy group and similar to that in HD patients. The 10% rate of psychotic disorder in the cerebellar group was also quite high, suggesting that cerebellar degeneration might be a risk for psychotic disorder as predicted by the "cognitive dysmetria" hypothesis. Personality change was present in both disease groups, but was significantly more common in the HD group than the cerebellar group.

Each subject was rated with instruments, including the Neuropsychiatric Inventory, designed to establish the severity of current psychopathology. As expected, psychiatric symptoms were elevated in both cerebellar and HD groups compared to the healthy group, though only modestly. Depression scores were only mildly elevated in the disease groups, suggesting that most of the individuals were not acutely depressed at the time of the interview, and that affective abnormalities in HD and cerebellar degeneration (CD) may have both chronic and episodic forms. Irritability, and especially apathy, were substantially higher in the cerebellar and HD groups than the healthy group, consistent with the modulatory effect of both the basal ganglia and the cerebellum on affective states thought to be modulated by the frontal cortex.

The similar rate of mood disorder but lower rate of personality change in patients with cerebellar degenerative disease compared to patients with HD suggests both similarities and differences of the cerebellum and the basal ganglia on mood and executive functioning. This distinction is consistent with the similar but not identical neuroanatomic connections of the cerebellum and the basal ganglia to the frontal cortex and other brain regions. In addition, part of the similarity in the psychopathology of the two patient groups in this study may stem from degenerative factors common to the groups, particularly cortical degeneration. Cortical involvement is certainly part of the neuropathology of HD, and may occur in some of the diseases that affect the cerebellum. Determining the relative contribution of the cerebellum itself to the psychopathology of degenerative diseases affecting the cerebellum will require investigation of genetic forms of cerebellar degeneration that do not also involve the cerebral cortex.

We performed a second study to determine how frequently psychiatric disorders were detected in patients with cerebellar disease during routine clinical evaluation by neurologists, and to determine if basal ganglia involvement modified psychiatric disorders in patients with cerebellar disease *(75)* (Fig. 4). Neurological records of 213 consenting patients referred to the Neurogenetics Testing Laboratory at Johns Hopkins were reviewed. Those cases that met the following criteria for CD were included in the study: (a) an MRI scan documenting cerebellar atrophy, (b) a clinical diagnosis of spinocerebellar ataxia (SCA) or cerebellar degeneration, or (c) the presence of both ataxia and dysmetria on clinical examination. Exclusion criteria included the presence of predominantly parkinsonian presentation or evidence of strokes. A subgroup of the CD cases was identified that also had clinical or MRI evidence of basal ganglia involvement. Psychiatric symptoms and diagnoses noted in the neurological records were categorized using a conservative scheme: a notation of "major depression" or depression with suicide attempt was considered evidence of major depression; "depression" or "depressed mood" evidence of nonmajor depression; and "psychosis" and "schizophrenia" evidence of a psychotic disorder. Anxiety, obsessive-compulsive disorder, or panic disorder were symptomatic of anxiety syndrome whereas dementia, memory disturbance, or cognitive impairment signified cognitive impairment. Notations reflecting persistent changes in temperament or behavior were considered evidence of personality change.

One hundred thirty-three cases met both inclusion and exclusion criteria for cerebellar disease, and 59 of these cases also met criteria for basal ganglia involvement. Forty-one percent of all patients had

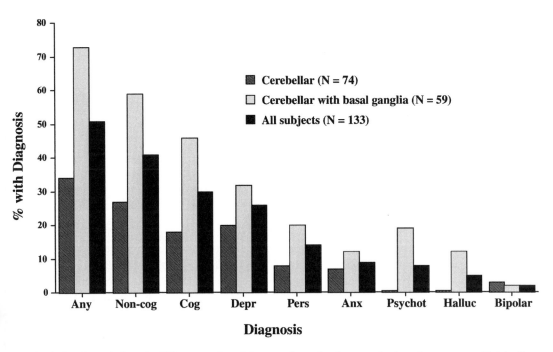

Fig. 4. Psychopathology in 133 cases referred for genetic testing by neurologists. Any, any psychiatric diagnosis or notation of cognitive ; Noncog, non-cognitive psychopathology; Cog, cognitive abnormality; Depr, any depressive disorder; Pers, personality change; Anx, anxiety-related syndromes; Psychot, schizophrenia or other nonaffective psychotic disorders; Halluc, isolated hallucinations; Bipolar, biopolar affective disorder. (Reprinted with permission from American Psychiatric Publishing, copyright © 2004 *[75]*.)

psychiatric symptoms and 30% had cognitive impairment. The most common psychiatric manifestation was depression (28%). Depression and depressive symptoms were the most commonly observed noncognitive psychiatric phenomena, but personality change, anxiety, and psychosis were also detected at a relatively high rate. Rates of both cognitive impairment and noncognitive psychopathology were higher in cases with basal ganglia involvement. This may reflect the increased risk for psychopathology conferred by basal ganglia involvement, or that cases with both basal ganglia and cerebellar involvement were generally more severe. Overall, this study indicated that psychopathology is commonly detected in routine neurological evaluation of patients with disorders affecting the cerebellum.

In summary, focal and diffuse diseases that affect the cerebellum increase the risk of both chronic and intermittent psychiatric disorders. Involvement of regions beyond the cerebellum, particularly the basal ganglia, may change the nature and severity of the psychopathology. Little can yet be said about the long-term prognosis of psychopathology in the context of cerebellar disease.

TREATMENT

Determining the cause of the underlying disorder is essential because cerebellar degeneration secondary to nutritional, dietary, and some metabolic disorders may be treatable and at least partially reversible. Surgical intervention may be important for tumors and vascular malformations. There is no treatment for sporadic or genetic degenerative diseases of the cerebellum.

It is essential that a neurologist perform a psychiatric history and mental status examination, assessing various aspects of mood, as well as self-attitude, sense of physical well-being, appetite, libido, sleep, suicidality, hallucinations, delusions, obsessions, compulsions, and anxiety. A bedside cognitive exam should be performed that includes brief tests of executive function. Opinions about the patient's cognition, mood, and behavior should be sought from the family.

Cognitive treatments are supportive and educational, as in other dementias. In the case of cerebellar disease, education may be particularly important, as patients, families and referring clinicians may not be aware of the association between cerebellar disease and cognitive deficits, and the relative sparing of declarative memory may mask more subtle executive deficits. As with any impairment affecting executive dysfunction, it is of great value to help family members avoid blaming the patient or each other for behavioral idiosyncrasies. Neuropsychological evaluation may prove valuable in pinpointing cognitive strengths and weaknesses over time, and in providing the patient and family with objective data that may explain difficulties otherwise attributed to "laziness" or a "bad attitude." Establishing routines, finding outside sources of support such as day programs, and adjusting cognitive demands on the patient to match his or her capacity can vastly improve quality of life for both the patient and their family.

Little is known about the treatment of noncognitive psychiatric disorders in patients with diseases of the cerebellum. Psychotherapy is likely to be of help, both as a specific treatment for the psychiatric symptoms and to help the demoralized patient adapt to the psychiatric disorders and the underlying cerebellar disease. Pharmacotherapy of psychiatric syndromes secondary to cerebellar disease has not been systematically assessed. In a very small nonblinded study in which patients with SCA3 were treated with fluoxetine for movement abnormalities, depression ratings were incidentally found to have improved (although not to the point of statistical significance) even though the patients had not been selected for depression. Anecdotal accounts indicate that patients respond to standard psychotropic medicines, including various classes of antidepressants and electroconvulsive therapy *(76)*. Caution is necessary with agents that may increase ataxia. However, the main point is to avoid undertreatment, as psychiatric disorders may be life-threatening and lead to major morbidity, while medicines can be quickly stopped should untoward side effects develop. Above all, it is vital that the clinician not automatically accept the explanations offered by patients and their family that psychiatric symptoms merely reflect an understandable psychological reaction to functional disability.

REFERENCES

1. Fadda F, Rossetti ZL. Chronic ethanol consumption: from neuroadaptation to neurodegeneration. Prog Neurobiol 1998; 56:385–431.
2. Raco A, Caroli E, Isidori A, Salvati M. Management of acute cerebellar infarction: one institution's experience. Neurosurgery 2003;53:1061–1065.
3. Pandolfo M. Friedreich ataxia. Semin Pediatr Neurol 2003;10:163–172.
4. Margolis RL. The spinocerebellar ataxias: order emerges from chaos. Curr Neurol Neurosci Rep 2002;2:447–456.
4a. Sadock BJ, Sadock VA, eds. Comprehensive Textbook of Psychiatry, Eighth Edition. Baltimore, MD: Lippincott Williams & Wilkins; 2004.
5. Brodal P. The corticopontine projection in the rhesus monkey. Origin and principles of organization. Brain 1978;101: 251–283.
6. Glickstein M, May JG III, Mercier BE. Corticopontine projection in the macaque: the distribution of labelled cortical cells after large injections of horseradish peroxidase in the pontine nuclei. J Comp Neurol 1985;235:343–359.
7. Schmahmann JD, Pandya DN. Anatomical investigation of projections to the basis pontis from posterior parietal association cortices in rhesus monkey. J Comp Neurol 1989;289:53–73.
8. Schmahmann JD. An emerging concept. The cerebellar contribution to higher function. Arch Neurol 1991;48:1178–1187.
9. Schmahmann JD, Pandya DN. Prelunate, occipitotemporal, and parahippocampal projections to the basis pontis in rhesus monkey. J Comp Neurol 1993;337:94–112.
10. Schmahmann JD, Pandya DN. Prefrontal cortex projections to the basilar pons in rhesus monkey: implications for the cerebellar contribution to higher function. Neurosci Lett 1995;199:175–178.
11. Brodal P. The pontocerebellar projection in the rhesus monkey: an experimental study with retrograde axonal transport of horseradish peroxidase. Neuroscience 1979;4:193–208.
12. Middleton FA, Strick PL. Dentate output channels: motor and cognitive components. Prog Brain Res 1997;114:553–566.
13. Middleton FA, Strick PL. Basal ganglia output and cognition: evidence from anatomical, behavioral, and clinical studies. Brain Cogn 2000;42:183–200.

14. Alexander GE, DeLong MR, Strick PL. Parallel organization of functionally segregated circuits linking basal ganglia and cortex. Annu Rev Neurosci 1986;9:357–381.

15. Dempesy CW, Tootle DM, Fontana CJ, Fitzjarrell AT, Garey RE, Heath RG. Stimulation of the paleocerebellar cortex of the cat: increased rate of synthesis and release of catecholamines at limbic sites. Biol Psychiatry 1983;18:127–132.

16. Marcinkiewicz M, Morcos R, Chretien M. CNS connections with the median raphe nucleus: retrograde tracing with WGA-apoHRP-Gold complex in the rat. J Comp Neurol 1989;289:11–35.

17. Haines DE, Dietrichs E, Mihailoff GA, McDonald EF. The cerebellar-hypothalamic axis: basic circuits and clinical observations Int Rev Neurobiol 1997;41:83–107.

18. Brodal A. Neurological Anatomy. New York: Oxford University Press; 1981:1053–1053.

19. O'Hearn E, Molliver M. Organizational principles and microcircuitry of the cerebellum. Int Rev Psychiatry 2001;13:232–246.

20. Christian KM, Thompson RF. Neural substrates of eyeblink conditioning: acquisition and retention. Learn Mem 2003;10:427–455.

21. Thompson RF, Bao S, Chen L, et al. Associative learning. Int Rev Neurobiol 1997;41:151–189.

22. Miller MJ, Chen NK, Li L, et al. fMRI of the conscious rabbit during unilateral classical eyeblink conditioning reveals bilateral cerebellar activation. J Neurosci 2003;23:11,753–11,758.

23. Lee T, Kim JJ. Differential effects of cerebellar, amygdalar, and hippocampal lesions on classical eyeblink conditioning in rats. J Neurosci 2004;24:3242–3250.

24. Colombel C, Lalonde R, Caston J. The effects of unilateral removal of the cerebellar hemispheres on spatial learning and memory in rats. Brain Res 2004;1004:108–115.

25. Lalonde R, Strazielle C. The effects of cerebellar damage on maze learning in animals. Cerebellum 2003;2:300–309.

26. Middleton FA, Strick PL. Basal ganglia and cerebellar loops: motor and cognitive circuits. Brain Res Brain Res Rev 2000;31:236–250.

27. Snider RS, Maiti A. Cerebellar contributions to the Papez circuit. J Neurosci Res 1976;2:133–146.

28. Berman AJ. Amelioration of aggression: response to selective cerebellar lesions in the rhesus monkey. Int Rev Neurobiol 1997;41:111–119..

29. Sacchetti B, Baldi E, Lorenzini CA, Bucherelli C. Cerebellar role in fear-conditioning consolidation. Proc Natl Acad Sci USA 2002;99:8406–8411.

30. Gebhart AL, Petersen SE, Thach W. Role of the posterolateral cerebellum in language. Ann NY Acad Sci 2002;978:318–333.

31. Raichle ME, Fiez JA, Videen TO, et al. Practice-related changes in human brain functional anatomy during nonmotor learning. Cereb Cortex 1994;4:8–26.

32. Ackermann H, Graber S, Hertrich I, Daum I. Categorical speech perception in cerebellar disorders. Brain Lang 1997;60:323–331.

33. Appollonio IM, Grafman J, Schwartz V, Massaquoi S, Hallett M. Memory in patients with cerebellar degeneration. Neurology 1993;43,1536–1544.

34. Desmond JE. Cerebellar involvement in cognitive function: evidence from neuroimaging. Int Rev Psychiatry 2001;13:283–294.

35. Gerwig M, Dimitrova A, Kolb FP, et al. Comparison of eyeblink conditioning in patients with superior and posterior inferior cerebellar lesions. Brain 2003;126:71–94.

36. Woodruff-Pak DS, Papka M, Ivry RB. Cerebellar involvement in classical eyeblink conditioning in humans. Neuropsychology 1996;10:443–458.

37. Thach WT. A role for the cerebellum in learning movement coordination. Neurobiol Learn Mem 1998;70:177–188.

38. Parsons LM, Bower JM, Gao JH, Xiong J, Li J, Fox PT. Lateral cerebellar hemispheres actively support sensory acquisition and discrimination rather than motor control. Learn Mem 1997;4:49–62.

39. Courchesne E, Townsend J, Akshoomoff NA, et al. Impairment in shifting attention in autistic and cerebellar patients. Behav Neurosci 1994;108:848–865.

40. Lang CE, Bastian AJ. Cerebellar damage impairs automaticity of a recently practiced movement. J Neurophysiol 2002;87:1336–1347.

41. Akshoomoff NA, Courchesne E, Townsend J. Attention coordination and anticipatory control. Int Rev Neurobiol 1997;41:575–598.

42. Gomez BM, Garcia-Monco JC, Quintana JM, Llorens V, Rodeno E. Diaschisis and neuropsychological performance after cerebellar stroke. Eur Neurol 1997;37:82–89.

43. Hausen HS, Lachmann EA, Nagler W. Cerebral diaschisis following cerebellar hemorrhage. Arch Phys Med Rehabil 1997;78:546–549.

44. Heyder K, Suchan B, Daum I. Cortico-subcortical contributions to executive control. Acta Psychol (Amst) 2004;115:271–289.

45. Schmahmann JD. The cerebrocerebellar system: anatomic substrates of the cerebellar contribution to cognition and emotion. Int Rev Psychiatry 2001;13:247–260.

46. Ito M. Cerebellar long-term depression: characterization, signal transduction, and functional roles. Physiol Rev 2001;81:1143–1195.

47. Ivry RB, Spencer RM. The neural representation of time. Curr Opin Neurobiol 2004;14:225–232.

48. Paradiso S, Johnson DL, Andreasen NC, et al. Cerebral blood flow changes associated with attribution of emotional valence to pleasant, unpleasant, and neutral visual stimuli in a PET study of normal subjects. Am J Psychiatry 1999;156:1618–1629.

49. Lee GP, Meador KJ, Loring DW, et al. Neural substrates of emotion as revealed by functional magnetic resonance imaging. Cogn Behav Neurol 2004;17:9–17.

50. Gunder H, O'Connoer MF, Littrell L, Fort C, Lane RD. Functional neuroanatomy of grief: an fMRI study. Am J Psychiatry 2004;160:1946–1953.

51. Parvizi J, Anderson SW, Martin CO, Damasio H, Damasio AR. Pathological laughter and crying: a link to the cerebellum. Brain 2001;124:1708–1719.

52. Schmahmann JD. The cerebellar cognitive affective syndrome: clinical correlations of the dysmetria of thought hypothesis. Int Rev Psychiatry 2001;13:313–322.

53. Schmahmann JD, Sherman JC. The cerebellar cognitive affective syndrome. Brain 1998;121(Pt 4):561–579.

54. Neau JP, Arroyo-Anllo E, Bonnaud V, Ingrand P, Gil R. Neuropsychological disturbances in cerebellar infarcts. Acta Neurol Scand 2000;102:363–370.

55. Hoffmann M, Schmitt F. Cognitive impairment in isolated subtentorial stroke. Acta Neurol Scand 2004;109:14–24.

56. Pollack I. Neurobehavioral abnormalities after posterior fossa surgery in children. Int Rev Psychiatry 2001;13:302–312.

57. Riva D, Giorgi C. The cerebellum contributes to higher functions during development: evidence from a series of children surgically treated for posterior fossa tumours. Brain 2000;123:1051–1061.

58. Kish SJ, el Awar M, Schut, L, Leach L, Oscar-Berman M, Freedman M. Cognitive deficits in olivopontocerebellar atrophy: implications for the cholinergic hypothesis of Alzheimer's dementia. Ann Neurol 1988;24:200–206.

59. Kish SJ, el-Awar M, Stuss D, et al. Neuropsychological test performance in patients with dominantly inherited spinocerebellar ataxia: relationship to ataxia severity. Neurology 1994;44:1738–1746.

60. Brandt J, Munro C. Memory Disorders in Subcortical Dementia. (Baddeley AD, Kopelman MD, Wilson BA, eds.), Hoboken, NJ: Wiley, 2001. 591–614.

61. Hirono N, Yamadori A, Kameyama M, Mezaki T, Abe K. Spinocerebellar degeneration (SCD): cognitive disturbances. Acta Neurol Scand 1991;84:226–230.

62. Brandt J, Leroi I, O'Hearn E, Rosenblatt A, Margolis RL. Cognitive impairments in cerebellar degeneration: a comparison with Huntington's disease. J Neuropsychiatry Clin Neurosci 2004;16:176–184.

63. Burk K, Globas C, Bosch S, et al. Cognitive deficits in spinocerebellar ataxia type 1, 2, and 3. J Neurol 2003;250:207–211.

64. Zawacki TM, Grace J, Friedman JH, Sudarsky L. Executive and emotional dysfunction in Machado-Joseph disease. Mov Disord 2002;17:1004–1010.

65. Schelhaas HJ, van de Warrenburg BP, Hageman G, Ippel EE, van Hout M, Kremer B. Cognitive impairment in SCA-19. Acta Neurol Belg 2003;103:199–205.

66. White M, Lalonde R, Botez-Marquard T. Neuropsychologic and neuropsychiatric characteristics of patients with Friedreich's ataxia. Acta Neurol Scand 2000;102:222–226.

67. Wollmann T, Barroso J, Monton F, Nieto A. Neuropsychological test performance of patients with Friedreich's ataxia. J Clin Exp Neuropsychol 2002;24:677–686.

68. Le Ber I, Moreira MC, Rivaud-Pechoux S, et al. Cerebellar ataxia with oculomotor apraxia type 1: clinical and genetic studies. Brain 2003;126:2761–2772.

69. Starkstein, SE, Robinson RG, Berthier ML, Price TR. Depressive disorders following posterior circulation as compared with middle cerebral artery infarcts. Brain 1988;111:375–387.

70. Woodworth JA, Beckett RS, Netsky MG. A composite of hereditary ataxias. Arch Int Med 1959;104:594–606.

71. Kutty IN, Prendes JL. Psychosis and cerebellar degeneration. J Nerv Ment Dis 1981;169:390–391.

72. Tashiro H, Suzuki SO, Hitotsumatsu T, Iwaki T. An autopsy case of spinocerebellar ataxia type 6 with mental symptoms of schizophrenia and dementia. Clin Neuropathol 1999;18:198–204.

73. Skre H. A study of certain traits accompanying some inherited neurological disorders. Clin Genet 1975;8:117–135.

74. Leroi I, O'Hearn E, Marsh L, et al. Psychopathology in degenerative cerebellar diseases: A comparison to Huntington's disease and normal controls. Am J Psychiatry 2002;159:1306–1314.

75. Liszewski CM, O'Hearn E, Leroi I, Gourley L, Ross CA, Margolis RL. Cognitive Impairment and Psychiatric Symptoms in 133 patients with diseases associated with cerebellar degeneration. J Neuropsychiatry Clin Neurosci 2004;16:109–112.

76. Weintraub D, Lippmann SB. Electroconvulsive therapy in the acute poststroke period. J ECT 2004;16:415–418.

V Other Topics

20

Childhood Disorders

Dorothy E. Stubbe

INTRODUCTION

Human development begins with genetic endowment and neurophysiological potential, and unfolds via the interaction between the individual and his or her nurturing environment. Psychosocial adversity, abuse, neglect, trauma and illness can adversely affect the developmental trajectory. The risk and protective influences of environment are interwoven with biological vulnerabilities and resilience to determine the complex aspects of psychiatric health or illness.

Although essentially all of the adult psychiatric disorders can occur in children, some disorders must be evident from a very early age for diagnosis (such as autism or attention deficit hyperactivity disorder [ADHD]). Development powerfully influences the nature of presenting symptoms of other disorders (such as mood disorders). Children often display more variability in symptom presentation. Irritability, hyperactivity and other nonspecific symptoms may be a diagnostic clue to a number of disorders. Additionally, the age of onset and chronicity of symptoms influences prognosis. Children may respond differently than adults to medications and psychosocial treatments. The evidence base is less robust for treatment efficacy of psychiatric disorders in children and adolescents, and the potential long-term side effects of medications largely unstudied.

This chapter reviews the essential components of evaluation and diagnosis of childhood psychiatric disorders. Developmental disorders and ADHD are discussed in detail. Other axis I disorders usually first diagnosed in infancy, childhood, or adolescence, including separation anxiety, selective mutism, reactive attachment disorder, elimination disorders, oppositional-defiant disorder and conduct disorder are summarized in table format. Tourette's syndrome is discussed in another chapter, and is not discussed here. Additionally, the unique aspects of early-onset psychiatric disorders are discussed.

EVALUATION OF CHILD AND ADOLESCENT PSYCHIATRIC DISORDERS

The ever-shifting and malleable nature of development makes the diagnostic evaluation more complex, and the potential for the child and family to benefit from early intervention more compelling. The assessment requires multiple informants (e.g., parents, teachers, medical care providers, child), as the child's behavior may be variable in different settings, a fact that is crucial to understanding the nature of the difficulties. Some behavioral symptoms (temper tantrums, transient phobias, etc.) may be within the scope of normal childhood development, and must be differentiated from those that have become functionally impairing and in need of intervention. The effectiveness of treatments will be contingent upon a comprehensive understanding of the child in his or her contextual environment, and must be based on a thorough assessment. Often, this assessment is ongoing, as the nature of the disorder only

From: *Current Clinical Neurology: Psychiatry for Neurologists*
Edited by: D.V. Jeste and J.H. Friedman © Humana Press Inc., Totowa, NJ

Table 1
Essentials of the Child and Adolescent Psychiatric Evaluation

1. History from multiple sources (parents, teachers, pediatrician, child)
   a. Reason for Referral
   b. History of Present Illness
   c. Review of Psychiatric Symptoms
   d. Prenatal, Developmental and Social History (including obstetrical and birth history, early temperament, developmental milestones, toilet training, history of trauma or abuse, risk-taking behaviors, substance abuse, friendships, sexual behaviors, legal difficulties)
   e. Psychiatry History
   f. Educational History
   g. Stress level/psychosocial adversity
   h. Medical History and Review of systems
   i. Family psychiatric/medical/genetic history
   j. Child and Family Strengths and Weaknesses
2. Mental Status Examination
   a. Appearance and grooming (including tics, mannerisms)
   b. Speech fluency, volume, rate and language skills
   c. Ability to cooperate and engage with assessment
   d. Motor activity level, attention, frustration tolerance, impulsivity
   e, Mood and affect, neurovegetative symptoms, manic symptoms
   f. Psychotic symptoms (hallucinations, delusions, thought disorder)
   g. Anxiety, fears and phobias, obsessions or compulsions, post-traumatic anxiety
   h. Oppositionality, conduct symptoms, aggression (verbal or physical)
   i. Clinical estimate of cognitive skills
   j. Insight and judgment
3. Screening physical and neurological examination
4. Diagnostic tests, where appropriate
   a. Lead level
   b. Thyroid and other screening laboratory tests
   c. ECG, EEG or neuroimaging procedures as indicated
   d. Psychoeducational testing to rule out learning disability and intellectual impairment (at times, neuropsychological testing, to assess executive functioning and more subtle or complex deficits)
5. Rating scales (such as Conners for ADHD, Beck Depression Inventory for depression, etc) to assess the number and severity of symptoms. Baseline and follow-up rating scales are helpful in monitoring the effectiveness of treatment interventions and medication regimens.

becomes clear with ongoing maturation, a more persistent pattern of symptoms, or environmental stabilization *(1)*. Table 1 outlines the components of a thorough child and adolescent psychiatric evaluation. Components may be added or omitted as clinically appropriate.

Early-onset psychiatric disorders may have a profound effect on development in multiple domains. Social, academic, and adaptive capacities are all vulnerable to disruption which may negatively affect the child's ability to function and damage self-esteem. Regardless of the etiology of the primary psychiatric disorder, the prognosis is multidetermined by biological, social, cultural, familial, economic, and interventional factors. Interventions that enhance the compensatory capacities and promote resilience may markedly improve the child's long-term functional capabilities and achievements *(2)*.

DEVELOPMENTAL DISORDERS

Pervasive Developmental Disorders/Autistic Disorder

The initial description by Leo Kanner in 1943 of children having "come into the world with innate inability to form the usual, biologically provided affective contact with people" *(3)* has remained the essential feature of children suffering from autistic disorder. These are children who from birth (and at least evident by the age of three) demonstrate functional disabilities in social interaction, social communication, and symbolic or imaginative play. Autistic disorder is one of the pervasive developmental disorders (PDDs), the others including Rett's disorder, childhood disintegrative disorder, Asperger's disorder, and PDD not otherwise specified (NOS). Co-existing mental retardation or learning difficulties are very common, but not essential for the diagnosis *(4)*.

Epidemiology

The overall prevalence estimates of the PDDs have been steadily increasing, probably because of changes in case definition and improved recognition. Autistic disorder is estimated to have a prevalence of 5–10 per 10,000 in the United States *(5)*. Broader autism spectrum disorders may occur at a rate of 20 per 10,000. Rett's disorder (estimated prevalence of 0.44 to 2.1 per 10,000 females) and childhood disintegrative disorder (fewer than 100 cases reported) are much less common. Except for Rett's disorder, which appears to affect predominantly girls, the PDDs are more common in boys (4–5 to 1). Girls who are affected tend to be more severely mentally retarded. These disorders are evenly distributed in all socioeconomic classes *(6)*.

Signs and Symptoms

PDDs are characterized by severe and pervasive impairment in the developmental areas of reciprocal social interaction skills, communication skills, or the presence of stereotyped behavior, interests, and activities. These disorders are usually evident in the first years of life and are often associated with mental retardation or learning disabilities (LDs). The PDDs are sometimes observed with a diverse group of other general medical conditions, including chromosomal abnormalities, congenital infections, or structural abnormalities of the central nervous system (CNS) *(4)*.

Etiology and Pathogenesis

Genetic Factors

Research (family studies, twin studies, and chromosome studies) indicates that genetic factors play a major contributory role in a subgroup of autistic individuals. Although the exact etiology of the autistic spectrum disorders remains unknown and is likely quite heterogeneous and multifactorial, there are a large number of studies identifying association with various and diverse chromosomal abnormalities (including deletions, duplications, translocations, trisomies, inversions, mosaicism, ring chromosomes, and complex chromosomal rearrangements). The prevalence of autism in siblings is 4.5%, a rate 50 times higher than the risk for autism in the general population *(7)*. A family study by Folstein and Rutter *(8)* found that although only 36% of monozygotic (MZ) twin pairs were concordant for autism, when a broader spectrum of related cognitive or social abnormalities was applied, 92% of the same MZ pairs were concordant for the spectrum, compared with 10% of dizygotic pairs. These findings suggest that autism is under a high degree of genetic control, with multiple genetic loci, and that a combination of genetic predisposition and environmental insult may be involved.

The search for candidate genes for autism has resulted in quite variable findings—genomewide screens for susceptibility genes have demonstrated limited concordance of linked loci. There may be numerous genes of weak effect and/or genetically heterogeneous factors contributing to the disorders. The 7q31-35, 15q11-13, and 16p13.3 chromosomes have perhaps demonstrated the most consistent evidence for a linkage with autism *(9)*. There is evidence of a link between the serotonin-transported gene (HTT) in the 15q11-13 region and autism (a genetic area known to cause Angelman's syndrome). Although a direct link between the *HTT* alleles alone may not directly convey risk for autism, they may modify the severity of autism in the social and communication domains.

Some known genetic syndromes are also associated with autism, including phenylketotonuria, fragile-X syndrome, tuberous sclerosis, and Angelman's syndrome.

Neurodevelopmental Factors

Researchers have reported an association between unfavorable events in prenatal, perinatal, and neonatal period and autism *(10)*. Nonspecific neurological abnormalities are common. In several series of studies with autistic patients, 30–50% were noted to display signs of dysfunction possibly associated with the basal ganglia and neostriatum, including hypotonia or hypertonia, coordination deficits, abnormal reflexes, posture and gait abnormalities, and movement disorders of various types *(6)*. Macrocephaly is a common finding (between 12 and 46%) *(11)*. Seizure disorders appear in 35–50% of patients by the age of 20 years, more commonly in the presence of concurrent mental retardation.

Neuroanatomical Factors

There is a great deal of variability in neuroanatomical findings in autism. Postmortem brain studies have revealed both negative and positive findings. Imaging studies demonstrate a wide range of abnormalities, as well. Computed tomography scans show variable nonspecific changes, such as porencephalic cysts, ventricular enlargement, and abnormal symmetry. Magnetic resonance imaging studies have reported cerebellar hypoplasia and small brainstem structures in autistic patients, as well as forebrain morphological abnormalities *(6)*.

Autoimmune Factors

Autoimmune abnormalities have been suggested as etiological in autistic disorder. Autoantibodies to serotonin-1A receptor, which are not present in brain-damaged non-autistic patients, have been reported in 40% of autistic patients *(12)*. Peripheral serotonin levels are also frequently elevated, possibly affecting CNS development via potentiation of synapses. Concerns about the link between the mumps, measles, and rubella vaccine and autism have not been substantiated.

Diagnosis

Autism and the autistic spectrum disorders are clinical diagnoses, with criteria for the diagnosis of autism in Table 2 *(4)*. Delayed social smile, poor eye contact, delayed speech, or suspected deafness are some of the earliest manifestations that may concern parents. The evaluation of a child with suspected autistic disorder should be a multidisciplinary collaborative process. In addition to standard assessment procedures, hearing testing is essential, as are assessments of cognitive, language, social, and adaptive functioning. Neurological examination is important to detect possible inborn metabolic, structural, or degenerative diseases or seizures. An electroencephalogram (EEG) (to rule out a seizure disorder or developmental regression), chromosome analysis (for fragile X, etc.), and labwork for lead level and other toxic/metabolic screeners may be indicated. Standardized diagnostic rating scales such as the Autistic Diagnostic Observation Schedule or the Childhood Autism Rating Scale may be utilized *(13)*.

The PDDs have unique diagnostic characteristics that should be differentiated. Asperger's disorder does not cause delays in language development, cognitive development, age-appropriate self-help skills, or adaptive behavior. The child typically develops intense but unusual interests and loses social skills. At times, there is a discrepancy in cognitive functioning, with language-related abilities superior to visuospacial skills. Rett's disorder occurs almost exclusively in females and includes deceleration of head growth, severe mental retardation, hand-washing stereotypical movements, and loss of purposeful motor skills. Childhood disintegrative disorder has a characteristic pattern of severe developmental regression beginning at age 2 years. PDD NOS includes individuals with a number of autistic behaviors, but not meeting full criteria or not as functionally impairing. The other psychiatric and medical diagnoses to be ruled out are given in Table 3.

There is a high degree of co-morbidity of autistic spectrum-disordered patients with mental retardation (approx 80% of autistic patients are mentally retarded). Occasionally, savant skills (special capacities) in drawing, music, mathematics, or calendar calculation is observed. Additionally, anxiety disorders (generalized anxiety or obsessive-compulsive features) and ADHD are frequently co-morbid.

Table 2
DSM-IV TR Diagnostic Criteria for Autistic Disorder

A. A total of six (or more) items from (1), (2), and (3), with at least two from (1), and one each from (2) and (3):
  1. Qualitative impairment in social interaction, as manifested by at least two of the following:
      a. marked impairment in the use of multiple nonverbal behaviors such as eye-to-eye gaze, facial expression, body postures, and gestures to regulate social interaction
      b. failure to develop peer relationships appropriate to developmental level
      c. a lack of spontaneous seeking to share enjoyment, interests, or achievements with other people (e.g., by a lack of showing, bringing, or pointing out objects of interest)
      d. lack of social or emotional reciprocity
  2. Qualitative impairment in communication as manifested by at least one of the following:
      a. delay in, or total lack of, the development of spoken language (not accompanied by an attempt to compensate through alternative modes of communication such as gesture or mime)
      b. in individuals with adequate speech, marked impairment in the ability to initiate or sustain a conversation with others
      c. stereotyped and repetitive use of language or idiosyncratic language
      d. lack of varied, spontaneous make-believe play or social imitative play appropriate to developmental level
  3. Restricted repetitive and stereotyped patterns of behavior, interests, and activities, as manifested by at least one of the following:
      a. encompassing preoccupation with one or more stereotyped and restricted patterns of interest that is abnormal either in intensity or focus
      b. apparently inflexible adherence to specific, nonfunctional routines or rituals
      c. stereotyped and repetitive motor mannerisms (e.g., hand or finger flapping or twisting, or complex whole-body movements)
      d. persistent preoccupation with parts of objects
B. Delays or abnormal functioning in at least one of the following areas, with onset prior to age 3 years: (1) social interaction, (2) language as used in social communication, or (3) symbolic or imaginative play
C. The disturbance is not better accounted for by Rett's disorder or childhood disintegrative disorder

Course and Prognosis

Autistic disorder is often apparent in early infancy, with delayed developmental milestones, delayed social smile, eye contact, and language and communication (pointing and shared attentional activities). Sometimes an initial period of seemingly normal development may be followed by arrested or regressed developmental trajectory.

Early diagnosis and multimodal intervention may markedly improve prognosis. Predictors of overall better adaptive outcome include later manifestation of symptoms, higher IQ, language skills (verbal communication by the age of 5 years), and less impaired social skills. The course of the disorder is quite variable, characterized generally by gradual but erratic improvement punctuated by intermittent regressions (often precipitated by environmental stress or illness). Some children may demonstrate self-abusive or aggressive behavior in the face of frustrations. The onset of adolescence may precipitate behavioral deterioration, with seizures more likely to appear during this time. Adults with autistic disorder typically continue to improve gradually but retain clinical evidence of organic impairment. Depending on the degree of mental retardation and severity of the autistic disorder, adults may achieve adaptive functioning within the normal range. About one-third are able to function independently as adults, although deficits in social skills, empathy, and rigid coping skills frequently persist.

Treatment

Initially thought to be resistant to treatment, autistic individuals with early rigorous multimodal treatment have demonstrated the potential for significant improvement. Essential interventions include

Table 3
Differential Diagnosis for Autism

Other Pervasive Developmental Disorders
   Rett's Disorder
   Asperger's Disorder
   Childhood Disintegrative Disorder
   Pervasive Developmental Disorder, NOS
Other Psychiatric Disorders
   Mental Retardation
   Juvenile onset Schizophrenia
   Reactive Attachment Disorder
   Selective Mutism/Anxiety Disorders
   Developmental Expressive and Receptive Language Disorders
Medical Disorders
   Congenital Deafness
   Congenital Blindness
   Seizure Disorder
   Genetic abnormalities (such as Fragile X)
   Degenerative neurological diseases
   Toxic/metabolic disorders
   Heavy metal poisoning

early and intensive speech and language therapy, special educational services, adaptive skill training, and behavioral therapy. The treatments should be integrated across settings (school and home, etc.), and include continual rewards for positive behavior, speech, social interaction, self-care skills, and adaptive functioning. Parent guidance is critical. Parenting children with autistic spectrum disorders is quite challenging, and parents require support to deal with emotional reactions such as denial or guilt. Additionally, psychoeducation about the nature of the disorder, how to access essential services, and the crucial nature of parental participation as a member of the treatment team is needed. Parents are extremely important collaborators in the child's learning of language and self-care skills. Training in behavior management skills is essential to the child's learning of more adaptive behaviors to cope with frustration and ensuring a safe home environment.

Long-term treatment and services are generally required. Vocational training is important as the autistic individual enters adolescence. Acute hospitalization or longer term residential treatment may be required if symptoms are serious and disabling. Co-morbid mood, anxiety disorders, attentional problems or the onset of seizures should be assessed in an ongoing way.

Medication Treatment

Although medications are not specific to the treatment of the autistic spectrum disorders, psychotropics may be used to target specific disabling psychiatric and behavioral symptoms, such as aggression or agitation, anxiety, depression, and attentional issues. Individuals with developmental disorders may be quite sensitive to the therapeutic, but also side effects of psychotropic medications. In general, beginning with very low doses of medication and increasing very gradually as needed for effectiveness is advised. The risk of tardive dyskinesia with antipsychotic medications may be higher in these patients because of the length of treatment and perhaps biological vulnerability. Additionally, irritability or activation with the antidepressants or stimulant medications may be seen.

The antipsychotic medications are the most widely studied of the medications used in children and adolescents with autistic spectrum disorders. Controlled studies (primarily with haloperidol and risperidone) demonstrate clinical effectiveness in the treatment of severe aggression, interpersonal withdrawal with paranoid or delusional thoughts and stereotypies. Low doses of less-sedating antipsychotic medications, in conjunction with a highly structured psychoeducational program, may help control behavioral symptoms, reduce excessive agitation and activity, and enhance the effectiveness of behavioral therapies.

Co-morbid ADHD is common in individuals with pervasive developmental disorders. Psychostimulant medications may decrease the symptoms of overactivity, impulsivity, and distractibility. However, these medications must be used cautiously and monitored carefully, as the dopamine agonist effects may exacerbate rituals, stereotypies, and agitation. The selective serotonin reuptake inhibitors (SSRIs) such as fluvoxamine may reduce obsessive-compulsive behaviors. Clomipramine may decrease the frequency of some self-abusive behaviors. Fluoxetine can relieve depressive symptoms in adolescents with autism.

β-blockers and the α-2-agdrenergic receptor agonist clonidine have demonstrated effectiveness for decreasing aggression in some individuals with autism. Clonidine is also used for sleep disturbance, which is common. However, tolerance often develops with longer term use. There is evidence that the opiate antagonist naltrexone may decrease the frequency of self-injurious behaviors in some patients with autistic disorder *(13)*.

Parental distress and the hope for a significant breakthrough in treatment has resulted in a barrage of unsubstantiated treatments for autism that are ineffective, toxic, or divert time and resources away from the more scientifically grounded treatments *(14)*. Parent education and discussion concerning these unconventional treatments is an ongoing process in the care of children with autism and their families.

MENTAL RETARDATION

The Diagnostic and Statistical Manual of Mental Disorders, Fourth Edition, Text Revision (DSM-IV-TR) diagnosis of mental retardation requires low intellectual functioning (IQ of 70 or below on an individually administered IQ test); deficits in adaptive functioning in at least two areas (communication, self-care, home living, social/interpersonal skills, use of community resources, self-direction, functional academic skills, work, leisure, health, and safety); with an onset before the age of 18 years *(4)*. Table 4 provides an overview of the features of mental retardation.

Epidemiology

The prevalence of mental retardation in the United States is estimated at about .8%, with by far the largest percent of individuals being in the mild mental retardation category. Associated medical, neurological, and sensory disorders are common. Seizure disorders occur in up to 30%, with an increase in associated seizures, physical, and sensory handicaps increasing with the increasing severity of the mental retardation.

Etiology and Pathogenesis

Insults to the CNS of any sort may result in cognitive and associated adaptive impairment. Alterations in fetal development, called errors in morphogenesis, may be caused by malformations (failure of tissue to form normally), deformations (alterations of normally forming tissue by abnormal mechanical forces), and disruptions (*in utero* injury to developing CNS tissue). Many of these disorders have a genetic etiology, although toxins (alcohol, illicit substances, medications, or other chemicals), viruses, and other intrauterine insults may contribute. Errors in metabolism (inborn or not), as well as extraordinary extrinsic events (such as hypoxia, trauma, or poisoning) may also result in irreversible cognitive impairments.

Diagnosis

Some genetic syndromes may be diagnosed via prenatal or postnatal screening. Poor muscle tone and developmental delay may be the earliest manifestation. However, by definition, both individualized cognitive testing and impairment in adaptive functioning are required for diagnosis. Mental

Table 4
Features of Mental Retardation

	Mild	Moderate	Severe	Profound
IQ level	50–55 to 70	35–40 to 50–55	20–25 to 35–40	Below 20–25
Population Prevalence	.5%	< .2%	< .1%	< .05%
Percentage of MR population	85%	10%	4%	1%
Educational Expectations	Educable	Trainable	Simple skills	Mostly Nonverbal
Functional Expectations	Independent Living	Sheltered Living	Supervised Living	Highly Supervised Living
	Independent ADLs	Minimal assistance ADLs	Supervised ADLs	Assisted ADLs
	Holds job	Supervised job	Minimal job skills	

retardation is not necessarily a lifelong disorder. Some individuals may acquire a high level of adaptive and independence skills to the level that they no longer meet diagnostic criteria.

The diagnostic evaluation of a child with developmental delay should include a detailed obstetrical and perinatal history, family history, and developmental history. Additionally, a thorough physical and neurological examination, and labwork (genetic testing, lead level, thyroid, study of metabolic disorders, etc.), an EEG, or neuroimaging may be indicated. Psychological testing by a psychologist experienced in working with young children or children with delays is important for early detection.

Children and adolescents with mental retardation are generally at higher risk for developing psychopathology. Thus, the diagnostic assessment should not only identify the cognitive and adaptive delays, but assess for concomitant PDD, ADHD, disruptive behavior disorders, mood disorders, and anxiety disorders. Poor frustration tolerance, inadequate coping and verbal skills may lead to a higher degree of behavioral symptoms. Aggression is one of the most common reasons for psychiatric referral for children and adolescents with mental retardation. Helping the child gain more adaptive methods of communicating wants, needs and frustrations may help in alleviating the aggressive behavior *(15,16)*.

Treatment

Early diagnosis and intervention is essential for children with developmental disorders of any type. The Individuals with Disabilities Education Act specifies that children who qualify for special education are entitled to a "free and appropriate public education" from birth to age 21 *(17)*. Birth-to-Three services to address motor and communication skill deficits are indicated. Additionally, children with disabilities are eligible for special preschool services from the age of 3.

Treatment approaches are designed to help improve overall level of functioning and quality of life. Coordination of medical, psychiatric, and educational services is crucial. Family support and psychoeducation is indicated. Behavioral modification and supportive therapies may be quite helpful in alleviating maladaptive behaviors. Individualized special educational services may include occupational therapy, physical therapy, speech and language therapy, and other special services, in addition to a curriculum that is adapted to the learning capabilities of the child. Mainstream classes or small, self-contained classes may be appropriate, as long as the child is able to learn and adapt socially in the environment provided. Medications may be utilized to target secondary symptoms of psychiatric illness or aggression, as needed.

DEVELOPMENTAL DISORDERS OF LEARNING, MOTOR SKILLS, AND COMMUNICATION

Learning, communication, and motor skills disorders are common developmental impairments that may negatively impact a child's mental health and ability to function academically and socially. Unlike mental retardation, the learning, communication, and motor skills disorders do not have deficient intellectual functioning as a diagnostic feature. Epidemiological and clinical research has demonstrated an association between ADHD and overlapping learning, language, and motor disorders, a constellation of impairments which is sometimes referred to as deficits in attention, motor control, and perception *(18)*.

Epidemiology

LDs are very common, with an estimated 1–20% of children and adolescents suffering from some level of learning and/or communication disorder. About 5.3% of all students in US public schools receive a special education designation and special services for LD. About 50% of these children have a co-morbid psychiatric disorder, making these disorders a very significant public health issue *(19)*.

Etiology and Pathogenesis

The etiology of LDs is unknown. However, the complexity of neural circuitry involved in higher cognitive processes suggests that functional neurocognitive deficits of multiple types that disrupt cognitive processing may lead to learning difficulties. Both hereditary and environmental factors have been implicated in reading disorders. Prematurity, perinatal adversity, poverty, malnutrition, poor schooling, early abuse, and neglect and parental substance abuse have all been described. Additionally, genetic loci on chromosomes 6 and 15 have been identified as linked to some familial cases of reading disability *(20)*. There is also a link between reading disability and ADHD on a hereditary basis.

Diagnosis

The diagnosis of LD involves establishing a discrepancy between academic skill and the child's intelligence, and then eliminating all other explanations for the discrepancy. To establish this discrepancy, a psychoeducational evaluation is performed by a qualified psychologist, using scores on standardized academic achievement tests as compared with standardized intelligence scores. A significant difference is set as 1 to 2 standard deviation discrepancy, with achievement level lower than IQ. The types of LDs include reading disorder, mathematics disorder, disorder of written expression, and LD NOS.

Psychiatric evaluation for concomitant psychiatric disorders is indicated because of the high degree of co-morbidity involved. ADHD is the most common co-occurring disorder, but significant issues of self-esteem with depression, anxiety, and disruptive behaviors are common as well.

Treatment

Early diagnosis and intervention is helpful in the treatment of the LD and avoiding the secondary morbidity associated with academic frustration and recurrent failures. Although the scope of the chapter does not allow a full discussion of therapeutic modalities used, multimodal approaches, direct treatment of visuomotor deficits, and enhancing attention and motivation are used. Identification for special education services, and an individualized educational program to provide interventions that directly address the LD, is indicated. Specialized tutoring or other types of educational support are individualized to the child's needs in the least-restrictive setting. The physician is often quite helpful in advocating for appropriate services for patients with special needs.

Children with LDs are often helped by a clear explanation of the nature of their difficulty. Children that understand that every person has areas that come easily or are much more difficult, and that this is part of each individual's uniqueness, may not be as self-conscious about the disorder. Framing the disability as an area in which the child needs to work harder than many peers may help increase motivation, decrease frustration, and improve self-esteem. Highlighting areas of strength and ability, as well as remediating difficulties, may also be quite helpful.

Psychotherapy, family counseling, and the judicious use of medications may be indicated for some children and adolescents with co-occurring psychiatric issues. Therapeutic interventions should be coordinated between the school, home, and therapist, and should be targeted to the child's individual needs. Tutoring and special assistance in the area of the disability is indicated *(19)*.

AXIS I DISORDERS USUALLY FIRST DIAGNOSED IN INFANCY, CHILDHOOD, OR ADOLESCENCE

Attention Deficit Hyperactivity Disorder

ADHD is the most commonly diagnosed psychiatric disorder of childhood, and is characterized by deficits in attention, concentration, activity level, and impulse control. The public health impact of ADHD on the child, his or her family, schools, and society is enormous, with billions of dollars spent annually for school services, mental health services, and increased use of the juvenile justice system. In contrast with historical notions, children do not typically "outgrow" ADHD. Morbidity and disability often persist into adult life *(21)*.

Epidemiology

ADHD is relatively common, affecting an estimated 3–12% of school-age children. The DSM-IV classification of ADHD into three categories—inattentive type, hyperactive-impulsive type, or combined type—has led to a broadening of the disorder to include more girls, preschoolers, and adults, and has impacted the educational services and treatment modalities utilized.

In community samples of children, boys are diagnosed with ADHD, combined type, in a frequency of 3:1 as compared with girls. Clinic samples tend to be higher, approaching a 9:1 male to female ratio, most likely as a result of the higher proportion of disruptive behaviors in boys with ADHD, combined type, which may promote referral for treatment. ADHD is diagnosed in as many as half of children referred for mental health services. The inattentive subtype of ADHD is not associated with an increase in disruptive behaviors, and is more nearly equal in prevalence between boys and girls.

Psychosocial correlates with ADHD include low income/poverty, urban residence, family dysfunction, and parents with psychiatric disorder. These psychosocial risk factors suggest that there may be multiple pathways leading to the clinical constellation of ADHD in vulnerable children.

Signs and Symptoms

ADHD is a syndrome consisting of symptoms in several categories—inattention, hyperactivity and impulsivity, or the combination of both sets of symptoms. A variety of other psychiatric disorders may present with difficulties with sustained attention (such as anxiety, depression, or psychotic disorders), high levels of activity (such as bipolar disorder or PDD), or both. Thus, the clinician must differentiate the core symptoms of ADHD from the secondary effects of the other psychiatric disorders or a primary medical disorder (e.g., fetal alcohol syndrome, atypical seizures, toxic/metabolic disorder) *(22)*.

Etiology and Pathogenesis

Genetic Factors

Although the exact etiology of ADHD remains unknown, data from family genetic, twin, adoption, and segregation analysis strongly suggest that there is genetic component in the etiology for the disorder.

ADHD is thought to be a complex genetic disorder resulting from the combined effects of several genes and interactions with the environment. Preliminary molecular genetic studies have implicated candidate genes associated with the dopamine system, including the dopamine D2 and D4 receptors and the dopamine transporter. There is also preliminary evidence that genes involved in norepinephrine modulation are affected in some patients. Given the importance of these catecholamines for the modulation of attentional circuits, it is not surprising that alterations in these systems would result in impaired attention regulation. However, there is a great deal of study left to be done on the role of genes and the gene–environment interaction in the etiology of ADHD *(21)*.

Neurodevelopmental Factors

Prefrontal, parietal, and temporal association cortices, and their projections to the striatum, make distinct contributions to the core ability to focus attention. In particular, the prefrontal cortex uses working memory to guide overt responses (movement) as well as covert responses (attention), allowing us to inhibit inappropriate behaviors and to attenuate the processing of irrelevant stimuli. The neurotransmitters of dopamine and norepinephrine are both intricately involved in modulating prefrontal cortical functioning. There is evidence that moderate amounts of these neurotransmitters are essential to prefrontal cortical functioning, but that high levels (as is found in extreme stress) may actually impair optimal functioning *(23)*.

Brown has argued that the common etiological deficit in all types of ADHD is one of impaired executive functioning. Developmental difficulties with activation, focus, sustaining effort, modulating emotions, utilizing working memory and regulating behaviors are all subsumed under the rubric of executive functioning impairment *(24)*.

Early neurodevelopmental problems such as obstetrical complications, prematurity, other genetic abnormalities (such as fragile X disorder and others), and exposure *in utero* to alcohol, cocaine, or other toxins, may predispose to ADHD. It is postulated that fetal insults may cause subtle functional abnormalities to the frontal cortex and other brain structures, resulting in the disorder. Early findings are also provocative regarding the neuronal–environmental interactions as related to brain functioning. Specifically, the efficiency of brain functioning may be molded in the perinatal period via neuronal pruning that is enhanced by appropriate levels of stimulation and nurturance. Severe psychosocial adversity in infancy, thus, may predispose to subtle neurodevelopmental disorders such as ADHD.

Neuroimaging Findings

Imaging studies of ADHD have focused on the prefrontal cortex, basal ganglia, and cerebellum. Although results have been mixed, there is evidence of structural and functional differences in the brains of children and adults with ADHD. Volumetric measures have detected smaller right-sided prefrontal regions overall in boys with ADHD. These reductions correlated with performance on tasks that require response inhibition. Girls with ADHD have been found to have smaller left and total caudate volumes. A consistent finding in ADHD has been reduced volume of the posterior–inferior cerebellar vermis, a region that exhibits a high degree of dopamine receptor reactivity.

Functional neuroimaging has demonstrated decreased metabolism in the regions of the prefrontal cortex and striatum in adults with ADHD by positron emission tomography (PET) scanning. Although functional MRI has not been conclusive, early results also indicate subtle deficits in frontal lobe activity. Preliminary results of PET imaging examining the neuropharmacology of ADHD support the notion that catecholamine dysregulation is central to the pathophysiology of the disorder, and not just to its treatment *(23)*.

Diagnosis

ADHD is a clinical diagnosis. There is no definitive diagnostic test or neuroimaging procedure for ADHD, but rather the diagnosis is established by clinical judgment based on a comprehensive assessment that involves multiple domains, informants, methods, and settings. Table 5 gives the DSM-IV diagnostic criteria for the disorder. Hyperactivity is a symptom of many disorders, and therefore the differential diagnosis of ADHD is quite extensive. The clinician must complete a thorough assessment to clarify the diagnosis and nature of the disabling symptoms. It is important to rule out a primary medical disorder (such as thyroid disorder, lead intoxication, seizure or other toxic/metabolic,

Table 5
DSM-IV-TR Diagnostic Criteria for Attention Deficit Hyperactivity Disorder

A. Either (1) or (2)
    1. Six (or more) of the following symptoms of inattention have persisted for at least 6 months to a degree that is maladaptive and inconsistent with developmental level:

Inattention
    a. often fails to give close attention to details or makes careless mistakes in schoolwork, work, or other activities
    b. often has difficulty sustaining attention in tasks or play activities
    c. often does not seem to listen when spoken to directly
    d. often does not follow through on instructions and fails to finish schoolwork, chores, or duties in the workplace (not due to oppositional behavior or failure to understand instructions)
    e. often has difficulty organizing tasks and activities
    f. often avoids, dislikes, or is reluctant to engage in tasks that require sustained mental effort (such as schoolwork or homework)
    g. often loses things necessary for tasks or activities (e.g., toys, school assignments, pencils, books, or tools)
    h. is often easily distracted by extraneous stimuli
    i. is often forgetful in daily activities
    2. Six (or more) of the following symptoms of hyperactivity-impulsivity have persisted for at least 6 months to a degree that is maladaptive and inconsistent with developmental level:

Hyperactivity
    a. often fidgets with hands or feet or squirms in seat
    b. often leaves seat in classroom or in other situations in which remaining seated is expected
    c. often runs about or climbs excessively in situations in which it is inappropriate (in adolescents or adults, may be limited to subjective feelings of restlessness)
    d. often has difficulty playing or engaging in leisure activities quietly
    e. is often "on the go" or often acts as if "driven by a motor"
    f. often talks excessively

Impulsivity
    g. often blurts out answers before questions have been completed
    h. often has difficulty awaiting turn
    i. often interrupts or intrudes on others (e.g., butts into conversations or games)
B. Some hyperactive-impulsive or inattentive symptoms that caused impairment were present before age 7 years.
C. Some impairment from the symptoms is present in two or more settings (e.g., at school [or work] and at home).
D. There must be clear evidence of clinically significant impairment in social, academic, or occupational functioning.
E. The symptoms do not occur exclusively during the course of a Pervasive Developmental Disorder, Schizophrenia, or other Psychotic Disorder and are not better accounted for by another mental disorder (e.g., Mood Disorder, Anxiety Disorder, Dissociative Disorder, or a Personality Disorder).

Code based on type:
    314.01 Attention-Deficit/Hyperactivity Disorder, Combined Type: if both Criteria A1 and A2 are met for the past 6 months
    314.00 Attention-Deficit/Hyperactivity Disorder, Predominantly Inattentive Type: if Criterion A1 is met but Criterion A2 is not met for the past 6 months
    314.01 Attention-Deficit/Hyperactivity Disorder, Predominantly Hyperactive-Impulsive Type: if Criterion A2 is met but Criterion A1 is not met for the past 6 months

Table 6
Differential Diagnosis for ADHD

Psychiatric Disorders
    Mood Disorders (depression and bipolar bisorder)
    Anxiety disorders
    Tic disorders
    Substance use disorders
    Oppositional defiant or conduct disorder
    Pervasive developmental disorder
    Learning disorders
    Post-traumatic stress disorder
    Mental retardation or borderline intellectual functioning
Psychosocial Conditions
    Abuse and/or neglect
    Poor nutrition
    Neighborhood violence
    Chaotic family situation
    Being bullied at school
Medical Disorders
    Partial deafness
    Poor eyesight
    Seizure disorder
    Fetal alcohol syndrome
    Genetic abnormalities (such as Fragile X)
    Sedating or activating medications
       (common are asthma medications and caffeine)
    Substance abuse
    Thyroid abnormality
    Heavy metal poisoning

or neurological disorders). Table 6 lists the differential diagnosis of ADHD to be considered. The onset of ADHD impairment must be in early childhood, at least before the age of 7, even if it was not diagnosed until later in life. There must be functional impairment in a variety of life settings (e.g., home, school, work). Milder forms of PDD may present with intractable hyperactivity as a primary symptom. ADHD should not be diagnosed separately if it presents only concomitantly with a PDD or psychotic disorder *(25)*.

A complete history and screening physical and neurological exam are necessary to provide accurate assessment of ADHD in children and adolescents. As with all psychiatric evaluations, the use of multiple informants is key. Teacher ratings are particularly essential in assessing ADHD. The structured setting, individualized attention, and novelty may mask ADHD symptoms during assessment in the physician's office.

Many parents will relate difficult early temperament and poor impulse control from an early age. Often, early gross motor development, with more delayed fine motor and language development are described. The psychiatric history should focus on presenting symptoms, the longitudinal timeline of symptoms development, and associated features and/or confounding factors (e.g., mood disorders, developmental problems, recent stress or traumas, substance abuse). Co-morbidity with other psychiatric disorders is frequent (40–60% of children with ADHD), and negatively affects treatment response and prognosis. The most common co-morbid conditions include oppositional defiant and conduct disorder (50%), anxiety disorders (25–33%), depression (around 30%), and bipolar disorder (around 10–20% of clinical populations). Thus, both the ADHD and concomitant disorders must be the focus of treatment. Rating scales of symptoms (Conners scale *[26]* or others) is essential in quantifying the symptom severity and response to treatment.

Psychoeducational testing to assess intellectual ability, academic achievement, and possible learning disabilities is a crucial component of a thorough assessment. At times, more complete neuropsychological testing, to assess executive functioning and more subtle deficits of the disorder, may be indicated. The Continuous Performance Task is a computerized test that assesses attentional abilities and impulsivity of response style. Although not specifically diagnostic, it may help in the complete diagnostic assessment. Children with ADHD frequently have learning issues, and these must be well delineated to ensure appropriate educational services.

Course and Prognosis

Although many of the symptoms of ADHD may remit, it has become clear that ADHD is frequently a chronic disorder, which leads to a negative impact on functioning throughout the life cycle. About three-quarters of these children continue to show symptoms of ADHD into adolescence, and pervasive academic, social, self-esteem and conduct difficulties are common.

Follow-up studies into adulthood suggest that up to 33% of ADHD vs 1–9% of controls drop out of high school. ADHD children go on to have less education overall (by 2–3 years) and fewer go on to complete a graduate degree. Likewise, the ADHD cohort demonstrates significantly lower occupations rankings at the age of 25. Children with ADHD are also at increased risk for developing antisocial personality disorder and substance abuse disorders in adulthood. An estimated 40–50% continue to suffer from clinically significant symptoms of ADHD *(22)*.

Treatment

ADHD is a complex disorder affecting every area of functioning, and thereby requires a comprehensive treatment program. Psychosocial interventions, medication treatment, and ensuring an appropriate educational plan are all part of the effective treatment for ADHD *(22,25)* (*see* Table 7).

The Multimodal Treatment Study of ADHD (MTA) was a large ($N = 579$) study sponsored by the National Institute of Mental Health investigating the effects of various treatment modalities on children with ADHD-combined type over a 14-month time period. The aim of the MTA was to compare the effectiveness of medication treatment combined with intensive and broad-based psychosocial treatment with medication management or psychosocial treatment alone, and to compare these treatment programs with regular community care. In the MTA, the psychosocial treatments provided included an 8-week, all-day summer treatment program that utilized contingency management and included social skills training. Additionally, parent training and teacher consultation on classroom behavior management were included. The medication used was methylphenidate adjusted on a monthly basis with monthly teacher feedback and family interview. Children in the community-care arm of the study also frequently received medication, but overall on a lower dosage than the children in the study.

The study found that for the core symptoms of ADHD, intensive medication management was superior to behavioral treatment and treatment in the community. However, for non-ADHD areas of functioning, the combined treatment was superior to the other groups in the treatment of oppositional and aggressive symptoms, internalizing symptoms, teacher-rated social skills, parent–child relations, and reading achievement *(27)*.

Psychosocial Treatments

Psychosocial treatments may include psychoeducation, parent training in behavioral management skills, classroom interventions, contingency management, social skills training, cognitive-behavior therapy, and individual psychotherapy of the child. Of these, parent training, classroom interventions, contingency management, and social skills training have demonstrated efficacy. Psychoeducation, which includes intensive support and education of the family, is essential in developing an ongoing therapeutic alliance between the therapist, the child and his or her family to ensure collaboration in the complex task of helping the child achieve optimal functioning.

Table 7
Essentials of Treatment for ADHD

1. Treatment should include more than just medication management. Parental guidance and counseling and psycho-education are cornerstones of treatment.
2. Unsuccessful treatment of ADHD often occurs when comorbid diagnoses, hyperactivity associated with another psychiatric disorder (such as PDD), or primary medical diagnoses are not identified and addressed.
3. Collaboration with a child's school is usually critical to ensure academic progress.
4. Medication holidays should be individualized to the child's unique situation, and utilized only if the child's social functioning and safety will not be severely compromised. Medication holidays over the summer or during weekends do not decrease the effectiveness of stimulants.
5. Treatment with stimulants does not increase the likelihood of substance use disorders, and may actually lower the risk.
6. In general, failure of an initial stimulant trial should be followed with one or two subsequent stimulant trials before treating with a different class of psychotropic medication.

School is where ADHD symptoms may be most disabling, as the demands to sit quietly, pay attention, and work cooperatively are inherent in the school setting. School interventions include ensuring that learning needs are appropriately assessed and addressed. Additionally, contact with teachers regarding the diagnosis and effectiveness of treatment is required. It is crucial that the teacher understands the disorder, and that he or she provides a classroom environment that optimizes the child's learning. Preferential seating (seating within the class to optimize paying attention and minimize distractions), a behavioral management plan that highlights positive reinforcement for desired work habits and behavior, social skills groups, and other interventions may help the child gain school success. More intensive interventions (a small self-contained classroom, special educational services, or a more intensive therapeutic educational plan) may be required for children who are more impaired by the disorder and/or co-morbidities *(21,22)*.

Medication Treatment

As highlighted in the MTA study, medication treatment may be highly effective in addressing the core symptoms of ADHD *(27,28)*. There is a large body of literature documenting the efficacy of stimulants on core features of ADHD (motoric overactivity, impulsivity, and inattentiveness) as well as their substantial effects on cognition, social function, and aggression. The stimulant medications are the most thoroughly studied medications in child and adolescent psychiatry, and have demonstrated safety and efficacy in more than 200 controlled studies. Despite concerns of many families about the abuse potential of the medication, and the risk of precipitating an addictive personality, use of stimulant medication treatment may actually decrease a child's risk for substance abuse, legal difficulties, and other sequelae of poor impulse control. Finally, concerns that stimulant medication might be responsible for the smaller brain structures found in ADHD children do not appear supported *(29)*.

At times, medication "holidays" may be indicated. This is when the child does not take ADHD medication during non-school periods of time. Although this practice may be helpful for children for whom appetite and sleep are disturbed with the medication, many children may require the medication even when not in school to maintain appropriate social behavior, to be able to enjoy and benefit from group activities, and to decrease highly impulsive behavior that may pose a safety issue.

In general, the stimulant medications are considered first line in the treatment of the core symptoms of ADHD. Atomoxetine is an antidepressant that has recently been marketed as a long-acting, noncontrolled medication monotherapy for ADHD, and some clinicians are beginning to use this medication first line, although the body of data on efficacy and effectiveness remains small. Common side effects of the stimulant medications are appetite suppression, sleep disturbances, and some changes in pulse and blood pressure. Stimulants may precipitate or exacerbate tics. At times, stimulant medications may

272

Stubbe

Table 8
Medication Algorithm for Treating ADHD

Considered first-line
    Methylphenidate: Ritalin*, Ritalin SR*, Concerta*, Metadate*, Focalin*,
    Dextroamphetamine: Dexedrine*, Dextrostat*
    Amphetamine Salts: Adderall*
Second-line
    Atomoxetine (Straterra)*
    Bupropion (Wellbutrin)
    Venlafaxine (Effexor)
    Tricyclic Antidepressants (TCAs): nortriptyline, desipramine, imipramine
    Guanfacine (Tenex)
    Clonidine (Catapres)
Considered when most other medications are ineffective
    Atypical Antipsychotics: risperidone, olanzapine, quetiapine, ziprasidone
    Typical Antipsychotics: haloperidol*, thioridazine*, chlorpromazine*,
    Pemoline (Cylert)*

*FDA approved for treatment of ADHD.

cause more serious side effects, such as dsyphoria, irritability, or even hallucinations. These symptoms may be more common in very young children. Clonidine or guanfacine or the tricyclic antidepressants may be considered first line in the treatment of patients with ADHD and tics. However, stimulant medications have been used successfully in some patients with tic disorders, if the dosages are started low and increased slowly. *See* Table 8 for an algorithm for the use of medications in the treatment of ADHD.

The antipsychotic medications may be helpful in treating the agitation and aggression of children and adolescents with ADHD, but are used only third line and usually in low dose in combination with other ADHD medications. General principles of pharmacotherapy should be followed in the medication treatment of children, adolescents and adults with ADHD. These include beginning with one medication and slowly titrating medication dosages up as needed until optimal effectiveness is achieved with minimal side effects. At times, changing dosage timing may help decrease such side effects as appetite suppression or sleep disturbance. Routine monitoring of vital signs (blood pressure and pulse), height, and weight are indicated. If stimulant medications successfully treat ADHD, but co-morbid symptoms (such as depression) persist, addition of an antidepressant medication may be indicated. Several studies have described safety and efficacy of combined SSRIs and stimulant pharmacotherapy. Alternatively, the use of an antidepressant medication with secondary ADHD effects (such as bupropion or venlafaxine) may be considered. However, venlafaxine has been recently implicated in increased suicidal behavior for children and youth. Pemoline has been associated with hepatitis, and should be used only when other medications have been tried, and only with close blood monitoring of liver function every 2 weeks.

OTHER AXIS I DISORDERS USUALLY FIRST DIAGNOSED IN INFANCY, CHILDHOOD, OR ADOLESCENCE

Oppositional defiant disorder and conduct disorder are disorders of behavior that may resolve, but incur increased risk in adulthood of antisocial behavior, substance abuse, and mood disorders. Separation anxiety disorder, pica, rumination, encopresis, enuresis, and selective mutism nearly all remit by adulthood. Children with reactive attachment disorder remain impaired into adulthood, although more research is needed into the types and levels of disability of psychiatric disability. Table 9 gives an overview of the clinical manifestations, treatments, and prognosis for these disorders.

Table 9

Axis I Disorders Usually First Diagnosed in Infancy, Childhood or Adolescence

Disorder	Diagnosis	Epidemiology	Etiology	Differential diagnosis	Treatments
Separation anxiety disorder (SAD)	• Developmentally inappropriate anxiety concerning separation from home or significant others • Duration of 4+ weeks • Onset prior to 18 years • Functionally impairing	• 2–5% of children • ¾ of children with SAD are school avoidant	• Genetic inheritance of anxiety disorders generally • Temperament • Family dynamics • Multi-determined	• Normal separation fears • Other anxiety disorders • Pervasive developmental disorder • Autism • Schizophrenia • Trauma history • Medical etiology of somatic symptoms (headache, stomachache, etc)	• Multimodal treatment • Psychosocial treatments of cognitive behavioral, supportive, educational/psychodynamic treatment • Parent guidance and family therapy • Behavior modification • School consultation (especially for school avoidance) • Medication to treat anxiety (especially if associated school "phobia"—including brief use of benzodiazepines and SSRIs)
Selective Mutism	• Not speaking in one or several important settings • Having the ability to comprehend spoken language and to speak • Symptoms for at least one month • Functional disability (education and interpersonal)	• <1% of school children • Usually ages 3–8 • Female > male by 2:1	• Anxiety disorders • Family instability and loss • Emotional or physical trauma • Often have delayed onset of speech or articulation difficulties • Neuro-developmental disorders	• Frequently co-morbid with anxiety disorders • Speech and language disorder • Other concurrent neurological disorders • Oral-facial abnormalities • Hearing delay • Mental Retardation • PDD • Schizophrenia • Conversion disorder	• Multimodal treatment • Behavioral therapy and shaping • School consultation • Family systems therapy • Play therapy • Speech and language therapy • Medication for anxiety disorder

(continued)

Table 9 (*continued*)

Disorder	Diagnosis	Epidemiology	Etiology	Differential diagnosis	Treatments
Reactive Attachment Disorder (RAD)	• Inability to form normal interpersonal relationships • Before the age of 5 • History of severe maltreatment • Inhibited type with hypervigilance and social distance • Disinhibited type with inappropriate sociability	• Unknown prevalence • Increased incidence in children with multiple foster placements	• Pathogenic care • Abuse, neglect, or impaired parenting • Multiple changes of caregivers • Parental psychopathology	• Pervasive developmental disorders • Depression (for inhibited type) • ADHD (for disinhibited type)	• Provision of consistent adequate nurturance and ensuring the safety of the child • Treat parental psychopathology • Regular longer-term supportive psychotherapy with consistent treater to gain sense of stability and trust • Medication treatment of secondary disorders
Pica	• Eating nonfood materials • Most commonly lead, clay, soil or ice	• Up to ⅓ of children • Ages 1–2 most common • Risk factors include low SES, MR, parent mental illness	• May be culturally normative • Nutritional deficiencies • Parent-child relationship problems • Poor stimulation • Poor supervision	• Consider pica in all cases of mental retardation, learning problems, or chronic constipation • Rule out lead poisoning • Check for parasites • Rule out inadequate supervision	• Increased supervision • Behavioral therapy (reward eating of nutritive foods) • Education about the difference between edible and nonedible behaviors (especially for the cognitively limited child)
Rumination Disorder of Infancy	• Infants that regurgitate and rechew their food • Absence of an associated GI illness • Induction of vomiting • Apathetic and irritable when not ruminating	• Rare • Potentially fatal	• Unknown • Adverse psychosocial factors implicated • Maternal eating disorder implicated • Increased incidence with MR or developmental disorders	• Esophageal or gastric disorders	• Parent training • Behavioral interventions • Increased positive stimulation • Hospitalization for malnutrition, medical workup and intensive parent and child treatment

Functional Enuresis	• Urinary incontinence after developmental age of 5 • Twice weekly for 3 months • Causing distress or impairment • Primary—bladder control never achieved • Secondary—wetting reappears after continence	• 5–10% of 5-year-olds • 3–5% of 10-year-olds • Boys > girls	• Genetics • Maturational • Poor ability to concentrate urine • Medication side-effect	• Diabetes insipidus • Diabetes mellitus • Urinary tract abnormalities • UTI • Renal disease • Urethritis • Seizure disorder • Sickle cell trait • Neurogenic bladder • Urinary obstruction	• Behavioral plan and charts • Maturation • Restricting fluid or waking child to urinate • Bladder training exercises • Urine alarm ("bell and pad") • Medications such as DDAVP or tricyclic antidepressants at bedtime • Psychotherapeutic treatment if associated psychiatric disorder
Functional Encopresis	• Fecal soiling or excretion in inappropriate places • At least once monthly for 3 months • Child at least 4 • Medical workup negative • Primary—bowel control never achieved • Secondary—regression to soiling after 1 yr	• 2% of 6 year olds • Primary encopresis more common with delayed development • Secondary encopresis associated with psychosocial adversity • Boys > girls 3–4:1	• Chronic constipation and "retentive encopresis" with overflow incontinence • Stress-induced diarrhea • Psychosocial stress	• Hirschsprung's disease (congenital megacolon) • Medical causes of fecal incontinence (thyroid, hypercalcemia, lactose intolerance, cerebral palsy, pseudo-obstruction, rectal stenosis, anal fissure/trauma, myelomeningocele, • Anxious children avoiding public toilets	• Treatment of constipation • Bowel cleaning and bowel retraining • Behavioral shaping for toilet use • Parent management training in behavior management techniques • Stress reduction training
Oppositional-defiant Disorder	• Often loses temper • Often argues • Defies adults' rules • Deliberately annoys people • Blames others for his/her mistakes • Easily annoyed • Spiteful • Functional impairment	• 3–15% • Boys > girls • Often occurs with ADHD • ⅓ go on to develop Conduct Disorder	• Inconsistent parental discipline and limit-setting • Parents with oppositionality • Lack of parental emotional availability • Temperamental factors • Possible genetic factors	• Panic and anxiety leading to oppositionality • Mood disorder • Psychotic disorder • Adjustment disorder • ADHD	• Multimodal treatment • Parent management training in behavior modification techniques • Social skills, conflict management and problem-solvinggroups • Token economy • Medications for associated disorders (e.g., ADHD) • Educational interventions

(continued)

Table 9 (*continued*)

Disorder	Diagnosis	Epidemiology	Etiology	Differential diagnosis	Treatments
Conduct Disorder (CD)	• Behavior violates rights of others and social norms • Aggression to people and animals • Destruction of property • Deceitfulness or theft • Serious violation of rules • Functional Impairment • At least one criterion within past 6 months	• 1–16% • Boys > girls 3–4 : 1 • Childhood onset (prior to age 10), boys > girls, more aggression and ADHD • ⅓ go on to develop Antisocial Personality	• Genetic predisposition • Other psychiatric disorders (ADHD, learning disorders, mood disorders, substance abuse, PTSD, ODD) • Neurobiological factors with low autonomic arousal and possibly executive functioning deficits • Temperamental factors • Poor parenting skills • Psychosocial adversity	• Almost all psychiatric disorders can present with disturbance of conduct (especially mood disorders, psychotic disorders, intermittent explosive disorder, adjustment disorder) • Neurological disorders with poor impulse control or seizures	• Early intervention is critical • Multimodal treatment • Parent management training in behavior modification techniques • Problem-solving skills training, anger management • Multisystemic therapy • Behavior modification • Legal sanctions • Educational interventions • Pharmacotherapy of target symptoms and associated disorders

CHILD AND ADOLESCENT MANIFESTATIONS OF AXIS I DISORDERS

Children may suffer from any of the psychiatric disorders (except antisocial personality disorder, which by definition requires an age of 18). Some disorders have a peak incidence in adolescence and early adulthood, including anorexia and bulimia nervosa, substance-related disorders, schizophrenia, and mood disorders. In general, the earlier the onset of the disorder then the more urgent the need for treatment to decrease the intensity and chronicity of the disorder. Early-onset disorders are more common in families with strong genetic loading for the disorder, and/or for children with serious psychosocial adversity. The prognosis for early-onset psychiatric disorders tends to be worse, as normal development is interrupted.

REFERENCES

1. King RA, Schwab-Stone M, Peterson B, et al. Psychiatric assessment of the infant, child and adolescent. In: Kaplan HI, Kaplan VA, eds. Kaplan and Sadock's Comprehensive Textbook of Psychiatry, Seventh Edition, Vol 2. Baltimore, MD: Lippincott, Williams & Wilkins; 2000:2558–2586.
2. Dulcan MK, Martini DR, Lake MB. Concise Guide to Child and Adolescent Psychiatry, Third Edition. Washington, DC: American Psychiatric Publishing Inc; 2003.
3. Kanner L. Autistic disturbances of affective contact. Nerv Child 1943;2:217–250.
4. American Psychiatric Association. Diagnostic and Statistical Manual of Mental Disorders, Fourth Edition, revision. Washington, DC: American Psychiatric Association; 2000.
5. Fombonne E. Epidemiology of autism: a review. Psychol Med 1999;29:769–786.
6. Tsai LY. Autistic disorder. In: Wiener JM, Dulcan MK, eds. Textbook of Child and Adolescent Psychiatry, Third Edition. Washington, DC: American Psychiatric Publishing Inc; 2004.
7. Ritvo ER, Jorde LB, Mason-Brothers A, et al. The UCLA-University of Utah epidemiologic survey of autism: recurrence risk estimate and genetic counseling. Am J Psychiatry 1989;146:1032–1036.
8. Folstein S, Rutter M. Infantile autism: a genetic study of 21 twin pairs. J Child Psychol Psychiatry 1977;18:297–321.
9. Lauritsen M, Ewald H. The genetics of autism. Acta Psychiatr Scand 2001;103:411–427.
10. Juul-Dam N, Townsend J, Courchesne E. Prenatal, perinatal, and neonatal factors in autism, pervasive developmental disorder-not otherwise specified, and the general population. Pediatrics 2001;107:E63.
11. Fidler DJ, Bailey JN, Smalley SL. Macrocephaly in autism and other pervasive developmental disorders. Dev Med Child Neurol 2000;42:737–740.
12. Todd RD, Hickok IM, Anderson GM, Cohen DJ. Antibrain antibodies in infantile autism. Biol Psychiatry 1988;23:644–647.
13. American Academy of Child and Adolescent Psychiatry. Practice parameters for the assessment and treatment of children, adolescents, and adults with autism and other pervasive developmental disorders. J Am Acad Child Adolesc Psychiatry 1999;38(Suppl):32S–54S.
14. Herbert JD, Sharp IR, Gaudiano BA. Separating fact from fiction in the etiology and treatment of autism: a scientific review of the evidence. Scientific Review of Mental Health Practice 2002;1:23–43.
15. King RA, State MW, Shah B, et al. Mental retardation: a review of the past 10 years: part I. J Am Acad Child Adolesc Psychiatry 1997;36:1656–1663.
16. State MW, King RA, Dykens E. Mental retardation: a review of the past 10 years: part II. J Am Acad Child Adolesc Psychiatry 1997;36:1664–1671.
17. US Congress. Amendments to the Individuals with Disabilities Education Act. Washington, DC: US Government Printing Office; 1997.
18. Tannock R. Language, reading, and motor control problems in ADHD: a potential behavioral phenotype. In: Greenhill L, ed. Learning Disabilities: Implications for Psychiatric Treatment. Washington, DC: American Psychiatric Press; 2000: 129–168.
19. American Academy of Child and Adolescent Psychiatry. Practice parameters for the assessment and treatment of children and adolescents with language and learning disorders. J Am Acad Child Adolesc Psychiatry 1998;37:46S–62S.
20. Grigorenko EL, Wood WB, Meyer MS, et al. Susceptibility loci for distinct components of developmental dyslexia on chromosomes 6 and 15. Am J Hum Genet 1997;60:27–39.
21. Stubbe DE. Attention-deficit/hyperactivity disorder. Child and Adolescent Psychiatric Clinics of North America 9(3), Philadelphia: WB Saunders Company; 2000.
22. Dulcan M, Benson RS. Practice parameters for the assessment and treatment of children, adolescents and adults with attention-deficit/hyperactivity disorder. J Am Acad Child Adolesc Psychiatry 1997;36(Suppl 10):85S–121S.
23. Faraone SV, Biederman J. The neurobiology of attention deficit hyperactivity disorder. In: Charney DS, Nestler EJ, Bunney BS, eds. Neurobiology of Mental Illness. New York: Oxford University Press; 1999:788–801.
24. Brown TE. Attention-Deficit Disorders and Comorbidities in Children, Adolescents and Adults. Washington, DC: American Psychiatric Press; 2000.

25. Barkley RA. Attention Deficit Hyperactivity Disorder: A Handbook for Diagnosis and Treatment, Secondnd Edition. New York, NY: Guilford; 1998.

26. Conners CK. Conners ADHD DSM-IV Scales for Parents and Teachers: Technical Manual. North Tonowanda, New York: Multi Health Systems; 1997.

27. MTA Cooperative Group. Moderators and mediators of treatment response for children with attention-deficit/hyperactivity disorder. Arch Gen Psychiatry 1999;56:1088–1096.

28. MTA Cooperative Group. National Institute of Mental Health Multimodal Treatment Study of ADHD follow-up: changes in effectiveness and growth after the end of treatment. Pediatrics 2004;113:762–769.

29. American Academy of Child and Adolescent Psychiatry. Practice parameter for the use of stimulant medications in the treatment of children, adolescents and adults. J Am Acad Child Adolesc Psychiatry 2002;41(Suppl):26S–49S.

21

Geriatric Disorders

Colin A. Depp and Jody Corey-Bloom

INTRODUCTION

At one time, the psychiatry of old age was believed to be "the darkest area of psychiatry." The often confounding nature of psychiatric disorder in the elderly is illustrated by the large number of terms used over the years to address the diversity among geriatric psychiatric patients, including "late paraphrenia," "vascular depression," "pseudodementia," and "masked depression." Many of these labels grew out of efforts to distinguish "organic" syndromes from "functional" psychiatric disorders. However, a growing number of studies employing neuroimaging and other state-of-the-art techniques have revealed new insights into the role of brain changes in the etiology of depression and schizophrenia in late life, shedding light on these disorders and yielding hope for new treatment paradigms.

There is good reason for the increased emphasis on psychiatric disorders in the elderly. The absolute number of elderly individuals with psychiatric disorders in the United States will increase dramatically as the "baby boom" population ages, from 4 million in 1970 to an estimated 15 million by the year 2030 *(1)*. Moreover, psychiatric disorders often show unique features in the elderly, are difficult to diagnosis and treat, and more frequently accompany neurological and medical co-morbidity. Previous chapters have reviewed "secondary" psychiatric manifestations of neurological disorders and "primary" psychiatric disorders in younger people. This chapter is a review of the epidemiology, presentation, etiology, course, diagnosis, and treatment of psychiatric disorders in the elderly, with emphasis on the biological aspects of these disorders.

For both the clinician and the researcher, there are several inherent challenges to geriatric psychiatry that cut across the different diagnoses. First, aging brings heterogeneity in presentation and etiology. Thus, elderly people with the same psychiatric disorder may have widely disparate illness histories. For instance, an individual may have a long-standing psychiatric illness and has survived to old age, or has developed new symptoms in association with neurological changes, such as a stroke or "silent" cerebrovascular lesions. Second, co-morbidity with medical disorders is both highly common and complex. Psychiatric symptoms may arise as a direct result of medical conditions, many of which are more prevalent in elderly people (e.g., hypothyroidism), or as part of complex interaction with medical illness (e.g., cardiovascular disease [CVD]), or exacerbate or predate an existing illness (e.g., Alzheimer's disease [AD]), or as a reaction to pharmacotherapy (e.g., corticosteroids). The bidirectional influence exerted by either psychiatric or medical problems may be direct (e.g., some strokes appear to cause depressive symptoms) or indirect (e.g., depression may reduce adherence with cardiac treatment).

From: *Current Clinical Neurology: Psychiatry for Neurologists*
Edited by: D.V. Jeste and J.H. Friedman © Humana Press Inc., Totowa, NJ

Third, as opposed to some neurological disorders such as Huntington's disease and AD, we do not have at our disposal pathognomonic signs, biological markers, or definitive neurobiological models for schizophrenia or depression. For example, lesions in the brain's white matter co vary with late-life depression in a number of ways, but are also present in elderly people with progressive dementia and those with no psychiatric disorder. This means that a major task for the neurologist is to discern, in probabilistic terms, the specificity of neurobiological findings to symptoms *(2)*. Fourth, although elderly people can and do suffer from nearly any mental illness found in younger people, much of the existing knowledge base concerns depression and schizophrenia. Therefore, much of this chapter is devoted to depression and schizophrenia, which is a reflection of the lack of data on personality disorders, bipolar disorder, and anxiety disorders in the elderly.

DEPRESSION AND BIPOLAR DISORDER

Epidemiology

Depression, particularly depressive symptoms, is among the most common psychiatric disorders in the elderly. However, despite folklore about the despair inherent to old age, epidemiological surveys consistently report a lower prevalence in those over age 65 compared to younger groups. The Epidemiological Catchment Area (ECA) survey *(3)* reported that the 1-month prevalence of major depression was 0.7% in the elderly, which was substantially lower than that reported for individuals aged 25 to 44 (3.0%). Prevalence of bipolar disorder in the elderly ECA sample was even lower than depression, estimated to be 0.1%, compared to 1.4% in those between ages 25 and 44. Lower rates of major depression among the elderly are consistent across other epidemiological surveys as well *(4)*. Reasons for the lower prevalence in elderly in the ECA may reflect an actual decline in depression, factors related to aging (increased mortality resulting from depression; cohort differences in reporting of symptoms), and/or factors related to data collection (bias in instruments used to detect depression, failure to adequately survey institutionalized populations) *(5)*.

However, less severe forms of depression appear to be frequent in the elderly. It is estimated that about 10% of elderly people in the community have minor depression. About 13.5% of elderly community-dwellers have clinically significant depressive symptoms without meeting criteria for a depressive disorder *(6)*. Furthermore, higher rates of major depression are seen in medical settings, where about 6.5% of elderly outpatients and about 11.5% in elderly medical inpatients have major depression *(6)*. Residents of nursing homes or other residential facilities also appear to have a higher frequency of depression than that seen in the community (4–15%) *(5)*. Finally, bipolar disorder accounts for 8–10% of elderly psychiatric inpatients *(7)*.

In the ECA data *(3)*, major depression was about three times more common in females in the elderly, as is the case with younger individuals. Among ethnicities, African-American elderly reported fewer depressive symptoms than Latino or Caucasian elderly. The prevalence of bipolar disorder is also higher among women in the elderly (2:1), whereas in younger age groups the gender ratio is about equal *(7)*.

Although there are several ways to interpret the prevalence of depression in the elderly, there is little debate that depression is a major public health problem in late life. In addition to reduced well-being and poorer social adjustment, depression in late life is associated with increased disability, higher risk of falls, exacerbation of medical illness, poorer compliance with medical treatment, and increased health care utilization *(5)*. Depression is the leading cause of suicide in the elderly and appears to be an independent risk factor for early nonsuicidal mortality. Finally, depression seems to be associated with poorer functioning whether or not criteria for major depression are met *(8)*.

In summary, elderly community-dwelling people appear less likely than younger adults to have a diagnosis of major depression. However, rates of subsyndromal symptoms of depression are much higher than ECA estimates, and upwards of one-fourth of elderly persons in medical settings, particularly nursing homes, appear to experience clinically significant depression. Depression is strongly associated with disability in late life.

Signs and Symptoms

Geriatric Depression Compared to Younger Patients

In comparison to younger patients, elderly depressed patients more often report somatic and cognitive symptoms than depressed mood, which has led some to describe a geriatric-specific subtype of "depression without sadness" or a "depletion syndrome." Study of depressive symptoms over the life span shows that symptoms of lack of vigor, apathy, and social withdrawal appear to increase in prevalence with age, whereas archetypical dysphoric depressive symptoms decline with increasing age *(9)*. Thus, depression in the elderly may present with loss of interest, with accompanying symptoms of weight loss, guilt, suicidal ideation, and somatic symptoms, yet without a subjective sense of sadness. Lower prevalence of depressed mood in the elderly has been linked, at least theoretically, to the under recognition of depression by clinicians. Sleep disturbance has also been found to be a risk factor for depression in the elderly in prospective study, and depression and aging are independently associated with reduced sleep efficiency, more time awake in bed, and rapid eye movement disturbances *(10,11)*. Only a few studies have examined changes in manic symptoms with aging, and they generally indicate that mania becomes less intense with age *(12,13)*.

Subtypes of Geriatric Depression

Research has examined the validity of late-onset geriatric depression as a separate "phenotype" (onset of illness after age 60). Late-onset depression is associated with a higher rate of cognitive dysfunction. In contrast, early-onset depression often has a greater personal history of personality and relationship dysfunction than late-onset depression *(14)*. A subset of elderly late-onset depressives may have primarily vascular etiology, so-called "vascular depression," which is covered in more detail later. In late-life bipolar disorder, similar attempts have been made to differentiate late-onset form early-onset bipolar disorder. Limited data suggests that later onset is associated with a higher frequency of neurological illnesses, although the evidence for lower family history in late-onset groups is mixed *(7)*.

Features of depression that may indicate higher severity are co-morbid anxiety, psychosis, and cognitive impairment *(14)*. In older adults, anxiety more often presents as subjective symptoms, such as tension, fearfulness, irritability, and worry, as opposed to somatic symptoms, such as rapid heart rate or difficulty breathing. Anxiety disorders are present in about 40% of elderly patients with major depression *(15)*. When co-morbid, anxiety and depression co vary in severity, and anxiety in combination with depression appears to increase suicidality. Psychosis is present in 25–40% of hospitalized elderly depressed patients, and presence of psychosis is associated with a higher rate of recurrence and reduced response to antidepressants *(5)*.

Cognitive dysfunction is among the more clinically challenging and disabling aspects of depression in older adults, with estimates of 20–50% of geriatric patients showing impairment on neuropsychological tests *(15)*. Memory problems, reduced attention, and executive dysfunction (i.e., the ability to organize and plan behavior) are all present in geriatric depression, which may cause depression to be mistaken for progressive dementia (i.e., "pseudodementia"). Different profiles of cognitive impairment may have utility in predicting later course in geriatric depression. Memory impairment in the context of depression is more likely to relate to later development of AD. In contrast, impairment in executive function less often predates progressive dementia, yet often relates to poorer treatment response *(14)*.

Neurobiology of the Psychiatric Manifestations

The causes of depression in the elderly are likely to be idiosyncratic to the individual, with relative and interactive contributions from vascular and neurodevelopmental brain changes, psychosocial factors, and genetic vulnerability. Although a comprehensive neurobiological model that explains all causes of depression is unrealistic, neuroimaging, clinical, and neuropathological study has uncovered a wealth of data on abnormalities in brain circuits believed to be related to the expression of depressive symptoms in the elderly.

Genetic Factors

Elderly depressed patients appear to have reduced genetic loading of familial affective disorder than younger patients with depression. In addition, late-onset depression may have a lower rate of family history of affective disorder compared to elderly early-onset depressives, although family history is higher in this group compared to the general population. The differences in family history among early- and late-onset bipolar disorder are equivocal. Across 10 clinical studies of late-life bipolar disorder, family history of affective disorder was present in 39% of patients (ranging from 25 to 57%) (7). Thus, genetic vulnerability may be lesser among geriatric affective disorders compared to younger patients, yet is still higher than in the general population.

Structural Abnormalities

A growing number of studies have used magnetic resonance imaging (MRI) to examine the structural brain changes in geriatric depression. Decreased frontal volume in the orbital frontal cortex a brain area implicated in the emotional valence of reward in behavior as well asthe dorsolateral prefrontal cortex has been noted by several research groups (16,17). Decreased bilateral frontal volume appears to be related to increased depression severity. Late-life minor depression shows lower prefrontal volumes than controls but less reduction than those with late-onset major depression, further validating the relationship between depression and brain changes (18). Volume loss in subcortical structures has also been found, particularly in the basal ganglia and hippocampus (2).

Among the more robust findings in geriatric depression are the presence of lesions in the preiventricular areas, deep white matter and subcortical gray matter. These signal hyperintensities are detected by T2-weighted MRI (2). The most replicable finding is that white matter hyperintensities (WMH) are more common in geriatric depression than in normal controls, and they correlate with depression severity. These WMH are not typically observed in younger depressive patients, and they are more often seen in late-onset depression, suggesting that they may have a role in the pathology of depression in the elderly. Although location is somewhat inconsistent across studies, WMH appear to cluster in the frontal lobes and basal ganglia in late-onset groups. Importantly, subcortical WMH appear to relate to higher rates of executive dysfunction, as well higher functional impairment (15). Greater change in WMH volume over the course of 2 years related to a lower likelihood of remission from late-life depression (19). WMH also appear to relate to cerebrovascular disease, as well as cerebrovascular risk factors in general (e.g., coronary artery disease [CAD]) (15).

Late-onset bipolar disorder may also be associated with focal neurological signs. WMH have been found in older adults with bipolar disorder as well, and more frequently in late-onset patients compared to early-onset patients (20,21). In addition, using computed tomography, Young et al. found increased cerebral sulcal widening in a sample of geriatric bipolar patients (22).

Functional Neuroimaging

Fewer studies have utilized functional techniques in late-life depression, such as functional MRI, single photon emission computed tomography (SPECT), and positron emission tomography (PET), and most have been conducted in the resting state (23). Using SPECT, reduced activity in the frontal lobes has been found, and PET study has indicated generalized reduced cerebral blood flow and glucose metabolism in late-life depression (23). Diffusion tensor imaging, which is a variant of MRI that provides an indication of the integrity of white matter tracts, is a particularly promising technique for geriatric depression research (2).

Neurobiological Models of Geriatric Depression

As is evident from the neuroimaging studies reviewed above, mounting evidence points toward vascular lesions in late-life depression. The "vascular depression" hypothesis, advanced by Alexopolous et al. (24) and Krishnan et al. (25), posits that a subset of late-onset elderly depressives develop depression in response to cerebrovascular changes. It is hypothesized that WMH may produce depression by interrupting cortico-subcortical neural circuits involved in mood regulation and psychomotor activity (e.g., connections between frontal, limbic, and striatal structures). Disruption in the frontal cortex may explain neuropsychological deficits in processing speed and executive functioning in vascular depression. Clinical signs differentiating vascular from nonvascular depression may be increased executive dysfunction, as well as lower interest, greater psychomotor retardation, impaired insight, but comparatively less guilt *(14)*.

The next logical question is: what causes these vascular lesions? Two nonmutually exclusive candidate areas of investigation are activation of the hypothalamic–pituitary–adrenal (HPA) axis and genetic vulnerability. Overactivity in the HPA axis has long been associated with depression, as well as stress in general. It is theorized that HPA overactivity, and subsequent hypercortisolism, may produce inflammatory processes, subsequently increasing cellular adhesion and ischemia. Elevated cortisol levels may also increase vulnerability to glutamate neurotoxicity and/or glial cell loss, although these factors would be more germane to depression in general (i.e., not restricted to vascular depression) *(10)*.

Another possibility is that cerebrovascular disease and depression share a common genetic pathway. Platelet activation was higher in a group of elderly depressed patients with the serotonin-linked promoter region polymorphism, which could translate to a higher risk of heart disease *(5)*. However, two other polymorphisms, the very low-density lipoprotein receptor (VLDL-R) encoding for the VLDL cholesterol-receptor and DCP-1 encoding for the angiotensin-converting enzyme were not found to relate to increased depression in older adults *(26)*. Interestingly, the e4 allele of the apolipoprotein E gene was found to be more prevalent in elderly depressives with WMH, even though e4 and depressive symptoms do not appear to relate in geriatric depression in general *(5,26)*. The search for other genes that are involved in vascular lesions will yield more information about the etiological link between depression and vascular disease.

Other Etiopathological Factors Contributing to Morbidity

Medical Co-Morbidity

About 80% of elderly individuals have a chronic medical illness, and there appears to be a complex reciprocal relationship between medical illness and depression in late life. As stated in the introduction, teasing apart whether depression is a cause, consequence, or source of "excess disability" in medically ill geriatric patients is a major clinical challenge. Whatever the direction, depression appears to account for a significant proportion of disability in the elderly, and depression is associated with higher number of medications, more hospital days, and subsequently higher health care costs in those with medical illnesses. Furthermore, diseases that have higher prevalence in the elderly appear to have higher-than-normal rates of depression in studies of younger people (e.g., heart disease, cancer).

In elderly persons with CVD, previous depression is associated with higher risk for myocardial infarction *(27)*. In addition, major and minor depression are common in those with CAD, each are present in approximately one-fifth of patients. Depression is also co-morbid with diabetes, twice as common than in those without diabetes, and is even more frequent in those after myocardial infarction and congestive heart failure. Mortality may be up to four times higher in patients with CAD with depression *(15,27)*.

The etiological link between depression and vascular disease is unclear, although direct causes may derive from neuroendocrine dysfunction, low heart rate variability in depression, increased platelet aggregation, and/or immune dysfunction. Indirect causes of morbidity may be nonadherence to medications and rehabilitation, as well as increased behavioral risk factors (e.g., smoking, alcoholism) *(15,27)*.

Which older patients with cardiovascular and other medical illnesses are most likely to become depressed? Previous episodes of major depression are the greatest risk factor for current depression in combination with CAD, and women and younger age also appear to be risk factors for depression. In addition, depression appears to confer a risk for later CVD, particularly CAD, vascular dementia, and stroke *(27)*. However, it is unclear which symptoms of depression are most likely to relate to later vascular disease.

Psychosocial Factors

Environmental risk factors for depression in the elderly were reviewed recently by Bruce *(28)*. Perhaps the most powerful risk factor for geriatric depression of all may be death of a spouse, which increased risk for depression by a factor of 24 over 1 year. Other identified risk factors are lack of social contact, being unmarried, and having low income. Beekman et al. *(8)* examined the prevalence of environmental risk factors with regard to depression severity. In the Longitudinal Aging Study Amsterdam (LASA) sample, recent stressful life events were more related to risk of minor depression, whereas major depression was more likely to represent long-standing vulnerability factors. Diminished social support is a risk factor for depression in late life, and protective effects of social support on mitigating depression have been demonstrated. In particular, the presence of a confidant appears to confer protective benefits in avoiding depression, which may partially account for higher rates of depression in nursing homes *(15)*.

Diagnosis and Differential Diagnosis

It is frequently held that geriatric depression goes undiagnosed and untreated in about 60–80% of the estimated number of cases *(5,15)*. The failure to detect depression in the elderly is of particular concern in the primary care setting, where elderly depressed patients are most likely to present. In part, this under recognition can be attributed to the greater somatic and cognitive complaints in older depressed patients, and the lower frequency of complaints of depressed mood. Another cause is likely that too often depression is seen as a normal aspect of aging by clinicians, as opposed to a treatable disease. Elderly men may be particularly at risk for under recognition.

Clinicians can avoid under diagnosis by casting a wide net in screening for depression in the elderly. A general rule of thumb is that depression should be suspected in those older adults who complain of anhedonia, hopelessness, anxiety, psychomotor retardation, or unexplained weight or energy loss. In addition, those older adults who utilize a great deal of health services, particularly for unexplained symptoms of pain, sleep problems, or appetite loss should be assessed for depression. In nursing home settings, signs of apathy and/or agitation, nonadherence to rehabilitation, or changes in social behavior, dependency, or functioning may signify depression as well.

Diagnostic procedures in detecting depression consist of history, physical, and laboratory tests. Accuracy may be improved through the use of standardized clinical measures. Several screening instruments are available; the most commonly used are the Geriatric Depression Scale *(29)* and the Center for Epidemiological Studies—Depression Scale *(30)* These measures have approx 80% sensitivity and slightly lower specificity in detecting major depression in those without severe cognitive impairment. Once depression is suspected, cognitive status, nutritional status, and activities of daily living should be assessed.

Finally, suicide is twice as common in the elderly, and elderly white men are the highest risk group in terms of completed suicide (six times more likely than the general population) *(14)*. The majority of elderly patients who commit suicide had visited a physician in the month preceding, suggesting that many clinicians may fail to query patients about suicidal ideation. Care should be taken to assess ideation, availability of means, and the presence of a plan. Depression severity appears to correlate with suicidal ideation, and identified risk factors for suicide in the elderly are being male, a widow or widower, living alone, experiencing stress, and having poor sleep *(14)*.

Course and Prognosis

It is generally believed that prognosis for elderly persons with depression are worse than that for younger individuals. A recent meta-analysis indicated that at 2 years of follow-up of community-dwelling elderly with depression, 33% were well, 33% were still depressed, and 21% were deceased *(31)*. Chronicity has been found in about one-third of elderly with major depression and in half of those with dysthymic disorder, the majority of those with dysthymic disorder have onset earlier in life. Furthermore, the importance of assessing subsyndromal symptoms is highlighted by the fact that

25% of elderly patients with clinically significant symptoms but without major depression will go on to develop major depression within 2 years *(32)*. Thus, depression must be considered a persistent illness in the elderly. Patients at high risk for relapse include those with deficits in executive functioning (more so than those with memory impairment), those with psychosis, and those with anxiety co-morbidity *(2)*. Finally, it is not clear what the course of bipolar disorder in late life is because of a dearth of longitudinal data. However, retrospective studies of late-life bipolar disorder indicate that a subset of elderly manic inpatients develop mania after up to 15 to 20 years of recurrent depression *(7)*. Therefore, elderly depressed patients are at some risk of mania, a needed area of further study.

Treatment

The best empirical evidence for efficacy and safety in biological treatment of geriatric depression is with selective serotonin reuptake inhibitors (SSRIs) and tricyclic anti-depressants (TCAs). Across studies in older adults, the average efficacy of these medications is 50–60% compared to 30% in placebo *(5)*. The rate of response to antidepressants in elderly people is similar to younger adults, and antidepressants have shown efficacy in older adults across settings (e.g., nursing home, primary care). SSRIs do not likely show greater efficacy than TCAs, and there do not appear to be higher rates of adverse events in comparison trials, but there are fewer coronary side effects of SSRIs, a greater risk anti-cholinergic effects, and under treatment with TCAs. Therefore, SSRIs are thought to be a first-line treatment, with no particular SSRI (e.g., paroxetine, fluoxetine, sertraline, citalopram) showing greater efficacy. Consensus guidelines *(33)* recommend citalopram as the first choice, followed by sertraline, and then paroxetine. In addition, venlafaxine and mirtazapine have shown efficacy in recent study with older adults *(5)*. Although there is good cause to be optimistic about depression treatment in the elderly, older adults may have a more "brittle" response to medications, in that they are more prone to recurrence and relapse. Furthermore, Blazer *(5)* noted that the results of antidepressant efficacy studies often exclude elderly patients with significant cognitive and medical impairment, such that response in "high co-morbidity" patients is unclear.

Because of the often relapsing or chronic nature of depression in late life, treatment should be considered long term. It is recommended that after a first episode of depression, treatment should continue for 12 months after remission. Clinicians should add 1 year of continuation therapy for each additional prior depressive episode. If medications do not appear to be working after the first 3 to 6 weeks, clinicians may decide to switch to another class or type of antidepressant, augment with another medication, or combine with psychotherapy.

There is substantial support for the efficacy of certain forms of psychotherapy in treating depression in older adults, either as a stand-alone treatment or in combination with medication. Manualized cognitive-behavioral therapy (CBT), interpersonal therapy, and problem-solving therapy qualify as evidence-based treatments in reducing depressive symptoms in older adults *(34)*. Indeed, combined medication and psychotherapy may produce the greatest remission rate. A remission rate of 80% was found in a sample of elderly depressed patients receiving both interpersonal psychotherapy and a TCA *(35)*. Despite the established efficacy of psychotherapy in older people, clinicians are less likely to refer elderly patients for psychotherapy compared to younger patients.

Other strategies have been tried in psychotic or treatment-resistant depression. Electroconvulsive therapy (EC) may be helpful in those with more severe depression and particularly in elderly with psychotic depression *(5,33)*. In psychotic depression, it is recommended to try an SSRI along with either risperidone or olanzapine; if efficacy is not shown, ECT is indicated *(33)*. In persistent nonpsychotic geriatric depression, less support is available for medication augmentation strategies, such as the addition of lithium or methylphenidate. In light of the relationship between depression and vascular disease, recent research has investigated the use of medications with vascular benefit to augment antidepressant therapy in patients with vascular depression (e.g., calcium channel blockers) *(36)*. According to Alexopolous *(2)*, future medications may target the dopamine (D2), acetylcholine, and opioid neurotransmission systems because of their heavy involvement in the frontosubcortical circuits that may underlie vascular depression.

There have been no randomized controlled studies of the efficacy of medication for mania in elderly patients with bipolar disorder. Open-label trials with older manic inpatients have shown clinical improvement with the use of lithium, valproate, and newer anticonvulsants, including gabapentin and lamotrigine *(37)*. The increasing use of valproate for mania in the elderly *(38)*, probably reflects clinicians' preference for the better safety profile of valproate compared to lithium. However, in a retrospective case-note study, older bipolar inpatients on lithium monotherapy more often showed improvement than those on valproate monotherapy, especially in those with classic symptoms of mania vs mixed features *(39)*.

What is the relationship of cognitive functioning and vascular disease to treatment response? Elderly patients with vascular depression and/or evidence of frontal lobe impairment (e.g., lower performance on executive functioning tests) appear to be more treatment-resistant *(40)*. However, having cerebrovascular risk factors in and of themselves appear not to affect treatment response *(41)*, and although treatment resistance may be more common among those with WMH, antidepressants are still efficacious. Finally, there is mixed evidence whether cognition is improved as a result of treatment, although it is likely that cognitive abilities do not reach normal functioning.

In summary, antidepressants and psychotherapy appear to be safe and effective treatments for geriatric depression, even in patients with medical and/or cerbrovascular burden. In general, a major principle of treatment is that if medical and depressive symptoms are present and are suspected to interact, it is best to treat both. Medical factors that are known contributors to depression, such as sensory impairment, as well as health habits, such as smoking, should be vigorously treated as well. Finally, in light of the growing evidence that vascular lesions contribute to some proportion of depressive symptoms in the elderly, it may be that interventions that reduce vascular burden/risk factors in combination with antidepressants may be of special benefit to geriatric depression.

SCHIZOPHRENIA

Prevalence

As with depression, evidence from the ECA suggests a lower rate of schizophrenia among people over age 65. The 1-month prevalence in the ECA was 0.3%, compared with 1.5% in the entire population and 0.6% in those between ages 44 and 64 *(42)*. However, it is hypothesized that the ECA data underestimated the true prevalence of schizophrenia in the elderly. At the time of the ECA, diagnoses were based on the DSM-III, which required onset of schizophrenia to occur prior to age 45. Also, sampling from long-stay psychiatric institutions and nursing homes was limited. Therefore, the true prevalence in the elderly may be around 1%. In the elderly ECA data, the ratio of females to males with schizophrenia is three to two, and Latinos and African Americans were more at risk for schizophrenia *(42)*. The prevalence of psychotic symptoms in the elderly is between 4 and 10% *(42)*, yet the majority of psychotic symptoms in elderly are likely attributable to dementia. About 75% of elderly patients with schizophrenia reside in the community *(43)*, and the remainder reside in institutions. The vast majority of institutionalized elderly patients with schizophrenia reside in nursing homes.

Signs and Symptoms

How do symptoms of schizophrenia in the elderly compare with younger adults with schizophrenia? On one hand, older age is associated with reduced psychopathology, largely attributable to fewer positive symptoms. The association of old age with lower levels of positive symptoms has been found in outpatients as well as chronically institutionalized patients *(44)*. Furthermore, with the possible exception of chronically institutionalized or extremely low functioning patients, cognitive functioning in geriatric patients does not appear to deteriorate more than age-matched peers. On the other hand, extrapyramidal symptoms (EPS) and medical co-morbidity become more apparent in comparison to normal controls, and negative symptoms appear to persist into older age. And, even if cognitive impairment does not increase more than associated with aging alone, up to 85% of older patients with schizophrenia show significant neuropsychological impairment *(45)*.

Recent findings about the relationship between symptoms and disability in older adults with schizophrenia are somewhat surprising. Cognitive impairment and affective symptoms appear to be more disabling than positive and negative symptoms. Cognitive testing of patients with schizophrenia has revealed a number of reliable deficits in attention/information-processing speed, working memory, and executive functioning *(46)*. In memory domains, key deficits are those that involve efficiency of encoding and retrieval of information, such as the failure to use strategies in organizing information. Relative to psychotic symptoms, these cognitive deficits appear to confer greater reductions in social and community-living skills. In reports on middle-aged and older outpatients from the University of California, San Diego (UCSD) Center on Late-Life Psychosis, depressive symptoms *(47)* and anxiety symptoms *(48)* also appear to relate to substantially reduced health-related quality of life in middle-aged and older outpatients with schizophrenia.

As in depression, researchers have attempted to distinguish late-onset variants of schizophrenia from early-onset schizophrenia. In a review by Harris and Jeste *(49)*, approx 23.5% of inpatients with schizophrenia had their first episode after age 40, and 7% after age 50. In general, there are more similarities than differences between early- and late-onset groups. However, there is higher proportion of women among late-onset patients, and late-onset schizophrenia is more often associated with positive symptoms than negative symptoms. Thought disorder and the disorganized subtype appear to be less frequent in late-onset patients, whereas the paranoid subtype may be more common. Family history of psychosis is higher in both early- and late-onset schizophrenia compared to normal controls, yet rates may be higher in early- than late-onset. The pattern of cognitive deficits appears to be roughly equivalent between early- and late-onset groups, although late-onset patients appear to have better, perhaps more persevered, learningand abstraction skills.

Neurobiology of the Psychiatric Manifestations

The majority of brain changes that are evident in schizophrenia are present at first episode, perhaps even earlier. Furthermore, brain changes in schizophrenia, even among the elderly, are surprisingly subtle, given the severity of the cognitive deficits and behavioral manifestations of the disorder. Probably the most consistent finding in the many neuroimaging studies of the brains of patients with schizophrenia across the life span is enlarged ventricular spaces *(46)*. These enlargements are more commonly seen in the lateral and third ventricles, particularly the temporal horns. However, it is unclear what the relationship of ventricular enlargement is to the pathogenesis of schizophrenia.

Structural and functional neuroimaging via MRI in mixed-age patients with schizophrenia have also identified abnormalities in a number of brain areas, including the frontal, temporal, and parietal lobes *(46)*. There is some evidence that abnormalities in specific brain regions may "map on" to particular syndromes of schizophrenia. Reduced volume in prefrontal regions has been more often related to negative syndromes, whereas individuals with more prominent positive symptoms may have reduced volume in the temporal lobes. Subcortical structures showing volume loss on MRI are the amygdala, thalamus, and hippocampus. Researchers have questioned whether late-onset schizophrenia is more associated with brain abnormalities than early-onset groups. Symonds et al. *(50)* found no evidence for higher prevalence of volume changes, strokes, or WMHs in a group of patients with late-onset schizophrenia. Finally, studies employing functional neuroimaging techniques have revealed age-related reduction in frontal lobe activity in schizophrenia, although it has not been shown that the trajectory of this change is more than that seen in normal aging *(44)*.

Several studies have examined possible neurodegenerative bases for the cognitive deficits observed in elderly patients with schizophrenia. Postmortem study of the brains of 100 geriatric patients with schizophrenia showed no neuropathological evidence that cognitive deficits are casued by plaque and neurofibrillary tangle formation as in AD *(51)*. Furthermore, WMH or other lesions do not appear to be more prevalent in late-onset schizophrenia, at least not to the extent seen in late-onset depression. Accordingly, recent thought has focused on schizophrenia as a neurodevelopmental disorder; specifically, that patterns of neural connectivity are abnormal. Evidence supporting this hypothesis include the finding of a lower number of neural projections and dendritic spines in hippocampal, thalamic, and cortical areas in younger patients with schizophrenia *(46)*.

Finally, the neurochemistry of schizophrenia has been an active research area for decades, although less so with geriatric patients. The early predominant view was that higher than normal dopamine neurotransmission underlies the positive symptoms of schizophrenia *(46)*. Interestingly, fewer D2 receptors have been found in older patients with schizophrenia in postmortem study compared to younger patients, which may relate to the decrease in positive symptoms in elderly patients. However, elevated dopamine does not account for negative and cognitive symptoms of schizophrenia, leading researchers to consider the role of other neurotransmitters, particularly 5HT and, more recently, glutamate. The affinity of atypical antipsychotics to 5HT2A receptors, coupled with their relatively higher efficacy in the treatment of negative symptoms, has stimulated interest in 5HT. Furthermore, drugs that block a subtype of glutamate receptor induce schizophrenia-like behaviors. Future treatments for schizophrenia may include compounds that stimulate glutamate receptor function, as well as cognitive enhancers that target frontal-subcortical circuits involved in the cognitive deficits of schizophrenia *(52)*.

Other Etiopathological Factors Contributing to Morbidity

Medical conditions are common in older patients with schizophrenia, and the number of medical conditions correlates with depression and psychotic symptoms *(53)*. Older patients with schizophrenia may have more severe medical illnesses than normal controls. However, older adults with schizophrenia do not appear to have a higher number of medical problems than patients with other psychiatric diagnoses in late life, including those with AD or major depression *(53)*. This finding may be the result of a "survivor effect," whereby less healthy schizophrenia patients die before they reach old age. Similarly, mortality is likely higher in older schizophrenia patients relative to the general population, yet lower than in other psychiatric disorders.

Unhealthy lifestyles are common in schizophrenia *(53)*. Lower levels of exercise, poorer diet, and higher rates of smoking are characteristics of patients with schizophrenia. On balance, older schizophrenia patients appear to have a lower rate of substance abuse disorder compared to younger patients, although it is unclear whether lower substance abuse represents a cohort effect. In addition to worse health habits, it is felt that patients with schizophrenia often receive suboptimal treatment for medical illnesses. It is hypothesized that clinicians may overlook medical problems in favor of treating psychiatric symptoms, and that symptoms of schizophrenia may interfere with the medical evaluation and treatment process *(54)*. In addition, antipsychotic medications confer a risk of metabolic changes and other side effects (*see* section on side effects).

Diagnosis and Differential Diagnosis

Diagnosis begins with a process of exclusion of neuropsychiatric syndromes and other causes of psychosis. Particularly in patients with no history of psychosis, results of brain imaging should be obtained. Furthermore, assessing the presence of sensory impairments and social isolation is important, as they may be associated with psychotic symptoms in the elderly. Because some older patients with schizophrenia can present with severe cognitive deficits, differential diagnosis with progressive dementia may be difficult. However, compared to AD, schizophrenia is more often associated with delusions of thought control, more auditory hallucinations, less word-finding and short-term memory loss, and more social impoverishment *(55)*. However, geriatric schizophrenia patients who have marked functional deficits may have memory impairment that is roughly equivalent to AD patients, showing severe impairment in delayed recall and recognition memory *(44)*.

Once schizophrenia is suspected, the evaluation should be broad, with care to assess psychiatric, social, functional, cognitive, and medical domains. Because schizophrenia is associated with lack of insight, history should be obtained from family, friends, treating clinicians, and medical records. In older patients, screening with instruments measuring cognitive functioning is helpful, and useful validated instruments include the Dementia Rating Scale *(56)* or the Mini-Mental State Exam *(57)*. In addition, gaining a sense of the patient's ability to perform self-care, their social contacts/skills, and their medication-management skills is important in structuring a treatment plan. The presence of mood symptoms should be part of the psychiatric evaluation, and measures such as the Hamilton Depression Rating Scale *(58)* can be used (although the construct validity of depression in schizophrenia has yet to be established). Finally, as in depression, the presence of suicidal ideation should be evaluated, as schizophrenia appears to have among the highest rates of suicide among psychiatric illnesses. In schizophrenia, it seems that the highest risk age group for suicide is shortly after onset of the illness.

Course and Prognosis

In comparison to other psychiatric disorders, chronicity is more frequent in schizophrenia. The majority of early-onset patients will continue to experience psychiatric symptoms and functional impairment in old age, although remission of symptoms occurs in 20–40% of early-onset patients prospectively followed into later life *(59)*. A major question is whether schizophrenia involves a decline in cognitive functioning over the life span, in line with a neurodegenerative process. Studies conduced at UCSD on primarily outpatients have found no evidence that cognitive impairment increases with age in comparison with normal comparison subjects *(60)*. However, another research group in New York has identified significant declines in measures of cognitive functioning among chronically institutionalized patients with schizophrenia *(44)*. The discrepancy between these sets of findings has been attributed to different patient populations; the UCSD patients were higher functioning than the patients in the New York group. However, when both groups of patients were studied longitudinally (1–5 years), less evidence for cognitive deterioration was seen within individuals. Harvey *(44)* reported that those "poor-outcome" patients who do show deterioration are more often older, with lower education and more severe positive symptoms.

Treatment

As with younger adults, antipsychotic medication is the mainstay of treatment for older patients with schizophrenia. Although no double-blind controlled trials have been reported, open-label studies indicate that 48–61% of patients show full remission of psychosis *(61)*. However, lower doses are recommended. Elderly patients have been found to take about 40% of the dosage (chlorpromazine equivalent) provided to younger patients *(62)*. Late-onset patients may respond to dosages that are 25–50% of those taken by early-onset patients *(62)*. Atypical antipsychotics are the first-line choice in elderly patients because of reduced risk of side effects and their relatively greater efficacy in reducing negative symptoms. Except in circumstances of demonstrated clinical stability and lack of significant side effects in patients with history of long-term treatment with conventional antipsychotics, a carefully monitored switch to an atypical antipsychotic is recommended. A general rule in antipsychotic treatment is to minimize the life-time exposure to the medication, by maintaining a patient at the lowest effective dose and avoiding unnecessary usage.

Risperidone is the most widely used medication for psychosis in the elderly, followed by quetiapine and olanzapine. In younger patients, recent reviews indicate no differences between these medications in efficacy *(34)*. An open-label trial of risperidone in 23 patients with schizophrenia showed an 85% response rate in patients receiving an average dose of 4.5 mg, although the maximum dose is generally less than 3 mg *(63)*. A similar conclusion with regard to safety and efficacy was reached for quetiapine in a trial of 152 elderly patients with psychosis and in several smaller trials with olanzapine *(63)*. Clozapine is used infrequently, owing to its potential for toxicity and need for frequent lab testing *(34)*.

Side Effects

EPS are common with conventional antipsychotic medications. Older adults are at substantially higher risk of extrapyramidal symptoms, and of serious concern, tardive dyskinesia (TD). TD is a disabling syndrome consisting of abnormal involuntary movements, which may be choreatic or stereo-typic (not including tremor). Often, TD involves a facial and oral dyskinesia, such as writhing of the tongue. Understandably, TD can be disabling and unpleasant for the patient. Older age is the single most potent risk factor for TD (more so than duration of treatment); prevalence of TD in conventional antipsychotic treatment in older adults is 29% within the first year and 60% after 3 years *(46)*. Moreover, older adults display greater severity of TD. Older women may be at greatest risk for TD, and they may experience more severe forms.

The pathophysiology of TD is unclear. Beyond an increased sensitivity of striatal neurons to dopamine, it is likely that multiple neurotransmitter systems are involved. Fortunately, atypical antipsy-chotics confer lowerrisk of TD compared to conventional antipsychotics, and a switch to atypicals may reduce the incidence of TD symptoms in those with pre-existing TD. However, atypical antipsy-chotics, including risperidone and olanzapine, do produce parkinsonian side effects in some older patients, particularly those more frail and/or cognitively impaired *(64)*. Clinicians may fail to recog-nize medication-induced Parkinsonism, as it often occurs in the absence of tremor. Thus, monitoring motor effects of antipsychotic medications is essential in the elderly, even among those treated with atypical antipsychotics.

Other side effects of antipsychotic medication include sedation, hypotension, and dry mouth. Emerging evidence suggests that these agents produce weight gain, and thus increase the risk of obesity, hypertension, and CAD *(63)*. Risk of weight gain may be lower in the elderly, but mor-bidity associated with heightened risk of CVD is clearly greater. In addition, olanzapine and cloza-pine in particular also appear to confer a risk of new-onset type 2 diabetes that may be independent from weight gain *(63)*. In light of the sedentary lifestyle of many patients with schizophrenia, mon-itoring and treating cardiovascular functioning and glucose levels are important facets of antipsy-chotic treatment.

Although antipsychotic medications appear to be fairly efficacious in reducing positive symptoms of schizophrenia, negative symptoms and functional disability often persist. In addition, cognitive func-tioning, including working memory, may show only slight improvement. Furthermore, about 40% of mixed-age patients with schizophrenia are fully or partially nonadherent to antipsychotic medications. Thus, adjunctive psychosocial treatments are often required, with the different modalities sharing the goal of engaging patients in treatment and compensating for their cognitive, social, and functional deficits. Treatments with empirical support include social skills training, family therapy, and CBT, and promising approaches include adaptive skill training and cognitive rehabilitation *(65)*. Each of these has at its core the teaching of skills in independent functioning, and emphases include teaching adaptive skills, including taking medications as prescribed, and acquisition of social skills, such as assertiveness. Particularly for older patients without involved caregivers, community-based interven-tions, such as assertive community treatment and case management, should be considered as well. Thus, the treatment of the pervasive deficits in cognitive, psychiatric, and functional domains in older patients with schizophrenia often involves multiple clinicians and treatment modalities.

ANXIETY DISORDERS

Prevalence

Anxiety disorders in late life have received less empirical attention, yet anxiety is surprisingly common among older adults. Anxiety disorders include a broad spectrum of diagnoses, including panic disorder, generalized anxiety disorder, social phobia, specific phobia, posttraumatic stress disorder (PTSD), and obsessive-compulsive disorder (OCD). In the ECA data *(3)*, the prevalence of any anxi-ety disorder in those over age 65 was 5.5%; thus, anxiety disorders were more common than major depression and dementia in those over age 65. The prevalence of any anxiety disorder was lower than in younger adults, and elderly women (6.8%) more frequently met criteria than men (3.6%). In the ECA, the most common anxiety disorder in those over age 65 was phobic disorder. Although not assessed in the ECA, generalized anxiety disorder (GAD) is likely the most common anxiety disorder in the elderly, estimated at 2–7% *(4)*. Panic disorder, PTSD, and OCD are each present in about 1% of community-dwelling elderly *(4)*. Similar to depression, the prevalence of clinically significant anxiety symptoms is higher than the prevalence of anxiety disorder. As in late-life depression, anxiety disorders and symptoms are about twice as common among older women than older men. In the LASA study, both subsyndromal anxiety and anxiety disorder had significant negative impact on quality of life and disability *(66)*. Furthermore, rates of anxiety disorders are higher among patients in nursing homes and in mental health clinics *(4)*.

Signs and Symptoms

It is suspected, although not confirmed empirically, that anxiety in the elderly presents more cognitively and subjectively than physiologically. Excessive worry, fearfulness, and tension occur more frequently than racing heart or feelings of choking, and these cognitive/subjective symptoms are easier to separate from the direct effect of medical problems. It is also suspected that anxiety and depressive symptoms have a higher co-morbidity in the elderly compared to younger adults, with less differentiation. In the LASA study, 26.5% of those with anxiety disorders also met criteria for major depression *(8)*. Co-morbidity with depression was higher in panic and OCD than in GAD, yet in those with both GAD and major depression, higher severity of GAD corresponded to higher severity of major depression. Accordingly, it has been proposed that "mixed-anxiety depression" disorder may be a useful diagnosis in the elderly *(67)*. Finally, anxiety disorders, particularly panic disorder and GAD, can present for the first time in late life.

Neurobiology of the Psychiatric Manifestations

No studies have examined the neurobiology of anxiety in the elderly. In younger adults (as described in Chapter 5), the brain circuitry involved in fear and anxiety behaviors have been described in great detail, and specific models of PTSD, social anxiety, and panic disorder have been proposed. These models postulate a central role for the amygdala in basic fear conditioning, and its projections to the hippocampus, temporal and frontal cortices, and other subcortical areas in sensitization to fear and learned fear responses (e.g., avoidance) *(52)*. From this standpoint, simple phobia may be a function of the amygdala and hippocampus, whereas more complex anxiety disorders (e.g., GAD), may involve connections with multiple brain structures. Neurotransmitters believed to be involved in anxiety disorders are norepinephrine, 5HT, γ-aminobutyric acid (GABA), and glutamate *(52)*.

Other Etiopathological Factors Contributing to Morbidity

As with depression and schizophrenia, medical co-morbidity likely impacts the course of anxiety. The directional influence of medical disorders on anxiety in the elderly is uncertain, yet anxiety appears to be more common in older patients with hypothyroidism, heart disease, diabetes, chronic obstructive pulmonary disorder, and gastrointestinal distress. In the LASA study, risk factors for "pure" anxiety disorder were different from depression; anxiety was more related to environmental factors, particularly stressful live events, lower education, and a smaller social network *(68)*.

Diagnosis and Differential Diagnosis

Elderly persons with anxiety, as in those with depression, most often present in the primary care setting. Much of the same concern for under diagnosis in depression is likely true for anxiety disorders—physicians may not recognize anxiety because of the high co-morbidity with medical disorders and co-occurrence of symptoms such as insomnia, gastrointestinal distress, and dizziness. Specific anxiety disorders may differ with regard to difficulty of detection. For example, agoraphobia and unwillingness to leave the house may be intermixed with functional disability, whereas panic symptoms are more clearly self-evident. Screening instruments are available, although studies examining sensitivity in detecting anxiety disorders in late life are rare.

Course and Prognosis

The long-term course and prognosis of anxiety disorders is unknown, owing to the dearth of longitudinal study in geriatric populations. In the LASA study, neuroticism and female gender predicted a higher probability of chronicity over 3 years *(68)*.

Treatment

Despite their widespread and often long-term use in the elderly, no controlled trials of antianxiety medications have been reported in late-life anxiety disorders. Existing data on the efficacy and safety of benzodiazepines derive from studies of other more generalized syndromes in the elderly (e.g., insomnia, agitation) *(34)*. It is clear that benzodiazepenes should be used cautiously in the elderly because of their tendency to produce a higher risk of falls and negative effects on cognition *(67)*.

Other more promising treatment options are antidepressants and CBT. Antidepressants, particularly SSRIs, are indicated for anxiety disorders in younger people. A recent pooled analysis of older adults from multiple studies of Venlafaxine SR showed equivalent efficacy in those over, vs those under, age 60 (average response in older adults was 66% *[69]*). In addition, anxiety symptoms in older adults, when co-morbid with depression, appear to respond to antidepressant treatment *(70)*. An emerging literature suggests that CBT, focusing on skills to cope with the physiological and cognitive aspects of stress, shows promise in reducing anxiety in late life *(34)*. A clear benefit of psychotherapy in late-life anxiety is the lack of medical side effects associated with treatment.

CONCLUSION

Psychiatric disorders in older people are a growing public health problem. These disorders present in heterogeneous fashion in the elderly, with complex interactive contributions from medical, psychosocial, neurobiological, and genetic factors. Although data is accumulating rapidly on geriatric psychiatric disorders, there remains little empirical understanding of the neurobiology and optimal treatment of schizophrenia, bipolar disorder, and anxiety in older people. However, with careful differential diagnosis and comprehensive assessment of biological and environmental factors, existing evidence suggests that psychiatric disorders among older adults respond about as well to treatment as among younger adults. Future treatments that directly target brain circuits that regulate mood and certain cognitive abilities, as well as psychosocial treatments that augment pharmacological strategies, will hopefully further reduce the substantial morbidity associated with these disorders.

REFERENCES

1. Jeste D, Alexopoulos GS, Bartels SJ, et al. Consensus statement on the upcoming crisis in geriatric mental health: research agenda for the next 2 decades. Arch Gen Psychiatry 1999;56:848–853.
2. Alexopoulos G. Frontostriatal and limbic dysfunction in late-life depression. Am J Geriatr Psychiatry 2002;10:687–695.
3. Weissman M, Leaf P, Tischler G, et al. Affective disorders in five US communities. Psychol Med 1988;18:141–153.
4. Hybels C, Blazer D. Epidemiology of late-life mental disorder. Clin Geriatr Med 2003;19:663–696.
5. Blazer D. Depression in late life: review and commentary. J Gerontol A Biol Sci Med Sci 2003;58:249–265.
6. Beekman A, Copeland J, Prince M. Review of community prevalence of depression in later life. Br J Psychiatry 1999; 174:307–311.
7. Depp C, Jeste DV. Bipolar disorder in older adults: a critical review. Bipolar Disord 2004;6:343–367..
8. Beekman A, Deeg D, van Tilberg T, Smit J, Hooijer C, van Tilberg W. The natural history of late life depression. Arch Gen Psychiatry 2002;59:605–611.
9. Newman J, Engel R, Jensen J. Changes in depressive-symptom experiences among older women. Psychol Aging 1991;6:212–222.
10. Krishnan K. Biological risk factors in late life depression. Biol Psychiatry 2002;52:185–192.
11. Cole M, Dendukuri N. Risk factors for depression among elderly community subjects: a systematic review and meta-analysis. Am J Psychiatry 2003;160:1147–1156.
12. Broadhead J, Jacoby R. Mania in old age: a first prospective study. Int J Geriatr Psychiatry 1990;5:215–222.
13. Young RC, Falk J. Age, manic psychopathology, and treatment response. Int J Geriatr Psychiatry 1989;4:73–78.
14. Alexopoulos G, Borson S, Cuthbert B, et al. Assessment of late life depression. Biol Psychiatry 2002;52:164–174.

15. Alexopoulos G, Buckwalter K, Olin J, Martinez R, Wainscott C, Krishnan K. Comorbidity of late life depression: an opportunity for research on mechanisms and treatment. Biol Psychiatry 2002;52:543–558.

16. Kumar A, Bilker W, Jin Z, Udupa J. Atrophy and high intensity lesions: Complementary neurobiological mechanisms in late-life depression. Biol Psychiatry 2000;55:390–397.

17. Taylor W, Steffens D, McQuoid D, Payne M, Lee S, Lai T. Smaller orbital frontal cortex volumes associated with functional disability in depressed elders. Biol Psychiatry 2003;53:144–149.

18. Kumar A, Bilker W, Lavretsky H, Gottlieb G. Volumetric asymmetries in late onset mood disorders: an attenuation of frontal asymmetry with depression severity. Psychiatry Res 2000;100:41–47.

19. Taylor W, Steffens D, MacFall J, et al. White matter hyperintensity progression and late-life depression outcomes. Arch Gen Psychiatry 2003;60:1090–1096.

20. McDonald W, Krishnan KR, Doraiswamy M, Blazer D. Occurence of subcortical hyperintensities in elderly subjects with mania. Psychiatry Research Neuroimaging 1991;40:211–220.

21. Fujikawa T, Yamawaki S, Touhouda Y. Silent cerebral infarctions in patients with late-onset mania. Stroke 1995;26:946–949.

22. Young R, Nambudiri D, Jain H, de Asis H, Alexopoulos G. Brain computed tomography in geriatric manic disorder. Biol Psychiatry 1999;45:1063-1065.

23. DeAsis J, Silbersweig D, Pan H, Young RC, Stern E. Neuroimaging studies of fronto-limbic dysfunction in geriatric depression. Clin Neurosci Res 2003;2:324–330.

24. Alexopoulos GS, Meyers B, Young RC, Campbell S, Silbersweig D, Charlson M. The 'vascular depression' hypothesis. Arch Gen Psychiatry 1997;54:915–922.

25. Krishnan K, Hays J, Blazer D. MRI-defined vascular depression. Am J Psychiatry 1997;154:497–501.

26. Cervilla J, Prince M, Joels S, Russ C, Lovestone S. Genes related to vascular disease (APOE, VLDL-R, DCP-1) and other vascular factors in late-life depression. Am J Geriatr Psychiatry 2004;12:202–210.

27. Thomas A, Kalaria R, O'Brien J. Depression and vascular disease: what is the relationship? J Affect Disord 2004;79:81–95.

28. Bruce M. Psychosocial risk factors for depressive disorders in late life. Biol Psychiatry 2002;52:175–184.

29. Yesavage J, Brink T, Rose T. Development and validation of a geriatric depression screening scale: a preliminary report. J Psychiatr Res 1983;17:37–49.

30. Radloff L. The CES-D scale: a self-report depression scale for research in the general population. J Appl Psychol Meas 1977;1:385–401.

31. Stoudemire A. Recurrence and relapse in geriatric depression: a review of risk factors and prophylactic treatment strategies. J Neuropsychiatry Clin Neurosci 1977;9:208–221.

32. Lyness J, King D, Cox C, Yoediono Z, Caine E. The importance of subsyndromal depression in older primary care patients: prevalence and associated functional disability. J Am Geriatr Soc 1999;47:647–652.

33. Alexopoulos GS, Streim J, Carpenter D, Docherty JP; Expert Consensus Panel for Using Antipsychotic Drugs in Older Patients. Using antipsychotic agents in older patients. J Clin Psychiatry 2004;65:5–99.

34. Bartels S, Dums A, Oxman T, et al. Evidence-based practices in geriatric mental health care: an overview of systematic reviews and meta-analyses. Psychiatr Clin North Am 2003;26:970–990.

35. Reynolds CF, Frank E, Perel J, Mazumdar S, Kupfer D. Maintenance therapies for late-life recurrent major depression: research and review circa 1995. Int Psychogeriatr 1995;7:27–39.

36. Taragano F, Allegri R, Vicario A, Bagnatti P, Lyketsos C. A double blind randomized clinical trial assessing the efficacy and safety of augmenting standard antidepressant therapy with nimodipine in the treatment of 'vascular depression'. Int J Geriatr Psychiatry 2001;16:254–260.

37. Eastham J, Jeste DV, Young R. Assessment and treatment of bipolar disorder in the elderly. Drugs Aging 1998;12:205–224.

38. Shulman K, Rochon P, Sykora K, et al. Changing prescription patterns for lithium and valproic acid in old age: shifting practice without evidence. BMJ 2003;326:960–961.

39. Chen ST, Altshuler L, Melnyk K, Erhart S, Miller E, Mintz J. Efficacy of lithium vs. valproate in the treatment of mania in the elderly: a retrospective study. J Clin Psychiatry 1999;60:181–186.

40. Alexopoulos G, Meyers B, Young RC, et al. Executive dysfunction and long-term outcomes of geriatric depression. Arch Gen Psychiatry 2000;57:285–290.

41. Miller M, Lenze E, Dew M, et al. Effect of cerebrovascular risk factors on depression treatment outcome in later life. Am J Geriatr Psychiatry 2002;10:592–598.

42. Regier D, Narrow W, Rae D, Manderscheid RW, Locke BZ, Goodwin FK. The de facto US mental and addictive disorders service system. Epidemiologic catchment area prospective 1-year prevalence rates of disorders and services. Arch Gen Psychiatry 1993;50:85–94.

43. Meeks S, Depp C. What are the service needs of elderly people with schizophrenia? In: Cohen C, ed. Schizophrenia into Later Life. Washington DC: American Psychiatric Association Press; 2003.

44. Harvey P. Cognitive impairment in elderly patients with schizophrenia: age related changes. Int J Geriatr Psychiatry 2001;16(Suppl 1):S78–S85.

45. Palmer B, Heaton R, Paulsen J, Perry W, Jeste DV. Is it possible for schizophrenia to be neuropsychologically normal? Neuropsychology 1997;11:437–447.

46. Twamley EW, Dolder CR, Corey-Bloom J and Jeste DV: Neuropsychiatric aspects of schizophrenia. In: Schiffer RB, Rao SM, Fogel BS, eds. Neuropsychiatry, Second Edition. Philadelphia: Lippincott Williams & Wilkins; 2003:776-798.

47. Wetherell J, Palmer B, Thorp S, Patterson T, Golshan S, Jeste DV. Anxiety symptoms and quality of life in middle-aged and older outpatients with schizophrenia and schizoaffective disorder. J Clin Psychiatry 2003;64:1476–1482.

48. Jin H, Zisook S, Palmer B, Patterson T, Heaton R, Jeste DV. Association of depressive symptoms with worse functioning in schizophrenia: a study in older outpatients. J Clin Psychiatry 2001;62:797-803.

49. Harris M, Jeste DV. Late-onset schizophrenia: an overview. Schizophr Bull 1988;14:39–55.

50. Symonds L, Olichney J, Jernigan T, Corey-Bloom J, Healy R, Jeste DV. Lack of clinically significant structural abnormalities in MRI's of older patients with schizophrenia and related psychoses. J Neuropsych Clin Neurosci 1997;9:251–258.

51. Powchik P, Davidson M, Haroutunian V, et al. Postmortem studies in schizophrenia. Schizophr Bull 1998;24:325–341.

52. Krystal J, D'Souza D, Sanacora G, Goddard A, Charney D. Current perspectives on the pathophysiology of schizophrenia, depression, and anxiety disorders. Med Clin North Am 2001;85:559–571.

53. Jeste DV, Gladsjo J, Lindamer L, Lacro JP. Medical comorbidity in schizophrenia. Schizophr Bull 1996;22:413–430.

54. Cohen C. Medical comorbidity in older persons with schizophrenia. In: Cohen C, ed. Schizophrenia into Later Life. Washington DC: American Psychiatric Association Press 2003, 113–138.

55. Desai A, Grossberg G. Differential diagnosis of psychotic disorders in the elderly. In: Cohen C, ed. Schizophrenia into Later Life. Washington DC: American Psychiatric Association Press 2003, 55–75.

56. Gardner R, Oliver-Munoz S, Fisher L, Empting L. Mattis Dementia Rating Scale: internal reliability using a diffusely impaired population. J Clin Neuropsych 1981;3:271–275.

57. Folstein M, Folstein S, McHugh P. Mini-mental state. A practical method for grading the cognitive state of patients for the clinician. J Psychiatric Res 1975;12:189–198.

58. Hamilton M. Development of a rating scale for primary depressive illness. Br J Soc Clin Psychol 1967;6:278–296.

59. Tsuang M, Woolson R, Fleming J. Long-term outcome of major psychoses. I. Schizophrenia and affective disorders compared with psychiatrically symptom-free surgical conditions. Arch Gen Psychiatry 1979;36:1295–1301.

60. Palmer B, Bondi MW, Twamley E, Thal L, Golshan S, Jeste DV. Are late-onset schizophrenia spectrum disorders neurodegenerative conditions? Annual rates of change in two dementia measures. J Neuropsychiatry Clin Neurosci 2003; 15:45–52.

61. Tune L, Salzman C. Schizophrenia in late life. Psychiatr Clin North Am 2003;26:103–113.

62. Howard R, Rabins P, Seeman M, Jeste DV. Late-onset schizophrenia and very-late-onset schizophrenia-like psychosis: an international consensus. Am J Psychiatry 2000;157:172–178.

63. Kaskow J, Mohamed S, Zisook S, Jeste DV. Use of novel antipsychotics in older patients with schizophrenia. In: Cohen C, ed. Schizophrenia into Late Life. Washington DC: American Psychiatric Association Press 2003, 195–204.

64. Friedman J, Fernandez H, Trieschmann M. Parkinsonism in a nursing home: underrecognition. J Geriatr Psychiatry Neurol 2004;17:39–41.

65. Pilling S, Bebbington P, Kuipers E, et al. Psychological treatments in schizophrenia: I. Meta-analysis of family intervention and cognitive behaviour therapy. Psychol Med 2002;32:763–782.

66. de Beurs E, Beekman A, van Balkom A, Deeg D, van Dyck R, van Tilberg W. Consequences of anxiety in older persons: its effect on disability, well-being and use of health services. Psychol Med 1999;29:583–593.

67. Palmer B, Jeste DV, Sheikh J. Anxiety disorders in the elderly: DSM-IV and other barriers to diagnosis and treatment. J Affect Disord 1997;46:183–190.

68. Beekman A, de Beurs E, van Balkom A, Deeg D, van dyck R, van Tilberg W. Anxiety and depression in later life: co-occurrence and communality of risk factors. Am J Psychiatry 2000;157:89–95.

69. Katz I, Reynolds CF, Alexopoulos G, Hackett D. Venlafaxine ER as a treatment for generalized anxiety disorder in older adults: pooled analysis of five randomized placebo-controlled clinical trials. J Am Geriatr Soc 2002;50:18–25.

70. Lenze E, Mulsant B, Dew M, et al. Good treatment outcomes in late-life depression with comorbid anxiety. J Affect Disord 2003;77:247–254.

22

Fatigue

Christopher Christodoulou, William S. MacAllister, and Lauren B. Krupp

INTRODUCTION

Fatigue is a common symptom in neurological, psychiatric, and general medical disorders and often causes difficulties for both patients and health care providers. As a result of fatigue, individuals with medical illnesses experience limitations in their daily living and coping, and clinicians become frustrated by management uncertainties. This chapter reviews current efforts to understand, measure, and treat fatigue.

DEFINITION

Fatigue can be broadly characterized as either a subjective feeling or a decrement in a person's ability to perform up to standard. The subjective feelings make take the form of excessive, uncharacteristic feelings of exhaustion, while the performance decrements may appear as a reduction in muscle strength after a period of exertion, or an increase in error rate over time on tasks requiring constant vigilance.

Fatigue is a frequent experience in our society. Although it exists as a pathological feature of various medical conditions, large numbers of otherwise healthy individuals also complain of fatigue. Pathological fatigue can be distinguished from its nonpathological counterpart by its greater intensity, longer duration, and more disabling effects on functional activities. Fatigue in healthy persons generally follows a period of exertion or sleep deprivation, and can be reduced if not eliminated by rest or sleep. In contrast, pathological fatigue can remain after rest as a severe chronic condition that disrupts an individual's ability to carry out important daily social and occupational activities and obligations.

Self-report measures of fatigue can help the clinician to quantify the severity of fatigue, characterize its specific features (e.g., mental vs physical fatigue), and judge its impact on the life of the patient. Many scales were designed for use in particular medical conditions, but items are often general and applicable to a wider range of disorders. A variety of self-report measures are available, ranging from single item scales to longer multidimensional assessments (see Table 1). Multidimensional scales allow for the assessment of the complex pattern of fatigue experienced by the individual patient. However, it might also be argued that pure measures of fatigue should be more homogeneous, perhaps including only the core feelings of fatigue, and excluding the measure of other aspects such as affective feelings, which might best be assessed by separate instruments (depression scales). Common fatigue measures include the Fatigue Severity Scale for an overall level of severity, and the Multidimensional Fatigue Inventory for the specification of fatigue subscales.

From: *Current Clinical Neurology: Psychiatry for Neurologists*
Edited by: D.V. Jeste and J.H. Friedman © Humana Press Inc., Totowa, NJ

Table 1
Fatigue Scales

Name of scale	Initial population	Specified fatigue subscales
Piper Fatigue Scale *(1)*	Cancer	Behavioral/severity, Affective meaning, Sensory, Cognitive/mood
Fatigue Severity Scale *(2)*	MS, lupus, healthy	Global measure
Single Item Visual Analogue Scale of Fatigue *(2)*	MS, lupus, healthy	Single item
Fatigue Assessment Instrument *(3)*	Lyme, CFS, lupus, MS, dysthymia, healthy	Fatigue severity, Situation-specificity, Consequences of fatigue, Responds to rest/sleep
Fatigue Scale *(4)*	Primary care patients	Physical, mental
Checklist Individual Strength *(5)*	CFS	Subjective experience of fatigue, Concentration, Motivation, Physical activity
Modified Fatigue Impact Scale *(6)*	MS	Physical, cognitive, psychosocial
Myasthenia Gravis Fatigue Scale *(7)*	Myasthenia gravis	Perception of fatigue, task avoidance, observable motor signs or symptoms
Multidimensional Assessment of Fatigue *(8)*	Rheumatoid arthritis	Degree, Severity, Distress, Impact on activities of daily living
Mulitidimensional Fatigue Inventory *(9)*	Students, physicians, cancer, CFS, soldiers	General fatigue, physical fatigue, mental fatigue, reduced motivation, reduced activity
Multidimensional Fatigue Symptom Inventory *(10)*	Cancer	Global, somatic, affective, behavioral, cognitive symptoms of fatigue
Fatigue Descriptive Scale *(11)*	MS	Spontaneous mention of fatigue, antecedent conditions, frequency, impact on life
Fatigue Symptom Inventory *(12)*	Cancer	Intensity, duration, impact on quality of life
IOWA Fatigue Scale *(13)*	Primary care patients	Cognitive, fatigue, energy, productivity
Child Fatigue Scale *(14)*	Children with cancer (also versions for parents and staff)	Lack of energy, not able to function, altered mood

MS, multiple sclerosis; CFS, chronic fatigue syndrome. (Adapted from ref. *15*.)

Aside from self-report scales, the other general approach to measuring fatigue involves the direct measurement of performance decrement. The degree to which a person's performance declines over time is posited to result from fatigue. Almost any behavioral or cognitive performance can conceivably be assessed (e.g., muscular contractions, eye blinking, overall motoric activity, and various cognitive tasks). Although performance-based measures are useful research tools, their clinical applicability is fairly limited, as they tend to be more specialized, less widely available, and can require expensive equipment and extensive training to administer.

PATHOPHYSIOLOGY

The pathophysiology of fatigue is multifactorial and complex. Fatigue can result from dysregulation of the immune system, from changes in the nervous system related to the disease process, and from neuroendocrine and neurotransmitter changes. Other illness co-factors can also influence fatigue, including pain and deconditioning. It is hoped that further delineation of the pathophysiological mechanisms and co-factors leading to fatigue will lead to improved treatments.

Central Nervous System Mechanisms

Specific central nervous system (CNS) regions have been implicated in the pathophysiology of fatigue, including the premotor cortex, the limbic system, the basal ganglia, and the brainstem. Dysfunction here may be the result of neuronal injury secondary to immune changes, and axonal destruction. Hypofunction in these areas may lead to fatigue.

Functional neuroimaging has been applied to the study of fatigue. Although this line of research is in the preliminary stages, the results are promising. For example, one investigation in patients with multiple sclerosis (MS) fatigue utilizing functional magnetic resonance imaging linked fatigue to lower levels of activation in the thalamus, possibly relevant in its role as a relay station between the motor cortex and prefrontal regions to the basal ganglia. MS fatigue has also been studied with positron emission tomography (PET) scanning that has shown reductions in glucose uptake in the frontal lobe. In Parkinson's disease (PD), fatigue has also been associated with reduced frontal lobe activity, characterized by deficits in perfusion and glucose uptake.

Neurotransmitter Disruption

Dopaminergic, histaminergic, and serotonergic pathways may partially mediate fatigue. It has been suggested that disruption of serotonergic pathways can adversely affect attention and secondarily produce cognitive fatigue. Furthermore, the hypothalamus may contribute to fatigue through its related pathways affecting decreased arousal. Modafinil, a medication used to treat sleep disorders, may act through mechanisms mediated by the hypothalamus.

Neuromuscular Mechansims

Neuromuscular fatigue refers to fatigue produced by changes in peripheral motor conduction, muscle changes, or a combination of both. Fatigue of this type is usually defined as any reduction of maximal muscle force or motor output. Neuromuscular fatigue has been associated with disorders of motor control including impaired muscular excitation, contraction, and metabolism. For example, in post-polio syndrome fatigue, it is assumed that premature exhaustion of anterior horn cells contribute to a peripheral muscle fatigue. However, motor fatigability does not appear to correlate to perceived or subjective fatigue. For example, the muscle fatigue experienced by individuals with amyotrophic lateral sclerosis is not associated with self-reported fatigue. Likewise, measures of intracellular metabolism and muscle neurophysiology during maximum voluntary contraction of the tibialis anterior muscle are also not significantly different in patients with severe fatigue and unfatigued healthy controls. At present, it is unclear how abnormalities in motor pathways contribute to subjective or perceived fatigue.

Immunological Dysregulation

There are several lines of evidence that suggest that immune system dysregulation plays a role in fatigue. First, medications that are products of the immune system, such as cytokines, clearly produce fatigue as a side effect when given to patients with various disorders. For example, high-dose interleukin-2 administration causes fatigue, fever, and myalgia. In addition, both interferon (IFN)-α and IFN-β can induce fatigue as well as other neuropsychiatric complications. The fatigue effects of IFNs may be mediated via interactions with the endocrine system and in particular thyroid function.

Second, fatigue is a prominent symptom in disorders of autoimmune etiology such as systemic lupus erythematosus (SLE) and MS. In both disorders, patients may experience episodes of severe fatigue as part of a disease exacerbation or relapse, and fatigue can develop prior to signs of organ damage.

Finally, a range of different perturbations in the immune response have been identified in individuals with persistent and severe fatigue. For example, in fatigued patients with chronic fatigue syndrome (CFS), several changes consistent with a decreased cellular immunity and alterations in cytokine levels have been identified. Some reported changes in cytokines such as interleukin 1 and tumor necrosis factor-α, which have effects on sleep regulation, may produce fatigue through disorders such as sleep apnea and idiopathic hypersomnia. Evidence also suggests that these cytokines accumulate during periods of wakefulness, and promote fatigue.

An association between perceived fatigue and circulating markers of immune activation has also been observed in some but not all studies of MS patients. Despite the possible contribution of activation of the immune system and fatigue, immune changes are not specific enough for diagnostic purposes and are not correlated with end-organ damage in chronically fatigued individuals.

Fatigue Co-Factors

There are numerous factors that can secondarily influence fatigue in medical, psychiatric, and neurological conditions. Such co-factors are especially relevant to individuals with chronic illness. They include deconditioning, sleep problems, pain, and depression.

Physical Deconditioning

Deconditioning results from the failure to get adequate exercise. Illness often leads to weakness and decreased mobility. For many patients, this results in a decline in aerobic capacity. Unfortunately, lack of exercise tends to further exacerbate fatigue. Furthermore, in severely disabled patients who have difficulty with mobility, respiratory muscles often become weakened. This causes an increase in the amount of energy required to breathe.

Sleep Disorders

Daytime fatigue is often a co-existent feature of sleep disorders that accompany a variety of medical problems. For example, as many as two-thirds of SLE patients report poor sleep quality, and sleep problems correlate with fatigue in these patients. Excessive daytime sleepiness is also common in patients with movement disorders. In both PD and post-polio syndrome, abnormal movements such as restless leg syndrome and periodic limb movements can disrupt sleep at night and lead to daytime fatigue. Disrupted sleep patterns (e.g., difficulty falling asleep, early morning awakening) also commonly accompany depression and depressive states.

Pain

Pain and fatigue have a high degree of overlap, and it is often difficult for patients to determine which of these two symptoms has the greatest effect on their functioning. There are a number of ways in which pain can contribute to fatigue. Physically, pain can cause deconditioning by limiting activity. The presence of nighttime pain can also disrupt normal sleep patterns causing excessive daytime sleepiness and fatigue. Pain also has a high degree of association with psychological factors. It can contribute to depression and other affective disorders, and these can, in turn, can increase feelings of fatigue. Finally, it is likely that the experience of moving and functioning in pain is energy consuming and leads to a depletion of reserves.

Depression and Affective Disorders

Affective disorders such as depression are very common among fatigued patients. Fatigue is a typical symptom of depression, and is often reported as a lack of motivation or energy. Depression can be brought on by fatigue, and it can in turn engender additional fatigue.

An association between fatigue and depressive states has been reported in many medical disorders, including CFS, SLE, MS, PD, postoperative states, and epilepsy. Fatigue is a major component of a number of affective disorders, including major depression, seasonal affective disorder, and dysthymia. The role of depression in fatigue is complex and may differ between disorders. For example, a recent study found that successful treatment of depression in MS patients also reduced their fatigue, although a similar study in oncology patients did not find any improvement in fatigue.

There are a number of theories as to why depression is common in persons with fatigue. In disorders such as MS and PD, where there is a clear insult to the neurological system, depression and fatigue may stem from damage to the same neurological pathways. Depression in CFS has been linked to changes in neurohormonal or immunological function. Depression can also be the result of the stresses associated with chronic illness, as has been reported in SLE. These stresses can increase depression, to the point that depression can replace the underlying disease as the patient's primary concern.

Psychosocial Factors

Psychosocial factors can also contribute to fatigue severity. For example, in persons with post-polio syndrome, fatigue has been associated with low levels of social support. For example, in patients with SLE, fatigue has been associated with higher levels of perceived "helplessness," as well as the lack of health insurance. Similarly in MS, feelings of control lessen fatigue, whereas focusing on bodily sensations can exacerbate fatigue. Individuals who feel they can create environments appropriate to their psychological and physical needs experience less fatigue and fatigue-related stress.

Diagnostic Workup

A workup for fatigue is essential to diagnosing and determining the most effective course of treatment. Essential elements in the workup are a detailed medical health history, including family history and psychosocial history, thorough examination, and selected laboratory tests.

The medical history is a key element in the fatigue evaluation. Fatigue is often associated with other symptoms and in order to fully assess fatigue it is important to understand the patient as fully as possible, both physically and psychologically. Specific questions about onset, severity, and presence of any triggering factors are helpful. The interview should be designed to inquire about medical and psychiatric disorders that may contribute to fatigue. Table 2 provides a list of medical conditions in which fatigue is common.

It is also important to inquire about the patient's professional activities including level of stress at work, as well as any changes in family status, alcohol use, or close relationships. During the interview, the clinician should observe the patient carefully for signs of negative affect, mood disturbance, or anxiety that may be indicative of psychiatric disorders.

As part of the evaluation there should be an assessment of what other medications the patient may be taking, with an emphasis on any recent changes. As shown in Table 3, many medications used to treat other symptoms in chronic illness, may actually contribute to fatigue. For example, several pain medications (such as opioids) have fatigue as a major side effect. Antispasticity agents, such as baclofen and tizanidine, can also produce fatigue, as do sedatives, anticonvulsants, and antihistamines. Reduction or discontinuation of agents known to produce fatigue as a side effect may help to reduce fatigue in some individuals.

A number of routine laboratory tests may be useful in the evaluation of the fatigued individual (*see* Table 4). Laboratory tests can also be used to exclude causes of fatigue such as anemia, hypothyroidism, infection, and metabolic disease. Of note, immune assays, such as viral titres to Epstein-Barr virus, are not recommended in the workup of the fatigued patient.

It is important to be aware of the presence of possible sleep disorders, in which case the patient may be referred to a sleep clinic to rule out idiopathic sleep disorders, obstructive sleep apnea (OSA), or movement disorders that interfere with the sleep cycle. Specialized breathing tests include spirometry to rule out chronic obstructive pulmonary disorder (COPD). In cases of suspected peripheral muscular fatigue, neurological referral and neuromuscular testing can be performed.

Table 2
Medical Conditions Commonly Associated
With Fatigue

Anemia
Anxiety disorder
B_{12} deficiency
Cancer
Cerebrovascular disease
Chemotherapy
Chronic fatigue syndrome
Chronic obstructive pulmonary disease
Cushings syndrome
Deconditioning
Diabetes
Dysthymia
Fibromyalgia
HIV infection
Hypothyroidism
Lyme disease
Major depression
Mixed connective tissue disease
Multiple sclerosis
Myasthenis gravis
Obstructive sleep apnea and other sleep disorders
Parkinson's disease
Postoperative states
Post-polio syndrome
Pregnancy
Rheumatoid arthritis
Somatization disorder
Systematic lupus erythematosus
Viral illness

As with any workup, the clinician should use his or her best judgment in the workup for fatigue, ordering appropriate laboratory tests and specialized testing when indicated.

THERAPY FOR FATIGUE

A management algorithm for fatigue is shown in Fig. 1. The clinician should first seek to eliminate or reduce factors that may contribute to fatigue, including mood disturbance, sleep disruption, and medications that may produce fatigue as a side effect. If fatigue persists, more specific interventions must be considered. These may include nonpharmacological and pharmacological interventions, or a combination of both.

Nonpharmacological Approaches to the Treatment of Fatigue

Nonpharmacological interventions to improve fatigue in MS include education and reassurance, exercise programs, nutritional improvements, and energy-conservation strategies. Each has at least some empirical support, but all share common sense features that make them palatable to patients who might be reluctant to add another medication to their regimen.

Education

Fatigue in chronic illness differs from the fatigue that healthy individuals experience on occasion. The fatigue experienced by persons with post-polio syndrome, PD, or MS differs from that of friends

Table 3
Medications That Can Produce Fatigue as an Adverse Event

Drug	Used for	Examples
Analgesics	Pain control	Butalbital, hydrocodone (Vicodin®), oxycodone (Oxycontin®)
Interferon therapies	Reducing MS exacerbations	IFN β-1a (Avonex®, Rebif®); IFN β-1b (Betaseron®)
Muscle relaxants	Spasticity, muscle strain, anxiety disorders	Tizanidine (Zanaflex®), baclofen (oral or through an intrathecal pump); carisoprodal (Soma®)
Sedatives/antihypnotics	Sleep aids, anxiety, muscle relaxation	Alprazolam (Xanax®), clonazepam (Klonopin®); diazepam (Valium®); zolpidem (Ambien®)
Anticonvulsants	Seizure control; pain control; depression or anxiety	Carbamazepine (Tegretol®); divalproex (Depakote®); gabapentin (Neurontin®)
Antidepressants	Depression and anxiety disorders	Clomipramine (Anafranil®); nefazodone (Serzone®); sertraline (Zoloft®)
Antihistamines	Allergies, hay fever	Diphenhydramine (Benadryl® or other over-the-counter allergy medicines); cetirizine (Zyrtec®)
Antipsychotics	Schizophrenia, psychoses	Clozapine (Clozaril®); risperidone (Risperdal®)
Hormone therapies	Hormone replacement, contraception	Medroxyprogesterone (Depo-Provera®)

MS, multiple sclerosis; IFN, interferon. (Adapted from ref. 6.)

Table 4
Laboratory Tests That Are Useful in the Fatigue Workup

Laboratory test	Assesses for
Serial temperatures	Infection, malignancy
Complete blood count with differential	Infection, malignancy
Erythrocyte sedimentation rate	Abscesses, osteomyelitis, endocarditis, cancer, tuberculosis, mycosis, collagen-vascular disease
Electrolytes	Adrenal insufficiency, tuberculosis
Glucose	Diabetes mellitus
Blood urea nitrogen/ Creatinine	Renal failure
Calcium	Hyperparathroidism, cancer, sarcoidosis
Total bilirubin	Hepatitis, hemolysis
Serum glutamic oxalocetic transaminase	Hepatocellular disease
Serum glutamic pyruvic transaminase	Hepatocellular disease
Alkaline phosphatase	Obstructive liver disease
Creatine phosphokinase	Muscle disease
Urinalysis	Renal disease, proteinuria
Posteroanterior lateral chest radiograph	Cardiopulmonary disease
Antinuclear antibodies	Systemic lupus erythematosus, other collagen-vascular disease
Thyroid stimulating hormone	Hypothyroidism
HIV antibody test	HIV/AIDS
Purified protein derivative	Tuberculosis
Hepatitis screen	Hepatitis
Lyme serologies	Lyme disease/post-Lyme syndrome

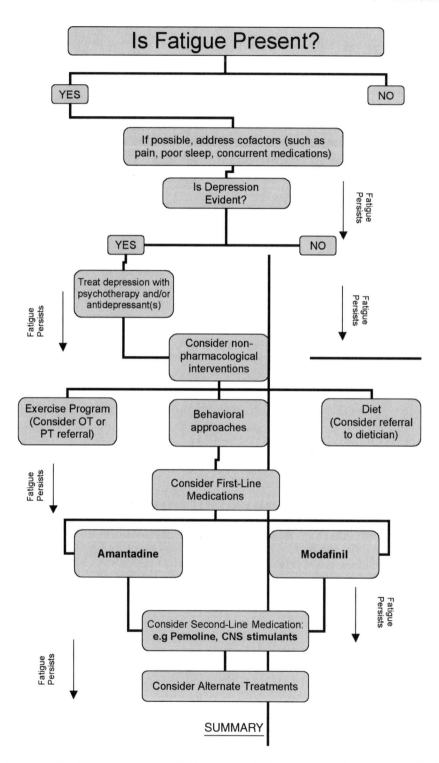

Fig. 1. An approach to fatigue management that incorporates both nonpharmacological and medication strategies for fatigue. Addressing other disease symptoms and remaining vigilant to the possibility of depression of co-existent depression or psychological distress are all features critical for successful management.

of families. Fatigue is sometimes wrongly attributed to a lack of effort or laziness. Both patient and family need to be educated that the fatigue is an intrinsic part of the disease process.

Exercise Programs

An exercise regimen developed in accordance with a patient's level of physical ability can be of clear benefit in terms of overall effects on aerobic functioning and strength. An exercise plan can be incorporated into an overall wellness plan for the majority of neurological , medical, and psychiatric disorders associated with fatigue. Even individuals with advanced illness, such as cancer patients under hospice care, can benefit from exercise programs.

Exercise can help reduce fatigue, as well as increase quality of life, endurance, and aerobic capacity in a variety of disorders, including MS, cancer, and COPD. Exercise may also help upregulate cortisol levels, which are implicated in fatigue pathophysiology, and may be chronically low in states of deconditioning.

Psychological Interventions

Several randomized, controlled trials have evaluated cognitive-behavioral therapy (CBT) in CFS populations, showing various degrees of long-term benefit. For example, CBT was more likely than relaxation therapy improve fatigue in individuals with CFS following participating in a clinical trial. Both "behavioral therapies," and graded exercise therapy, are the main therapies to benefit individuals with CFS.

Diet

There is no specific diet that will combat fatigue, however, developing a healthy nutrition program can be of some benefit for patients with significant fatigue. For example, it has been recommended that such patients should avoid foods that contain refined sugars, as erratic blood glucose levels can contribute to fatigue. Adequate hydration is also essential, and patients should avoid caffeine and alcohol. Eating smaller meals throughout the day, rather than three large meals can also be helpful. The meals should be balanced, being high in vitamins, minerals, protein, and complex carbohydrates

Energy Conservation

A few studies to date have shown empirical support for the use of energy-conservation techniques to reduce fatigue in patients with MS. One study, for example, assessed the effectiveness of a 2-hour per week energy course, led by occupational therapists. This intervention resulted in reductions in fatigue, as well as improvements in quality of life and perceived self-efficacy. Smaller investigations have found similar results. Although these results are preliminary at this point and require replication, they do suggest that referrals to an occupational therapist with expertise in this area may be helpful.

Medications

There are a several potential pharmacological approaches to the problem of fatigue in various diseases. Some treatments are quite specific. For fatigue caused by anemia, iron supplementation and exogenous erythropoietin have been found to be effective in both improving hemoglobin levels and lessening fatigue.

Other pharmacological agents are used in a more general fashion to reduce fatigue, including dopaminergic medications, psychostimulants, wake-promoting agents, and antidepressants and antianxiety agents. Much of the work with pharmacological therapy has been performed in the field of MS. However, positive results in treating fatigue and/or hypersomnolence with pharmacological therapies have also been demonstrated in other disorders, such as post-polio syndrome (bromocriptine and amantadine), sleep disorders (modafinil), cancer (methylphenidate), and HIV disease (testosterone replacement, methylphenidate, and pemoline).

Table 5 lists the pharmacological agents most often used for fatigue. One potentially effective agent is amantadine, an antiviral agent and medication used in PD that is believed to act along dopaminergic

Table 5
Medications Used to Treat Fatigue (Adult Doses)

Drug	Starting dose	Usual maintentance dose	Usual maintenance dose	Side effects
Amantadine (Symmetrel®)	100 mg per day in the morning	100 mg twice per day	300 mg per day	Insomnia, vivid dreams, livedo reticularis
Modafinil (Provigil®)	100 mg per day in the morning	200 mg per day in the morning, or 100 mg in the morning and 100 mg at lunchtime	200 mg per day (some people might respond to higher doses)	Headache, insomnia
Pemoline (Cylert®)	18.75 mg per day in the morning	18.75–56.25 mg per day	93.75 mg per day	Irritability, restlessness, insomnia, potential liver problems
Bupropion, sustained release (Wellbutrin SR®)	150 mg per day in the morning	150 mg twice per day	200 mg twice per day	Agitation, anxiety insomnia, seizures
Fluoxetine (Prozac®)	20 mg per day in the morning	20–80 mg per day	80 mg per day	Weakness, nausea insomnia
Venlafaxine (Effexor-XR®)	75 mg per day in the morning	140–180 mg per day	225 mg per day	Weakness, nausea, dizziness

Adapted from ref. *16.*

pathways. It has shown benefits in fatigue therapy for about one-third of patients with MS. Given its favorable safety profile and the fact that it is inexpensive, it is a worthwhile medication to try in the individual with fatigue. In the case of MS, some but not all experts have suggested that amantadine be considered as first-line therapy for mild fatigue, whereas other agents are used for severe fatigue.

Another potentially effective medication to treat fatigue is modafil, which has a favorable side-effect profile. It has been approved for the treatment of excessive daytime sleepiness associated with narcolepsy. Modafinil is not a stimulant. It is believed to be a unique "wake-promoting" medication that exerts effects through pathways of "normal wakefulness." It has been shown to reduce fatigue scores on several different fatigue scales in a range of neurological disorders including MS, and hypersomnolence states in PD, depression, and OSA.

There are a number of CNS stimulants, including pemoline and methylphenidate, that are generally approved for use in the treatment of attention deficit hyperactivity disorder. These medications act to produce wakefulness along the mesocorticolimbic pathways (the pathways involved in the vigilance, or "fight or flight" response). Pemoline has been best studied with regard to fatigue treatment, and has been assessed in several trials of MS patients. Results of these trials have been mixed, with higher doses (>75.5 mg per day) tending to show a limited degree of benefit. However, adverse events such as irritability may limit use.

Given the documented association between fatigue, depression, and anxiety, use of antidepressant and and/or antianxiety agents may be advantageous in the treatment of fatigue. Antidepressants may also help stimulate the appetite in persons who are not meeting their nutritional needs. Antianxiety agents may help conserve energy otherwise being dissipated by maladaptive energy-consuming affective states. However, some antianxiety agents may be sedating and therefore must be used cautiously.

SUMMARY

Fatigue is a significant factor in the lives of many patients. In many disease states it is among the most commonly reported symptoms. Fatigue is an important symptom to consider as it can disrupt patient's social lives, occupations, and activities of daily living. Efforts to predict fatigue have been mixed, but it is often related to overall quality of life and mood. From a pathophysiological perspective, fatigue is multifactorial and complex, involving, changes in the nervous system related to the disease process, neuroendocrine and neurotransmitter changes, dysregulation of the immune system as well as other factors, such as physical deconditioning, sleep disturbance, pain, and medication side effects. Various attempts to assess fatigue have been made, and now many measures are available for use in clinical practice and research. In clinical practice, measures will help guide treatment considerations.

Recent research has provided valuable strategies to ameliorate fatigue and, many patients receive substantial relief. Nonpharmacological approaches are considered the first step in treatment. These include education and reassurance, exercise programs, dietary considerations, and energy-conservation strategies. For patients who continue to experience significant fatigue, several medications, although not specifically approved for use in the reduction of fatigue, appear to be efficacious. First-line agents include amantadine and modafinil. Second-line agents include pemoline and antidepressant medications. Other pharmacological agents have also shown some promise.

ACKNOWLEDGMENTS

The authors wish to thank Andrew Sobel for his editorial and technical assistance.

REFERENCES

1. Piper BF, Dibble SL, Dodd MJ, Weiss MC, Slaughter RE, Paul SM. The revised Piper Fatigue Scale: psychometric evaluation in women with breast cancer. Oncol Nurs Forum 1998;25:677–684.
2. Krupp LB, LaRocca NG, Muir-Nash J, Steinberg AD. The fatigue severity scale. Application to patients with multiple sclerosis and systemic lupus erythematosus. Arch Neurol 1989;46:1121–1123.
3. Schwartz JE, Jandorf L, Krupp LB. The measurement of fatigue: a new instrument. J Psychosom Res 1993;37:753–762.
4. Chalder T, Berelowitz G, Pawlikowska T, et al. Development of a fatigue scale. J Psychosom Res 1993;37:147–153.
5. Vercoulen JH, Bazelmans E, Swanink CM, et al. Physical activity in chronic fatigue syndrome: assessment and its role in fatigue. J Psychiatric Res 1997;31:661–673.
6. Multiple Sclerosis Council for Clinical Practice Guidelines. Fatigue and multiple sclerosis: evidence-based management strategies for fatigue in multiple sclerosis. Washington DC: Paralyzed Veterans of America; 1998.
7. Kittiwatanapaisan W, Gauthier DK, Williams AM, Oh SJ. Fatigue in Myasthenia Gravis patients. J Neurosci Nurs 2003;35: 87–93,106.
8. Belza BL. Comparison of self-reported fatigue in rheumatoid arthritis and controls. J Rheumatol 1995;22:639–643.
9. Smets EM, Garssen B, Bonke B, De Haes JC. The Multidimensional Fatigue Inventory (MFI) psychometric qualities of an instrument to assess fatigue. J Psychosom Res 1995;39:315–325.
10. Stein KD, Martin SC, Hann DM, Jacobsen PB. A multidimensional measure of fatigue for use with cancer patients. Cancer Pract 1998;6:143–152.
11. Iriarte J, Katsamakis G, de Castro P. The Fatigue Descriptive Scale (FDS): a useful tool to evaluate fatigue in multiple sclerosis. Mult Scler 1999;5:10–16.
12. Hann DM, Denniston MM, Baker F. Measurement of fatigue in cancer patients: further validation of the Fatigue Symptom Inventory. Qual Life Res 2000;9:847–854.
13. Hartz A, Bentler S, Watson D. Measuring fatigue severity in primary care patients. J Psychosom Res 2003;54:515–521.
14. Hockenberry MJ, Hinds PS. Barrera P, et al. Three instruments to assess fatigue in children with cancer: the child, parent and staff perspectives. J Pain Symptom Manage 2003;25:319–328.
15. Christodoulou C. The assessment and measurement of fatigue. In: DeLuca J, ed. Fatigue as a Window to the Brain. New York: MIT Press. In press.

16. Krupp LB. Fatigue in Multiple Sclerosis: A Guide to Diagnosis and Management. New York: Demos Medical Publishing Inc; 2004.

SUGGESTED READINGS

Adinolfi A. Assessment and treatment of HIV-related fatigue. J Assoc Nurses AIDS Care 2001;12(Suppl):29–34.

Bakshi R. Fatigue associated with multiple sclerosis: diagnosis, impact and management. Mult Scler 2003;9:219–227.

Bartley SH, Chute E. Fatigue and Impairment in Man. New York: McGraw-Hill; 1947.

Chaudhuri A, Behan PO. Fatigue in neurological disorders. Lancet 2004;363:978–988.

Deale A, Husain K, Chalder T, Wessely S. Long-term outcome of cognitive behavior therapy versus relaxation therapy for chronic fatigue syndrome: a 5-year follow-up study. Am J Psychiatry 2001;158:2038–2042.

DeLuca J. (Ed.) Fatigue as a window to the brain. New York: MIT Press. In press.

Dimeo FC. Effects of exercise on cancer-related fatigue. Cancer 2001;92:1689–1693.

Dittner AJ, Wessely SC, Brown RG. The assessment of fatigue: a practical guide for clinicians and researchers. J Psychosom Res 2004;56:157–170.

Friedman JH, Chou KL. Sleep and fatigue in Parkinson's disease. Parkinsonism Relat Disord 2004;10(Suppl 1):S27–S35.

Krupp LB. Fatigue. Philadelphia, PA: Elsevier Science; 2003.

Roelcke U, Kappos L, Lechner-Scott J, et al. Reduced glucose metabolism in the frontal cortex and basal ganglia of multiple sclerosis patients with fatigue: a 18F-fluorodeoxyglucose positron emission tomography study. Neurology 1997;48:1566–1571.

Stasi R, Abriani L, Beccaglia P, Terzoli E, Amadori S. Cancer-related fatigue: evolving concepts in evaluation and treatment. Cancer 2003;98:1786–1801.

Wessely S, Hotopf M, Sharpe D. Chronic Fatigue and its Syndromes. New York: Oxford University Press; 1998.

John C. M. Brust

DEFINITIONS

Consciousness requires both arousal and attentiveness; one is conscious *of something*. Arousal is mediated by the reticular activating system of the brainstem and diencephalon. Attentiveness depends on the cerebral cortex, especially polymodal association areas.

Different states of arousal—lethargy, obtundation, stupor, coma—are defined clinically in terms of response to stimuli. Coma is lack of response to any stimulus, including pain. (An exception to this definition would be someone alert but receiving total neuromuscular blockade.) The cardinal feature of delirium, on the other hand, is impaired attentiveness.

Delirium is a syndrome, less easily defined than stupor or coma. A number of terms have been used to describe the symptoms and signs of delirium, including clouding of consciousness, acute brain syndrome, acute confusional state, acute encephalopathy, metabolic encephalopathy, and toxic psychosis. The essential features of delirium are listed in the American Psychiatric Association's Diagnostic and Statistical Manual (DSM) of Mental Disorders (Table 1).

SYMPTOMS AND SIGNS

Delirium evolves rapidly, over hours or days, rarely longer, and it fluctuates in severity from minute to minute or hour to hour. There may be brief periods of lucidity. Either over- or under-stimulation can exacerbate symptoms, which tend to worsen at night. Mild inattentiveness may consist of distractibility and difficulty focusing, maintaining, or shifting attention. Severe inattentiveness may preclude any meaningful interaction with the environment, including verbal and nonverbal exchange with the examiner. The term *confusion* (which carries a number of different clinical connotations) in the context of delirium refers to disorganized thinking; intruding thoughts seem to compete with one another, and an inability to express thoughts in a directed, coherent fashion. Speech is tangential, rambling, and punctuated by stops, starts, and perseverations.

Alterations in arousal usually accompany delirium. The stereotypic delirious patient has increased psychomotor activity or agitation, yet lethargy and decreased arousal are actually more common. Many patients fluctuate between hypo- and hyper-alertness. In either state they do not fully register the events occurring around them, and they substitute perceptual misrepresentations of their own. Hyper-alert patients are likelier to have illusions or hallucinations, usually visual and three-dimensionally formed (e.g., animals or people). Such perceptual disturbances are usually unpleasant, but auditory hallucinations as encountered with psychosis (e.g., accusing voices) are unusual. Some patients, although not frankly hallucinating, misperceive their surroundings, for example, declaring that they are at home

From: *Current Clinical Neurology: Psychiatry for Neurologists*
Edited by: D.V. Jeste and J.H. Friedman © Humana Press Inc., Totowa, NJ

Table 1
Criteria for Delirium in Diagnostic and Statistical Manual of Mental Disorders, Fourth Edition

1. Disturbance of consciousness (i.e., reduced clarity of awareness of the environment with reduced ability to focus, sustain, or shift attention).
2. A change in cognition (such as memory deficit, disorientation, language disturbance) or the development of a perceptual disturbance that is not better accounted for by pre-existing, established, or evolving dementia.
3. The disturbance develops over a short period (usually hours to days) and tends to fluctuate during the course of the day.
4. There is evidence from the history, physical examination, or laboratory findings that the disturbance is caused by the direct physiological consequences of a general medical condition.

despite obvious visual evidence to the contrary. The sleep–wake cycle is often disturbed, with lethargy during the day and agitation at night ("sundowning"), and it is possible that some hallucinations represent dream-like phenomena intruding into wakefulness.

To the extent that they can be tested, delirious patients display an array of cognitive abnormalities, including disorientation to time and place and abnormal ordering of events in time. Inability to register information limits testing of recent memory by standard means (e.g., repeating three unrelated words and then recalling or recognizing them after a few minutes). The same limitations apply to language and spatial testing, which are often abnormal. Delusions, paranoid or otherwise, tend to be fleeting, not fixed as in psychosis, and they are often strikingly triggered by sensory input. Emotional swings and depression are common.

PREVALENCE

Delirium is common, especially among patients on general medical/surgical services, in surgical intensive care units, and in coronary care units. Up to one-fourth of hospitalized patients aged 65 or older have delirium on admission, and one-third more develop delirium during hospitalization.

HISTORY AND EXAMINATION

History-taking often depends on the observations of others. Pre-existing dementia is present in nearly half of all patients hospitalized with delirium, and pre-existing milder cognitive disturbance is present in many more. Delirium and dementia have different time courses, but in already demented patients it may be difficult for family members to pinpoint the earliest symptoms of delirium. Cognitive or behavioral performance in dementia can vary from day to day, and greater-than-usual difficulty in performance might be interpreted as progression of the dementing process. Other early easy-to-misinterpret symptoms include insomnia and frightening dreams. In addition to pre-existing cognitive disturbance, risk factors for delirium include advanced age, systemic illness (especially metabolic, multiple, or severe), infection, malnutrition, medication (especially sedative, analgesic, or anticholinergic), ethanol or drug abuse, sensory impairment (especially visual), sensory overstimulation (e.g., "ICU psychosis"), fever, hypothermia, dehydration, and depression (which can itself produce symptoms that overlap with those of "quiet delirium"). Patients undergoing surgery, especially cardiac, orthopedic, ophthalmological, and urological, are also at risk for delirium.

A DSM criterion for delirium is that the condition is caused by "a general medical condition." That term would include primary disorders of the central nervous system (CNS), and physical/neurological examination must be comprehensively directed at identifying such a condition. Funduscopy might suggest increased intracranial pressure (ICP) or hypertensive encephalopathy. Meningismus might suggest CNS or subarachnoid hemorrhage. Focal neurological signs might suggest structural lesions such as stroke, neoplasm, or abscess. Asterixis plus myoclonus is seen with uremia; asterixis without myoclonus is seen with hepatic encephalopathy. Intermittent focal twitching (e.g., of the fingers or the corner of the mouth) might reflect nonconvulsive seizures. Tetany suggests hypocalcemia or hypomagnesemia. Limitation of eye movement might signify thiamine deficiency and Wernicke encephalopathy. Extreme hyperthermia might reflect heat stroke, neuroleptic malignant syndrome, thyrotoxic crisis, or cocaine intoxication. Hypothermia suggests exposure, sepsis, hypotension, myxedema, ethanol or other intoxication, or hypoglycemia. Fever, dry skin, and dilated unreactive pupils suggest anticholinergic poisoning (including tricyclic antidepressants). Tremor is a feature of a number of drug intoxications (including lithium, psychostimulants, and valproate) as well as drug withdrawal syndromes (including ethanol and sedatives). Intermittent "burst" nystagmus is seen with phencyclidine ("angel dust") poisoning. Cerebellar ataxia is a feature of ethanol or sedative intoxication. Asymmetric cranial neuropathy and radiculopathy might reflect meningeal carcinomatosis.

In patients capable of cooperating, specific tests for attentiveness include digit-span recitation (normal five to seven), reverse recitation of serial digits (normal four to five), counting backward from 20, reciting the months backward, or spelling backward a word such as world. The ability to follow sequential tasks might include the "palm-side-fist" maneuver or folding a piece of paper in a particular way and then putting in a particular place. Abnormalities on these tasks might reflect impairment of working memory rather than attentiveness *per se*. Inattentiveness is usually identified during the course of history-taking and general examination; its presence may be especially evident during visual field or proprioceptive testing.

LABORATORY STUDIES

Laboratory evaluation is individualized. Medications and their side effects are identified; blood or urine toxicological studies (including the identification of illicit drugs) are based on index of suspicion. Psychoactive medications are discontinued. A search for infection includes chest radiograph, urinalysis, and appropriate cultures. Complete blood count, serum electrolytes, blood urea nitrogen, creatine, glucose, calcium, phosphate, liver enzymes, arterial blood gases, and electrocardiography are indicated in most patients. If a cause is not readily identified, a spinal tap (preferably preceded by brain imaging) is necessary to exclude meningitis/encephalitis. Brain computed tomography or magnetic resonance imaging is performed in patients with neurological focal signs, history or evidence of trauma, or signs of increased ICP. Although pharmacotherapy is best avoided in delirium, it may be necessary when brain imaging is performed. Additional laboratory tests include serum levels of cobalamin, ammonia, and magnesium, and thyroid function tests.

The electroencephalogram (EEG) in delirium demonstrates slowing and disorganization (reflecting the pathophysiological kinship of delirium to stupor and coma). Its principal usefulness is in diagnosing occult seizures and in identifying nondelirious psychiatric disorders (normal EEG).

Many delirious patients, especially the elderly, have more than one causal disorder. Among the elderly the commonest causes of delirium are metabolic disease, infection, stroke, and drugs, especially sedative, analgesic, and anticholinergic medications. Among younger patients the commonest causes are drug intoxication and withdrawal.

DELIRIUM TREMENS

A special case is *delirium tremens*, most often identified with alcohol withdrawal but also sometimes caused by withdrawal from other sedatives, especially barbiturates. Within the first 2 or 3 days, ethanol withdrawal produces tremor, seizures, or hallucinations, but the sensorium is usually clear. By contrast, *delirium tremens* usually emerges after several days of abstinence, and tremor and hallucinations are accompanied by delirium (usually agitated) and autonomic instability (tachycardia, fever, blood pressure swings, profuse sweating). Fluid loss can be marked, and mortality is as high as 15%. The treatment of *delirium tremens* includes sedation with benzodiazepines (often in huge titrated doses), cardiac and respiratory monitoring, and careful attention to fluid and electrolyte balance in an intensive care unit.

Delirium is not a feature of withdrawal from benzodiazepines, opioids, cocaine, other psychostimulants, marijuana, hallucinogens, phencyclidine, or anticholinergic agents.

DELIRIUM IN SURGICAL PATIENTS

Another special situation is delirium in surgical patients. Postoperative delirium can be caused by multiple factors, including residual drug and anesthetic effects, hypoxia, infection, electrolyte imbalance, psychological stress, and disrupted sleep patterns. Delirium occurs in up to 40% of patients receiving open heart or coronary bypass surgery, in some cases consequent to microemboli to the brain. Orthopedic procedures also carry risk, especially femoral fractures and knee replacements, in some cases related to fat emboli. Sensory deprivation probably contributes to delirium following cataract surgery and hyponatremia to delirium following prostate surgery.

DELIRIUM AND STROKE

Agitated delirium can be a feature of stroke in a variety of locations, especially infarction involving the right parieto-temporal convexity. Similar symptoms are described with infarcts or hemorrhages involving the inferior temporal lobe (left, right, or bilateral), the thalamus, the medial frontal lobe, and the caudate nucleus.

DIFFERENTIAL DIAGNOSIS

Distinguishing delirium from dementia, aphasia, and psychiatric disorders can be difficult, and diagnosing one condition does not exclude the possible co-occurrence of another. Dementia is usually insidiously progressive over months or years, but it can make an abrupt appearance after a stroke. Day-to-day fluctuations in behavior or performance are usually not striking in demented patients, but dementia with cortical Lewy bodies can produce marked fluctuations in cognition and hallucinations. The great majority of patients with Alzheimer-type dementia have early memory impairment, followed by language and spatial difficulties; grossly abnormal behavior usually makes a late appearance. Floridly abnormal behavior is often the initial feature of other dementing illnesses, however, including neurosyphilis, Huntington's disease, and the frontotemporal dementias involving τ protein.

Aphasia most often follows stroke or head trauma and is thus usually of sudden onset. Paranoia and agitation are not unusual in aphasic patients, especially when speech comprehension is disrupted. Empty speech or prominent paraphasias and neologisms provide helpful clues, as do additional focal signs on the neurological examination or appropriately located lesions on neuroimaging.

Schizophrenia is usually of insidious onset, but acute psychotic episodes with agitation and delusions can be superimposed. Speech is disorganized, but often a bizarre on-going theme is identifiable. Hallucinations are usually auditory with self-reference, including commands and accusations. Delusions tend to be systematized and fixed, and inattentiveness is a component of more elaborate bizarre behavior.

Depression is also usually gradual in onset, but patients with bipolar disorder can undergo rapid shifts, and both depression and mania can produce agitation and paranoia. Depressed or manic patients can have impaired attentiveness, delusions, hallucinations, and disturbed sleep patterns. On the other hand, many hospitalized patients referred to psychiatrists for depression turn out to have delirium. Broadly speaking, features that are encountered in both delirium and psychosis (whether a schizophrenic or a mood disorder) include agitation, delusions, hallucinations, and language disturbance. In delirium, however, in contrast to psychosis, symptoms fluctuate and are fragmented and unsystematized. They occur in the setting of difficulty either maintaining or shifting attention. There is often impaired memory. The EEG is usually abnormal. Finally, there is a plausibly causal underlying medical disorder, medication use, or substance intoxication or withdrawal.

TREATMENT

Treatment of delirium is divided into nonpharmacological and pharmacological interventions. Nonpharmacological management for any delirious patient includes avoidance of over- or under-stimulation, encouraging family members to be present, using "sitters" to provide orientation, and placing patients in single rooms or near the nurses' station. Frequent communication, including eye contact, is important and can progress to reorientation and therapeutic activities programs. Sleep should be uninterrupted, and immobilization should be as brief as possible. Attempts should be made to compensate for impaired vision or hearing. Underlying medical or neurological illnesses are addressed, and adequate nutrition and hydration are provided.

Pharmacological interventions should be used only when absolutely necessary (i.e., the patient cannot be safely managed otherwise). No drug is ideal, and reduction of agitation carries the cost of masking the patient's level of alertness. Barbiturates and benzodiazepines, moreover, can cause paradoxical excitement. (Benzodiazepines remain the treatment of choice for ethanol and sedative withdrawal, however.) If neuroleptic agents (e.g., haloperidol or risperidone) are used, they should be given in the lowest effective dose. Agents with anticholinergic properties are avoided. Physical restraints should also be considered a last resort. Whether they are more dangerous than pharmacological restraints is controversial, and in most hospitals regulatory guidelines discourage the use of both.

COURSE AND PROGNOSIS

In those patients whose causative condition is rapidly corrected, the prognosis for delirium is usually good. In many cases, however, delirium is a protracted state, lasting 30 days or longer, and it is estimated that at 6 months up to 80% of patients continue to have some symptoms. Especially in the elderly, an acceleration in cognitive decline can follow delirium, interfering with activities of daily living and hastening the need for nursing home placement. Depression is also a frequent aftermath.

SUGGESTED READINGS

Brust JCM, Caplan LR. Agitation and delirium. In: Bogousslavsky J, Caplan LR, eds. Stroke Syndromes, Second Edition. New York: Cambridge University Press; 2001:222–231.

Carnes M. Howell T, Rosenberg M, Francis J, Hildebrand C, Knuppel J. Physicians vary in approaches to the clinical management of delirium. J Am Geriatr Soc 2003;51:234–239.

Diagnostic and Statistical Manual of Mental Disorders, Fourth Edition. Washington DC: American Psychiatric Association; 1994:129.

Elie M, Cole MG, Primeau FJ, Bellavance F. Delirium risk factors in elderly hospitalized patients. J Gen Intern Med 1998; 13:204–212.

Farrell KR, Ganzini L. Misdiagnosing delirium as depression in medically ill elderly patients. Arch Intern Med 1995;155: 2459–2464.

Inouye SK, Bogardus ST, Charpentier PA, et al. A multicomponent intervention to prevent delirium in hospitalized older patients. N Engl J Med 1999;340:669–676.

Jacobson SA. Delirium in the elderly. Psychiatr Clin North Am 1997;20:91–110.

Marcantonio ER, Simon SE, Bergmann MA, Jones RN, Murphy KM, Morris JN. Delirium symptoms in post-acute care: prevalent, persistent, and associated with poor functional recovery. J Am Geriatr Soc 2003;51:4–9.

Roche V. Southwestern Internal Medicine Conference. Etiology and management of delirium. Am J Med Sci 2003;325:20–30.

Taylor D, Lewis S. Delirium. J Neurol Neurosurg Psychiatry 1993;56:742–751.

Trzepacz PT. Delirium. Advances in diagnosis, pathophysiology, and treatment. Psychiatr Clin North Am 1996;19:429–448.

24

Psychopharmacology
A Pharmacodynamic Approach

Christian Dolder and Beatriz Luna

INTRODUCTION

The modern era of psychotropic medications has supplied providers and patients with substantial ammunition in the treatment of psychiatric disorders. Despite the variety of psychotropic medications available for the treatment of common psychiatric conditions, room for improvement exists. Antipsychotics, antidepressants, and anxiolytics with enhanced efficacy, refined pharmacological profiles, and reduced side effects would be welcomed. In addition to improvements in the pharmacological treatment of the most common psychiatric disorders, pharmacological treatment of other psychiatric illnesses should be enhanced. Psychotropic medications are commonly used for many disorders besides schizophrenia, depression, bipolar disorder, and anxiety disorder. The prescription of antipsychotics for aggression associated with dementia and anxiolytics for sleep disturbances are examples. Medications not classically considered to be psychotropics are also used for psychiatric conditions (e.g., anticonvulsant medications for mood stabilization). This diverse use of medications with psychotropic properties, both indicated and off-label, is accompanied by evidence that varies widely in terms of its quality and quantity of support. All of these factors can create confusing therapeutic situations for psychiatrists and nonpsychiatrists when prescribing psychotropic medications.

Knowledge of the pharmacokinetics and pharmacodynamics of psychotropic medications can aid clinicians in the rational use of these medications. Pharmacokinetics, the study of drug movement within biological systems (e.g., absorption, distribution, metabolism, and excretion), provides clinicians with an understanding of how the body acts on medication. A pharmacokinetic understanding of psychotropic medications can assist with such therapeutic considerations as minimizing drug–drug interactions, choosing appropriate dosage forms, and selecting patient-specific medication doses. Pharmacodynamics, the study of pharmacologically active molecules at their site of action (i.e., how a drug acts on the body), provides clinicians with a plethora of useful information. For example, understanding basic pharmacodynamic aspects of medications can assist prescribers by applying the mechanisms of action of psychotropic medications to the indicated uses, off-label uses, side effects, and selection of medication. Whereas pharmacokinetic considerations of psychotropic medications are important, this chapter focuses on the pharmacodynamics of psychotropic medications. The purpose of this chapter is to examine common psychotropic medications (i.e., anticonvulsants [mood stabilizers], antidepressants, antipsychotics, and anxiolytics) from a pharmacodynamic perspective. In illustrating the mechanism of action of these medications, psychotropic utility and related side effects are illuminated. Special emphasis is placed on the neurological side

From: *Current Clinical Neurology: Psychiatry for Neurologists*
Edited by: D.V. Jeste and J.H. Friedman © Humana Press Inc., Totowa, NJ

effects of psychotropic medications. In addition, we review psychiatric side effects associated with common somatic medications.

PSYCHOTROPICS: PHARMACODYNAMIC CONSIDERATIONS

Anticonvulsants

Anticonvulsants, especially the newer agents, are a heterogeneous group of compounds with a variety of mechanisms of action. This mechanistic variety has led to diverse psychotropic, anticonvulsant, and adverse effect profiles. Mechanistic and clinical differences also create difficulty when trying to predict, for example, psychotropic activity. Thus, despite the utility of many anticonvulsants for psychiatric conditions (e.g., bipolar disorder, depression, and anxiety disorder), the level of evidence supporting these assorted uses differ.

Some individuals (*1*), based on the general profiles of anticonvulsants, have categorized these agents as "sedating" (benzodiazepines, carbamazepine, oxcarbazepine, gabapentin, valproate), "mixed" (topiramate, zonisamide), and "activating" (felbamate, lamotrigine). In addition to the antimanic and anxiolytic potential for many agents classified as sedating, these medications generally are limited by sedative, cognitive, and weight gain-related side effects. Anticonvulsants with an activating profile have potential to relieve fatigue, cause weight loss, and improve depression symptoms. Agents with a mixed profile have a greater ability to cause sedation while potentially also possessing the ability to produce weight loss and antidepressant effects.

The different efficacy and side-effect profiles of sedating, activating, and mixed anticonvulsants can to some extent be explained by their effects on γ-aminobutyric acid (GABA), the main inhibitory neurotransmitter in the human brain, as well as glutamate, the main excitatory neurotransmitter in the human brain. In a simplistic sense, many anticonvulsants are thought to produce a reduction in seizures via an increase in GABA and/or decrease in glutamate activity. GABA is also thought to be involved with mood disorders. Enhancement of GABA neurotransmission, directly or indirectly, is thought to produce anxiolysis. Several medications (valproate, gabapentin) have structural similarities to GABA and GABAergic effects. Lithium, carbamazepine, and valproate have effects on GABA (i.e., GABA receptors, GABA turnover). These agents' relationship with GABA may explain their "sedating" profile. The somewhat muted anxiolytic effects of these medications may be explained by their indirect activity on GABA. Medications such as valproate and carbamazepine exert their therapeutic effects primarily via sodium channel modulation. The inhibition of voltage-gated ion channels may indirectly lead to increased synthesis and release of GABA. The anticonvulsant tiagabine, on the other hand, has direct effects on GABA and may be a more robust anxiolytic. Tiagabine, in a manner similar to selective serotonin reuptake inhibitors (SSRIs), inhibits presynaptic GABA reuptake (*1–3*).

Glutamate has also been implicated in the pathophysiology of mood disorders, negative symptoms of schizophrenia, and to some extent symptoms of depression. Several anticonvulsants classified as "activating" (lamotrigine, felbamate) have antiglutamatergic effects. Medications with a "mixed" profile (topiramate, zonisamide) have effects on both GABA and glutamate. Thus, when taking into consideration the potential mechanism of action of the above listed medications, psychotropic and side-effect potential is illuminated (*1,2*).

Although a number of anticonvulsants have psychotropic potential based on their mechanism of action, only a handful of agents have clearly demonstrated efficacy. Focus is placed on these agents (i.e., carbamazepine/oxcarbazepine, valproate, lamotrigine). Carbamazepine, valproate, and lamotrigine have demonstrated efficacy in bipolar disorder. Lamotrigine is considered to be first-line therapy for bipolar depression. Carbamazepine is effective in bipolar mania and valproate has demonstrated efficacy in bipolar depression and mania (*4*). These agents are limited by side effects. For example, the rash potential of lamotrigine, including Stevens-Johnson syndrome, requires careful attention to dose titration and drug interactions. The ability of carbamazepine to cause hematological irregularities and valproate to cause hepatotoxicity and pancreatitis requires the clinician to carefully monitor patients treated with these medications. A number of other agents, including felbamate, gabapentin, and topiramate may have psychotropic utility but their use is currently limited by side effects or lack of proven efficacy *(5–7)*.

Antidepressants

The introduction of reserpine as an antihypertensive in the 1950s and the subsequent finding of its ability to induce depression by inhibiting the storage of amine neurotransmitters in presynaptic nerve endings led to the amine hypothesis of depression. This discovery led to the development of medications with activity on neurotransmitters at the synaptic cleft. Despite the large number of antidepressants that have been introduced into the market since the 1950s, the vast majority of antidepressants are classified as having their primary actions on the metabolism, reuptake, or selective receptor antagonism of serotonin, norepinephrine, or both. Whereas these agents' immediate actions with one or more monoamine neurotransmitter receptors or enzymes have led to the current classification of antidepressants, these simplistic classifications do not adequately explain the mechanism of action of antidepressants. In actuality, the long-term effects resulting from changes in neurotransmitter activity (e.g., post-synaptic receptor desensitization/downregulation, alteration in gene expression, and hormonal alterations) may more completely depict antidepressant mechanisms of action and the ability of many antidepressants to treat more than just depression *(6,8)*.

All of the currently marketed antidepressants, regardless of class, have similar efficacy for most types of depression. What differentiates these agents are their pharmacodynamic actions, which lead to efficacy profiles that may extend beyond depression and to different side effect potentials. For example, tricyclic antidepressants (TCAs) such as amitriptyline and imipramine are effective antidepressants that are believed to act by blocking the reuptake transporters for both serotonin and norepinephrine (and dopamine to a lesser degree). Unfortunately, all TCAs have at least three other actions: blockade of muscarinic cholinergic receptors, blockade of histamine type-1 (H1) receptors, and blockade of α-1 adrenergic receptors. These "other" actions account for many of the bothersome side effects associated with TCAs (e.g., sedation, blurred vision, urinary retention, and orthostasis). TCAs also affect sodium channels in the heart and brain, which leads to the cardiac toxicity and seizure profile of these medications. SSRIs such as fluoxetine, sertraline, and citalopram differ from TCAs in that they produce selective and potent inhibition of serotonin reuptake, which is more powerful than their actions on norepinephrine reuptake or on α-1, histaminic, or muscarinic cholinergic receptors. In addition, SSRIs have almost no ability to block sodium channels. The pharmacodynamic profile of SSRIs explains the therapeutic benefits and drawbacks of these agents in ways other than merely comparing SSRIs with TCAs. The potent and widespread effect of SSRIs on serotonin results in a number of side effects specific to these agents and to an efficacy profile that extends beyond depression. Whereas serotonergic projections to the frontal cortex are thought to play an important role in terms of antidepressant efficacy, serotonergic projections to the limbic cortex are thought to be important in explaining SSRI utility in a number of anxiety disorders (e.g., panic disorder, generalized anxiety disorder, social anxiety disorder). Conversely, the stimulation of a variety of serotonin receptors (5HT) is thought to be associated with numerous SSRI-related side effects. For instance, stimulation of 5HT2A receptors in brainstem sleep centers may lead to nocturnal awakenings; stimulation of 5HT2A receptors in the spinal cord may inhibit spinal reflexes involved with orgasm and ejaculation and cause sexual dysfunction; stimulation of 5HT2A receptors in the basal ganglia may produce neurological side effects; and stimulation of 5HT3 and 5HT4 receptors in the gastrointestinal tract may cause increased bowel motility, cramps, and diarrhea commonly associated with SSRI treatment *(6,8)*.

A number of other antidepressants have been developed with mechanisms of action that are different than SSRIs. Although the similarities between these newer agents and SSRIs (i.e., serotonergic activity and lack of muscarinic cholinergic and histaminic effects) explain the antidepressant and anxiolytic efficacy, mechanistic differences also explain some of the toxicity and potential efficacy variations. For instance, bupropion is believed to produce some of its therapeutic effects via reuptake inhibition of dopamine. This is thought to explain the generally activating profile of bupropion and the lower reported prevalence of sexual side effects. Venlafaxine inhibits the reuptake of serotonin and norepinephrine. Unlike the relatively flat dose–response curve of SSRIs, venlafaxine has primarily serotonergic activity at low doses and both serotonergic and noradrenergic effects at higher doses. This can result in a side-effect profile that varies by dose. Not all newer antidepressants are void of muscarinic cholinergic or histaminic effects. Mirtazapine, although possessing a unique mechanism of action (i.e., presynaptic α-2 receptor antagonist), has substantial histaminic properties *(6,8)*.

Antipsychotics

With the discovery of chlorpromazine's neuroleptic effects in the 1950s, the modern era of antipsychotics emerged. The ability of chlorpromazine and other conventional antipsychotics to block postsynaptic dopamine type 2 (D2) receptors prompted the dopamine hypothesis of schizophrenia. Plainly stated, the dopamine hypothesis postulates that an excess of dopamine in the mesolimbic pathway of the brain is associated with positive symptoms of schizophrenia (i.e., delusions, hallucinations) and a deficiency of dopamine in the mesocortical pathway of the brain is associated with negative symptoms of schizophrenia (i.e., anhedonia, avolition, alogia). Although simplistic, the dopamine hypothesis has in part driven the development of antipsychotic medications. All currently approved antipsychotics block D2 receptors. The potency and specificity of D2 blockade and effects at other receptors differentiate antipsychotics. Conventional antipsychotics (e.g., haloperidol, fluphenazine, chlorpromazine) block D2 receptors in a widespread manner but with varying levels of potency. Low-potency conventional antipsychotics such as chlorpromazine also have significant effects on muscarinic cholinergic, histaminic, and α-1 receptors. High-potency conventional antipsychotics such as haloperidol produce more motor side effects as opposed to the muscarinic cholinergic, histaminic, and α-1 effects of low-potency conventional antipsychotics. D2 receptor antagonism is responsible for the therapeutic effects of conventional antipsychotics but also a number of side effects. Conventional antipsychotic's blockade of postsynaptic receptors in the mesolimbic pathway is associated with improvements in the positive symptoms of schizophrenia. In contrast, the ability of these older antipsychotics to block postsynaptic dopamine receptors in the nigrostriatal pathway, mesocortical pathway, and tuberoinfundibular pathway is associated with motor side effects, detrimental cognitive effects, and negative effects related to hyperprolactinemia, respectively *(6,8)*.

Atypical (or second-generation) antipsychotics were developed in response to the previously mentioned drawbacks of conventional antipsychotics. All atypical antipsychotics are thought to act via D2 receptor antagonism and 5HT2A receptor antagonism. This "dual" mechanism of action led to three important features: reduced risk of causing extrapyramidal symptoms (EPS); reduced ability (as a group) to raise prolactin levels; and improved negative symptoms when compared to conventional antipsychotics. These mechanism-related benefits of atypical antipsychotics are related to the fact that serotonin opposes the release of dopamine in the nigrostriatal and tuberoinfundibular pathways but not mesolimbic pathway. Thus, the more specific modulation of dopamine has resulted in the previously mentioned benefits. In addition, the serotonergic activity is thought to have increased the range of psychotropic efficacy of atypical antipsychotics. For example, the atypical antipsychotics risperidone, olanzapine, enetiapine, and aripiprazole are indicated for the treatment of acute mania. The lower dopaminergic binding affinity of many atypical antipsychotics compared to their conventional antipsychotic counterparts has also been hypothesized to have an important mechanistic role. Despite the therapeutic benefits of atypical antipsychotics, the mechanism of action of these medications is also thought to be responsible for a number of side effects that are discussed later *(6,8,9)*.

The only atypical antipsychotic that does not fit the usual D2 and 5HT2A receptor antagonist mold is aripiprazole. Whereas aripiprazole is an antagonist at 5HT2A receptors, it is a D2 partial agonist with low-intrinsic activity. Aripiprazole acts as an agonist in situations of low dopamine-receptor stimulation, whereas it acts primarily as an antagonist in situations of high dopamine stimulation. Thus, aripiprazole is thought to produce its antipsychotic actions by being functionally selective *(10)*.

Anxiolytics

Anxiolytics are another frequently prescribed class of medications used in a broad spectrum of patients. The evolution of anxiolytics has seen a progression to agents with more specific pharmaco-dynamic actions in an attempt to produce a more targeted effect with a narrower side-effect profile. The classic definition of a sedative agent involves a substance that can reduce anxiety and produce a calming effect with hopefully little effect on motor skills or mental function. This blending of efficacy and toxicity in the previous definition resulted from the activity of classic anxiolytics (i.e., barbiturates and to a lesser extent benzodiazepines). Benzodiazepines produce their effects by acting as a positive allosteric modulator of the GABA type A receptor. By enhancing GABAs actions, the associated chloride ion channel is modulated to produce neuronal hyperpolarization. This leads to the therapeutic effects seen with benzodiazepines. Unfortunately, there are also a number of pharmacodynamically related side effects. As the dose of benzodiazepines increases, a range of potential therapeutic uses (i.e., sedative, anxiolytic, hypnotic, anticonvulsant, and muscle relaxant) are possible; however, a variety of potential side effects (e.g., drowsiness, impaired judgment, diminished motor skills, lethargy) can also occur. Thus, although benzodiazepines are effective anxiolytics (and hypnotics), the side-effect profile and abuse potential of these agents seriously limit the utility of benzodiazepines *(6,8)*.

Despite the common use of benzodiazepines, there remains a great need for safe and effective anxiolytics and hypnotics. Buspirone, a 5HT1A partial agonist, was created to be an anxiolytic without the drawbacks of benzodiazepines. The mechanistic differences associated with buspirone has led to a somewhat effective anxiolytic that has a delayed onset of action (more analogous to that of antidepressants); a lack of hypnotic, anticonvulsant, or muscle relaxant properties; and a reduced potential for abuse. Similarly, zolpidem and zaleplon were designed to act as hypnotic agents without the drawbacks of benzodiazepines. The more selective receptor activity of these agents (i.e., specificity for benzodiazepine type 1 receptor instead of activity at benzodiazepine type 1 and type 2 receptor) and their short half-life has created effective hypnotic medications with fewer effects on cognition and motor function *(6,8)*.

SIDE EFFECTS

Effects of Psychotropic Medications on Seizure Threshold

Reports of epileptic seizures exist for almost all psychotropic medications. Thus, the potential of psychotropic medications to provoke epileptic seizures is a common concern among providers. Whereas all classes of psychotropic medications have been implicated, antidepressants and antipsychotics are the psychotropics of most concern. In a review of psychotropic medications and their ability to produce seizures, Pisani and colleagues *(11)* reported that seizure incidence rates, derived from large investigations, have ranged from 0.1 to 1.5% in patients treated with therapeutic doses of common antidepressants and antipsychotics. In comparison, the authors noted that the incidence of the first unprovoked seizure in the general population is 0.07 to 0.09%. The authors concluded that the antidepressants maprotiline, clomipramine, and bupropion and the antipsychotics chlorpromazine and clozapine had a relatively high seizure potential. On the other hand, fluoxetine, paroxetine, sertraline, venlafaxine, fluphenazine, haloperidol, and risperidone were reported to have a relatively low seizure risk. Other investigators consider antidepressants such as amitriptyline, nortriptyline, imipramine, and desipramine to have an intermediate likelihood of seizures as an adverse effect. Interestingly, monoamine oxidase inhibitors (MAOIs) such as phenelzine and tranylcypromine have been considered to have anticonvulsant activity *(12)*.

Medication dose is an important consideration when examining the seizure potential of psychotropic agents. In patients who have taken an overdose of psychotropic medications, the reported incidence of seizures has ranged from 4 to 30% *(11)*. Whereas the variability in results likely reflects methodological differences among studies, the dose-dependent phenomenon of this adverse effect is clear. Bupropion and imipramine are medications with apparent dose-dependent seizure risk. For example, the seizure incidence in patients receiving bupropion is reported to be as high as 0.9% in doses greater than 450 mg per day and less than 0.1% in lower doses. Furthermore, the incidence of seizures with imipramine at daily doses of 200 mg or less has been reported to be 0.1 and 0.6% at daily doses above 200 mg *(11)*.

The relationship between psychotropics and epileptic seizures is more complicated than merely avoiding the use of certain antidepressants or antipsychotics in patients with psychiatric illness. For example, seizure potential might need to be addressed in patients with psychiatric disorders treated with therapeutic doses of psychotropic medications, in patients diagnosed with epilepsy and concomitant psychiatric disorders, in patients with an inherited low seizure threshold, in drug toxicity situations, and in pathological conditions such as neuroleptic malignant syndrome. Therefore, although evidence demonstrates the ability of some psychotropic medications to lower the seizure threshold, clinicians must account for both drug- and patient-related factors when prescribing psychotropic medications, especially antidepressants and antipsychotics. Specifically, each individual's seizure susceptibility should be considered. For example, the presence of "seizurogenic" conditions such as epilepsy, brain damage, or febrile convulsions should be gauged. In terms of drug-related factors, it is necessary to look beyond merely the intrinsic seizure potential of a medication. The use of high doses, rapid-dose escalations, sudden discontinuations, and combinations of psychotropic medications should be considered when trying to minimize the risk of epileptic seizures *(11)*. Furthermore, a psychotropic medication's seizure risk within the context of the benefits of associated with treatment when determining the need, intensity, and duration of therapy.

Other Neurological Effects of Psychotropic Medications

Antipsychotics

As previously discussed, the ability of antipsychotics to block D2 receptors in the central nervous system (CNS) is thought to be a critical component of these agents' mechanism of action. Dopamine blockade, however, is also thought cause a number of neurological side effects of antipsychotics including acute dystonia, parkinsonism, akathisia, tardive dyskinesia (TD), and neuroleptic malignant syndrome.

ACUTE DYSTONIA

Acute dystonic reactions that develop in conjunction with the use of antipsychotic medications result in a muscle contraction or spasm. It is hypothesized that a hypercholinergic state, resulting from dopamine blockade, is responsible for antipsychotic-induced dystonia. The frequency of this antipsychotic-induced side effect has been reported to range from 2 to 12% of patients taking conventional antipsychotic medications. Antipsychotic-induced acute dystonia most frequently results in torticollis, glossal dystonia, trismus, and oculogyric crisis. High doses and abrupt dose escalations of high-potency conventional antipsychotics appear to be the most important risk factors for the development of a dystonic reaction. Acute dystonia is considerably less likely to occur with atypical antipsychotic medications (i.e., less than 5% of individuals).

Although antipsychotic-induced acute dystonia typically subsides within hours after onset, the intense distress experienced by patients requires treatment. The standard approach to treatment is the immediate administration of an anticholinergic or antihistaminic agent (orally, intramuscularly, or intravenously). In refractory severe cases, an intramuscular or intravenous anticholinergic or antihistaminic can be used at more frequent dosing intervals. Intramuscular benzodiazepines, such as lorazepam, may also be administered *(4,13,14)*.

PARKINSONISM

Parkinsonian-like symptoms can develop in association with the use of an antipsychotic medication as a result of postsynaptic (D2) receptor blockade in the corpus striatum. Symptoms (i.e., tremor, muscle rigidity, and akinesia) may develop at any time but generally manifest 2 to 4 weeks after antipsychotic initiation. The clinical presentation of drug-induced parkinsonism is indistinguishable from Parkinson's disease, although drug-induced parkinsonism is more likely to be symmetric and less likely to be associated with tremor *(14)*. The incidence of "clinically significant" parkinsonism with conventional antipsychotics is 10 to 15%. Rates of parkinsonism induced by atypical antipsychotics are considerably lower. Achieving a balance of dopaminergic blockade to achieve therapeutic efficacy while minimizing parkinsonian-like side effects is important. Using positron emission tomography and other technologies, the relationship between D2 receptor blockade in the basal ganglia with antipsychotic efficacy and antipsychotic-induced parkinsonism has been examined. Clinically effective doses of conventional antipsychotics have been shown to block 70–90% of D2 receptors in the basal ganglia. Furthermore, with conventional agents at least 60% occupancy is needed for satisfactory antipsychotic response but parkinsonism tends to occur with 80% or greater occupancy of the D2 receptors *(13,14)*. The lower affinity and/or rapid dissociation from the D2 receptor (except for aripiprazole) seen with atypical antipsychotics at recommended dosages and the serotonergic blockade seen with these medications are believed to lead to the reduced risk of antipsychotic-induced parkinsonism *(4)*.

The signs and symptoms of antipsychotic-induced parkinsonism typically improve by reducing the antipsychotic dose, discontinuing the antipsychotic, switching to an atypical antipsychotic in patients previously receiving a conventional antipsychotic, or switching from the offending atypical antipsychotic to another atypical antipsychotic. Improvement is also seen with the addition of anti-parkinsonian agents. The lower incidence of extrapyramidal symptoms associated with atypical antipsychotics compared to that of conventional agents represents a substantial side-effect advantage *(5)*.

Akathisia

Antipsychotic-induced acute akathisia is a relatively common side effect of antipsychotic treatment. Akathisia tends to occur within the first 4 weeks of initiating or increasing the dose of antipsychotic medication. It is estimated to occur in 20 to 75% of all patients treated with conventional antipsychotics. Although atypical antipsychotics are less likely to cause akathisia compared to typical agents, prevalence rates have varied. The subjective feelings of restlessness and the intensely unpleasant need to move that may occur secondary to antipsychotic treatment is problematic and bothersome to patients. Unfortunately, akathisia can be mistaken for worsening psychosis rather than a medication side effect, a mistake that may lead to a worsening of akathisia as a result of treating presumed psychotic symptoms rather than side effects *(4)*.

The pathophysiological mechanism of akathisia remains unknown; however, a number of hypotheses have been proposed including dopamine blockade in the mesocortical system, excessive noradrenergic activity, and abnormal serotonergic activity. The variety and uncertainty regarding the mechanism of akathisia may result in difficulties when treating akathisia. The best initial approach is to try and reduce the chance of developing akathisia by minimizing the dosage of antipsychotic medication. The use of atypical antipsychotics is important as a result of their lower risk of akathisia. Consideration may also be given to prescribing an antiakathisic medication. A number of agents have been reported to be effective, including β-adrenergic blockers, anticholinergic drugs, benzodiazepines, and clonidine; although a lipophilic β-blocker such as propranolol appears to be the best choice *(4)*.

Tardive Dyskinesia

Antipsychotic-induced TD is a syndrome consisting of abnormal, involuntary movements caused by long-term treatment with antipsychotic medication. The movements are typically choreoathetoid in nature and principally involve the mouth, face, limbs, and trunk. TD, by definition, occurs late in the course of drug treatment. The etiology and pathophysiology are unclear, although it is thought that several separate neurotransmitter systems are involved in the pathogenesis of TD. What is clear regarding TD is its seriousness and relationship with conventional antipsychotics *(15)*. Yassa and Jeste *(16)* reviewed 76 studies of the prevalence of TD published from 1960 to 1990. In a population of approx 40,000 patients, the overall prevalence of TD was 24.2%, although it was much higher (about 50%) in studies of elderly patients treated with antipsychotics. In comparison with the risk that antipsychotic type and age place on developing TD, other risk factors are relatively unclear. Additional potential risk factors that have been reported include gender, presence of mood disorders, ethnicity, diagnosis of diabetes mellitus, existing dementia, and total exposure to antipsychotics.

TD may occur at any age and typically has an insidious onset. It may develop during exposure to antipsychotic medication or within 4 weeks of withdrawal from an oral antipsychotic (or within 8 weeks of withdrawal from a depot antipsychotic). There must be a history of at least 3 months of antipsychotic use (or 1 month in the elderly) before TD may be diagnosed (4). In terms of the course of TD, one-third of patients with TD experience remission within 3 months of discontinuation of antipsychotic medication, and approximately half have remission within 12 to 18 months of antipsychotic discontinuation (4). When TD patients must be maintained with antipsychotics, TD seems to be stable in 50%, worsen in 25%, and improve in the rest. Another related dyskinesia is a withdrawal dyskinesia following abrupt discontinuation of antipsychotics. This is most likely experienced when switching patients from conventional to atypical antipsychotics. Withdrawal dyskinesia can occur in the form of a new movement disorder or a worsened existing disorder (14).

No consistently reliable therapy for TD currently exists. As a result, the clinician must focus efforts toward prevention of the disorder. The use of atypical antipsychotics is recommended due to their lower risk of TD. A number of investigations have demonstrated a lower risk of developing TD with the use of atypical antipsychotics (i.e., clozapine, risperidone, olanzapine, quetiapine) than that of conventional antipsychotics (15). Regardless of antipsychotic type, antipsychotic use should be minimized in all patients. Patients with nonpsychotic mood or other disorders who need antipsychotics should receive the minimum necessary amount of antipsychotic treatment and should have the medication tapered and then stopped once the clinical need is no longer present. In general, there must be enough clinical evidence to show that the benefits of treatment outweigh the potential risks of side effects (5).

A number of experimental studies have attempted to treat TD with alternative strategies. Agents such as vitamin E, diltiazem, verapamil, nifedipine, clonazepam, and melatonin have been studied with mixed or unimpressive results. Although the results are far from conclusive, vitamin E remains a reasonably safe treatment modality for a patient with recently diagnosed TD (17).

Neuroleptic Malignant Syndrome

Neuroleptic malignant syndrome (NMS) is a potentially fatal reaction to antipsychotic medications that is characterized by muscle rigidity, fever, autonomic instability, and changes in level of consciousness. A clear understanding of the frequency of NMS is unclear; however, a number of retrospective and prospective studies have found between 0.02 and 3.2% of patients treated with antipsychotics develop NMS. This syndrome usually presents in the first month of antipsychotic treatment but may develop at any time. Two-thirds of the cases manifest within the first week of treatment.

The pathophysiological mechanism of NMS remains unclear. Nevertheless, a popular hypothesis involves reduced dopaminergic activity secondary to antipsychotic-induced dopamine blockade. This reduced dopamine activity in different parts of the brain (hypothalamus, nigrostriatal system, and corticolimbic tracts) may serve to explain the various clinical features of NMS. Nevertheless, the dopaminergic-blocking theory does not adequately explain all of the important aspects of NMS. The dopaminergic-blocking theory is, however, supported when considering antipsychotic-related risk factors. Higher doses of antipsychotic, rapid increases in dosage, and intramuscular injections of high-potency conventional agents (e.g., haloperidol and fluphenazine) have been reported to be risk factors for NMS. NMS can occur (but rarely) in patients prescribed atypical antipsychotics. A review of atypical antipsychotic-induced NMS concluded that symptoms appear similar to NMS induced by conventional antipsychotics (18).

In terms of treating NMS, the most critical step is to recognize the clinical features of the syndrome and rapidly discontinue the antipsychotic. Once the antipsychotic has been stopped, supportive care remains the foundation of treatment (5). At present, the appropriate course is to begin with antipsychotic discontinuation and supportive care and to consider antidote therapy only if improvement in symptoms is not seen within the first few days.

Mood Stabilizers

The use of traditional anticonvulsant medications as mood stabilizers is common in psychiatry. Unfortunately, commonly used mood stabilizers such as carbamazepine, valproic acid, and lithium can cause a variety of neurological side effects. Carbamazepine has a number of fairly common neurological side effects such as drowsiness, vertigo, diplopia, ataxia, and blurred vision. When such side effects occur during dose titrations, the rate of dose escalation can be slowed in order to reduce potential side effects. In addition, neurological side effects experienced during stable dosage periods may necessitate a dosage reduction of carbamazepine. Confusion has also been reported with carbamazepine use, although it does not appear to have as great an effect on memory or other cognitive functions as some older antiepileptic medications *(5)*.

Sedation is a common and problematic side effect of valproic acid (VA) and related medications (i.e., divalproex sodium, sodium valproate). Hand tremor has been reported as the most common long-term neurological side effect. Dose reduction of VA, if feasible, represents a successful method to reduce both sedation and tremor. Ataxia has been noted with higher doses of VA. Asterixis, stupor, coma, and behavioral stereotypies have been rarely reported, usually in association with medication toxicity *(5)*.

Lithium has been associated with a number of neurological side effects, effects that vary in terms of likelihood, severity, duration of therapy, and medication dose. Mild neurological side effects such as lethargy, fatigue, weakness, and action tremor can be seen at the start of therapy, during periods of dose escalation, or at times of peak daily levels during chronic, stable therapy. The tremor is similar to essential tremor rather than the pill-rolling tremor associated with Parkinson's disease. Reduction of lithium dose, limitation of caffeine intake, reduction in anxiety, or addition of a β-blocker such as propranolol, represent potential treatments. In a small number of patients, lithium may cause EPS or worsen antipsychotic-induced EPS. The presence of new neurological symptoms or worsening existing minor neurological symptoms should make clinicians consider the possibility of lithium toxicity, especially because of lithium's narrow therapeutic window. Moderate to severe neurological symptoms, including neuromuscular irritability, ataxia, coarsening of tremor, dysarthria, incoordination, visual disturbances, and mental cloudiness can be experienced at lithium levels only somewhat higher than therapeutic serum concentrations. Severe neurological toxicity with lithium can lead to ataxia, seizures, hallucinations, delirium, coma, and death *(5)*.

A number of other anticonvulsant medications, with varying levels of supporting evidence, are used as mood stabilizers. Many of these agents also have neurological side effects. Lamotrigine, for instance, has been associated with diplopia, ataxia, and blurred vision. Topiramate has been reported to cause sedation, dizziness, ataxia, and paresthesias *(5)*.

Antidepressants

Antidepressant drug therapy has been associated with a variety of neurological side effects such as tremor, akathisia, myoclonus, dyskinesias, and delirium. The risk of such neurological side effects varies among individual antidepressant medications but is generally uncommon. The ability of antidepressants to cause some neurological effects can often be predicted based on antidepressant mechanism of action. Possible clinical consequences of the reuptake inhibition of norepinephrine and dopamine are tremors and psychomotor activation, respectively. Therefore, agents with relatively potent activity at these sites such as TCAs (e.g., desipramine, imipramine) and bupropion may be expected to potentially cause the previously mentioned neurological side effects. Potent blockade of serotonin reuptake is associated with EPS. For this reason, SSRIs such as paroxetine and sertraline may cause EPS. Other potential neurological effects of antidepressants may be pharmacodynamically related. For instance, muscarinic cholinergic antagonists such as imipramine, desipramine, and paroxetine can lead to memory disturbances and blockade of H1 receptors by agents such as mirtazapine and TCAs may lead to sedation and drowsiness *(19)*.

In addition to the neurological side effects of antidepressants that may be experienced under common therapeutic conditions, serotonin syndrome, a condition usually related to intentional or unintentional overdose is also an important therapy consideration. Serotonin syndrome is a condition associated with increased serotonergic stimulation in the presence of medications that elevate serotonin levels. Neurological symptoms include confusion, myoclonus, tremor, and incoordination. This serious and potentially life-threatening syndrome can result from the combination of SSRIs with other serotonergic medications such as TCAs, meperidine, buspirone, dextromethorphan, and MAOIs. Because of this potential for toxicity, a number of medication combinations with additive serotonergic effects are contraindicated or only used in situations with adequate monitoring and follow-up *(19)*.

Other Psychotropics

Benzodiazepines may also cause neurological side effects. In addition to fatigue and drowsiness, these agents can cause motor incoordination and cognitive impairment, including memory and recall deficits. Transient anterograde amnesia, which may or may not be desirable depending on the intended use, is also associated with benzodiazepine use.

Non-Neurological Side Effects of Psychotropic Medications

Sexual Dysfunction

Sexual dysfunction is frequently reported in the general population and in those with psychiatric disorders. Sexual dysfunction is a complex disorder with a variety of influencing factors such as age, gender, mood, general health, and medications. Lifestyle factors such as smoking, alcohol, and obesity, common problems among persons with psychiatric illness, may also negatively impact sexual function. Whereas a variety of lifestyle factors exist that may influence sexual function, medications, especially some psychotropics, have been implicated in sexual dysfunction. Conventional antipsychotics, anticonvulsants, and antidepressants have been reported to cause sexual dysfunction to varying degrees. The mechanism of sexual dysfunction with psychotropic medications can be direct or indirect. For instance, sexual dysfunction noted with conventional antipsychotics is thought to be related to hyperprolactinemia, a secondary effect of central dopamine receptor blockade. Another example of secondary sexual dysfunction is that an improvement in depressive symptoms following antidepressant therapy may unmask a pre-existing sexual dysfunction as a result of an increase in patient expectations. In contrast, the prescription of SSRIs may worsen existing or cause sexual dysfunction as a consequence of alterations in serotonin in the CNS (i.e., spinal reflexes) *(20)*.

Antidepressants, especially those with primarily serotonergic activity, have been reported to cause sexual dysfunction more frequently (e.g., 25–65%) than other psychotropic medications. Unaddressed sexual dysfunction can severely hamper medication adherence, therapeutic alliance, and treatment outcomes. In the presence of antidepressant-induced sexual dysfunction, the most prudent treatment options include dosage adjustments, antidepressant medication changes, or the addition or substitution of existing therapy with bupropion, nefazodone, or mirtazapine. Although these three antidepressants possess their own drawbacks, all have been associated with lower rates of sexual dysfunction. A variety of other treatment modalities have been examined (e.g., yohimbine, sildenafil, ginkgo biloba, granisetron, amantadine) but with a variety of results, many not positive *(20)*.

Weight Gain

For a long time, weight gain has been a recognized side effect of psychotropic medications. Traditionally, attention was focused on the changes in weight experienced with anticonvulsants and antidepressants. More recently, substantial attention has been directed toward the growing evidence surrounding weight gain associated with second-generation antipsychotics. Regardless of psychotropic type, any chronic medication with the ability to cause substantial increases in weight should catch the attention of clinicians. Overweight patients are at risk for coronary heart disease, hypertension, dyslipidemia, some types of cancer, decreased quality of life, and reduced adherence to the offending medication.

A variety of psychotropics have been linked to weight gain; however, elucidating the causative role of individual agents and determining clinical significance can be complicated. For example, weight loss and anorexia are symptoms of depression, symptoms that must be accounted for when trying to obtain a clear understanding of whether, with antidepressant therapy, weight gain can be accounted for by recovery from depression or extra weight gain. Accounting for this important consideration, a number of more recent studies have contradicted previous investigations by reporting that SSRIs may not be associated with significantly greater weight gain when compared to placebo. Nonetheless, weight gain among antidepressants appears to vary. For instance, the considerable histamine-blocking activity of mirtazapine is believed to account for this agent's association with weight gain, whereas venlafaxine and bupropion have been occasionally associated with weight loss. The ability of antidepressants to cause weight gain can be conceptualized (from highest to lowest): mirtazapine > TCAs and MAOIs > SSRIs > bupropion, nefazodone, and venlafaxine *(20)*.

Weight gain and obesity have been noted to be more common in patients with schizophrenia than the general population prior to the development of atypical antipsychotics. Nonetheless, weight gain appears to be more substantial with the use of particular atypical antipsychotics, especially clozapine and olanzapine. Antipsychotic-associated weight gain appears to stem from an increase in body fat as a result of increased appetite and food intake. It is hypothesized that central H1 receptor antagonism is responsible for weight gain. In addition, the 5HT2C receptor antagonism of atypical antipsychotics may cause weight gain synergistically by creating hyperphagia. Although a lot of attention has been paid to the ability of atypical antipsychotics to cause weight gain, there do appear to be differences among individual agents. Based on a number of studies, the weight-gain potential appears to be (from lowest to highest) ziprasidone, aripiprazole < risperidone, quetiapine < clozapine and olanzapine *(21)*.

Diabetes

The relationship among diabetes, schizophrenia, and antipsychotic medications is not a new topic. For decades, suggestions that schizophrenia patients were at an increased risk for diabetes have existed. The relationship between diabetes and schizophrenia is clouded by a number of confounding factors such as poor diet, physical inactivity, and obesity. In addition, there have been previous suggestions that antipsychotic medications may lead to glucose intolerance or diabetes. This variety of evidence has led to the belief that the prevalence of type 2 diabetes is approximately two to three times greater in patients with schizophrenia than that of the general population *(21)*. Furthermore, there appears to be a greater risk for diabetes with certain atypical antipsychotics. Atypical antipsychotics, especially clozapine and olanzapine, have been associated with an increased risk of new-onset type 2 diabetes or diabetic ketoacidosis. Ample evidence exists to displace previous suggestions that antipsychotics merely worsen existing diabetes via weight gain. Jin and colleagues *(22)* reviewed the published cases of new-onset diabetes, ketoacidosis, and non-ketotic hyperosmolar coma for atypical antipsychotics. Forty-two percent of cases presented with diabetic ketoacidosis and 84% presented with glucose intolerance within 6 months of initiating antipsychotic therapy. Whereas the majority of patients were overweight, 50% of patients had not experienced any weight gain while prescribed the offending medication. Despite the relative rarity of new-onset diabetes or ketoacidosis associated with antipsychotics, the seriousness and potential long-term outcomes of diabetes warrants proactive care. The Food and Drug Administration, after reviewing the available data, recommended that all manufacturers of atypical antipsychotics include warnings in the prescribing information about the possibility of hyperglycemia, diabetes, and associated consequences. The American Diabetes Association has recommended baseline assessment and follow-up monitoring of serum glucose when starting patients on atypical antipsychotics *(23)*. Recommendations for baseline and follow-up monitoring of weight and cholesterol accompany the glucose monitoring guidelines. Although there is a relationship between atypical antipsychotics and diabetes, the mechanism of action for this relationship is unclear. It appears that more than mere insulin resistance is involved because the development of ketoacidosis usually requires impaired β-cell function and severe insulin deficiency. In addition to antipsychotics causing insulin resistance, it has been proposed that atypical antipsychotics' effect on serotonin and serotonin's effect on β-cell function may be implicated in the development of diabetes and diabetic ketoacidosis.

PSYCHIATRIC SYMPTOMS WITH COMMON SOMATIC MEDICATIONS

Psychiatric side effects of medications prescribed to treat somatic illnesses are not uncommon. Medications used to treat various medical conditions are often reported to cause psychiatric symptoms, but these symptoms are not always well characterized. Descriptions in the literature about the CNS effects of somatic medications include mood disturbances (anxiety, depression, mania), perceptual disturbances (hallucinations, delusions), cognitive disturbances (delirium, confusion, dementia), and behavioral disturbances (agitation, insomnia) *(24–27)*. Such effects have been reported to occur in a variety of situations including at therapy initiation, during chronic therapy, during medication dose changes, at therapeutic doses, and at high medication doses *(25)*.

Certain patient populations have been identified to be at higher risk for developing drug-induced psychiatric disorders. These include patients with a history of organic brain disease, underlying dementia, or a history of mental illness, and elderly patients *(25,26)*. Although there are limited data concerning the psychiatric side effects of somatic medications, certain agents have been described more thoroughly in the literature.

Corticosteroids

Corticosteroids (e.g., prednisone, dexamethasone) are routinely prescribed medications for the management of allergic and immunological disorders. These agents are known to cause a number of serious systemic adverse effects including psychiatric side effects. Psychiatric symptoms such as mania and psychosis have been described in the literature *(27–29)*. In patients receiving prednisone for the management of systemic lupus erythematosus, the incidence of psychiatric side effects has been reported to be up to 57% *(29)*. Although the corticosteroid most frequently implicated in the literature to cause such symptoms is oral prednisone, other corticosteroids including inhaled formulations have been associated with psychiatric symptoms *(29)*. Whereas the exact dose and duration of corticosteroid therapy responsible for causing psychiatric symptoms has not been defined, the risk of these effects appears to increase with higher corticosteroid doses. The Boston Collaborative Drug Surveillance Program reported a direct dose and effect relationship between prednisone and psychiatric side effects. The incidence was reported to be 1.3, 6, and 18.4% in patients receiving prednisone doses of 40 mg or less per day, 41 mg to 80 mg per day, and 80 mg or more per day, respectively *(29)*. Smaller studies have reported mania in up to 26% of patients taking 80 mg of prednisone per day for 5 days *(28)*. Brown and colleagues described significant mood changes, particularly symptoms of mania, in asthma patients receiving short bursts of prednisone (40 mg for an average of 5 days) *(27)*. In all cases, symptoms resolved after therapy discontinuation.

Antibiotics

Antibiotics are a commonly prescribed group of medications with potential effects on the CNS. Since their introduction, psychiatric side effects including depression, psychosis, and delirium have been reported. Sternbach and colleagues *(30)* conducted a scholarly review of the neuropsychiatric effects of specific antibiotic classes. The following is a summary of their findings.

Psychosis during therapy with the combination of sulfamethoxazole and sulfamethorazol and "trimethoprin," a commonly used sulfonamide agent, has been reported. The onset of symptoms usually occurred 3 to 10 days after therapy initiation. Symptoms included confusion, disorientation, euphoria, depression, and hallucinations. It has been suggested that the degree of psychiatric manifestations may depend on the patient's pretreatment state. The mechanism of this effect is unknown.

β-Lactam antibiotics, including the penicillins, cephalosporins, and monobactams have all been associated with psychiatric side effects. The penicillins are the oldest generation of β-lactams and most penicillins have been associated with neurotoxicity. Possible risk factors for developing neurotoxicity include advanced age, impaired renal function, and route of administration. Hoigne's syndrome is a collection of psychiatric symptoms that have been described in patients receiving procaine penicillin, an intramuscular form of penicillin. This syndrome consists of a sudden onset of apprehension, fear of imminent death, excitation, agitation, or hallucinations. This syndrome has been described in both adult and pediatric patients with a rapid onset and usually a spontaneous resolution. Although the exact mechanism of this syndrome is unknown, it has been hypothesized that procaine penicillin's role as a prostaglandin antagonist or procaine induced limbic kindling may play a role. Other agents in the penicillin class have also exhibited psychiatric reactions to a lesser extent, particularly in patients with impaired renal function (30). Psychiatric side effects with the cephalosporins, although rare, have been reported. These cases primarily involved patients with underlying renal dysfunction. Symptoms included euphoria, hyperreactivity, delusions, depersonalization, and visual hallucinations. A postulated mechanism for this effect involves cephalosporin-mediated inhibition of GABA activity (30).

Isoniazid and cylcoserine, agents used to treat tuberculosis, have both been associated with significant CNS stimulatory effects. Psychosis has been reported with isoniazid therapy and agitated depression and personality changes have been observed with cycloserine therapy. The onset of activity has been reported to range from 2 weeks to 8 months from the start of therapy (30).

CNS effects related to fluoroquinolone antibiotics are reported to occur in approx 1–4% of patients. Symptoms such as hallucinations, depression, and severe confusion have been described. Although such effects have been reported with most of the fluoroquinolones, ofloxacin has been implicated frequently in the literature as the cause of significant psychiatric effects. Hall and colleagues (31) described cases of ofloxacin-induced psychiatric side effects after patients received doses of ofloxacin 400 mg twice daily. Symptoms, including altered cognition and delusions, occurred within 12 hours of taking the first dose and resolved immediately after medication discontinuation. The antagonistic effect of fluoroquinolones on GABA receptor binding has been proposed as a possible mechanism (30,31).

Metronidazole, an antibiotic used in the treatment of anaerobic infections, has been implicated in causing depression, insomnia, and feelings of estrangement. In patients with underlying psychiatric disease, metronidazole has been shown to worsen pre-existing hallucinations and delusions (30).

Psychiatric side effects with the use of the macrolide antibiotics have also been reported, although the mechanism for this remains unknown. Risk factors include advanced age, renal or hepatic dysfunction, concomitant disease states, low body weight, and high medication doses. Psychiatric symptoms reported with erythromycin include nightmares, confusion, abnormal thinking, and labile mood. Acute psychosis in patients with advanced AIDS receiving high-dose clarithromycin for the treatment of *Mycobacterium avium complex* infection has also been reported (30).

Interferons

Interferons (IFNs) possess both antiviral and antitumor properties. With the increased use of IFNs for the treatment of multiple medical conditions, there are growing concerns regarding the psychiatric side effects of these agents. Psychiatric side effects of IFN therapy have been reported to occur shortly after therapy initiation or later during continued treatment (32,33). Memory loss, depression, cognitive slowing, acute delirium, visual and auditory hallucinations, delusions, feelings of personal inadequacy, and a reduction in goal-directed behavior are some of the reported side effects. The majority of these effects occurred in elderly patients receiving higher doses of drug, although case reports have identified patients of all ages (32,33). In a minority of patients, IFN therapy results in confusion, lethargy, impaired mental state, depression, mania, and suicidal tendencies. Trask and colleagues (32) reported a prevalence rate of psychiatric side effects that ranged from 0 to 70% and identified risk factors such as increased IFN dose, severity of disease, and prolonged length of IFN treatment. Although the exact mechanism of action is unknown, several mechanisms have been hypothesized and include IFN's effects on the neurotransmitters dopamine, serotonin, and norepinephrine; IFN's effects on endogenous opioid systems; and IFN's effects on the thyroid (32).

Nonsteroidal Anti-Inflammatory Drugs

Nonsteroidal anti-inflammatory medications (NSAIDs) are widely used to treat pain and inflammation. Psychiatric symptoms, although frequently reported in the prescribing information of such agents, have seldom been studied or reported systematically. Additionally, information regarding psychiatric adverse effects comes from very limited data. Anecdotal reports of paranoid psychosis (sulindac, ibuprofen), depression (sulindac, ibuprofen), mania (tolmetin), and paranoid ideation (naproxen) have been described in the literature *(34)*. Perhaps most noted are the psychiatric effects observed with indomethacin. A retrospective study of psychiatric reactions following the administration of indomethacin to postpartum women suggested that side effects most often occurred within 1 hour of a 100 mg dose administered rectally. Dizziness, agitation, anxiety, and fear were among the highest reported adverse effects. More severe but less common effects included hallucinations, fear of dying, and depersonalization. Proposed mechanisms for such side effects include the structural similarity of indomethacin and serotonin and an increased sensitivity to dopamine exacerbated by prostaglandin inhibition *(35)*. Limited data also suggest that the NSAIDs diclofenac, ibuprofen, and naproxen can induce or exacerbate depressed or paranoid symptoms including if used in patients with underlying psychiatric disease *(34)*.

Other Medications

Many other somatic medications have been implicated in causing psychiatric symptoms. Antihistamines used to treat acid reflux (i.e., histamine type-2 receptor antagonists) such as cimetidine and ranitidine have been associated with confusion, delirium, depression, hallucinations, and mania. The incidence of such effects has been reported to be higher in the elderly, patients who are seriously ill, and those with underlying hepatic or renal insufficiency. Symptoms have occurred anywhere from 24 hours to weeks after therapy initiation and usually subside within days after therapy discontinuation *(25)*. Antihistamines administered in combination with anticholinergic agents, found frequently in over the counter allergy and cold preparations, have also been reported to cause symptoms manifesting as confusion, hallucinations, disorientation, agitation, and memory deficits *(25,36)*.

Several agents used in the management of Parkinson's disease have been implicated in causing psychiatric side effects. The psychiatric manifestations of levodopa are numerous, including but not limited to depression, hypomania, delusions, euphoria, delirium, hallucinations, and paranoid psychosis. Symptoms severe enough to warrant discontinuation of the medication occur in approx 10% of patients. The anticholinergic agent benztropine has been shown to induce confusion, and less frequently hallucinations and delirium, especially in elderly patients. Visual hallucinations have been reported in patients taking the dopamine agonists bromocriptine and pergolide with or without concomitant levodopa. Insomnia, disorientation, nervousness, and confusion have been reported with amantadine, a dopamine agonist with antiviral properties. Data suggest that these effects are more prevalent in the elderly population and at higher doses but can be observed in adults of all ages *(36)*.

Limited data along with anecdotal experience report severe CNS effects with the antiretroviral medications zidovudine and efavirenz. Mania, visual and auditory hallucinations, and confusion are among some of the psychiatric side effects reported with these agents. Investigators have suggested that the effects with zidovudine are idiosyncratic, whereas the effects observed with efavirenz are related to plasma concentrations *(37–40)*.

CONCLUSION

Psychotropic medications, as a group, offer an array of pharmacological options for the treatment of a number of medical disorders. Unfortunately a range of side effects including neurological, non-neurological, minor, severe, acute, and long term are associated with the use of these agents. Understanding and applying pharmacodynamic aspects of psychotropic medications can assist with the rational use of these medications, which may result in improved patient outcomes. Additionally, a wide variety of somatic medications may cause psychiatric side effects. The ability of somatic medications to cause such effects should be considered when diagnosing and treating psychiatric manifestations.

REFERENCES

1. Ketter TA, Wang PW, Becker OV, Nowakowska C, Yang Y. The diverse roles of anticonvulsants in bipolar disorders. Ann Clin Psychiatry. 2003;15:95–108.
2. Krystal JH, Sanacora G, Blumberg G, et al. Glutamate and GABA systems as targets for novel antidepressant and mood-stabilizing treatments. Mol Psychiatry. 2002;7(Suppl 1):S71–S80.
3. Stahl SM. Tiagabine and other anticonvulsants with action on GABA. J Clin Psychiatry 2004;65:291–292.
4. American Psychiatric Association. Diagnostic and Statistical Manual of Mental Disorders, Fourth Edition, revision. Washington DC: American Psychiatric Association; 2000.
5. Arana GW, Rosenbaum JF. Handbook of Psychiatric Drug Therapy, Fourth Edition. Philadelphia, PA: Lippincott Williams & Wilkins; 2000.
6. Katzung BG. Basic and Clinical Pharmacology, Ninth Edition. New York: McGraw-Hill; 2003.
7. Evins AE. Efficacy of newer anticonvulsant medications in bipolar spectrum mood disorders. J Clin Psychiatry 2003; 64(Suppl 8):9–14.
8. Stahl SM, Muntner N. Essential Psychopharmacology, Second Edition. New York: Cambridge University Press; 2000.
9. Seeman P. Atypical antipsychotics: mechanism of action. Can J Psychiatry 2002;47:27–38.
10. Gründer G, Carlsson A, Wong DF. Mechanism of new antipsychotic medications. Arch Gen Psychiatry 2003;60:974–977.
11. Pisani F, Oteri G, Costa C, Di Raimondo G, Di Perri R. Effects of psychotropic drugs on seizure threshold. Drug Saf 2002;25:91–110.
12. Baldessarini RJ. Current status of antidepressants: clinical pharmacology and therapy. J Clin Psychiatry 1989;50:117–126.
13. Tarsy D, Baldessarini RJ, Tarazi FI. Effects of newer antipsychotics on extrapyramidal function. CNS Drugs 2002;16: 23–45.
14. Blanchet PJ. Antipsychotic drug-induced movement disorders. Can J Neurol Sci 2003;30(Suppl 1):S101–S107.
15. Correll CU, Leucht S, Kane JM. Lower risk of tardive dyskinesia associated with second-generation antipsychotics: a systematic review of 1-year studies. Am J Psychiatry 2004;161:414–425.
16. Yassa R, Jeste DV. Gender differences in tardive dyskinesia: a critical review of the literature. Schizophr Bull 1992;18: 701–715.
17. Simpson GM. The treatment of tardive dyskinesia and tardive dystonia. J Clin Psychiatry 2000;61(Suppl 4):39–44.
18. Hasan S, Buckley P. Novel antipsychotics and the neuroleptics malignant syndrome: a review and critique. Am J Psychiatry 1998;155:113–1116.
19. Fann JR. Neurological effects of psychopharmacological agents. Semin Clin Neuropsychiatry 2002;7:196–205.
20. Masand PS, Gupta S. Long-term side effects of newer-generation antidepressants: SSRIs, venlafaxine, nefazodone, bupropion, and mirtazapine. Ann Clin Psychiatry 2002;14:175–182.
21. Lebovitz HE. Metabolic consequences of atypical antipsychotic drugs. Psychiatr Q 2003;74:277–290.
22. Jin H, Meyer JM, Jeste DV. Phenomenology of and risk factors for new-onset diabetes mellitus and diabetic ketoacidosis associated with atypical antipsychotics: an analysis of 45 published cases. Ann Clin Psychiatry 2002;14:59–64.
23. American Diabetes Association. Consensus development conference on antipsychotic drugs and obesity and diabetes. Diabetes Care 2004;27:596–601.
24. Hubbard JR, Levenson JL, Graham PA. Psychiatric side effect associated with the ten most commonly dispensed prescription drugs: a review. J Fam Pract 1991;33:177–186.
25. Levy S, Abaza MM, Hawkshaw MJ, Sataloff RT. Psychiatric manifestations of medications commonly prescribed in otolaryngology. Ear Nose Throat J 2001;80:266–271.
26. Smith DA. Psychiatric side effects of non-psychiatric drugs. S D J Med 1991;44:291–292.
27. Brown ES, Suppes T Khan DA, Carmody TJ. Mood changes during prednisone bursts in outpatients with asthma. J Clin Psychopharmacol 2002;22:55–61.
28. Brown ES, Khan DA, Nejtek VA. The psychiatric side effects of corticosteroids. Ann Allergy Asthma Immunol 1999;83: 495–504.
29. Kershner P, Wang-Cheng R. Psychiatric side effects of steroid therapy. Psychosomatics 1989;30:135–139.
30. Sternbach H, State R. Antibiotics: neuropsychiatric effects and psychotropic interactions. Harv Rev Psychiatry 1997;5: 214–526.
31. Hall CE, Keegan H, Rogstad KE. Psychiatric side effects of ofloxacin used in the treatment of pelvic inflammatory disease. Int J STD AIDS 2003;14:636–637.
32. Trask PC, Esper P, Riba M, Redman B. Psychiatric side effects of interferon therapy: prevalence, proposed mechanism, and future directions. J Clin Oncol 2000;18:2316-2326.
33. Goeb JL, Cailleau A, Laine P, et al. Acute delirium, delusion, and depression during INF-beta-1a therapy for multiple sclerosis: a case report. Clin Neuropharmacol 2003;26:5–7.
34. Browning CH. Nonsteroidal anti-inflammatory drugs and severe psychiatric side effects. Int J Psychiatry Med 1996;26: 25–34.
35. Clunie M, Crone L, Klassen L, Yip R. Psychiatric side effects of indomethacin in parturients. Can J Anesth 2003;50:586–588.

36. Saint-Cyr JA, Taylor AE, Lang AE. Neuropsychological and psychiatric side effects in the treatment of Parkinson's disease. Neurology 1993;43(Suppl 6):S47–S52.
37. Juethner SN, Seyfried W, Aberg JA. Tolerance of efavirenz-induced central nervous system side effects in HIV-infected individuals with a history of substance abuse. HIV Clin Trials 2003;4:145–149.
38. Marzolini C, Telenti A, Decosterd LA, Greub G, Biollaz J, Buclin T. Efavirenz plasma levels can predict treatment failure and central nervous system side effects in HIV-1-infected patients. AIDS 2001;15:71–75.
39. Wright JM, Sachdev PS, Perkins RJ, Rodriguez P. Zidovudine-related mania. Med J Aust 1989;150:339–341.
40. Maxwell S, Scheftner WA, Kessler HA, Busch K. Manic syndrome associated with zidovudine treatment. JAMA 1988;259:3406–3407.

25

Electroconvulsive Therapy

Eric J. Christopher and Warren D. Taylor

INTRODUCTION

Electroconvulsive therapy (ECT) is the oldest somatic treatment still used in modern psychiatric practice, but is also laden with controversy. Although there are effective antidepressant medications, ECT continues to be widely used and may effectively treat depression in patients who have not responded to psychotherapy or medications. However, some patient advocacy groups lobby for bans on this treatment, claiming it is "inhumane" and citing possible cognitive and memory side effects. Regardless of the debate, it is an important treatment option for severely ill patients.

HISTORY OF ELECTROCONVULSIVE THERAPY

ECT is one of psychiatry's first somatic therapies, initially developed by Ladiaslas Joseph von Meduna in 1934. Von Meduna theorized that patients with epilepsy were protected from the development of psychotic symptoms seen in schizophrenia, a hypothesis eventually proven wrong. He tested his theory by using pharmacological agents to cause seizures in psychotic patients. The use of electricity to evoke seizure activity began with the experiments of Ugo Cerletti and Lucio Bini (1). Their success with ECT put it into widespread use.

ECT was the pre-eminent treatment for depression until the discovery of effective pharmacological antidepressants, at which time the use of ECT declined. This decline was further hastened by inaccurate depictions of ECT's use in the popular media not as a therapeutic treatment but rather as a means of behavioral control, such as seen in the movie *One Flew Over the Cuckoo's Nest*. Images of unwilling participants being held down and treated with resultant grand mal seizures are compelling, but it does not accurately depict the reality of modern ECT.

ECT has also been a focus of patient advocacy groups and others attempting to ban its use. Over the course of the last three decades, legislation has been introduced in many states, including Texas, California, and Vermont, attempting to either severely curtail its use or ban it entirely. ECT was briefly banned in Berkeley, California in 1983; this action was quickly overturned by the courts on the basis of it being an unwarranted local infringement of a statewide concern. Opponents often cite its effect on memory and mortality risk as two major concerns. It should be noted that the mortality risk has not been supported by careful monitoring (2–4), and others have proposed that the well-organized ECT opponents, many of whom received ECT, are so highly functional and effective that it raises questions of just how severely ECT actually does affect memory or cognition (5).

The decline of ECT's use has been gradually reversing. From 1987 to 1992, the rate of ECT use per 10,000 Medicare beneficiaries grew from 4.2 to 5.1 (6). Current estimates place ECT usage to

From: *Current Clinical Neurology: Psychiatry for Neurologists*
Edited by: D.V. Jeste and J.H. Friedman © Humana Press Inc., Totowa, NJ

be 65,000 patients, totaling 500,000 treatments per year *(7)*. Interestingly, the elderly are overrepresented in the patient population receiving ECT, which may reflect that they are at risk for more severe, anhedonic depression or a more emergent need for recovery owing to refusal to eat, suicidality, or psychosis.

INDICATIONS FOR ELECTROCONVULSIVE THERAPY

The second edition of the American Psychiatric Associations (APA) recommendations for ECT *(8)* outlines the indications for this therapy (Table 1). It is important to recognize that current recommendations identify no absolute contraindications to ECT, although there are certainly patients who are at increased risk for adverse events and so require a more intensive pre-ECT evaluation and closer monitoring. The use of ECT is an appropriate treatment for these primary indications at any time during the illness, although depression and bipolar disorder comprise the majority of illnesses treated. ECT should not be regarded as a treatment of "last resort," but as a successful and primary treatment modality in the appropriate patient.

The most common indication for ECT is major depression. ECT in depression is superior to placebo, sham or simulated ECT, and antidepressant medications as demonstrated in meta-analyses *(9,10)*. Although ECT is more effective than medications, there are limited data comparing ECT with newer antidepressant medications.

ECT is also used for other psychiatric indications, albeit less commonly. It appears to effectively treat mania, as seen in bipolar disorder *(11,12)*, with a response rate as high as 80%. It is also useful in the management of schizophrenia *(13)*, although the response rate is best in patients with schizophrenia and concomitant affective symptoms. Catatonia is particularly responsive to ECT *(14)*, even when it is secondary to medical rather than psychiatric illness. ECT's use in neurological disorders is discussed in more detail later in the chapter.

POTENTIAL MECHANISMS OF ACTION

Although the exact mechanism of how ECT results in improvement in depression is unknown, it is known that a generalized seizure is necessary to produce an antidepressant effect. One possibility is that successful ECT involves the recruitment of neurons from deep brain structures implicated in mood regulation, such as the thalamus and basal ganglia. As not all generalized seizures necessarily recruit neurons from these regions, this could also explain some variability in response.

Potential mechanisms may include the influence of ECT on neurotransmitters and their receptors, hormones and neuropeptides, and neurotrophic factors *(15)*. Evidence does not support that ECT alters brain structure *(16)*. ECT has an effect on almost every neurotransmitter system. Although this is a controversial area, ECT appears to affect the transmission of neurotransmitters thought to be involved in the pathophysiology of depression, including serotonin, dopamine, glutamate and γ-aminobutyric acid. Neuropeptide and hormone concentrations are also affected; the most consistently seen result of ECT is a substantial increase in serum prolactin levels, which return to baseline several hours after ECT. Cortisol, adrenocorticotropic hormone, thyroid-stimulating hormone, and oxytocin levels have also been shown to increase with ECT, however the extent of the increase in concentration in response to ECT may fall over a course of ECT. It is unclear how they may be related with seizure adequacy or treatment outcomes. Additionally, animal studies have demonstrated that ECT increases neurotrophic factors, such as brain-derived neurotrophic factorand nerve growth factor. This may increase neurogenesis and also enhance synaptic connectivity in regions implicated in mood regulation, including the hippocampus, amygdala, and prefrontal areas.

PRE-ECT EVALUATION AND TREATMENT

The ECT procedure is comprised of a consultation, pre-ECT evaluation, treatment or "index" course, and the decision whether to discontinue ECT and maintain remission of depression through

Table 1
Indications for Electroconvulsive Therapy

Primary diagnostic indications	Secondary diagnostic indications
Major depression	Mental disorders resulting from medical conditions
• Single episode or recurrent	• Catatonia
• Unipolar	• Delirium
• Bipolar I, depressed	Neurological disorders
• Bipolar mixed	• Status epilepticus
Mania	• Parkinson's disease
• Bipolar I, mania	• Neuroleptic malignant syndrome
• Bipolar I, mixed	
Psychotic disorders	
• Schizophrenia	
• Schizophreniform	
• Schizoaffective	

Note: Indications taken from the 2001 report from the American Psychiatric Association Task Force on Electroconvulsive Therapy *(8)*.

psychopharmacology, or to continue therapy through a maintenance phase. Consultation with a trained ECT provider is the first step.

Directed laboratory testing as determined by a treating psychiatrist and anesthesia provider is necessary prior to ECT. The current recommendations *(8)* specify that a minimum battery would include a complete blood count, measurement of serum electrolytes, and an electrocardiogram. Recent data evaluating the validity of this approach proved it to be sound *(17)*. Neuroimaging (either computed tomography or magnetic resonance imaging) or electroencephalography may be warranted where there is a suspicion of neurological disease. A chest x-ray is often included in this evaluation, but this should depend on the clinical situation and physical examination.

CONCOMITANT MEDICATIONS

The patient's medication regimen should be carefully evaluated as part of the pre-ECT evaluation. Particular focus should be paid to medications that affect, either positively or negatively, the seizure threshold. This is of particular importance given the role of anticonvulsants in the treatment of bipolar disorder. The use of most antidepressants and some antipsychotics are generally thought to be acceptable, although most antipsychotics can lower the seizure threshold to varying degrees.

There are several agents commonly used in psychiatry that raise particular concerns. Lithium is known to increase the risk of post-ictal delirium, as well as prolonging seizure activity. Some agents, such as bupropion (Wellbutrin) and clozapine (Clozaril) significantly lower the seizure threshold. Benzodiazepines, which increase the seizure threshold, may also be problematic, however, in some instances their use is continued with the effects reversed using the benzodiazepine receptor antagonist flumazenil *(18)*. It is unclear if this strategy has any effect on ECT outcomes.

ELECTROCONVULSIVE THERAPY TREATMENTS

Each ECT treatment is brief. The main goal of ECT is the application of an electrical stimulus to induce a generalized tonic-clonic seizure with no or minimal side effects. When ready to proceed, an ultra-brief acting anesthetic and a muscle relaxant are administered along with bag/mask ventilation. This combination of medicines provides brief motor paralysis, sedation, and amnesia.

The stimulus is applied to the head either bilaterally or unilaterally. Unilateral treatment is given over the nondominant hemisphere, and is the placement associated with less cognitive side effects *(19)*.

Bilateral placement, although associated with more confusion, provides more rapid improvement and is used either for ineffectiveness of unilateral placement or for emergent treatment.

There are four stages of change within the autonomic nervous system during ECT. The first, just after the application of the electrical stimulus, is a generalized discharge of neurons within brainstem nuclei causing a parasympathetic response. The ensuing seizure then activates the sympathetic nervous system with a rapid surge in catecholamines. This, in turn, is counterbalanced with another surge of the parasympathetic system. Finally, as the patient awakens from anesthesia, a smaller sympathetic discharge is noted. It is during these times of physiological change that pharmacotherapy can blunt or alter these autonomic responses. With the pharmacological modification of these effects, ECT can generally be used to treat any patient.

Electroconvulsive Therapy Course of Treatment

The first ECT treatment involves determining the seizure threshold, which may involve several stimuli that do not result in a seizure. This determines which stimulus dose is appropriate for a given patient. During the initial series of treatments, or the index course, ECT is typically provided three times a week initially up to 6–12 treatments. It may be continued until a plateau of improvement is reached, until the providers and patient determine they are not obtaining a sufficient response to the treatment, or until limiting side effects occur. Following a successful course of ECT, antidepressant treatment of some sort will still be required to prevent relapse of depression. Such maintenance treatment may either be a transition to a pharmacological agent or maintenance ECT.

Maintenance ECT may provide the benefit of continuing remission with less side effects than seen in an index course, although patients may still have cognitive side effects immediately following treatment. There is little evidence guiding how to space ECT maintenance treatments in individuals in a fashion that will minimize the risk of relapse. Many groups may initially start by transitioning to weekly treatment, then if that is successful, moving to bi-weekly treatments. Some patients may do well receiving treatments every 3 or 4 weeks. Maintenance treatments can be indefinite per the results of treatment or patient preference.

SIDE EFFECTS ASSOCIATED WITH ELECTROCONVULSIVE THERAPY

The most common side effects of ECT include headache and muscle soreness. These can typically be addressed either through premedications or adjustments to the muscle relaxant dose used in treatment.

An immediately concerning side effect is the development of ECT-induced delirium. As they awaken from anesthesia, all patients experience some post-ictal confusion that may last from minutes to a few hours. A variety of factors may increase the risk and length of confusional periods (Table 2). With repeated ECT treatments, this may develop into inter-ictal confusion. In these situations, ECT should be held, the patient should be closely monitored, and other potential contributions to the development of delirium should be investigated.

One side effect that is particularly troubling to the patient is the development of memory impairment. Memory impairment typically includes both anterograde and retrograde amnesia, varies significantly in severity and duration, and is influenced by the same factors influencing confusion (Table 2). This impairment typically disappears over days to weeks following a course of ECT, although anterograde amnesia often resolves more quickly than does retrograde amnesia *(20)*.

Some patients have reported that more remote memories have been permanently affected and some report that their memory never returns to normal following ECT *(16)*. Opponents often cite this as a primary concern about ECT. The cause of such a phenomenon is unclear, and although memory loss experienced by individuals cannot be concretely confirmed nor dismissed, a global effect does not appear to be present. It appears that long-term memories are preserved *(21)* and that personal and autobiographical memories are less affected by ECT than are impersonal memories about world events *(22)*. Clearly, more research is needed in this area, along with further investigation of techniques that would minimize this risk.

Table 2
Risk Factors for Development of Post-Ictal and Inter-Ictal Confusion

Patient characteristics	Electroconvulsive therapy characteristics
Older age	Stimulus waveform (sine wave)
Pre-existing cognitive deficits	Higher stimulus intensity
Other pre-existing neurological disease	Bilateral treatment
	Greater number of treatments
	More frequent treatments

ELECTROCONVULSIVE THERAPY IN PATIENTS WITH NEUROLOGICAL DISEASE

There are a multitude of other medical conditions present in patients receiving ECT, and one particular area of interest is of ECT in patients with complicated neurological conditions. Because the APAs recommendations now reflect no absolute contraindications to ECT, case reports are now being published in the ECT literature of successful treatment in patients with neurological disorders.

The greatest concern about treating individuals with neurological disease is the dramatic increase in intracranial pressure (ICP) seen during ECT. This increased ICP may be substantial: ECT is associated with an increase in cerebral perfusion at 300% normal *(23)*. However, modification of the hemodynamic response and decrease of mass edema may allow ECT to be safely performed in this population with neurological disorders. The attempt to reduce cerebral blood flow, and hence ICP, has been studied in the anesthesiology literature with varying results *(24,25)*. Whereas the systemic use of antihypertensives does not affect the increased cerebral blood flow, nitroglycerine may significantly decrease right middle cerebral artery flow as compared with alprenolol or nicardipine *(24)*.

Case reports exist for the successful use of ECT in patients with brain tumors and cerebral edema *(26)*, tumors and encephalomalacia *(27)*, intracranial vascular masses *(28)*, status post-vitrectomy *(29)*, metallic skull plates *(30)*, and brain-stimulating electrodes *(31)*. One should remember that isolated case reports might not capture the true risks of ECT in the larger population of patients with these problems. In patients with these conditions, it is important to individually evaluate the size and stability of lesions, and determine if the potential benefit is proportional to the risk of adverse outcomes.

Movement disorders in patients who do or do not have a co-existing psychiatric condition have also been reported to improve with ECT. Parkinson's disease (PD) is the most studied movement disorder in the ECT literature, but there are currently no published randomized, controlled clinical trials using ECT as a therapy for PD. A recent review found that 41 cases had been reported of treatment of PD without any associated psychiatric illness; there was motor improvement in 88% of patients *(32)*. The motor benefits associated with ECT lasted anywhere from days to years. Although improvement can be seen, patients with PD may be at greater risk for developing post-ECT delirium *(33)*. Possible treatment strategies to address this concern include decreasing dopaminergic medications prior to treatment or spreading out treatment sessions. ECT may also be highly effective in treating depression associated with PD *(33)*. Other movement disorders reportedly improved by ECT include tardive dyskinesia, progressive supranuclear palsy, Wilson's disease, and Huntington's disease.

There is little information on the efficacy or safety of ECT in patients with dementia or mild cognitive impairment. Despite the paucity of information, this is a particularly important topic given the association between subcortical ischemic disease, Alzheimer's disease, and depression. Naturalistic and retrospective studies report high rates of response in patients with these disorders, however the concern is that ECT will worsen already impaired cognitive function. Overall, it appears that elderly patients tend to have greater and prolonged cognitive side effects with ECT than do younger patients *(8)*, although other reports examining the elderly population show that ECT may have fewer side effects and greater efficacy than pharmacological antidepressant management *(34)*. Although ECT is effective in this population, modifications of treatment technique may be necessary to minimize cognitive side effects.

ECT may be used in individuals with co-existing seizure disorders, however this requires close consultation between psychiatry and neurology providers. These patients often have their anticonvulsant regimens adjusted or have anticonvulsant medications held the morning of ECT and given after treatment, although this would increase the risk of a prolonged seizure or status epilepticus (SE). Such events, whether they occur in patients with or without a pre-existing history of seizures, may require pharmacological management. There are algorithms for management of prolonged seizures in the ECT suite, and include re-administration of the anesthetic, short-acting benzodiazepines, and if the seizure continues, phenytoin *(35)*. It is also possible that the presence of excessive post-ECT confusion may represent nonconvulsive SE.

Interestingly, ECT has also been used to successfully terminate SE *(36)*. The question arises of how can ECT be a treatment for something that is a potential complication of its use? One theory is that using ECT in patients with SE may recruit inhibitory actions from healthy tissue, thus terminating the seizure *(36)*. Further research in this area is needed.

ELECTROCONVULSIVE THERAPY IN MEDICALLY ILL POPULATIONS

Cardiovascular Disorders

The majority of serious ECT complications arise from cardiovascular diseases (CVDs). Recent data from the state of Texas, which mandates reporting of all ECT treatments and complications, found in 41,660 treatments no immediate deaths and 6 deaths secondary to CVDs occurring from 1 to 4 days after treatment *(2)*. Two deaths occurred within 24 hours of ECT: a 48-year-old male died from a myocardial infarction and a 50-year-old female had a cause of death listed as a cardiac arrythmia secondary to interstitial fibrosis of the conducting system. No information was provided on pre-ECT workups, cardiac consultations, or pretreatment pharmacological interventions. Another brief report from the Texas databank examining 49,048 treatments over 5 years found no deaths at the time of treatment *(3)*. They concluded that ECT has a mortality rate of less than 2 per 100,000 treatments, which may reflect the risks of anesthesia rather than any risk of ECT itself.

ECT has been safely performed in almost all cardiac conditions. The American College of Cardiology/American Heart Association guidelines identify ECT as a low-risk procedure *(37)*. The main concern with ECT treatment in patients with CVD is the rapid autonomic fluctuations. The first parasympathetic rush that occurs with the electrical stimulus and tonic phase of the seizure can cause numerous arrhythmias including bradycardia, supraventricular arrhythmias, hypotension, and asystole *(38)*. The risk of asystole cannot be predicted, but increases with continued subseizure stimuli; this is more likely to occur during the first treatment wherein the seizure threshold is determined by "dose titration," which may involve several subseizure stimuli *(39)*. After the seizure's clonic phase, there is a brief flood of catecholamines, followed by another smaller parasympathetic discharge. Attention needs to be paid to these relatively rapid physiological changes.

ECT in patients with cardiac often poses a variety of concerns that must be addressed in consultation with a cardiologist. Although the risk of developing depression after a myocardial infarction has clearly been documented, the safe and efficacious use of ECT has not. Additional pre-ECT investigative studies beyond the routine might be required, such as stress testing or echocardiograms. Patients with atrial fibrillation should be anticoagulated at a therapeutic level for 3–4 weeks before beginning a course of treatment because of the possibility that they will convert to sinus rhythm after ECT *(40)*. There are also continuing developments in the field of electrophysiology, with patients being treated with pacemakers and automatic implantable cardiac defibrillators *(41)*. It appears that ECT may be safely used in these populations, but more study is needed.

Respiratory Disorders

The primary respiratory disorders encountered in the ECT suite are chronic obstructive pulmonary disease (COPD) and asthma, both of which are impacted by autonomic system responses during ECT. Both groups of patients should always receive pretreatment with their usual pulmonary medications. In patients with severe COPD, consideration should be given to additionally pretreating the patient with systemic anticholinergics (as opposed to just ipratroprium bromide) because of the possibility of increased respiratory secretions produced by the parasympathetic response.

In the pre-ECT evaluation, patients with COPD should have their medications carefully reviewed. Although less popular now than before, theophylline is still widely used in the treatment of some patients with COPD and asthma. It has the potential to decrease the seizure threshold and induce SE, although there are reports of successful ECT performed on patients with COPD who were concurrently using theophylline *(42)*. A rare side effect of seizures is postictal pulmonary edema. This "neurogenic" pulmonary edema has been reported on multiple occasions in the ECT, pulmonary, and epileptology literature *(43–45)*.

Other Medical Disorders

There are a multitude of other medical conditions present in patients receiving ECT but there is little information on its safety in these populations. One area of potential interest is in patients with hematological disorders, particularly disorders that increase bleeding risk. Successful ECT has been described in patients with thrombocytopenia *(46)*, being treated with an anticoagulant *(47)*, and with von Willebrand's disease *(48)*.

The treatment of patients with diabetes mellitus (DM), either type 1 or 2, has also been the focus of some controversy. Previous studies have associated ECT with hyper- and hypoglycemia in patients with diabetes *(49–51)*. A recent study refutes any complications of glycemic control in patients with type 2 DM who are on insulin therapy alone *(52)*. No such comprehensive reviews exist showing the effect of glycemic control on patient's with type 1 DM or those with type 2 DM who are taking oral hypoglycemic agents.

CONCLUSIONS

ECT has been used successfully in patients with psychiatric disorders and neurological conditions. With judicious attention to the physiology of generalized seizures and its modification in the ECT suite, the treatment of depression, bipolar, and some types of schizophrenia can be effectively treated in almost any clinical situation. Although the literature documents multiple successful treatments in the medically ill patient, no methodologically rigorous double-blind, comparisons exist on treatment procedures and outcomes in these groups. More studies will need to be completed in this area as the field moves into the realm of evidence-based psychiatry. Because ECT can provide rapid improvement in psychiatric diseases in the medically ill population, the use of ECT should receive a higher priority in the treatment of these patients.

REFERENCES

1. Accornero F. An eyewitness account of the discovery of electroshock. Convuls Ther 1988;4:40–49.
2. Scarano VR, Felthous AR, Early TS. The state of electroconsvulsive therapy in Texas. Part I: reported data on 41,660 ECT treatments in 5971 patients. J Forensic Sci 2000;45:1197–1202.
3. Shiwach RS, Reid WH, Carmody TJ. An analysis of reported deaths following electroconvulsive therapy in Texas, 1993–1998. Psychiatr Serv 2001;52:1095–1097.
4. Tomac TA, Rummans TA, Pileggi TS, Li H. Safety and efficacy of electroconvulsive therapy in patients over age 85. Am J Geriatr Psychiatry 1997;5:126–130.
5. Isaac RJ, Armat VC. Madness in the streets: how psychiatry and the law abandoned the mentally ill. New York: The Free Press, Macmillan; 1990.

6. Rosenbach ML, Hermann RC, Dorwart RA. Use of electroconvulsive therapy in the Medicare population between 1987 and 1992. Psychiatr Serv 1997;49:1537–1542.

7. Kelly KG, Zisselman M. Update on electroconvulsive therapy in older adults. J Am Geriatr Soc 2000;48:560–566.

8. APA Task Force on Electroconvulsive Therapy. A Task Force Report of the American Psychiatric Association: The Practice of Electroconvulsive Therapy Recommendations for Treatment, Training, and Privileging. Washington DC: American Psychiatric Association; 2001.

9. Janicak PG, Davis JM, Gibbons RD, Ericksen S, Chang S, Gallagher P. Efficacy of ECT: a meta-analysis. Am J Psychiatry 1985;142:297–302.

10. Pagnin D, de Queiroz V, Pini S, Cassano GB. Efficacy of ECT in depression: a meta-analytic review. J ECT 2004;20:13–20.

11. Small JG, Klapper MH, Kellams JJ, et al. Electroconvulsive treatment compared with lithium in the management of manic states. Arch Gen Psychiatry 1988;45:727–732.

12. Mukherjee S, Sackeim HA, Schnur DB. Electroconvulsive therapy of acute manic episodes: a review of 50 years' experience. Am J Psychiatry 1994;151:169–176.

13. Fink M, Sackeim HA. Convulsive therapy in schizophrenia? Schizophr Bull 1996;22:27–39.

14. Krystal AD, Coffey CE. Neuropsychiatric considerations in the use of electroconvulsive therapy. J Neuropsychiatry Clin Neurosci 1997;9:283–292.

15. Wahlund B, von Rosen D. ECT of major depressed patients in relation to biological and clinical variables: a brief overview. Neuropsychopharmacology 2003;28(Suppl 1):S21–S26.

16. Devanand DP, Dwork AJ, Hutchinson ER, Bolwig TG, Sackeim HA. Does ECT alter brain structure? Am J Psychiatry 1994;151:957–970.

17. Lafferty JE, North CS, Spitznagel E, Isenberg K. Laboratory screening prior to ECT. J ECT 2001;17:158–165.

18. Krystal AD, Watts BV, Weiner RD, Moore S, Steffens DC, Lindahl V. The use of flumazenil in the anxious and benzodiazepine-dependent ECT patient. J ECT 1998;14:5–14.

19. Squire SR, Slater PC. Bilateral and unilateral ECT: effects on verbal and non verbal memory. Am J Psychiatry 1978;135:1316–1320.

20. Weiner RD, Rogers HJ, Davidson JR, Squire LR. Effects of stimulus parameters on cognitive side effects. Ann N Y Acad Sci 1986;462:315–325.

21. Rami-Gonzalez L, Salamero M, Boget T, Catalan R, Ferrer J, Bernardo M. Pattern of cognitive dysfunction in depressive patients during maintenance electroconvulsive therapy. Psychol Med 2003;33:345–350.

22. Lisanby SH, Maddox JH, Prudic J, Devanand DP, Sackeim H. The effects of electroconvulsive therapy on memory of autobiographical and public events. Arch Gen Psychiatry 2000;57:581–590.

23. Nobler M, Sackeim H. Mechanisms of action of electroconvulsive therapy: functional brain imaging studies. Psychiatr Ann 1998;28:23–29.

24. Saito S, Kadoi Y, Iriuchijima N, et al. Reduction of cerebral hyperemia with antihypertensive medication after electroconvulsive therapy. Can J Anaesth 2000;47:767–774.

25. Wajima Z, Yoshikawa T, Ogura A, et al. Intravenous verapamil blunts hyperdynamic responses during electroconvulsive therapy without altering seizure activity. Anesth Analg 2002;95:400–402.

26. Patkar AA, Hill KP, Weinstein SP, Schwartz SL. ECT in the presence of brain tumor and increased intracranial pressure: evaluation and reduction of risk. J ECT 2000;16:189–197.

27. Kohler CG, Burock M. ECT for psychotic depression associated with a brain tumor. Am J Psychiatry 2001;158:2089.

28. Salaris S, Szuba MP, Traber K. ECT and intracranial vascular masses. J ECT 2000;16:198–203.

29. Saad DA, Black JL, Krahn LE, Rummans TA. ECT post eye surgery: two cases and a review of literature. J ECT 2000;16:409–414.

30. Madan S, Anderson K. ECT for a patient with a metallic skull plate. J ECT 2001;17:289–291.

31. Moscarillo FM, Annunziata CM. ECT in a patient with a deep brain-stimulating electrode in place. J ECT 2000;16:287–290.

32. Kennedy R, Mittal D, O'Jile J. Electroconvulsive therapy in movement disorders: an update. J Neuropsychiatry Clin Neurosci 2003;15:407–421.

33. Rasmussen KG, Rummans TA, Richardson JW. Electroconvulsive therapy in the medically ill. Psychiatr Clin North Am 2002;25:177–193.

34. Manly DT, Oakley SP, Bloch RM. Electroconvulsive therapy in old-old patients. Am J Geriatr Psychiatry 2000;8:232–236.

35. Beyer JL, Weiner RD, Glenn MD. Electroconvulsive therapy a programmed text. Washington DC: American Psychiatric Press; 1998.

36. Lisanby SH, Bazil CW, Resor SR, Nobler MS, Finck DA, Sackeim HA. ECT in the treatment of status epilepticus. J ECT 2001;17:210–215.

37. Eagle KA, Brundage BH, Chaitman BR, et al. Guidelines for perioperative cardiovascular evaluation for noncardiac surgery. Report of the American College of Cardiology/American Heart Association Task Force on Practice Guidelines. Committee on Perioperative Cardiovascular Evaluation for Noncardiac Surgery. Circulation 1996;93:1278–1317.

38. McCall WV. Asystole in electroconvulsive therapy: report of four cases. J Clin Psychiatry 1996;57:199–203.

39. Burd J, Kettl P. Incidence of asystole in electroconvulsive therapy in elderly patients. Am J Geriatr Psychiatry 1998; 6:203–211.
40. Ottaway A. Atrial fibrillation, failed cardioversion, and electroconvulsive therapy. Anaesth Intensive Care 2002;30: 215–218.
41. Lapid M, Rummans T, Hofmann V, Olney BA. ECT and automatic internal cardioverter-defibrillator. J ECT 2001;17: 146–148.
42. Rasmussen KG. Electroconvulsive therapy in patients taking theophylline. J Clin Psychiatry 1993;54:427–431.
43. Buisseret P. Acute pulmonary oedema following grand mal epilepsy and as a complication of electric shock therapy. Br J Dis Chest 1982;76:194–198.
44. Sinom RP. Physiologic consequences of status epilepticus. Epilepsia 1985;26:S58–S66.
45. Terrence CF, Rao GR, Perper JA. Neurogenic pulmonary edema in unexpected, unexplained death of epileptic patients. Ann Neurol 1981;9:458–464.
46. Gonzalez-Arriaza HL, Mueller PS, Rummans TA. Successful electroconvulsive therapy in an elderly man with severe thrombocytopenia: case report and literature review. J ECT 2000;17:198–200.
47. Petrides G, Fink M. Atrial fibrillation, anticoagulation, and electro convulsive therapy. Convuls Ther 1996;12:91–98.
48. Sincoff RC, Giuffra LA, Blinder MA, Isenberg KE. Successful electroconvulsive therapy given to a patient with von Willebrand's disease. J ECT 2000;16:68–70.
49. Normand PS, Jenike MA. Lowered insulin requirements after ECT. Psychosomatics. 1984;25:418–419.
50. Reddy S, Nobler MS. Dangerous hyperglycemia associated with electroconvulsive therapy. Convuls Ther 1996;12:99–103.
51. Finestone DH, Weiner RD. Effects of ECT on diabetes mellitus. An attempt to account for conflicting data. Acta Psychiatr Scand 1984;70:321–326.
52. Netzel PJ, Mueller PS, Rummans TA, Rasmussen KG, Pankratz VS, Lohse, CM. Safety, efficacy, and effects on glycemic control of electroconvulsive therapy in insulin-requiring type 2 diabetic patients. J ECT 2002;18:16–21.

26

Neurosurgical Treatments for Psychiatric Indications

Lawrence T. Park, Darin D. Dougherty, and Scott L. Rauch

INTRODUCTION

Neurosurgery for psychiatric indications is perhaps the strongest statement to date that psychiatric disorders, like neurological disorders, are grounded in brain dysfunction. The premise underlying the effectiveness of these procedures is that altering brain structure will change mental functioning. As we learn more about how biological states serve as a substrate for complex mental phenomena, the practice of psychiatry approaches that of other medical specialties, such as neurology. Psychiatric disorders are increasingly conceptualized as an alteration of brain processing and treatments are designed to intervene on a neurobiological level. Although the pull to connect mind and brain has been evident throughout the history of medicine, it has only been recently that we have begun to understand how and why brain-based interventions affect mental functioning in a clinically meaningful way.

The use of neurosurgery for psychiatric conditions has had a checkered past. Initial attempts to treat psychiatric and behavioral conditions with surgical interventions lacked scientific precision on a number of levels. Though these attempts were in large part empirically guided, they did not identify specific diagnostic indications, they utilized relatively large, crude lesions, and they often did not assess outcomes with standardized measurement instruments. These reasons, coupled with egregious overuse of "psychosurgery" in some instances in the past, have contributed to its controversial nature. Over the past century, many of these shortcomings have been addressed as indications have become more refined, lesion location has become more precise, and standardized, quantitative instruments are being used to assess effects. Current research has been able to focus on specific psychiatric disorders and has been rigorous about measuring outcomes and attending to ethical considerations. This has led to the creation of a body of coherent data on which clinical decision making can be based. Still, it is important to recognize that even the best data to date is of a case series or open nature; it has not been possible to design a randomized controlled trial that is able to assess nonspecific (placebo) effects.

Neurosurgery is rarely employed to treat psychiatric disorders in the present day. The main indications for these surgeries are the most severe and refractory cases of major depressive disorder (MDD) and obsessive-compulsive disorder (OCD). Some patients are so afflicted by their illnesses, that at the prospect of alleviating their suffering, they would choose to undergo such a procedure. It is of important note that these procedures are never performed on patients against their will. Although only a handful of patients undergo neurosurgery for these indications each year in the United States, this treatment modality is an important one, as it may provide relief when all other treatments have failed, thus providing hope to those most seriously afflicted. Moreover, like so many decades of previous exploration, the study of cerebral lesions and their effects on mental states augments our understanding of the

From: *Current Clinical Neurology: Psychiatry for Neurologists*
Edited by: D.V. Jeste and J.H. Friedman © Humana Press Inc., Totowa, NJ

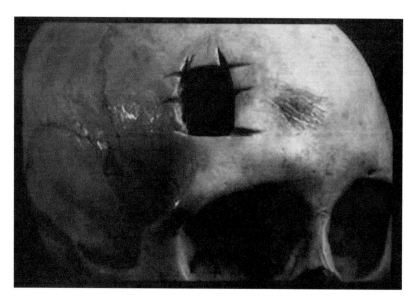

Fig. 1. Prehistoric example of rectangular trepanation lesion from Cinco Cerros, Peru. (Reprinted with permission from the San Diego Museum of Man.)

biological nature of psychiatric illness. This chapter examines the historical precedents of modern day neurosurgery for psychiatric indications, the development of different neurosurgical approaches, the current use of neurosurgery for psychiatric indications, the neurocircuitry models thought to underlie its effect, and future directions for the field.

HISTORICAL CONSIDERATIONS

A common motif throughout the history of medicine has been the idea that brain and mind are linked. Even preceding Déscartes, and across various cultures, attempts were made to manipulate the head (and its contents) to change mental states. One of the earliest attempts was called *trepanation* (Latin: to bore). Across many different cultures (including neolithic Europe, ancient Egypt, and Peru), the ancients performed trepanation, the practice of creating a craniotomy lesion using crude instruments, in an attempt to correct behavioral and mental conditions by releasing the demons or evil humors within (*see* Fig. 1).

In the late 1800s, during the "golden period" of classical neurology and psychiatry, empirical methods began to be applied to the study of the brain. These methods initially consisted of naturalistic observation and progressed to crude interventional studies on animals, and later humans. It was not until the later part of the 1900s, with the use of more precise lesions and the advent of more valid and reliable outcomes instruments, that full-fledged scientific inquiry into neurosurgery for psychiatric conditions began.

Observational studies of naturally occurring brain lesions confirmed the notion that damage to the brain resulted in changes in mental functioning. Perhaps the most famous case of a naturally occurring brain injury resulting in mental change was that of Phineas Gage. In a railway accident in Vermont, in 1848, Phineas Gage sustained a serious brain injury when an explosion drove an iron tamping rod through his skull (*see* Fig. 2). Damasio et al. *(1)* hypothesize that this accident led to significant injury to the left medial frontal lobe and possibly to the right medial frontal lobe as well. The change in Gage's mental state was profound. John Harlow, the physician who cared for Gage after this accident, offered a case report that described profound and lasting changes in personality. An entry on the 32nd day post-injury follows:

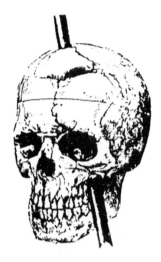

Frontal and lateral view of the cranium, representing the direction in which the iron traversed its cavity; the present appearance of the line of fracture, and also the large anterior fragment of the frontal bone, which was entirely detached, replaced, and partially re-united.

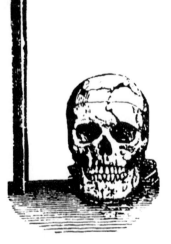

View of the tamping iron, and front view of the cranium, showing their *comparative* size.

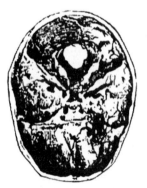

View of the base of the skull from within; the orifice caused by the passage of the iron having been partially closed by the deposit of new bone.

Fig. 2. Three views of the skull of Phineas Gage from Harlow's original report.

"Progressing favorably. Fungi disappearing; discharging laudable pus from openings. Takes more food, sleeps well, and says he shall soon go home. Remembers passing and past events correctly, as well before as since the injury. Intellectual manifestations feeble, being exceedingly capricious and childish, but with a will as indomitable as ever; is particularly obstinate; will not yield to restraint when it conflicts with his desires." Longer term, these cognitive changes persist. The equilibrium or balance, so to speak, between his intellectual faculties and animal propensities, seems to have been destroyed. He is fitful, irreverent, indulging at times in the grossest profanity (which was not previously his custom), manifesting but little deference for his fellows, impatient of restraint or advice when it conflicts with his desires, at times pertinaciously obstinate, yet capricious and vacillating, devising many plans of future operation, which are no sooner arranged than they are abandoned in turn for others appearing more feasible."

As described by Harlow, his mind was "radically changed"; he was "no longer Gage" *(2)*.

The case of Phineas Gage and other descriptions of brain-injured individuals led researchers to hypothesize that specific lesions result in specific functional deficits. Natural observation eventually led to active interventional studies. Unfortunately, the studies of this era offered woefully inadequate descriptions of treatment outcome. In a study of dogs, Friedrich Goltz *(3)* found that the surgical ablation of the temporal cortex made the animals more tame and less easily provoked. In an era where the ethical treatment of subjects (man or beast alike) was not emphasized, animal studies quickly led to ablative studies in humans. Gottlieb Burckhardt *(4)* was the first to perform surgical ablation of various cortical areas on humans with psychosis. Succinctly reporting on six cases, he qualitatively noted that three were "successes," two were "partial successes," and one ended in death. In another ablative series conducted on humans, Ludwig Puusepp *(5)* separated white matter tracts between frontal and parietal lobes. Again, without the use of standardized measures, Puusepp described his results as "failure."

One of the most significant events in the development of neurosurgical techniques for psychiatric indications occurred in 1935 at the Second World Congress in Neurology in London. Under serendipitous circumstances, the modern era of psychiatric neurosurgery was launched. At that gathering, Egas Moniz, the renowned Portuguese neurologist who invented cerebral ventriculography, had the opportunity to hear a presentation by John Fulton and Carlyle Jacobsen, two American researchers from Yale University. Fulton and Jacobsen were presenting their findings from their work creating ablative lesions in chimpanzees. They observed that after frontal cortical ablations, chimpanzees showed reduction in "experimental neurosis" and were less fearful, while retaining an ability to perform complex tasks *(6)*. Moniz hypothesized that similar effects might be seen in humans.

Upon his return to Portugal, Moniz, with his neurosurgical colleague, Almeida Lima, initiated the use of the pre-frontal leucotomy (referring to the separation of white matter tracts) as the first standardized neurosurgical approach for "certain psychoses" (note, *psychoses* in this context, following the Freudian influenced psychiatric nosology at that time, refers nonspecifically to severe psychiatric illness). Initially using absolute alcohol injected into frontal white matter tracts (centrum ovale), and subsequently using a specially designed instrument, the leucotome, to crush or sever white matter, Moniz and Lima treated severely mentally ill, chronically institutionalized patients *(see* Fig. 3). These patients are described as demonstrating psychotic symptoms (disorders of thought), affective symptoms (disorders of mood), or some combination of the two. Moniz describes the first patient that underwent the procedure, a 63-year-old woman with melancholia, anxiety, and paranoid delusions, and declared her "cured" *(7)*. Moniz *(8)* went on to describe a case series of 20 more patients, reporting that 7 were considered "cured," 7 were significantly improved, and 6 were unchanged. Significant complications, including long-term catatonia and mutism were seen in 11 of 20 patients. Other "minor" side effects included vomiting, urinary and fecal incontinence, diarrhea, nystagmus, and ptosis. For his work, Moniz was awarded the 1949 Nobel Prize in Medicine and Physiology.

Moniz was not the only neuroscientist in London impressed by Fulton and Jacobsen's work. Also in the audience was Walter Freeman, an American neuropathologist, who, after hearing Fulton and Jacobsen's presentation and conferring with Moniz, also became quite motivated to pursue such work. When he returned from London, Freeman collaborated with the neurosurgeon James Watts, and began

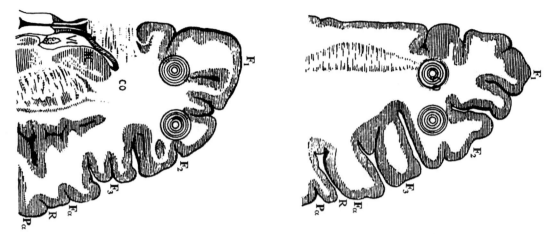

Fig. 3. Frontal lesion sites as described by Moniz. (Reprinted with permission from ref. 7.)

performing prefrontal leucotomies on psychiatric patients (9). Initially employing a lateral approach (following Moniz), Freeman soon developed a new procedure with what he considered to be a preferable approach. Employing a trans-orbital approach, Freeman effectively made similar lesions in frontal white matter tracts by inserting a slender leukotome through the supra-orbital ridge and sweeping across frontal white matter tracts (*see* Fig. 4). Because of the resemblance of the leukotome to the common ice-pick, this procedure, the trans-orbital leucotomy (in which orbital frontal cortex was essentially disconnected from the rest of the brain by virtue of severing its afferent and efferent tracts) came to be more commonly known as the "ice-pick lobotomy." In a nonstandardized study examining the effectivenss of this procedure, results among 74 patients demonstrated that 63% received "worthwhile benefit," 23% were "unchanged," and 14% were "worse." With symptoms reminiscent of Phineas Gage, psychiatric complications were characterized by "nonchalance, inability to carry out tasks, and loss of social control." Additionally, there was one reported case of hemiplegia and the mortality rate was 4% (10).

In an era of overflowing asylums and few effective treatments for chronic debilitating psychiatric illness (this was prior to the advent of early psychopharmacological agents such as lithium and chlorpromazine), the use of lobotomy and leucotomy spread across Europe and the United States. In the United States, the trans-orbital leucotomy became a common procedure for the treatment of the mentally ill in the 1950s, and thousands of these procedures were done annually. Freeman literally traveled around the United States performing trans-orbital leucotomies on thousands of patients. Watts, concerned about the liberal use of the procedure, lack of proper anesthetic techniques (Freeman used electroconvulsive therapy as "anesthesia"), and lack of sterile technique, distanced himself from Freeman.

DEVELOPMENT OF NEUROSURGICAL TREATMENTS FOR PSYCHIATRIC INDICATIONS

From the early procedures of Moniz and Freeman, other neuroscientists have continued to study and develop alternative neurosurgical approaches. While the initial leucotomy and lobotomy procedures had significant drawbacks (i.e., significant mortality, complications, and unclear indications), and despite the nonstandardized analysis of their effect, it was evident that some positive effects were noted. For example, in retrospective data from Tooth and Newton (11), 10,365 British patients who had undergone frontal lobe ablative procedures demonstrated a 70% improvement rate. However, the mortality rate was also 6% and other adverse events included a 1% incidence of seizures and 1.5% incidence of disinhibition syndromes.

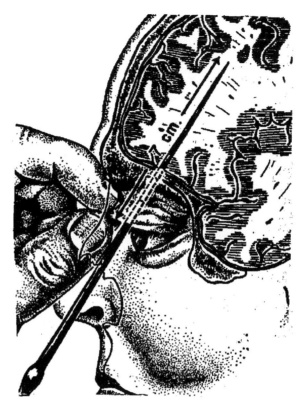

Fig. 4. Trans-orbital approach as diagrammed by Freeman. (Reprinted with permission from ref. *10.*)

Because of the high incidence of death and other significant adverse neuropsychiatric events associated with these early procedures, a more systematic and refined investigation between specific brain lesions and mental function was undertaken. Given initial experiences with prefrontal lobotomy, others attempted to refine the technique in an effort to minimize side effects. Lyerly and others *(12)* employed a more medial approach, as it was generally felt that increased psychological side effects were associated with more laterally placed lesions (*see* Fig. 5).

Wilder Penfield,who often studied epileptic patients and others with structural lesions, examined the effect of gray matter lesions (gyrectomies) of specific frontal lobe regions. Generally, he found the effect of such lesions on psychiatric symptomatology to be unsatisfactory, with a high incidence of adverse effects *(13)*. These patients were tested cognitively and found to have significant deficits in intelligence that could be accounted for by frontal lobe dysfunction *(14)*. William Scoville and colleagues *(15)* also focused on gray matter lesions, performing and reporting results of orbital undercutting, a procedure in which large portions of the orbitofrontal cortex were resected (*see* Fig. 6).

Following Scoville, Geoffrey Knight, a British neurosurgeon, performed 600 orbital undercuttings and concluded that the procedure demonstrated maximal efficacy if the lesions extended posteriorly into subcaudate structures *(16,17)*. Based on these findings, Knight refined this procedure, performing a subcaudate tractotomy (*see* Fig. 7), which targeted fronto-striato-thalamic pathway fibers in the region inferior to the caudate nucleus. Employing brachytherapy as a method of tissue ablation, Knight implanted seeds of Yttrium 90 (a γ radiation source) in the subcaudate target to create an approx 2 cm lesion around each seed (*see* Fig. 8).

Although brachytherapy proved to be effective, the size and location of the lesions were more difficult to control because the effect of radiation on surrounding tissues was difficult to predict and there

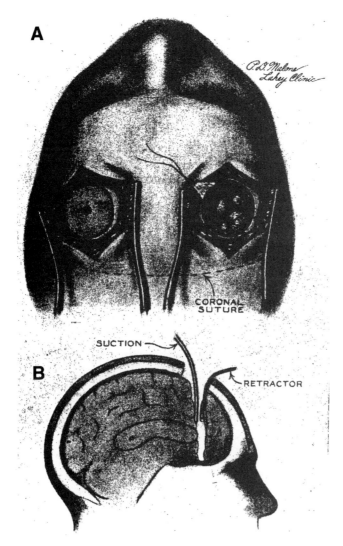

Fig. 5. Diagram by P. D. Malone of Lahey Clinic of bimedial approach. (Reprinted with permission from ref. *59.*)

was the risk that the implanted seeds could migrate. Bridges et al. *(18)* published a retrospective report of nearly 1300 patients with "non-schizophrenic affective disorders" at The Geoffrey Knight Unit in London. Of patients who underwent subcaudate tractotomy, 40–60% went on to live normal or near normal lives. Additionally, they also demonstrated that the suicide rate was reduced to 1% postoperatively, compared with 15% in uncontrolled affectively disordered patients. Another retrospective study of 208 patients with depression, anxiety, and obsessional neuroses with a mean follow-up period of 2.5 years demonstrated significant improvement in 68% of patients with depression, 50% of patients with obsessional neurosis, and 62.5% of patients with other anxiety disorders *(19)*. Patients with other psychiatric disorders, such as schizophrenia, substance abuse, or personality disorders responded poorly to the procedure. Adverse effects included short-term transient disinhibition syndromes, headache, confusion or somnolence; personality changes were seen in 6.7% of patients and seizures were seen in 2.2% of patients. In this study, there was one fatality resulting from migration of an Yttrium seed. Table 1 outlines early neurosurgical approaches for psychiatric indications.

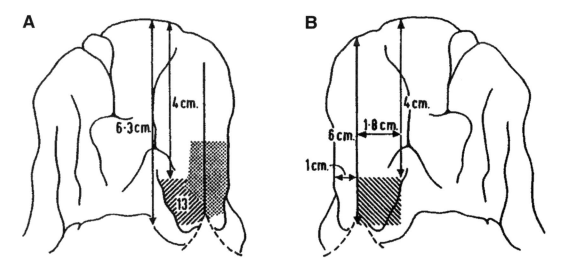

Fig. 6. Diagram of inferior aspect of orbitofrontal lobe. Area of restricted orbital undercutting as performed and described by Knight. (Reprinted with permission from ref. *16*.)

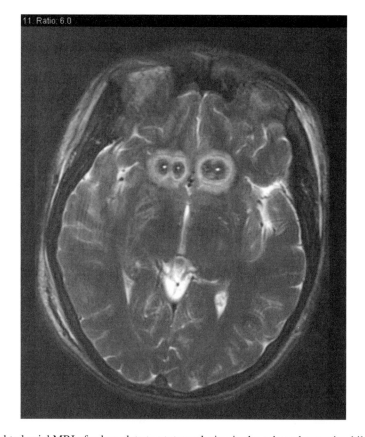

Fig. 7. T_2-weighted axial MRI of subcaudate tractotomy lesion in the subcaudate region bilaterally.

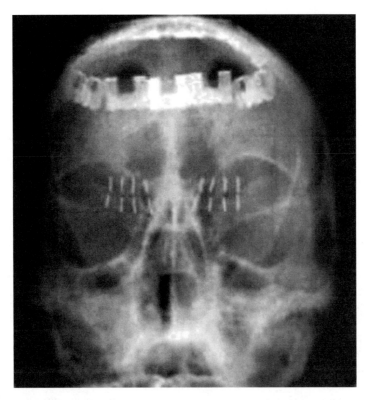

Fig. 8. STT brachytherapy. Anteroposterior radiograph, showing yttrium seeds used in Knight's original SST procedure. (Reprinted with permission from ref. *60*.)

One of the important technological advances that allowed for the development of more precise procedures was the ability to accurately position and localize targets in three-dimensional space. Initially done as unguided, free-hand procedures, lesion size and location were quite variable. This changed with the development of superior visualization and localization techniques. The stereotactic frame, initially designed by Sir Victor Horsley, represented an early localization system that led to marked improvement in the accuracy and precision of cerebral lesions. More sophisticated localization systems in current use employ computed tomography (CT)/magnetic resonance imaging (MRI) guidance and provide optimal lesion localization.

The development of an empirically based, statistically sound psychiatric nosology served as an equally important advance for psychiatric research. The earlier system of diagnosis based on Diagnostic and Statistical Manual of Mental Disorders, First Edition (DSM-I) (1952) and DSM-II (1968) served as a classification that embodied psychobiological theories of the time. DSM-III (1980) (and subsequently DSM-III R in 1987, and DSM-IV in 1994) represented a marked departure from a theoretically based nosology to a descriptive, empirically based system. Paralleling this evolution in psychiatric diagnosis was the development of quantitatively reliable and valid instruments for assessing the severity of psychiatric symptomatology.

Armed with these advances, researchers were able to study a range of different targets. As part of a posited "limbic system," the anterior cingulate gyrus was first mentioned by Fulton in 1947 as a possible target for neurosurgical intervention *(20)*. Dr. Thomas H. Ballantine, Jr. at Massachusetts General Hospital was one of the first to use this procedure clinically, and pioneered its application for treatment of MDD, chronic pain syndromes, and OCD. The surgery is typically conducted under local anesthesia; one to three contiguous lesions are made bilaterally via thermocoagulation through bilateral burr

Table 1
Early Neurosurgical Approaches for Psychiatric Indications

Procedure	Designers	Year	Main indications	Comment
Prefrontal lobotomy	Moniz/Lima	1936	"Psychosis"	Lateral approach, development of leukotome to sever white matter tracts
Bimedial lobotomy	Lyerly	1937	"Psychosis"	Medial approach thought to minimize cognitive complications
Trans-orbital leucotomy	Freeman	1946	"Anxiety, worry, nervousness"	Superior orbital approach, "ice-pick" leukotome
Orbital undercutting	Scoville	1948	Depression, anxiety	Orbito-frontal gray matter lesions

holes. The target is within dorsal anterior cingulate cortex (Brodmann areas 24 and 32), at the margin of the white matter bundle known as the cingulum. Originally, the placement of lesions was determined by ventriculography. Currently, however, anterior cingulotomy is performed stereotactically via MRI guidance (*see* Fig. 9). Given the use of relatively small lesions, one major advantage of anterior cingulotomy over the other procedures is the decreased incidence of significant complications. However, given the conservative nature of the lesions, efficacy may also be decreased, with approx 40% of patients returning for a second procedure to extend the first set of lesions.

Ballantine and colleagues *(21)* retrospectively reviewed 198 cases with mean follow-up of 8.6 years. They noted significant improvement in 62% of patients with affective disorders, 56% with OCD, and 79% with other anxiety disorders. A subsequent report reviewed a series of 34 patients who had undergone MRI-guided cingulotomy *(22)*. Among patients with unipolar depression, 60% responded favorably; among patients with bipolar disorder, 40% responded favorably; and among patients with OCD, 27% were classified as responders with another 27% categorized as possible responders. Most recently, a prospective report of 44 patients with OCD was published, based on a mean follow-up period of 32 months *(23)*. The investigators, employing stringent criteria, found that 45% had responded favorably, with no serious long-term adverse effects. Complications typically prove to be relatively minor, with short-term headache, nausea, difficulty with urination, and subjective transient problems with memory. Of the approx 1000 anterior cingulotomies performed by Ballantine, his successor G. Rees Cosgrove, and their colleagues at Massachusetts General Hospital, there have been no deaths, and the incidence of seizure remains approx 1%, with most occurring in patients with a pre-existing seizure history. Additionally, since the advent of MRI guidance, there has been only one case of stroke postoperatively. An independent analysis of a subset of these patients demonstrated no significant lasting intellectual or behavioral impairment or neurological or behavioral adverse effects *(24)*.

Another treatment strategy has involved a combination of two of the aforementioned lesions to maximize main effect. Desmond Kelley and colleagues *(25)* developed a procedure called limbic leucotomy, which combines anterior cingulotomy with subcaudate tractotomy (*see* Fig. 10). Theoretically, it was thought that an intervention at two different sites of the limbic system would improve efficacy. The lesions are made via thermo- or cryo-coagulation. Initially, localization of the lesion site was guided by intraoperative electrical stimulation (pronounced autonomic response designates the optimal lesion site); currently, lesion placement is stereotactically guided. The indications for limbic leukotomy include MDD, OCD, and other severe anxiety disorders. Retrospective review of patients undergoing this procedure *(26)* demonstrated an 89% improvement rate for OCD, 78% for MDD, and 66% for other anxiety disorders with mean follow-up of 16 months. Notably, improvement was only seen after a lag time of several months. Short-term side effects included headache, lethargy or apathy, confusion, and lack of sphincter control, which may last from a few days to a few weeks. Postoperative confusion was commonly seen, but typically resolved over several days. No seizures or deaths were reported, although

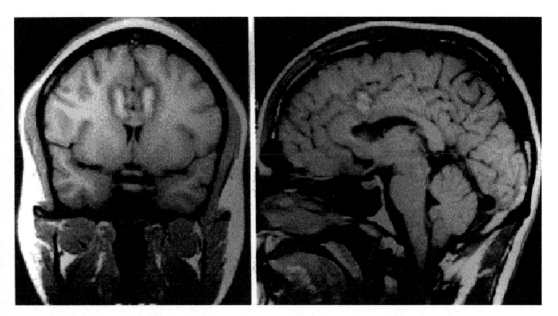

Fig. 9. Anterior cingulotomy. Early postoperative sagittal and coronal T1-weighted magnetic resonance images demonstrating radiofrequency thermocoagulation lesions created in the anterior cingulate gyrus bilaterally. (Reprinted with permission from ref. *55*.)

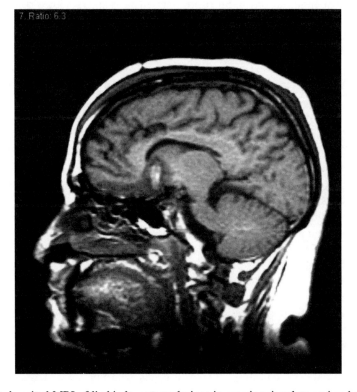

Fig. 10. T_1-weighted sagittal MRI of limbic leucotomy lesions in anterior cingulate gyri and subcaudate region.

one patient suffered severe memory loss as a result of improper lesion placement. More recently, another study of 21 patients who underwent limbic leukotomy for OCD or MDD demonstrated 36–50% response rate (using stringent response criteria) at mean follow-up of 26 months *(27)*. There is also some evidence (*n* = 5) that limbic leucotomy may be of benefit for patients with severe self-mutilation, in the context of repetitive, self-injurious, tic-like behaviors *(28)*.

Anterior capsulotomy targets white matter tracts in the anterior one-third of the anterior limb of the internal capsule at the level of the intercommissural plane, thereby interrupting fibers of passage between prefrontal cortex and subcortical nuclei *(see* Fig. 11). Initially designed in France, and further developed by Leksell and colleagues in Sweden, anterior capsulotomy utilizes much smaller lesions because the density of white matter tracts in the anterior capsule is much higher than white matter tracts closer to their neurons of origin. However, given that structures are functionally condensed, the need for precision of lesion placement is greater, as the possibility of side effects is relatively greater as well. Lesions were originally made in an open procedure via thermocoagulation. However, more recently the lesions have been made "noninvasively" through radiosurgery using the "Gamma Knife." Gamma Knife technology utilizes a γ-radiation source and focuses multiple rays through the use of a collimator helmet to converge on a single location to create a lesion. Indications for anterior capsulotomy include MDD, OCD, and other severe anxiety disorders. Herner *(29)* retrospectively reported on the first 116 patients that Leksell operated on. He noted a favorable response in 50% of those with OCD and 48% of those with MDD, whereas only 20% of those with anxiety and 14% of those with schizophrenia improved. In another prospective study of 35 patients with OCD, 70% had satisfactory outcomes *(30)*. The most significant complications include confusion, which typically resolves within 1 week postoperatively, permanent weight gain, and intracranial hemorrhage. Other short-term side effects can include transient headache, incontinence, fatigue, or memory difficulties. With the use of radiation ablation, recovery is typically quicker than open procedures (typical hospital stay is one night postprocedure), although there is an associated risk of cerebral edema, which may present as far out as 8–12 months postprocedure. No significant long-term cognitive problems or adverse personality changes have been noted in patients undergoing anterior capsulotomy.

Most recently, in an ongoing prospective study, the Butler Hospital and Rhode Island Hospital Group found that anterior capsulotomy was generally well tolerated and effective for patients with otherwise intractable OCD. Adverse events included cerebral edema and headache, small asymptomatic caudate infarctions, and possible exacerbation of pre-existing bipolar mania. There were no group decrements on cognitive or personality tests compared to presurgical baseline, although one patient developed a mild frontal syndrome, including apathy. A therapeutic response, defined conservatively, was seen in 10 of 16 patients receiving the most recent anterior capsulotomy procedure. Most therapeutic benefit was achieved by 1 year, and was essentially stable by 3 years (Rasmussen, personal communication).

CURRENT USE OF NEUROSURGERY FOR PSYCHIATRIC INDICATIONS

In the modern era of neurosurgery for psychiatric indications, four main procedures continue to be used; they are anterior cingulotomy, subcaudate tractotomy, limbic leucotomy, and anterior capsulotomy. All four procedures incorporate bilateral lesions and take advantage of modern stereotactic localization techniques *(see* Table 2).

These procedures have demonstrated the best balance to minimize adverse effects yet maximize beneficial effects. Informed by the abuses of the past, the use of these procedures is tightly controlled, usually by internal oversight by the institutions that perform them. Currently, only a handful of centers worldwide perform neurosurgery for psychiatric indications and the numbers of patients that receive this procedure in the United States annually ranges in the dozens. In the United States, centers in Boston, Massachusetts; Providence, Rhode Island; Gainesville, Florida; and Cleveland, Ohio have established interdisciplinary committees (consisting of neurosurgeons, neurologists, and psychiatrists) to evaluate patients for appropriateness for treatment. Criteria for appropriateness for surgery are quite stringent;

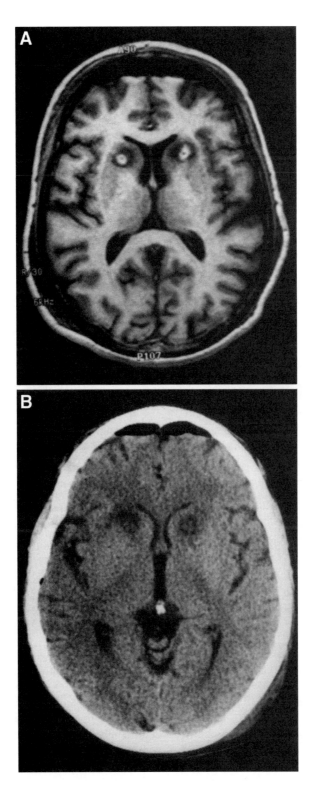

Fig. 11. **(A)** Axial T1 MRI of acute and **(B)** axial CT of chronic anterior capsulotomy lesions. (Reprinted with permission from BMJ Publishing Group. From JNNP, 63(6), 1997.)

Table 2
Current Stereotactically Guided Neurosurgical Approaches for Psychiatric Indications

Procedure	Designers	Year	Main indications	Comment
Anterior capsulotomy	Leksell	1950	OCD, anxiety, MDD	Anterior limb of the internal capsule, gamma knife
Subcaudate tractotomy	Knight	1964	Depression, anxiety, obsessions, schizophrenia	Subcaudate (ventral striatum) lesions, Yttrium 90 brachytherapy
Anterior cingulotomy	Fulton/ Ballantine	1967	MDD, OCD, chronic pain	Anterior cingulated gyrus and cingulum bundle
Limbic leukotomy	Kelley	1973	MDD, OCD, anxiety	Subcaudate tractotomy + cingulotomy

OCD, obsessive-compulsive disorder; MDD, major depression disorder.

patients must demonstrate nonresponsiveness to an exhaustive array of other available therapies. Additionally, patients are never forced or coerced into undergoing a procedure; in fact, patients (and their families) must petition these committees for consideration for surgery. International centers, in London and Stockholm, also employ the interdisciplinary committee approach, and in Britain additional formal approval from the Mental Health Act Commission is required.

Generally speaking, contemporary neurosurgical treatments across all psychiatric indications demonstrate significant improvement in 40–70% of cases and outstanding improvement in greater than 25% of cases. Response rates for MDD are slightly better than those for OCD. Side effects are minimal, with the most common severe complication being seizures that occur in 1 to 5% of cases. Frontal lobe syndromes, confusion or subtle cognitive deficits are relatively rare occurrences and typically mild when they do occur. In fact, overall cognitive function (as measured by standard intelligence quotient) often improves. This is attributed to the fact that cognitive compromise associated with primary psychiatric disorders resolves once the primary disease process remits. Studies have demonstrated that neurosurgery for psychiatric conditions may decrease suicide rates overall, although any individual patient who fails to respond to these "procedures of last resort" may be at higher risk for completed suicide (31).

Based on the current body of outcome data, the best established psychiatric indications for neurosurgery are MDD and OCD. Patients to be evaluated for neurosurgery must demonstrate extremely severe symptomatology, refractoriness to existing treatments, and willingness and capacity to consent for such a procedure. Furthermore, patients must also demonstrate access to and a willingness to participate in long-term psychiatric follow-up care. Symptoms must be chronic, severe and debilitating, and must be documented by quantifiable measures (i.e., patients with OCD typically have Yale-Brown Obsessive-Compulsive Scale scores ≥25; patients with MDD typically have Beck Depression Inventory scores of ≥30). Refractoriness to treatment refers to the failure of an exhaustive array of other available established treatment options. Patients must be free of other psychiatric conditions that would interfere with treatment effects. Psychoactive substance use or personality disorders are considered significant relative contraindications. Patients must be in good medical condition, and able to tolerate a procedure of this nature. A history of significant cardiopulmonary disease, age greater than 65 years, structural brain lesions, and significant central nervous system injuries are relative contraindications. A history of past seizures is a risk factor for perioperative seizures and must be weighed in the overall risk–benefit assessment. Preoperative work-up consists of standard blood and urine laboratory tests, electrocardiogram, brain MRI, electroencephalogram, and psychometric testing.

In the postoperative period, there is generally no immediate beneficial effect following the treatment; it may be several months before beneficial effects emerge. Side effects occur in less than one-half of all patients and are typically transient (lasting a few days to a few weeks). Short-term side effects may include altered mental status, headache, or urinary or fecal incontinence. Special care must be taken to monitor for potential surgical complications—including infection, hemorrhage, seizures, or altered mental status. Postoperatively, patients are typically monitored in the hospital setting for 1 to 2 days (this varies by procedure and surgical team). After the immediate postoperative phase, an MRI should be obtained to document the placement and extent of the lesions.

Because no immediate beneficial effect is typically observed, long-term comprehensive treatment, including psychopharmacology and psychotherapy, is required for all patients. Optimal response is thought to result from interplay between the neurosurgical intervention and traditional psychiatric therapies. Particularly for OCD, intensive behavior therapy should be initiated as soon as the patient is able, preferably within the first month postoperatively.

Given the history of use of neurosurgery for psychiatric conditions in the past, and given the potentially compromised nature of the mental state of the psychiatric patient, informed consent is a vital aspect of the evaluation process as well. Neurosurgery today is never performed on patients against their will, whether they are competent to refuse the procedure or not. All patients undergoing a neurosurgical procedure must be able to demonstrate competency to make such a decision, and must demonstrate their desire to proceed with the treatment. For this reason, age under 18 is seen as a relative contraindication, although there have been rare cases when procedures have been performed with the assent of the patient as well as the consent of the legal guardian.

NEUROCIRCUITRY MODELS

Evidence for neurobiological models of psychiatric conditions is gathered from various areas of research. The most basic source of information is the association between structural abnormalities in the brain and changes in mental functioning. The observation of neurosurgical lesions and their resulting functional effects is one example of this type of evidence. Additionally, the advent of neuroimaging has greatly increased our understanding of the underlying biology of mental states. Structural imaging techniques (CT and MRI) have been instrumental in associating certain biological changes with alterations in mental functioning. Improved neurochemical and neurohistological techniques have furthered our understanding of how the brain is wired and how it functions. Perhaps most importantly, the development of functional neuroimaging techniques has significantly advanced the field as in vivo functional physiological states can be linked with mental states.

Currently, there are two major neurocircuitry models that may serve as a conceptual framework for understanding psychiatric neurosurgery for OCD and MDD. One model focuses on cortico–striato–thalamo–cortical circuitry (CSTC) and provides us with a mechanism to explain how neurosurgery may help to treat OCD and other related disorders. The other model, a network model of limbic–cortical connectivity contributes insights into how neurosurgery effectively treats MD.

Cortico–Striato–Thalamo–Cortical Circuits: OCD and Related Disorders

The CSTC circuitry model has been elaborated by Alexander and colleagues *(32,33)*. This model describes five segregated CSTC circuit loops that are situated in parallel (with preservation of topological relationship to each other) and have been postulated to mediate specific types of human activity and behavior (*see* Fig. 12). Each circuit consists of a cortical area linked to a unique striatal area, which is in turn linked to a unique part of the thalamus and then returns in a feedback loop to the original cortical area. In addition to a main, or direct, pathway, there is also an associated indirect pathway. It is thought that the balance between direct and indirect pathway may serve as the mechanism for modulating the activity in each circuit. Each circuit is referred to by its associated cortical component. The five circuits include: motor cortex, oculomotor cortex, dorsolateral prefrontal cortex (DLPFC), orbitofrontal cortex (OFC), and anterior cingulate cortex (ACC). Interestingly, two of the circuits mediate motor activity,whereas the other three are thought to mediate aspects of mental activ-

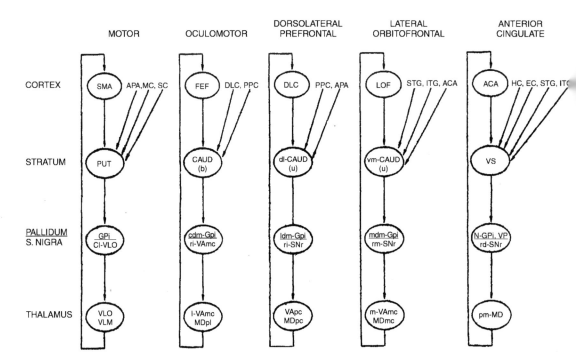

Fig.12. Parallel cortico–striato–thalamo–cortical circuits as diagrammed by Alexander. (Reprinted with permission from ref. *32*.)

ity. The DLPFC has been associated with executive function; the OFC and the ACC have been associated with attention modulation, and affective function.

Focusing on two of the five CSTC circuits, a theory of pathophysiology in OCD has been developed. Specifically, it has been proposed that the OFC circuit, ACC circuit, and the caudate nucleus play a central role in the pathophysiology of OCD *(34,35)*. Furthermore, there is a convergence of evidence to suggest that some primary pathological process within the striatum might underlie the CSTC dysfunction in OCD. The prevailing theory suggests that a relative imbalance favoring the direct vs. indirect pathways within this circuitry, leads to overactivity (i.e., amplification) within OFC and ACC, caudate nucleus and thalamus, resonant with failed striato-thalamic inhibition (i.e., filtration) within this same circuitry. There is hyperactivity at rest within the OFC-caudate CSTC circuit that is exaggerated during symptom provocation and attenuated following successful treatment. A similar profile is present within ACC, although this appears to be a more nonspecific finding across different types of anxiety states.

This basic scheme has been extended to provide a comprehensive model for a group of purportedly related disorders, called "obsessive-compulsive spectrum (OC spectrum) disorders." In addition to OCD, the OC spectrum also includes Tourette's syndrome, trichotillomania, and body dysmorphic disorder. The "striatal topography model" of OC-spectrum disorders suggests that these diseases share underlying CSTC dysfunction vis-à-vis primary striatal pathology. Moreover, each specific clinical presentation reflects the topography of pathology within the striatum and hence the constellation of dysfunction across CSTC circuits *(36,37)*. To elaborate, the notion is that OCD and body dysmorphic disorder (the OC spectrum disorders characterized by intrusive cognitive and visuospatial symptoms) involve caudate pathology; whereas Tourette 's syndrome and trichotillomania (principally characterized by intrusive sensorimotor symptoms), involve pathology within the putamen and dysfunction of sensorimotor CSTC circuitry.

Most recently, pioneering neuroanatomical research by Haber and colleagues *(38)* has provided a scheme for considering CSTC function that emphasizes a cascading spiral interaction, rather than segregation, across CSTC circuits. This model of normal CSTC function suggests a flow of information from motivation to cognition to motor behavior. This raises the possibility that OCD—as well as other OC spectrum disorders—may not reflect dysfunction within a single segregated CSTC circuit, but rather represent a failure in the smooth cascade of information across the various CSTC circuits. For instance, in the case of OCD, cognitions and motivations to act seem to persist (as obsessions with attendant anxiety, respectively), such that motor output fails to reset these thoughts and motivations, hence driving stereotyped motor repetition (compulsions).

Cortico–Limbic Network Model: Major Depression

Similar to OCD, CSTC circuitry has also been implicated as the biological substrate of MDD. However, in addition to CSTC mechanisms, prevailing models of MDD have focused on other critical elements of the limbic system, namely the amygdala and hippocampus, as well as the hypothalamic–pituitary–adrenal (HPA) axis *(39–43)*. Over the past several years, Helen Mayberg and colleagues *(41,44,45)* have been refining a theory of network dysfunction that theorizes that depression is mediated by dysregulation between different cortical, subcortical, and limbic components that have known anatomical and functional interconnections (*see* Fig. 13). As a work in progress, this model has been iteratively revised in order to assimilate and accommodate the body of research in this area as it accrues. In this model, specific brain areas are classified into three different main compartments: cortical (blue), limbic (red), and subcortical (green). Mayberg postulates that each of the compartments is related to different mental and physiological functions: cortical related to cognitive function, subcortical related to self-referential awareness, and limbic related to autonomic functioning. This theory fits well with the phenomenological quality of depressive episodes. As MDD is a syndrome, it is experienced as a constellation of various symptoms. In addition to emotional alteration, depressive episodes often are characterized by a combination of cognitive, motor, and neuroendocrinological manifestations. Following Mayberg, the cognitive and motor deficits of MDD may be explained by dysfunction within a cortical "dorsal compartment," including anterior, dorsal, and lateral prefrontal cortex, dorsal ACC, and parietal cortex as well as premotor cortex. The emotional symptoms of MDD may be related to dysfunction within a paralimbic "ventral compartment," including subgenual ACC, OFC, and anterior insular cortex. These dorsal and ventral compartments communicate with their striatal counterparts; the dorsal compartment is linked to the dorsal (cognitive/motor) striatum, and the ventral compartment is linked to the ventral (limbic) striatum. Interestingly, the dorsal and ventral compartments appear to be reciprocally inhibitory *(46–49)*. Thus, in MDD, generally there appears to be hypoactivity within the dorsal compartment and hyperactivity within the ventral compartment.

A triad of areas seem to play a critical role in mediating the balance of activity between the ventral and dorsal compartments, both in health and disease. The amygdala is positioned to assess the reward and threat value of external stimuli, and has the capacity to drive the balance of activity toward the ventral compartment. The pregenual ACC has the capacity to facilitate the restoration of dynamic equilibrium between the compartments, via its inhibitory influence over both dorsal and ventral elements *(46–49)*. Finally, the hippocampus, in addition to its role in cognition, has reciprocal connections with the amygdala, and projects to the hypothalamus to influence the HPA axis as well as other functions that are disturbed in depression such as sleep and appetite. Therefore, it is proposed that amygdala hyperactivity and hippocampal inefficacy may be central to the pathophysiology of MDD. Of note, it has been proposed that exposure to stress during early development or chronic exposure could represent a risk factor for evolving such a profile *(50)*. Thus, successful treatment of MDD (via any of a number of modalities) may rely on some combination of deactivation of the ventral compartment, inhibition of the amygdala, stimulation (or protection) of the hippocampus, and/or enhanced efficacy of the pregenual ACC.

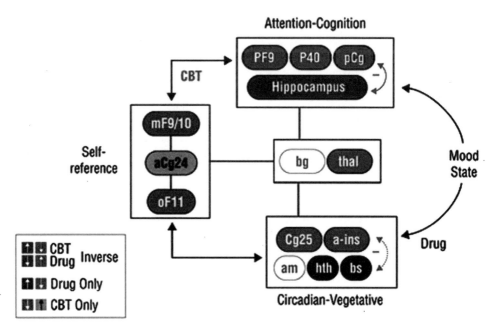

Fig. 13. Schematic model illustrating relationships among regions mediating cognitive-behavior therapy (CBT) and drug response. Regions with known anatomical and functional connections that also show significant metabolic changes following successful treatment are grouped into three compartments—cognitive, autonomic, and self-reference. Box labeled "Attention-Cognition" designates areas of change seen with both treatments. Box labeled "self-reference" designates changes unique to CBT. Box labeled "Circadian-Vegetative," except am (amygdala) and including thal (thalamus) in center box designates areas of change unique to paroxetine. Solid lines and arrows connecting these boxes identify known corticolimbic, limbic-paralimbic, and cingulate-cingulate connections. Lighter lines and arrows with "Attention-Cognition" and "Circadian-Vegetative" boxes indicate reciprocal changes with treatment. The model proposes that illness remission occurs when there is modulation of critical common targets ("Attention-Cognition" box), an effect facilitated by top-down (medial frontal, anterior cingulate) effects of CBT ("Self-reference" box) or bottom-up (brainstem, striatal, subgenual cingulate) actions of paroxetine ("Circadian-Vegetative" box and thal [thalamus] in center box). PF9 indicates dorsolateral prefrontal; p40, inferior parietal; pCg, posterior cingulate; mF9/10, medial frontal; aCg24, anterior cingulate; oF11, orbital frontal; bg, basal ganglia; thal, thalamus; Cg25, ventral subgenual cingulate; a-ins, anterior insula; am, amygdala; hth, hypothalamus; and bs, brainstem. Numbers are Brodmann area designations. (Reprinted with permission from ref. *62*.)

Mechanism of Action Underlying Neurosurgical Procedures

In the case of anterior cingulotomy, the lesions are placed within dorsal ACC and typically impinge upon gray matter in the cingulate gyrus as well as the white matter cingulum bundle. Thus, in addition to reducing cortical mass and activity within dorsal ACC, it is likely that these lesions modify cingulo-striatal projections, and also disinhibit pregenual ACC. Given the composition of the cingulum bundle, it is also possible that its disruption in cingulotomy could influence reciprocal connections between the ACC and several other structures, including OFC, the amygdala, the hippocampus, or posterior cingulate cortex *(51)*. Given the CSTC neurocircuitry model of OCD, these are all potential sites of therapeutic action. Given the cortico–limbic network model of MD, it might be more appealing to consider that lesions of dorsal ACC might produce disinhibition of pregenual ACC, which in turn, might render patients more responsive to antidepressant pharmacotherapy postsurgically. Alternatively, lesions of the cingulum bundle might interrupt ascending influences of the amygdala on the dorsal compartment.

In the case of subcaudate tractotomy, bilateral orbitomedial leucotomy lesions are made. The orbito-medial leucotomy lesions purportedly interrupt fibers of passage connecting OFC and subgenual ACC to the thalamus, and might also disrupt amygdalo-fugal fibers to OFC and subgenual ACC *(52)*. In OCD, interruption of reciprocal projections between OFC and thalamus would theoretically decrease reverberating (amplified) activity in the OFC-caudate CSTC, leading to a reduction of OCD symptoms. Likewise, in MDD, lesions of the subgenual ACC or OFC would directly reduce activity within the ventral compartment, which in turn would be hypothesized to reduce depressive symptoms.

In the case of anterior capsulotomy, lesions of the ventral portion of the anterior limb of the anterior capsule purportedly interrupt OFC and subgenual ACC pathways to the thalamus. Additionally, the placement of these lesions may also compromise areas of adjacent striatal territory. Striatal damage may occur if the lesions interrupt fronto-striatal projections, if the lesions themselves impinge on the striatum, or if infiltration of edema surrounding the lesions encroaches on the striatum itself or fronto-striatal projections. For OCD, disruption of pathological CSTC circuitry at the level of OFC-caudate or reciprocal OFC-thalamic communications could underlie the therapeutic effects of anterior capsulotomy. For MD, deactivation of subgenual ACC or disruption of interconnections between the elements of the ventral compartment are plausible modes of therapeutic action for anterior capsulotomy. Interestingly, an MRI study of anterior capsulotomy for OCD and other anxiety disorders indicated that appropriate placement of lesions within the right anterior capsule was critical to subsequent therapeutic response *(53)*. Furthermore, functional imaging data from a small cohort of patients with severe anxiety disorders undergoing anterior capsulotomy demonstrated reductions in activity within orbitomedial frontal cortex from presurgical to postsurgical scans *(54)*.

FUTURE DIRECTIONS

One current area of investigation based on neurocircuitry models has focused on predicting treatment response to neurosurgery. Given the serious nature of the intervention, such knowledge would be helpful in selecting candidates for neurosurgical invervention. Initial explorations in this area using preoperative positron emission tomography scans have demonstrated specific patterns of regional brain activity that may serve as predictors of response. Rauch et al. *(55)* demonstrated that preoperative hypermetabolism in right posterior cingulate cortex predicted superior treatment response in OCD (*see* Fig. 14). In the analogous study performed to examine correlates of treatment response in MD, Dougherty et al. *(56)* demonstrated that preoperative hypermetabolism in left subgenual cortex and left thalamus predicted superior treatment response (*see* Fig. 15). If treatment response can be reliably predicted by specific preoperative metabolic states, we may be able to more accurately determine the optimal candidate for a specific procedure.

Another exciting development is the application of neurosurgical devices in the treatment of psychiatric disorders. At this point in time, the most promising technology is deep brain stimulation (DBS). Originally developed as a treatment for movement disorders (such as Parkinson's disease), neurologists are quickly gaining experience with the operation of these devices. Recent preliminary reports have demonstrated the potential of DBS for treating OCD (using the capsulotomy target) *(57)* and for altering anxiety and mood states *(58)*. Further investigation will ultimately be needed to determine its efficacy and clinical value, however this modality of treatment offers many potential advantages. First and foremost, DBS offers a modality of treatment that is not inherently ablative in nature. In addition to avoiding the destruction of tissue, one has the theoretical flexibility of modulating treatment by varying such parameters as which combination of electrodes are activated, and stimulus characteristics such as polarity, intensity, and frequency. Thus, parameters could be optimized for each individual patient. As DBS does not permanently destroy brain tissue, electrodes could be inactivated or removed, with the presumed reversal of any effects. Additionally, from a research perspective, DBS provides an important opportunity to conduct studies with a crossover design, thus enabling trials comparing active treatment with sham control.

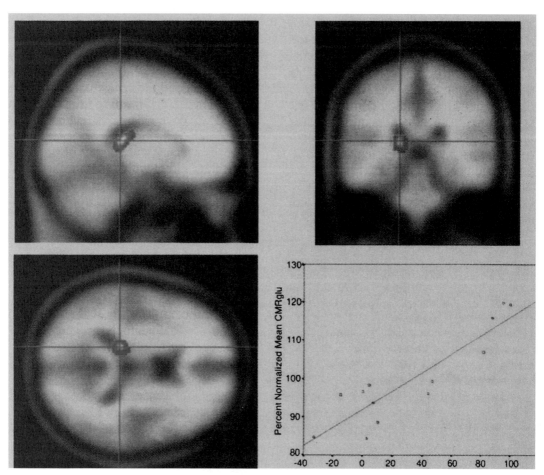

Fig.14. PET finding of a statistically significant correlation between preoperative cerebal metabolism within right posterior cingulate cortex and Y-BOCS improvement following cingulotomy. Upper left and right and lower left panels show the 9 voxel locus in brain of significant correlation, as viewed from the three conventional orthogonal perspectives. The correlation analysis is graphically illustrated in the lower right panel. The *y*-axis reflects % normalized rCMRglu values averaged over the 9 voxel ROI; 100% is equivalent to the grand mean of CMRglu for the entire acquired brain volume. The *x*-axis reflects perceent Y-BOCS improvement from preoperative to postoperative time points. rCMRglu, regional cerebral metabolic rates for glucose; ROI, region of interest; Y-BOCs, Yale-Brown Obsessive Compulsive Scale.

The use of neurosurgery for psychiatric indications remains one of the most powerful tools available both for clinical treatment of psychiatric disorders as well as for the exploration of the connection between mind and brain. Coupled with ever-developing neuro-investigative techniques, research into physical manipulations of the brain will not only expand our understanding of neurobiology, but also promises to lead to the development of increasingly safe and effective clinical interventions. In the near future, we hope to see refinement of lesion areas, identification of superior targets, individually tailored interventions for specific patient presentations (e.g., whereby targets are individually determined for each patient), development of predictive methods to determine likelihood of treatment response or complications, improved ability to utilize all treatment modalities in synergy, and the development of more efficacious and safer modalities of treatment.

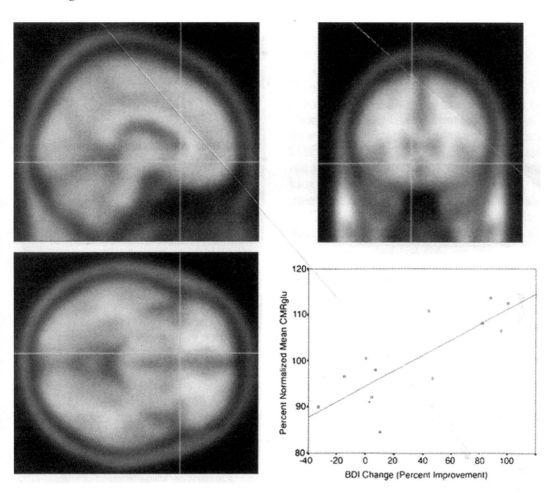

Fig. 15. Nominally structural MRI images transformed to MNI space illustrating the principal finding of a statistically significant correlation between preoperative rCMRG (CMRglu) within the left subgenual prefrontal cortex and BDI score imprvement following cingulotomy. These panels demonstrate the locus of significant correlation, as viewed from three conventional orthogonal perspectives. The intersection of the cross-hairs corresponds to the site of peak correlation (z score 3.32; MNI coordinates –8, 24, and –8); this defines the voxel of peak statistical significance used to generate the data depicted graphically (lower right). Specifically, for this voxel, the Pearson product-moment correlations between rCMRG and BDI score improvement yielded r^2 (11) = 0.81; $p = 0.001$.

REFERENCES

1. Damasio H, Damasio AR, Grabowski T, Frank R. The return of Phineas Gage: clues about the brain from the skull of a famous patient. Science 1994;264:1102–1105.
2. Harlow JM. Recovery From the Passage of an Iron Bar Through the Head. Publications of the Massachusetts Medical Society. Boston: David Clapp and Son; 1869.
3. Goltz F. Ueber die Verrichtungen des Grosshirns. Arch F nD ges Physiol 1890;26:1–49.
4. Burckhardt G. Über Rindenexcisionen, als Beitra zur operativen Therapie der Psychosen. Allegemaine Zeitschrift für Psychiatrie 1891;47:463–545.
5. Puusepp L. Alcune considerazioni sugli interventi chirurgici nelle malattie mentali. Giornale Della Accademia di Medicina di Torino. 1937;100:3–16.
6. Crawford MP, Fulton JF, Jacobsen CF, Wolfe JB. Frontal lobe ablation in chimpanzee: a resume of "Becky" and "Lucy." Res Publ Assoc Nerv Ment Dis 1948;27:3–58.

7. Moniz E. Tentatives Opératoires Dans Le Traitement De Certaines Psychoses. Paris: Masson and Cie; 1936.
8. Moniz E. Prefrontal leucotomy in the treatment of mental disorders. Am J Psychiatry 1937;93:1379–1385.
9. Freeman W, Watts JW. Prefrontal lobotomy in the treatment of mental disorders. South Med J 1937;30:23–31.
10. Freeman W. Transorbital leucotomy. Lancet 1948;2:371–373.
11. Tooth JC, Newton MP. Leucotomy in England and Wales 1942–1954. Reports on Public Health and Medical Subjects, No. 104. London: Her Majesty's Stationary Office; 1961.
12. Lyerly JG. Prefrontal lobotomy in involutional melancholia. J Fla Med Assoc 1938;25:225–229.
13. Penfield W. Symposium on gyrectomy. Part I. Bilateral frontal gyrectomy and postoperative intelligence. Proceedings of the Association of Research on Nervous and Mental Disease 1948;27:519–34.
14. Malmo RB. Symposium on gyrectomy. Part III. Psychological aspects of frontal gyrectomy and frontal lobotomy in mental patients. Proceedings of the Association of Research on Nervous and Mental Disease 1948;27:537–564.
15. Scoville WB. Selective cortical undercutting as a means of modifying and studying frontal lobe function in man: preliminary report of forty-three operative cases. J Neurosurg 1949;6:65–73.
16. Knight G. Stereotactic tractotomy in the surgical treatment of mental illness. J Neurol Neurosurg Psychiatry 1965;28: 304–310.
17. Knight GC. The orbital cortex as an objective in the surgical treatment of mental illness. The development of the stereotactic approach. Br J Surgery 1965;51: 114–124.
18. Bridges PK, Bartlett JR, Hale AS, Poynton AM, Malizia AL, Hodgkiss AD. Psychosurgery: stereotactic subcaudate tractotomy. An indispensible procedure. Br J Psychiatry 1994;165: 599–611.
19. Goktepe EO, Young LB, Bridges PK. A further review of the results of stereotactic subcaudate tractotomy. Br J Psychiatry 1975;126:270–280.
20. A Critical Assessment of Psychiatric Surgery. Past, Present and Future. American Handbook of Psychiatry, Vol. 8. Basic Books; 1986:1029–1047.
21. Ballantine HT, Bouckoms AJ, Thomas EK, Giriunas IE. Treatment of psychiatric illness by stereotactic cingulotomy. Biol Psychiatry 1987;22:807–819.
22. Spangler WJ, Cosgrove GR, Ballantine HT, et al. MRI-guided stereotactic cingulotomy for intractable psychiatric disease. Neurosurgery 1996;38:1071–1076.
23. Dougherty DD, Baer L, Cosgrove GR, et al. Update on cingulotomy for intractable obsessive-compulsive disorder: prospective long-term follow-up of 44 patients. Am J Psychiatry 2002;159:269–275.
24. Corkin S, Twitchell TE, Sullivan EV. Safety and efficacy of cingulotomy for pain and psychiatric disorders. In: Hitchcock ER, Ballantine HT, Myerson BA, eds. Modern Concepts in Psychiatric Surgery. Amsterdam: Elsevier; 1979;253–272.
25. Kelly D, Richardson A, Mitchell-Heggs N. Stereotactic limbic leucotomy: neurophysiologic aspects and operative technique. Br J Psychiatry 1973;123:133–140.
26. Mitchell-Heggs N, Kelley D, Richardson A. Stereotactic limbic leucotomy.A follow-up at 16 months. Br J Psychiatry 1991;128:283–291.
27. Montoya A, Weiss AP, Price BH, et al. Magnetic resonance imaging-guided stereotactic limbic leukotomy for treatment of intractable psychiatric disease. Neurosurgery 2002;50:1043–1049.
28. Price BH, Baral I, Cosgrove GR, et al. Improvement in severe self-mutilation following limbic leucotomy: a series of 5 consecutive cases. J Clin Psychiatry 2001;62:925–932.
29. Herner T. Treatment of mental disorders with frontal stereotactic thermal lesions. A follow-up study of 116 cases. Acta Psychiatrica Neurolog Scand 1961;158:36.
30. Bingley T, Leksell L, Meyerson BA, et al. Long-term results of stereotactic capsulotomy in chronic obsessive compulsive neurosis, In: Sweet WH, Obrador S, Martin-Rodriguez JG, eds. Neurosurgical Treatment in Psychiatry, Pain and Epilepsy. Baltimore: University Park Press; 1977:287–289.
31. National Commission for the Protection of Human Subjects of Biomedical and Behavioral Research. Report and Recommendations: Psychosurgery. Department of Health and Human Services, Pub No (OS) 77-002. Washington DC: US Government Printing Office; 1979.
32. Alexander GE, DeLong MR, Strick PL. Parallel organization of functionally segregated circuits linking basal ganglia and cortex. Ann Rev Neurosci 1986;9:357–381.
33. Alexander GE, Crutcher MD, DeLong MR. Basal ganglia-thalamocortical circuits: parallel substrates for motor, oculomotor, "prefrontal" and "limbic" functions. Prog Brain Res 1990;85:119–146.
34. Rauch SL, Whalen PJ, Dougherty DD, Jenike MA. Neurobiological models of obsessive compulsive disorders. In: Jenike MA, Baer L, Minichiello WE, eds. Obsessive-Compulsive Disorders: Practical Management. Boston: Mosby; 1998:222–253.
35. Saxena S, Brody AL, Schwartz JM, Baxter LR. Neuroimaging and frontal-subcortical circuitry in obsessive-compulsive disorder. Br J Psychiatry 1998;35:26–37.
36. Baxter LR, Schwartz JM, Guze BH, et al. Neuroimaging in obsessive-compulsive disorder: seeking the mediating neuroanatomy. In: Jenike MA, Baer L, Minichiello WE, eds. Obsessive Compulsive Disorder: Theory and Management., Second Edition. Chicago: Year Book Medical Publishers; 1990:167–188.
37. Rauch SL, Whalen PJ, Dougherty DD, Jenike MA. Neurobiological models of obsessive compulsive disorders. In: Jenike MA, Baer L, Minichiello WE, eds. Obsessive-Compulsive Disorders: Practical Management. Boston: Mosby; 1998: 222–253.

38. Haber SN, Fudge JL, McFarland NR. Striatonigrostriatal pathways in primates form an ascending spiral from the shell to the dorsolateral striatum. J Neurosci 2000;20:2369–2382.
39. Dougherty DD, Rauch SL. Neuroimaging and neurobiological models of depression. Harv Rev Psychiatry 1997;5:138–159.
40. Drevets WC. Neuroimaging studies of mood disorders. Biol Psychiatry 2000;48:813–829.
41. Mayberg HS. Limbic-cortical dysregulation: a proposed model of depression. J Neuropsychiatry Clin Neurosci 1997;9: 471–481.
42. Sheline YI. 3D MRI studies of neuroanatomic changes in unipolar major depression: the role of stress and medical comorbidity. Biol Psychiatry 2000;48:791–800.
43. Swerdlow NR, Koob GF. Dopamine, schizophrenia, mania and depression: toward a unified hypothesis of cortico-striato-pallido-thalamic function. Behav Brain Sci 1987;10:197–245.
44. Mayberg HS, Brannan SK, Tekell JL, et al. Regional metabolic effects of fluoxetine in major depression: Serial changes and relationship to clinical response. Biol Psychiatry 2000;48:830–843.
45. Mayberg HS, Liotti M, Brannan S, et al. Reciprocal limbic-cortical function and negative mood: converging PET findings in depression and normal sadness. Am J Psychiatry 1999;156:675–682.
46. Drevets WC, Raichle ME. Reciprocal suppression of regional cerebral blood flow during emotional versus higher cognitive processes. Implications for interactions between emotion and cognition. Cogn Emotion 1998;12:353–385.
47. Rauch SL, van der Kolk BA, Fisler RE, et al. A symptom provocation study of posttraumatic stress disorder using positron emission tomography and script-driven imagery. Arch Gen Psychiatry 1996;53:380–387.
48. Shulman GL, Corbetta M, Buckner RL, et al. Common blood flow changes across visual tasks: II. Decrease in cerebral cortex. J Cogn Neurosci 1997;9:647–662.
49. Whalen PJ, Bush G, McNally RJ, et al. The Emotional Counting Stroop paradigm: an fMRI probe of the anterior cingulate affective division. Biol Psychiatry 1998;44:1219–1228.
50. Kaufman J, Plotsky PM, Nemeroff CB, Charney DS. Effects of early adverse experiences on brain structure and function: clinical implications. Biol Psychiatry 2000;48:778–790.
51. Mufson EJ, Pandya DN. Some observations on the course and composition of the cingulum bundle in the rhesus monkey. J Comp Neurol 1984;225:31–43.
52. Amaral DG, Price JL. Amygdalo-cortical projections in the monkey. J Comp Neurol 1984;230:465–496.
53. Lippitz BE, Mindus P, Meyerson BA, Kihlstrom L, Lindquist C. Lesion topography and outcome after thermocapsulotomy or gamma knife capsulotomy for obsessive-compulsive disorder: relevance of the right hemisphere. Neurosurgery 1999;44:452–458.
54. Mindus P, Ericson K, Greitz T, Meyerson BA, Nyman H, Sjogren I. Regional cerebral glucose metabolism in anxiety disorders studied with positron emission tomography before and after psychosurgical intervention. A preliminary report. Acta Radiol Suppl 1986;369:444–448.
55. Rauch SL, Dougherty DD, Cosgrove GR, et al. Cerebral metabolic correlates as potential predictors of response to anterior cingulotomy for obsessive compulsive disorder. Biol Psychiatry 2001;50:659–667.
56. Dougherty DD, Weiss AP, Cosgrove GR, et al. Cerebral metabolic correlates as potential predictors of response to anterior cingulotomy for treatment of major depression. J Neurosurg 2003;99:1010–1017.
57. Gabriels L, Cosyns P, Nuttin B, Demeulemeester H, Gybels J. Deep brain stimulation for treatment-refractory obsessive-compulsive disorder: psychopathological and neuropsychological outcome in three cases. Acta Psychiatr Scand 2003;107: 275–282.
58. Kopell BH, Greenberg B, Rezai AR. Deep brain stimulation for psychiatric disorders. J Clin Neurophysiol 2004;21:51–67.
59. Poppen JL. Technique of prefrontal lobotomy. J Neurosurg 1948;5:514–520.
60. Knight GC. Bi-frontal stereotactic tractotomy: an atraumatic operation of value in the treatment of intractable psychoneurosis. Br J Psychiatry 1969;11:5257–5266.
61. Mindus P, Bergstrom K, Levander SE, Noren G, Hindmarsh T, Thuomas KA. Magnetic resonance images related to clinical outcome after psychosurgical intervention in severe anxiety disorder. J Neurol Neurosurg Psychiatry 1987;50:1288–1293.
62. Goldapple K, Segal Z, Garson C, et al. Modulation of cortical-limbic pathways in major depression: treatment-specific effects of cognitive behavior therapy. Arch Gen Psychiatry 2001;61:34–41.

27

Psychotherapy for Psychiatric Disorders

John R. McQuaid and Laura Campbell-Sills

INTRODUCTION

Psychotherapy has developed, in the past 100 or more years, from a theoretically derived intervention with little empirical support to a broad range of interventions for which there is an equally broad range of evidence. This chapter provides an overview of psychotherapy for psychiatric disorders. The goals of this chapter are to review the history of psychotherapy development, identify the primary efficacious approaches of psychotherapy, and describe the interventions currently used with specific disorders. This chapter focuses on evidence-based psychotherapies (with demonstrated treatment benefit in stringently controlled research trials) because it is our perspective that training and education in treatment should emphasize those interventions supported by scientific data. We hope to provide readers with an adequate understanding of the current literature to make effective treatment recommendations.

AN OVERVIEW OF THE HISTORY OF PSYCHOTHERAPY

Psychotherapy initially developed out of the models of Freud and his contemporaries in the form of psychoanalysis *(1,2)*. They proposed that disorder stemmed from unsuccessful attempts to control unconscious drives associated with sex and aggression. Freud argued that defenses, used to manage these drives, generated conflicts. Freudian theory stated that psychoanalysis provided insight into these drives, and that insight would lead to a reduction of the psychopathology. Interventions derived from Freudian models emphasized the use of the therapeutic relationship to uncover and develop insight into these unconscious processes. The analyst provided a neutral presence, upon which the patient's unconscious processes projected a range of assumptions and defenses. By interpreting these processes, the analyst aided the patient in becoming aware of unconscious drives and defenses against these drives, and aided the patient in developing insight. The model hypothesized that with insight patients would be able to engage in healthier behaviors in response to their drives.

Freud's theories were developmental in nature, attributing the presence of psychopathology to problems in coping with developmental milestones. Later psychodynamic models (such as object-relations theory) placed increasing emphasis on developmental influences and interpersonal relationships *(3)*. These models suggested that early relationships, by providing consistency, support, and nurturing, helped the developing individual gain a sense of self and the ability to differentiate between one's own needs and the needs of others. Psychopathology, according to these models, arose when early environments either did not provide appropriate boundaries (so that individuals had a poor ability to differentiate their own needs and those of others), or were inconsistent and unpredictable (leading to an experience of vulnerability and anxiety) *(3)*. The interventions remained similar to psychoanalysis in terms of an emphasis on examining the therapeutic relationship. On the other hand, there was a greater

From: *Current Clinical Neurology: Psychiatry for Neurologists*
Edited by: D.V. Jeste and J.H. Friedman © Humana Press Inc., Totowa, NJ

emphasis on the nurturing aspect of the relationship as a healing mechanism. Whereas in original psychoanalysis the role of the therapist was to provide an object to which the patient could react, and then serve as an interpreter of those reactions, in object-relations theory and self-psychology the therapist provided a "corrective emotional experience" by serving as a consistent, supportive relationship. These models propose that the positive relationship in itself improved functioning by allowing the patient to recognize old defenses and engage in new, more effective defenses.

In general, psychoanalytic and psychodynamic models proposed that therapy was a long-term process (in some cases, multiple sessions per week for years), requiring extensive examination of the therapeutic relationship to produce insight and change. Whereas these models dominated psychotherapy initially, the "behavioral revolution" particularly from the 1940s to 1960s, challenged several core tenets of psychoanalysis, including the validity of the underlying theory, the efficacy of the treatments, and the scientific merit of the interventions. Behavior therapy grew in popularity and sophistication, and benefited in particular from the application of scientific principles to assessing the effects of these treatments.

Behavioral therapies arose out of the theories of classical and operant conditioning. Behavior therapists rejected the reliance on unconscious (and therefore unobservable) processes to explain behavior, including pathological behavior *(4)*. Instead, they proposed that psychopathology could be explained by the same principles of learning that had been shown to explain how behaviors changed in response to positive and negative stimuli, and argued that only observable behaviors were appropriate targets for intervention. Behavioral therapists therefore developed interventions designed to modify problematic behaviors (e.g., avoidance resulting from anxiety, depressive withdrawal), by changing the reinforcers in the patient's life. This was done both through both operant conditioning (e.g., teaching assertiveness skills and activity scheduling, with the goal that the new behaviors would be reinforced by positive responses from the environment), and classical conditioning (e.g., systematically pairing feared stimuli with relaxation training). Behavioral therapy brought to psychotherapy the value of applying scientific principles to the study of psychotherapy. Because the interventions tended to focus on specific behaviors rather than broad personality change, behavior therapy tended to be much more short term, depending on the target of treatment *(5,6)*.

In the 1960s, researchers developed increasing sophistication in conceptualizing and studying cognitive processes. Whereas behaviorists had chosen to reject cognition as an appropriate target of intervention owing to its inherently unobservable nature, other scientists started to develop models that incorporated cognitive elements in the understanding of normal behavior as well as psychopathology. In particular, Albert Bandura developed social learning theory to explain scientific evidence of observational learning, in which behavior change occurred not through direct experience (as was the case in operant and classical conditioning) but through observing the behaviors of others *(7)*. Bandura and other cognitive researchers proposed that cognitive processes mediated between a stimulus and a learned response. These models implied that cognitive factors could serve as a target of treatment.

Cognitive therapy arose in part as a response to the developments in the understanding of cognition, and in part as a reaction to limitations of psychoanalytic/psychodynamic models of psychotherapy. Cognitive therapy, as conceptualized by Albert Ellis, Aaron Beck, and others, proposed that emotional responses arose from the cognitive interpretation of life experiences *(8,9)*. Individuals with mood and anxiety disorders had a tendency to interpret experiences in particularly negative or threatening ways. Based on this model, treatment involved retraining patients to notice their thinking, evaluate whether the thoughts were accurate or if there was some error contributing to the negative mood state, and then generate more accurate, healthy thoughts that helped improve mood. In contrast to psychodynamic models, cognitive therapy emphasized the present rather than exploration of early life history. In addition, therapy was structured, with the therapist actively teaching new skills and assigning homework. Over time, cognitive therapy has incorporated behavioral principles to such an extent that it is now frequently referred to as cognitive-behavior therapy (CBT), and this is the term that is used in the rest of the chapter.

Since the development of the cognitive therapies, there have been additional models elaborated and subjected to rigorous empirical validation. In particular, interpersonal psychotherapy (IPT) is a manualized intervention based on psychodynamic and attachment theories *(10)*. IPT was initially developed as a depression treatment, and focuses on interpersonal roles as contributors to depression. The treatment focuses on helping patients learn about these roles, and through their understanding develop healthier interpersonal relationships. Several studies have demonstrated that IPT is efficacious for the treatment and prevention of major depression *(11)*.

As researchers have advanced in their understanding of the mechanisms of treatments, some of the deficits in the standard treatments became apparent. In particular, researchers in cognitive and behavioral therapies identified that the emphasis on change at times did not address the reality of patients' lives. Therefore, therapy researchers began to develop modified interventions that included components designed to help patients with unchangeable situations. These interventions often drew on relaxation and meditation practices designed to allow patients to experience negative situations in a more "accepting" manner. Some examples of this are acceptance and commitment therapy *(12)*, dialectical behavior therapy *(13)*, and mindfulness-based cognitive therapy *(14)*. Several of these interventions have been subjected to randomized controlled trials and demonstrated to be effective for treatment of psychiatric disorders *(12–14)*.

This is a brief overview of major psychotherapeutic models. There are a variety of additional forms of therapy derived from each of these schools. In addition, many therapists describe themselves as eclectic (drawing techniques from different models) or integrationist (using an organizing theory that combines different theories to generate treatment approaches). An example of an integrationist model is biologically informed psychotherapy for depression (BIPD *[15]*). BIPD is based on a biological theory of the etiology and course of depression, and incorporates interventions derived from other models based on predictions generated by the biological model. Another model that is appearing to be more and more integrationist is "Eye Movement Desensitization and Reprocessing" *(16)* a controversial intervention that developed from a specific technique (i.e., having patients move their eyes back and forth while recalling traumatic events) to an elaborate model incorporating interventions from behavioral, cognitive-behavioral, and psychodynamic models.

Although there is extensive need for discussion of additional psychotherapy approaches, for the purposes of this chapter we emphasize the primary treatment models that have received scientific scrutiny. Several groups have recently put together guidelines for evaluating the efficacy and effectiveness of psychotherapy *(17,18)*. For the current chapter, we emphasize treatments that are efficacious or probably efficacious, based on the criteria established by Chambless and Hollon *(17)*. This requires that the intervention has been shown to be superior to placebo, or equivalent or superior to an established treatment, in at least two well-defined randomized controlled trials (RCTs). Probably efficacious therapies have either been shown superior to placebo or equivalent to a validated treatment in one well-designed RCT, or in several trials with significant limitations, or in a large series of case studies.

INTERVENTIONS FOR ADULT PSYCHOPATHOLOGY

Mood Disorders

A large number of studies have tested psychotherapies for unipolar major depressive disorder (MDD). Those that are currently known to be efficacious are behavior therapy (both group and individual), CBT, IPT, and behavioral marital therapy *(18–20)*. There are fewer studies for other mood disorders. There is some evidence for CBT as an intervention for bipolar disorder, as well as family therapy and a modified version of IPT *(21,22)*.

Behavior Therapy

Behavior therapy (BT) for depression emphasizes the importance of positive reinforcers and increasing rewards in the environment. As with any intervention, an initial assessment is necessary prior to treatment in order to determine whether the treatment is appropriate, and if so, what areas to target in therapy. However, given the behavioral framework on which this treatment is based, the assessment emphasizes quantifiable problems and target goals over more general terms such as diagnostic labels. Diagnosis is assessed with standardized measures, and then the components of the depressive symptomatology are detailed (e.g., specific problems associated with depression, behavioral changes, interpersonal difficulties). These data both improve the understanding of the diagnosis as well as provide initial targets for intervention.

Early treatment components include orientation and education about the model to facilitate patient involvement. At this point, the therapist conducts an extensive assessment of the reinforcers in the patient's environment, including pleasant or rewarding activities and social contacts. Patients learn to track their activities and rate the effect of their activities on their mood. They learn to set goals, schedule activities, and to problem solve when there are factors preventing the increase of rewarding activities.

The other major component of BT is interpersonal skills training. From a behavioral perspective, healthy relationships are a major resource for positive reinforcement. Patients in BT are taught skills specifically designed to improve relationships, including listening skills, assertive communication (e.g., learning to directly express opinions and desires in a clear but respectful manner), and effective agreeing and disagreeing. To aid in learning these skills, treatment can include role-playing, or be done in a group format so that other group members can provide feedback.

Cognitive-Behavior Therapy

As noted before, CBT interventions are short-term, problem-focused techniques designed to help patients notice their thoughts and behaviors, identify the costs and benefits of those thoughts and behaviors, try out new ones, and then assess whether the changes have improved the patient's target goals. We divide the interventions into three components, early, middle, and late interventions, for the purposes of review.

CBT is quite closely related to BT in many aspects, particularly early in therapy. Assessment is similar to BT assessment, emphasizing standardized assessment and quantifiable targets of intervention. However, there is a greater emphasis on assessing cognitive processes. As with BT, the CBT therapist wants to make sure that the patient is as informed as possible about the model of treatment. Both treatments are collaborative models, meaning that the patient is expected to play an active role in guiding the treatment, choosing the targets of intervention, and actually testing out exercises and providing feedback. To do so, the patient needs to understand the intervention.

In CBT, the therapist will describe the treatment to the patient, check in to make sure the patient understands the information presented, and provide patients with handouts describing the treatment. Critical components for the therapist to cover are the collaborative relationship between therapist and patient, the use of homework assignments, the role of behavioral experiments in testing patient beliefs and generating new behaviors, and the importance of feedback. As the patient comes to understand the treatment, the therapist and patient will develop a therapeutic agreement as to whether they will work together, and if so, for how long and toward what goals. Finally, the therapist attempts to provide the patient with some interventions both to demonstrate how therapy will work, as well as to help reduce some of the patient's current distress. One place where BT and CBT differ is perceived role of the behavioral activities in producing change. Whereas in BT the activities are an end to themselves, in CBT there is an emphasis on using activities to test beliefs that feed depression. For example, individuals who believe that others do not listen to them might be trained in assertive communication, and then asked to check how people respond when they communicate clearly. Such an intervention is directly beneficial, but also provides a chance to challenge the dysfunctional belief.

As the previous example indicates, thoughts and beliefs are a central target of CBT. Patients are taught how to differentiate thoughts (what they say to themselves) from feelings (emotional reactions). Patients learn to notice what they are thinking when in negative emotional states, identify flaws in the thoughts (e.g., whether the belief inaccurate or an exaggeration), and begin to learn how to change those unhelpful beliefs.

In the middle section, the therapist and patient work together to address the goals previously defined. The therapist trains the patient in skills of thought challenging, behavioral activation, and communication, depending on relevance to the goals. Therapy sessions tend to start with a review of previously assigned homework, and a discussion of the lessons learned. This is followed by application of CBT skills to any relevant issues that the patient has brought up for the week. As the session nears an end, the therapist assigns a new homework assignment, and then asks the patient for feedback on the session.

As therapy draws to an end, the primary goal of the therapist is to increase the patient's ability to apply learned skills in an independent manner, and to identify any future risks that may lead to symptom relapse. Therapy sessions continue in a similar structure. However, patients are now asked to generate homework assignments, assess their own progress, and start to serve as their own therapists.

Recent advances in CBT have incorporated the use of mindfulness meditation for prevention of relapse *(14)*. Mindfulness refers to teaching patients to observe their experiences, including thoughts, feelings, and body sensations, in a nonjudgmental manner. Following successful pharmacotherapy, mindfulness-based CBT has been shown to reduce depression relapse for individuals with a history of recurrent depression *(23)*.

CBT for bipolar disorder is not a stand-alone treatment, but rather an adjunctive intervention to appropriate medication. Whereas the therapist may directly attempt to reduce symptoms via CBT skills (e.g., using a thought record to examine distorted optimism in a hypomanic phase), there is a greater emphasis on relapse prevention for patients who are not experiencing acute mania or depression. Medication adherence is a central focus of treatment, including challenging thoughts about medications that may increase the risk of discontinuation. Patients also track changes in symptoms to identify evidence of impending relapse, with the goal of intervening early to prevent a full relapse. Given the difficulty of recognition of symptoms when manic, family members are often involved in treatment to aid the patient in recognizing symptom exacerbations and provide support for interventions.

Interpersonal Psychotherapy

IPT is based on the assumption that relationships play a critical role in the development and maintenance of depressive episodes. Treatment focuses on one or more of four major themes: grief (such as that stemming from the loss of a loved one), interpersonal disputes (e.g., marital conflict), role transitions (e.g., moving into a parenting role), and interpersonal deficits (e.g., lack of assertiveness skills). Therapy involves identifying the relevant deficits and then helping the patient address them using a variety of techniques. These can involve classic psychodynamic approaches (interpreting resistance, analysis of transference and countertransference), supportive interventions (empathic listening), and even cognitive and behavioral interventions (e.g., interpersonal skills training, examining problematic beliefs about relationships).

Couples Therapy and Family Therapy

Recent research has found that couples therapy for can be as effective for treating MDD as individual therapy, when the depressed individual is in a distressed relationship. In addition, couples therapy for depression also appears to decrease relationship distress. This intervention arose from the observation that approx 50% of depressed married individuals reported significant marital distress *(24)*. Behavioral marital therapy (BMT) for depression focuses on several target goals. After a broad assessment of the couples' relationship, the therapist helps the couple identify areas of change. Communication training is often a central focus of treatment, and includes teaching active listening skills, assertive communication, and effective agreeing/disagreeing. Patients also are taught problem-solving skills and are coached on applying these skills to the relevant problems in their relationship. Throughout the course of BMT, treatment emphasizes increasing the rewarding aspects of the relationship for each partner (e.g., scheduling enjoyable conjoint activities, increasing caring behaviors).

Family therapy for bipolar disorder *(25)* is primarily psychoeducational in nature. The intervention is based on the recognition that bipolar illness affects family members as well as the patient, and that the family can play a major role in either exacerbating symptoms or aiding in effective coping. Treatment generally involves teaching the family members (usually the spouse or parents) about the nature of bipolar disorder, including symptoms, course, treatment, and factors associated with relapse. Family members are trained to reduce stress in family environments through reducing hostile or critical communication, which has previously been associated with relapse.

Anxiety Disorders

Anxiety disorders include a wide range of diagnoses such as panic disorder (with or without agoraphobia), social phobia, specific phobia, obsessive-compulsive disorder (OCD), generalized anxiety disorder (GAD), and posttraumatic stress disorder (PTSD). Although symptoms vary across these disorders, efficacious treatments are generally cognitive-behavioral in nature and share several key components across the diagnoses.

Individuals frequently present to primary care and medical specialty settings with symptoms that are potentially manifestations of an anxiety disorder *(26,27)*. Anxiety is associated with somatic complaints as diverse as heart palpitations, shortness of breath, dizziness, nausea, trembling, chest pain, fatigue, and muscle tension *(28)*. Differentiating anxiety phenomena from cardiovascular, respiratory, neurological, and other medical disorders presents a diagnostic challenge to a wide range of health care professionals. Fortunately, once a clinician has determined a problem to be anxiety-related, effective treatment options are available.

The majority of psychosocial treatments for anxiety classified as efficacious or probably efficacious by the American Psychological Association employ cognitive and/or behavioral techniques *(17)*. The major "ingredients" of CBT for anxiety include psychoeducation, examination and countering of anxious thoughts, exposure to anxiety-producing stimuli, and homework practices. This section provides an overview of these treatment elements, along with examples of how they might be implemented for specific anxiety disorders.

Psychoeducation

The psychoeducational component of CBT for anxiety disorders serves multiple purposes. Educating clients about anxiety corrects distressing misconceptions, normalizes their experiences, instills hope, and creates healthy cognitive change. Teaching the cognitive-behavioral model of anxiety also fosters a collaborative therapeutic relationship in which clients and therapists have a shared language and conceptualization of anxiety.

Most cognitive-behavioral therapists treating clients with anxiety disorders begin by discussing the nature and purpose of anxiety and fear. Clients learn about the survival value of these emotions, and develop a basic understanding of their physiological basis. Therapists often emphasize the interactions between thoughts, feelings, and behaviors. Presentation of this model helps clients to understand how making changes in the areas of cognition and behavior might interrupt the cycle of anxiety. Psychoeducational interventions for anxiety also highlight the costs of avoidant coping strategies. In the short term, avoidance relieves anxiety and is therefore reinforced; however, avoidance ultimately maintains the anxiety disorder, decreases self-efficacy and life satisfaction, and creates other negative emotions (e.g., guilt). Recasting avoidance as a counterproductive strategy early in treatment provides a rationale for the exposure phase of treatment, in which clients are instructed to confront anxiety-provoking stimuli.

Beyond these basic elements of psychoeducation, the material covered in this phase of CBT varies based on the client's specific problems. For example, individuals suffering from panic disorder learn to interpret their panic symptoms as a harmless "misfiring" of their fight-or-flight system rather than as an indication that something terrible is happening (e.g., heart attack, "going crazy") *(29)*. In contrast, clients with OCD learn about the paradoxical effects of thought suppression *(30)*. Suppressing unwanted thoughts is a common coping mechanism for individuals with OCD; however, in CBT clients learn that this approach is likely to backfire and create a subsequent increase in the unwanted thought.

Cognitive Interventions

Cognitive techniques are similar to those described for mood disorders. In the case of anxiety disorders, typical cognitive distortions include "all or nothing thinking" (i.e., seeing things as either all good or all bad), "fortune telling" (i.e., predicting outcomes on the basis of little or no evidence), and "catastrophizing" (i.e., considering only the worst case scenario). Individuals with anxiety disorders tend to both overestimate the likelihood of negative events and underestimate their abilities to cope with unwanted or stressful outcomes. Therefore, the cognitive phase of treatment often revolves around correcting these types of misconceptions. Clients are taught to evaluate the realistic probability of catastrophic events occurring. For instance, an individual with a specific phobia of flying might be asked to research the probability of dying in a plane crash. In addition, CBT therapists encourage clients to consider how they might cope with difficult situations. An example would be encouraging a socially phobic client to think through how they might cope with not knowing the answer to a question during a work meeting.

Cognitive techniques are repeated frequently during sessions and homework practices, because it takes great effort for clients to "unlearn" the automatic, anxious way of thinking and to replace it with more balanced thinking. When cognitive techniques are employed effectively, clients are able to view situations as less threatening and to trust in their abilities to handle discomfort. These cognitive changes often lead to important behavioral changes as well.

Exposure

Exposure is a component of efficacious treatment for all of the anxiety disorders, with the possible exception of GAD *(31,32)*. This technique involves confronting anxiety-provoking stimuli in a repetitive fashion in order to facilitate habituation, or the natural abatement of the physiological fear reaction. Cognitive change also commonly results from exposure, as clients learn that their worst fears do not occur and that they can cope with anxiety more effectively than they predicted.

In collaboration with the therapist, clients first create a list of feared situations and rate them according to the degree of fear and avoidance they elicit. During each exposure practice, clients remain in the anxiety-provoking situation until subjective distress and physical symptoms decrease substantially. They also practice the same situation multiple times, until that situation no longer elicits a significant fear reaction. In some programs, a gradual approach is taken in which clients begin by confronting mildly anxiety-provoking stimuli. They gradually "move up" their hierarchy of feared situations and confront the most anxiety-provoking situations only after they have developed a sense of mastery with more manageable situations.

Exposures are tailored to the client's problem. For example, treatment of specific phobia of dogs would include exposures to dog-related stimuli (e.g., the sound of a dog barking, movie clips of dogs, actual dogs). In contrast, treatment of generalized social phobia would involve exposure to a wide variety of feared social situations (e.g., making eye contact, saying "hello" to a stranger, going on a date, giving a speech). Other examples of exposure practices might include touching "unclean" surfaces (OCD), having conversations with unfamiliar people (social phobia), and riding in an elevator (panic disorder or specific phobia).

Many CBT treatments also require clients to expose themselves to uncomfortable *internal* stimuli such as physical sensations, unwanted thoughts, and traumatic memories. In treatments for panic disorder, clients confront feared physical sensations through a series of symptom induction exercises called "interoceptive exposure" *(29)*. For example, a client might be asked to breathe through a thin straw in order to induce shortness of breath and dizziness. This exercise would be repeated until the client no longer experienced significant fear in the presence of the target sensation. The purpose of these exercises is to break the conditioned association between certain physical sensations and the panic response.

Individuals with OCD are asked to expose themselves to unwanted thoughts while refraining from maladaptive responses (e.g., rituals, thought suppression) *(31)*. They might be asked to hold a thought or image in their minds, or to listen to a "loop tape" that repeats an obsessional thought over and over. Again, clients practice these types of exercises until anxiety decreases in the presence of the previously feared stimulus (i.e., the unwanted thought). Individuals with PTSD also complete exposures to internal stimuli—namely, the memories of their traumatic experiences *(32)*. Imagery, writing assignments, and descriptions of the trauma to the therapist are used to facilitate exposure and promote habituation.

Exposure is one of the most powerful treatment strategies available for treating psychological distress. Some clients (and therapists) are hesitant to fully utilize exposure because it requires tolerance of significant distress. However, the rewards of skillfully conducted exposure are extensive: decreased fear and avoidance, increased confidence and mastery, and improved psychosocial functioning.

Homework Practices

As with all CBT interventions, anxiety treatment includes extensive practice at home. Only a limited amount of practice can be accomplished in weekly sessions; therefore, clients are regularly assigned tasks to do between sessions. In treatment of anxiety disorders, homework most often includes self-monitoring, practice in using the CBT model (e.g., analyzing anxiety in terms of thoughts, feelings, and behaviors), identifying and challenging anxious thoughts, and completing exposures to feared stimuli. Homework practices help the client take responsibility for their progress and allow treatment gains to generalize beyond the consultation room. Moreover, CBT is always undertaken with the idea that clients will eventually "become their own therapists." Homework practices assist the client in gradually attaining the independence that will allow them to make this transition.

Other Strategies

CBT for anxiety is not limited to the four major strategies outlined here. For example, relaxation techniques frequently have been included in treatment "packages" for anxiety disorders. Progressive muscle relaxation has proven to be useful for alleviating symptoms of GAD *(35)*, and diaphragmatic breathing may help some individuals with panic disorder *(29)*. Problem solving, time management, and assertiveness training also may help individuals cope with anxiety and stress *(36)*. Finally, mindfulness training and acceptance-oriented strategies have shown promising results and are increasingly being incorporated into anxiety treatments *(32)*.

Substance Use Disorder

There are several effective psychosocial interventions for substance use disorders, including CBT, motivational interviewing, and 12-step interventions. A recent multisite study designed to identify factors that predict treatment response found no differences between these three treatments on outcome *(37)*.

Cognitive-Behavior Therapy

CBT for substance use is similar to CBT for other disorders. However, there are several important modifications. When treating substance dependence, there is a strong emphasis on cognitions and behaviors associated with increasing the risk for use. This can include beliefs about use itself (e.g., "One drink won't hurt"), personal efficacy in coping with use ("I can handle it"), or beliefs about the benefits of use ("I need to get high to deal with this"). In terms of behaviors, patients are taught to identify "seemingly inconsequential decisions" that increase the risk of use (e.g., choosing to buy groceries in a liquor store as opposed to a supermarket).

Another emphasis is on relapse prevention. Patients learn to identify affective, cognitive, behavioral, interpersonal, and environmental risks for relapse and develop plans to cope with these risks. Therapy also addresses cognitions about relapse that can increase risk. For example, beliefs about relapse (e.g., "If I have one drink I might as well keep drinking, because I'm back to ground zero") can interfere with patients differentiating between lapse (an initial use of substances following treatment) and relapse (return to heavier levels of use).

Motivational Interviewing

Motivational interviewing is a brief intervention based on the stages of change model of substance abuse recovery *(38)*. The model proposes six stages associated with reducing substance use, including pre-contemplation (not considering change), contemplation (considering change), preparation (gathering information and resources necessary to make change), action (initiating change), maintenance, and termination. The goal of motivational interviewing is not necessarily to reduce substance use *per se*, but to facilitate patients recognizing discrepancies between goals and the behaviors associated with substance dependence. Interventions involve the therapist taking a neutral stance, asking patients to define their goals, and discussing the costs and benefits of continued substance use in the context of those goals. In the Project Match study *(37)*, motivational interviewing was as effective as CBT or 12-step facilitation (TSF) in reducing substance use. However, brief interventions such as motivational interviewing are likely more appropriate for patients with higher levels of functioning and without significant co-morbidity of social skills deficits.

12-Step Facilitation

As mentioned previously, TSF is the third treatment evaluated in the Project Match study *(37)*. This intervention is based on the Alcoholics Anonymous (AA) treatment model that utilizes a peer-led support group to treat addiction. Participants attend support meetings and work through a series of steps that include acknowledging powerlessness over alcohol, accepting a "higher power" and turning oneself over to that power, making a moral inventory, and making amends to individuals harmed in the past. There is some evidence of the efficacy of AA and other self-help models as a treatment. The goal of TSF is to aid patients in using the 12-step model.

Psychotic Disorders

There has been a recent upsurge in research regarding psychotherapy for psychotic disorders. Psychotherapy for psychotic disorders has currently only been validated as an adjunctive treatment to pharmacotherapy. Current psychotherapy treatments that have some evidence of efficacy are CBT and social skills training (SST).

Cognitive-Behavior Therapy

CBT for psychosis tends to be a longer term intervention when compared to treatments for other disorders. Interventions fall into two general types: coping skills training aimed at improving functioning and symptom-focused therapy. Both have been found to improve functioning as well as reduce both positive and negative symptoms.

CBT interventions for psychosis include many components of other CBT models, including the emphasis on skills training, the use of standardized assessments, the use of behavioral activities to improve functioning, and the examination of cognitions to reduce dysfunctional thinking. In coping focused treatment, the targets of cognitive interventions are beliefs that interfere with achieving improved functioning (e.g., thoughts such as "I'm crazy and can't do anything" or "my medications never help"). Treatment is focused on helping patients identify goals, develop problem-solving skills, and change beliefs that interfere with improving functioning.

Therapy that focuses on symptoms uses similar techniques, but actually targets the delusions and hallucinations associated with the disorder. When treating delusional beliefs, patients are taught to start gathering evidence that may dispute the beliefs just as they would for nonpsychotic dysfunctional thinking. In treating hallucinations, particularly voices, patients are taught to question the meaning and cause of the voices. For example, a patient who believes that the voice is the Devil and may be able to harm her might be encouraged to identify if there were times she did not obey the voice and was not harmed.

When dealing with psychotic symptoms, there is a strong emphasis on developing the therapeutic relationship. Patients are often quite defensive about their beliefs, and can find active CBT techniques distressing. In CBT for psychosis, therapists spend a great deal of time establishing trust through active listening and empathy skills prior to moving into the treatment phase.

Social Skills Training

SST is a behaviorally based, manualized treatment designed to maximize functioning for patients *(39)*. This group model provides training in social skills, symptom management (including identifying relapse signs and managing ongoing symptoms), problem solving, and medication adherence. Treatment is provided in a group format, and places a strong emphasis on experiential learning. Patients participate in role-plays of skills, and even review videotapes of their practice. The manualized nature of the treatment means it can be provided by therapists who do not possess advanced degrees.

TREATMENT OF CHILDHOOD DISORDERS

Efficacious psychosocial treatments exist for many disorders of childhood and adolescence. Many of these interventions incorporate behavioral strategies such as differential reinforcement of adaptive and problematic behaviors. Special considerations in treatment of children include tailoring interventions to the appropriate developmental level and involving parents and other significant adults (e.g., teachers).

Psychological disorders of childhood traditionally have been grouped according to "internalizing" and "externalizing" subtypes. Internalizing disorders are characterized by inhibited or withdrawal-oriented behavior. Internalizing disorders frequently encountered in children include specific phobia, social phobia, GAD, and separation anxiety disorder. In contrast, externalizing disorders are notable for behavior that is disruptive to the environment. Common externalizing disorders are attention deficit hyperactivity disorder (ADHD), conduct disorder, and oppositional defiant disorder (ODD). Many other disorders of childhood exist and may be amenable to psychosocial treatment. These other problems include tic disorders, elimination disorders (e.g., enuresis), learning disorders (e.g., reading disorder), communication disorders (e.g., stuttering), and pervasive developmental disorders (e.g., autism).

Effective treatments for children and adolescents are tailored to the client's developmental level. Clinicians must consider the child's level of language development, capacity for abstract thinking, ability to sustain attention, and age-appropriate interests before undertaking treatment. For example, cognitive techniques (i.e., identifying and challenging negative thoughts) may be very useful for some children and adults, but can be too abstract for children under the age of 9 or 10. Similarly, young children may not sustain interest in a therapy session that involves sitting in chairs and talking, but might be more engaged if invited to play a therapy-relevant game with the therapist. Psychosocial treatments for children also frequently employ parents and other family members to achieve treatment goals.

Some of the best-tested and widely utilized techniques for child therapy are based on principles of operant and classical conditioning. Behavioral treatments that employ these techniques have proven efficacious for reducing symptoms of conditions as varied as autism, anxiety disorders, enuresis, and ADHD *(40–43)*. Moreover, the conceptual basis of most behavior therapies for children is strikingly simple: adaptive behaviors are reinforced and maladaptive behaviors are not reinforced (and sometimes punished). Significant adults in the child's life including parents, teachers, and therapists can administer and withhold rewards and punishments.

Reinforcement involves applying a positive consequence after a desired behavior has occurred. Positive consequences or "reinforcers" may include praise, small tokens (e.g., stickers), or points toward larger benefits (e.g., points that accumulate toward a certain gift or privilege). Consistent application of reinforcers increases the likelihood that the desired behavior will be repeated. Examples of positive reinforcement might involve praising a child with ADHD for sitting through dinner without getting out of his chair, or giving a child with separation anxiety disorder a sticker for each night that he or she sleeps in his or her own bedroom.

In general, unwanted behaviors are curtailed in BT through the removal of reinforcers. Negative behaviors might be ignored or followed by a "time out," both of which involve removal of attention.

For example, if a child with ODD is being disruptive during a family game, the parents might first try ignoring the behavior by averting eye contact or turning away from the child. If the disruptive behavior persists, they might send the child to the "time-out chair," where the child is required to sit (without diversions or interaction) until the behavior subsides. Once the disruptive behavior ceases, the parents reward the child for self-regulation by inviting the child to rejoin the family activity. In limited cases, negative behaviors may be responded to with punishment or application of an aversive consequence. Punishment strategies are typically used as a last resort, but might include application of a loud "No!" or slap on the thigh following a highly disruptive behavior such as aggression *(42)*.

Common goals of BT include the development of social skills (autism, social phobia, ADHD), decreasing disruptive or inappropriate behaviors (ADHD, ODD, conduct disorder), decreasing fear and avoidance (anxiety and phobias), and building capacities for self-regulation (all disorders). As children advance in age, a wider range of therapeutic techniques can be used to achieve these goals. For instance, CBT that incorporates self-monitoring, cognitive restructuring, problem solving, relaxation techniques, and exposure has proven efficacious in children aged 9 and older with anxiety disorders *(41)*. In addition, habit-reversal treatments that teach children to implement a "competing response" when they have an urge to engage in an undesirable behavior are effective for treating tic disorders and trichotillomania *(44)*. In many cases, parents and other family members are taught behavioral principles that will help shape their child's behavior. Parents learn how to provide consistent reinforcement for adaptive behaviors and how to deal effectively with problematic behaviors. Therapists often explore with parents the possibility that they may be inadvertently reinforcing the behaviors they are seeking to change. For example, parents may be responding their child's fear of the dark by allowing the child to sleep in their room on nights when fear is greatest. Or parents might reinforce temper tantrums by giving the child what he or she wants once the tantrum reaches a certain level of severity. In these cases, parents are instructed to refrain from reinforcing maladaptive behaviors and provided with guidance about selectively reinforcing adaptive behaviors.

An example of a psychosocial treatment for childhood problems that targets parental behavior is parent–child interaction therapy (PCIT) *(45)*. This treatment focuses on improving the parent–child attachment and increasing parents' capacities for effectively managing maladaptive behavior. The first phase of PCIT teaches parents to engage in positive, nondirective play with their children. This treatment component is believed to strengthen the parent–child relationship and to provide a beginning introduction to behavior management for parents. Parents allow their children to direct a playtime interaction at least once a day, in which their main focus is mirroring the child, giving specific praise for adaptive behaviors, and ignoring problematic behaviors. PCIT's second phase assists parents in disciplining their children effectively. During this phase, parents practice the directing of interactions with their children. They learn skills for being clear in their requests and for applying suitable consequences for noncompliance (e.g., time out). Twelve-session PCIT protocols have been found to be effective in reducing disruptive behavior in preschool children *(45,46)*.

CONCLUSIONS

The data suggest that psychotherapy can be an important treatment, either as a primary intervention or as an adjunctive treatment, for the vast majority of psychiatric disorders.

In considering whether to refer patients for psychotherapy, questions to consider are as follows:

1. Is there an empirically validated intervention available for the disorder?
2. What is the patient's preference regarding treatment? (Patient preference is a strong predictor of both pharmacologic and psychotherapeutic response).
3. Is the patient physically and cognitively capable to participate in an intervention?

For major depression and anxiety disorders, efficacious psychotherapy interventions can serve as first-line, stand-alone treatments. There is evidence for these disorders that psychotherapy alone can lead to equivalent or superior response when compared to pharmacotherapy, and that psychotherapy interventions may lead to longer term benefits (e.g., reduced rates of relapse) *(47–49)*. However, for patients with more severe versions of depression or anxiety, adjunctive pharmacotherapy may be necessary for patients unable to engage in psychotherapy or at high risk of harming themselves or others. In the case of substance use disorders, psychosocial interventions, whether professional or peer-led, are generally the primary treatment of choice. Although there are some specific pharmacological interventions for substance disorders (e.g., methadone maintenance for opiate addiction), the standard of care is psychosocial treatment. In contrast, data at this time only supports psychotherapy as an adjunctive treatment to pharmacotherapy for bipolar disorder and schizophrenia.

Referring patients for psychotherapy can be a delicate issue, particularly if the patient perceives a stigma associated with having a mental health problem. Patients may be reassured to know that problems like anxiety, depression, and substance abuse are very common and treatable *(17,50)*. Normalizing mental health problems and instilling hope for improvement increases the likelihood that the patient will follow through with the referral. In addition, it is helpful to enhance a patient's sense of control by conveying that there are multiple options for treating some of the most common mental health problems (e.g., depression and anxiety). For example, the patient often will have a choice between medication treatment with a psychiatrist, psychotherapeutic treatment, or even self-help. Engaging the patient in discussion about his or her views of these different treatment modalities is another important aspect of making a successful referral. Patient preference can affect treatment expectancies, motivation, and compliance, which can in turn affect treatment outcome. Therefore, it is essential to consider the patient's preferences before making a referral.

One common question is who is a "candidate" for psychotherapy. One important consideration is the patient's likely diagnosis. If the patient is suffering from an anxiety disorder, unipolar depression, or a substance use disorder, then psychotherapy is a good option as long as the clinician is trained in efficacious treatments for those disorders. Beyond diagnosis, the patient characteristics most relevant for evaluating the appropriateness of psychotherapy are expectancies and level of motivation for a particular type of treatment. The referring clinician may ask: "Do you think psychotherapy might work for you?" "Can you see yourself giving it a chance?" "Are weekly therapy appointments feasible?" "Can you commit to completing assignments between sessions?" Patients who have positive expectancies for treatment and sufficient motivation to comply with treatment recommendations have better outcomes in psychotherapy *(51)*. Another consideration in referring patients for psychotherapy is their level of cognitive functioning. Most forms of psychotherapy are more cognitively challenging than taking medication every day. For instance, the abstract nature of challenging negative thoughts in cognitive therapy can prove frustrating for individuals with cognitive impairment. Pharmacotherapy or concrete BT programs might prove more useful for cognitively impaired individuals.

If a patient is interested in psychotherapy, there are a variety of disciplines (e.g., psychology, psychiatry, social work, marriage and family therapists) that can provide treatment. In our perspective, the particular discipline of the clinician is less critical in determining referrals for psychotherapy than whether the clinician has training and experience in an empirically supported treatment *(49)*. Empirically supported psychosocial treatments such as CBT are most often provided by psychologists but may also be offered by psychiatrists, social workers, marriage and family therapists, or other mental health professionals.

If a patient is being referred for treatment of a psychiatric disorder to a provider who is not a medical doctor, it is important that he or she has a physician conduct a general physical examination to rule out physical causes of the symptoms (e.g., hypothyroidism causing depressed mood). A referral should be made to a psychiatrist in the case of psychotic disorders, bipolar disorder, severe depression, or complex diagnostic presentations for consideration of pharmacotherapy in addition to any adjunctive psychotherapy.

As noted, specific populations will need treatments that are modified to their needs. There is a limited but growing body of literature on psychotherapy with children and adolescents. Most of these interventions logically place a large emphasis on involvement of family and other interpersonal influences (e.g., teachers), as well as an emphasis on behavioral approaches (as opposed to more cognitive/conceptual approaches). Psychotherapy with older patients incorporate multiple learning modalities to compensate with impairments related to cognitive decline and sensory problems, and address content specific to the patient's stage of life (e.g., loss, health, role-change, isolation). Psychotherapy interventions are also being modified to be more acceptable to different ethnic and cultural subgroups, which may have difficulty with some traditional models.

In conclusion, a number of forms of psychotherapy, particularly those with cognitive and/or behavioral components, are efficacious treatments for psychiatric disorders. Although additional research is required to identify specific patient and disorder characteristics that predict the best candidates for psychotherapy, pharmacotherapy, or combined treatment, the current validated models provide benefit to most patients who participate in them. Evidence also suggests that in some cases psychotherapy is as beneficial as pharmacotherapy, and may have benefits of long-term relapse prevention and cost-effectiveness. As we have moved past the decade of the brain and into the decade of behavior, the importance of psychotherapy as an option for patients continues to be demonstrated.

REFERENCES

1. Freud S. The origin and development of psychoanalysis. In: Munger MP, ed. The History of Psychology: Fundamental Questions. London: Oxford University Press; 2003:258–269.
2. Freud S, Strachey J. The Standard Edition of the Complete Psychological Works of Sigmund Freud. Oxford, England: Macmillan; 1964.
3. Fairbairn WRD. Synopsis of an object-relations theory of the personality. Int J Psychoanal 1963;44:224–225.
4. Skinner BF. Science and Human Behavior. New York: MacMillan; 1953.
5. Lewinsohn PM. A behavioral approach to depression. In: Friedman RJ, Katz MM, Martin M, eds. The Psychology of Depression: Contemporary Theory and Research. Oxford, England: John Wiley & Sons; 1974:xvii,318.
6. Lewinsohn PM, Clarke GN. The coping with depression course. Advances in Behavior Research and Therapy 1984;6: 99–114.
7. Bandura A. Social Learning Theory. Englewood Cliffs: Prentice-Hall; 1977.
8. Beck AT, Rush AJ, Shaw BF, Emery G. Cognitive Therapy of Depression. New York: The Guilford Press; 1979.
9. Ellis A. Reason and Emotion in Psychotherapy. Oxford, England: Lyle Stuart; 1962.
10. Klerman GL, Weissman MM, Rounsaville BJ, Chevron ES. Interpersonal Psychotherapy of Depression. New York: Basic Books; 1984.
11. Elkin I, Shea MT, Watkins JT, et al. NIMH Treatment of Depression Collaborative Research Program: I. General effectiveness of treatments. Arch Gen Psychiatry 1989;47:971–982.
12. Hayes SC, Strosahl KD, Wilson KG. Acceptance and Commitment Therapy: An Experiential Approach to Behavior Change. New York: Guilford Press; 1999.
13. Linehan MM. Cognitive-Behavioral Treatment of Borderline Personality Disorder. New York: Guilford Press; 1993.
14. Segal ZV, Williams JMG, Teasdale JD. Mindfulness-Based Cognitive Therapy for Depression. New York: Guilford Press; 2002.
15. Shuchter SR, Downs N, Zisook S. Biologically Informed Psychotherapy for Depression. New York: Guilford Press; 1996.
16. Shapiro F. Eye Movement Desensitization and Reprocessing: Basic Principles, Protocols, and Procedures. New York: Guilford Press; 1995.
17. Chambless DL, Hollon SD. Defining empirically supported therapies. J Consult Clin Psychol 1998;66:7–18.
18. Nathan PE, Gorman JM. A Guide to Treatments That Work, Second Edition. London: Oxford University Press; 2002.
19. Baucom DH, Shoham V, Mueser KT, Daiuto AD, Stickle TR. Empirically supported couple and family interventions for marital distress and adult mental health problems. J Consult Clin Psychol 1998;66:53–88.
20. DeRubeis RJ, Crits-Cristoph P. Empirically supported individual and group psychological treatments for adult mental health problems. J Consult Clin Psychol 1998;66:37–52.
21. Frank E, Swartz HA, Kupfer DJ. Interpersonal and social rhythm therapy: managing the chaos of bipolar disorder. Biol Psychiatry 2000;48:593–604.
22. Miklowitz DJ, George EL, Richards JA, Simoneau TL, Suddath RL. A randomized study of family-focused psychoeducation and pharmacotherapy in the outpatient management of bipolar disorder. Arch Gen Psychiatry 2003;60:904–912.
23. Ma SH, Teasdale JD. Mindfulness-based cognitive therapy for depression: replication and exploration of differential relapse prevention effects. J Consult Clin Psychol 2004;72:31–40.
24. Beach SR, O'Leary KD. Treating depression in the context of marital discord: outcome and predictors of response of marital therapy versus cognitive therapy. Behav Ther 1992;23:507–528.

25. Miklowitz DJ, Goldstein MJ. Bipolar Disorder: A Family-Focused Treatment Approach. New York: Guilford Press; 1997.

26. Kennedy BL, Schwab JJ. Utilization of medical specialists by anxiety disorder patients. Psychosomatics 1997;38:109–112.

27. Olfson M, Fireman B, Weissman MM, et al. Mental disorders and disability among patients in a primary care group practice. Am J Psychiatry 1997;154:1734–1740.

28. American Psychiatric Association. DSM-IV. Washington DC: American Psychiatric Association; 1994.

29. Craske MG, Barlow DH. Panic disorder and agoraphobia. In: Barlow DH, ed. Clinical Handbook of Psychological Disorders: A Step-by-Step Treatment Manual, Third Edition. New York: Guilford; 2001:1–59.

30. Rachman S. The treatment of obsessions. Oxford: Oxford University Press; 2003.

31. Barlow DH. Anxiety and its Disorders: The Nature and Treatment of Anxiety and Panic. New York: Guilford; 2002.

32. Roemer L, Orsillo SM. Expanding our conceptualization of and treatment for generalized anxiety disorder: integrating mindfulness/acceptance-based approaches with existing cognitive-behavioral models. Clinical Psychology: Science and Practice 2002;9:54–68.

33. Foa EB, Franklin ME. Obsessive compulsive disorder. In: Barlow DH, ed. Clinical Handbook of Psychological Disorders: A Step-by-Step Treatment Manual, Third Edition. New York: Guilford; 2001:209–263.

34. Resick PA, Calhoun KS. Posttraumatic stress disorder. In: Barlow DH, ed. Clinical Handbook of Psychological Disorders: A Step-by-Step Treatment Manual, Third Edition. New York: Guilford; 2001:60–113.

35. Borkovec TD, Costello E. Efficacy of applied relaxation and cognitive-behavioral therapy in the treatment of generalized anxiety disorder. J Consult Clin Psychol 1993;61:611–619.

36. Brown TA, O'Leary TA, Barlow DH. Generalized anxiety disorder. In: Barlow DH, ed. Clinical Handbook of Psychological Disorders: A Step-by-Step Treatment Manual, Third Edition. New York: Guilford; 2001:154–208.

37. Project Match Research Group (US). Matching alcoholism treatments to client heterogeneity: project MATCH post-treatment drinking outcomes. J Stud Alcohol 1997;58:7–29.

38. Miller WR, Rollnick S. Motivational Interviewing: Preparing People for Change, Second Edition. New York,: Guilford Press; 2002.

39. Liberman RP, DeRisi WJ, Mueser KT. Social Skills Training for Psychiatric Patients. Elmsford, NY: Pergamon Press, Inc; 1989.

40. Houts AC. Behavioral treatment for enuresis. In: Kazdin AE, ed. Evidence-Based Psychotherapies for Children and Adolescents. New York: Guilford; 2003:389–406.

41. Kendall PC. Treating anxiety disorders in children: results of a randomized clinical trial. J Consult Clin Psychol 1994;62: 100–110.

42. Lovaas OI. Behavioral treatment and normal educational and intellectual functioning in young autistic children. J Consult Clin Psychol 1987;55:3–9.

43. National Institutes of Health Consensus Development Conference Statement. Diagnosis and treatment of attention-deficit/hyperactivity disorder (ADHD). J Am Acad Child Adolesc Psychiatry 2000;39:182–193.

44. Peterson AA. Campise RL, Azrin NH. Behavioral and pharmacological treatments for tic and habit disorders: a review. J Dev Behav Pediatr 1994;15:430–441.

45. Hood KK, Eyberg SM. Outcomes of parent-child interaction therapy: mothers' reports of maintenance three to six years after treatment. J Clin Child Adolesc Psycho 2003;32:419–429.

46. Nixon RD, Sweeney L, Erickson DB, Touyz SW. Parent-child interaction therapy: a comparison of standard and abbreviated treatments for oppositional defiant preschoolers. J Consult Clin Psychol 2003;71:251–260.

47. Reynolds CF, Frank E, Perel JM, et al. Nortriptyline and interpersonal psychotherapy as maintenance therapies for recurrent major depression: a randomized controlled trial in patients older than 59 years. JAMA 1999;281:39–45.

48. Hollon SD, DeRubeis RJ, Shelton RC, et al. Prevention of relapse following cognitive therapy vs medications in moderate to severe depression. Arch Gen Psychiatry 2005;62:417–422.

49. DeRubeis RJ, Hollon SD, Amsterdam JD, et al. Cognitive therapy vs medications in the treatment of moderate to severe depression. Arch Gen Psychiatry 2005;62:409–416.

50. Kessler RC, McGonagle KA, Zhao S, et al. Lifetime and 12-month prevalence of DSM-III-R psychiatric disorders in the United States. Arch Gen Psychiatr 1994;51:8–19.

51. Fennell MJ, Teasdale JD. Cognitive therapy for depression: individual differences and the process of change. Cognit Ther Res 1989;11:253–271.

28

Psychiatric Emergencies and Crisis Management in a Neurological Practice

Sanjay Gupta

INTRODUCTION

The complexities of neurological practice have increased considerably in the 21st century. There is now greater awareness of links between neurological and psychiatric disorders as the branch of neuropsychiatry has moved ahead. It is well known, for example, that patients with dementia, Parkinson's disease, multiple sclerosis, and other disorders may have various behavioral problems well before the diagnosis is confirmed. This results in an increased need for having an understanding of psychological issues that neurological patients have. Depression commonly is associated with chronic pain and medical illnesses. This chapter focuses on these issues, as well as threatened violence and aggressive behavior in patients with traumatic brain injury (TBI).

In the hospital setting there is usually ready access to a psychiatric consult, which may not be always possible in the office setting. Having skills to deal with such issues can therefore be extremely helpful.

ACUTE GRIEF REACTION

One of the key tasks of an experienced clinician is breaking the news of a new illness to a patient for the first time. This task is one of the most difficult responsibilities in practice. Without prior thought or training, the discomfort and uncertainty associated with this task may result in the physician disengaging emotionally from the patient and the family. A common concern may be how the news will affect the patient and this is often used to justify withholding bad news. Hippocrates advised "concealing most things from the patient while you are attending on him. Give orders with cheerfulness and serenity . . . revealing nothing of the patient's future or present condition. For many patients . . . may have taken a turn for the worse . . . by forecast of what is to come" *(1)*. In 1847 the American Medical Association's first code of medical ethics stated "the life of a sick person can be shortened not only by the acts but also by the words or manner of a physician. It is therefore the sacred duty to guard himself carefully in this respect, and to avoid all things which have a tendency to discourage the patient and to depress his spirits." This involves a considerable amount of skill, as patients are already anxious, having undergone the investigative process, have fear as to how the diagnosis of a new illness is going to impact their life and that of their loved ones. The demonstration of empathy and compassion are key virtues, which help make this job easier *(2,3)*.

In a study in which verbal and nonverbal behavior of physicians was observed in videotaped interviews (actors role-playing as patients), it was noted that female physicians had superior communication

From: *Current Clinical Neurology: Psychiatry for Neurologists*
Edited by: D.V. Jeste and J.H. Friedman © Humana Press Inc., Totowa, NJ

skills compared with their male counterparts. They used more patient-centered communication techniques than their male counterparts (e.g., they were more likely to make empathy-building statements). The study suggested that training is beneficial for these occasions *(4)*. The definition of "bad news" usually refers to any news that drastically and negatively alters the patient's view of his or her future. Neurologists frequently give such information to their patients *(5)*.

The traditional paternalistic models of patient care have given way to an emphasis on autonomy and empowerment. A review of studies found that 50–90% of patients desired full disclosure *(6)*. Hence, the delivery of bad news has to be individualized to each patient. There are several impediments, such as the physician's own issues about the topic. It is an unpleasant task. Fear of reaction to the news, uncertainty of dealing with an intense emotional response, and lack of an appropriate setting can result in the physician emotionally disengaging from the situation *(2)*. The response of any patient to bad news is influenced by the psychosocial context (e.g., a diagnosis of epilepsy may not be compatible with current employment as well as may place a restriction on driving, and hence independence).

DELIVERY OF BAD NEWS

This process should occur in a compassionate manner in a proper setting with allotment of adequate time. Rabow and McPhee developed a practical and comprehensive model synthesized from multiple sources using the mnemonic ABCDE *(7)*. The original model has been modified with additional materials. These recommendations are to serve as a guide.

A: Advance Preparation

Familiarize yourself with relevant clinical information. Have the patient's chart and pertinent laboratory data on hand during the conversation. Be prepared to provide basic information about prognosis and treatment options.

Arrange for adequate time in a private setting and comfortable location. Instruct staff so there are no interruptions. Place the pager and or mobile on silent mode.

Mentally rehearse how you will deliver the news. You may wish to practice aloud as you prepare for public speaking. Script specific words and phrases to use or avoid. If you have limited experience, observe a more experienced colleague or role-play a variety of scenarios with colleagues before actually being faced with the situation. It is also important to prepare emotionally for such situations.

B: Build a Therapeutic Environment/Relationship

Determine the patient's preference for what and how much he or she wants to know. When possible, have family members or other supportive persons present. This should be at the patient's discretion. If bad news is anticipated, ask in advance whom the patient would like present and how the patient would like the others to be involved.

Introduce yourself to everyone present and ask names and relationships to the patient.

Foreshadow the bad news, e.g., "I am sorry but I have bad news."

Use touch where appropriate. Some patients and family members will prefer not to be touched. Be sensitive to cultural differences and personal preference. Avoid inappropriate humor or flippant comments; depending on your relationship with the patient, some discreet humor may be appropriate.

Assure the patient you will be available. Schedule follow-up meetings and make appropriate arrangements with your office. Advise appropriate staff and colleagues of the situation.

C: Communicate Well

Ask what the patient or family already know and understands. "Before you tell ask. . . Find out the patient's expectations before you give the information."

Speak frankly but compassionately. Avoid euphemisms and medical jargon. Use the words cancer or death. Allow silence and tears, and avoid the urge to talk to overcome your own discomfort. Proceed at the patient's pace.

Have the patient tell you his or her understanding of what you have said. Encourage questions. At subsequent visits, ask the patient if he or she understands, and use repetition and corrections as needed.

Beware that the patient will not retain much of what is said after the initial bad news. Write things down, use sketches or diagrams, and repeat key information.

At conclusion of each visit, summarize and make follow-up plans.

D: Deal With Patient and Family Reactions

Assess and respond to emotional reactions. Be aware of cognitive coping strategies (e.g., denial, blame, intellectualization, disbelief, acceptance). Be attuned to body language. With subsequent visits, monitor the patient's emotional status, assessing for despondency or suicidal ideations.

Be empathic; it is appropriate to say "I am sorry" or "I don't know." Crying may be appropriate, but be reflective—are your tears from empathy with your patient or are they reflection of your own personal issues?

Do not argue with or criticize colleagues; avoid defensiveness regarding your, or a colleague's, medical care.

E: Encourage and Validate Emotions

Offer realistic hope. Even if a cure is not realistic, offer hope and encouragement about what options are available. Discuss treatment options at the outset, and arrange follow-up meetings for decision making.

Explore what the news means to the patient. Inquire about the patient's emotional and spiritual needs and what support systems are in place. Offer referrals as needed. Use interdisciplinary services to enhance patient care (e.g., case management, counseling, hospice), but avoid using these as a means of disengaging from the relationship. On some occasions, the patient may begin to cry during this process. At this time, it might be prudent to wait. In some cases, it may be appropriate to acknowledge (e.g., "Let's just take a break now until you are ready to start again"). It is best not to assume the reason for the tears but explore (e.g., "what caused you to cry while we were talking"). It is always an empathic gesture to offer tissues (plan ahead for such a situation). It is also important to demonstrate that one is prepared to deal with such situations.

Attend to your own needs during and following the delivery of bad news. Issues of countertransference (feelings a therapist or provider may develop toward a patient) may arise, triggering poorly understood but powerful feelings. A formal or informal debriefing session with involved house staff, office, or hospital personnel may be appropriate to review the medical management.

Robert Buckman suggested a six-step protocol for breaking bad news.

Step 1. Getting started: The physical setting should be private and comfortable and the patient should be asked to choose whom he or she would like present. It is important to give the indication to the patient that this will be a two-way affair by a question "How are you feeling right now?"

Step 2: Finding out how much the patient knows: By asking a question such as "What have you already been told about your illness?", you can begin to understand what the patient has already been told or how much the patient understood of what he or she was told. It is important to know the patient's level of technical sophistication and emotional state.

Step 3: Finding out how much the patient wants to know: It is important to inquire from patients as to how detailed an explanation they want. A statement such as "Some patients want every detail while others want only the big picture—what would you prefer?" is appropriate. This establishes that there is no right answer but there are different individual styles. Also, this question establishes that the patient may ask for something different during the next conversation.

Step 4: Sharing the information: It is important to decide on the agenda before sitting down with the patient so you have access to the relevant information. The topics to consider include diagnosis, treatment, prognosis, and support or coping. An appropriate agent focuses on one or two topics. For a patient with a magnetic resonance imaging (MRI) scan suggesting multiple sclerosis (MS) it may be important to disclose the diagnosis of MS, the process of workup, and the treatment options. It is prudent to give the information in small chunks and ask if the patient is following you (e.g., "I am going to stop for a minute to see if you have any questions"). Long lectures are overwhelming. Remember to use simple English, and don't try to teach pathophysiology.

Step 5: Responding to patient feelings: If you don't understand the patient's reaction, you will leave a lot of unfinished business, and you will miss an opportunity to be a caring physician. Learning to identify and acknowledge a patient's reaction is something that definitely improves with experience, if you are attentive, but you can also simply ask (e.g., "Could you tell me a little bit about what you are feeling?").

Step 6: Planning and follow-through: At this point you need to synthesize the concerns of the patient and the medical issues into a concrete plan that can be carried out in the patient's system of health care. Outline a step-by-step plan that can be carried out in the patient's health care system. Be explicit about your next contact with the patient (e.g., "I will see you in a week") or the fact that you won't see the patient and Dr. Smith will. The patient must be given the phone number and other relevant information to contact the relevant medical caregiver.

Both these approaches have overlap and can be utilized in the office when informing patients or family about new neurological diagnosis or prognosis.

The limits of medicine assure that patients cannot always be cured. A growing body of evidence suggests that physicians' attitude and communications skills play a crucial role in how well patients cope with bad news. The task of delivering bad news to a patient in a neurological practice is a challenging one, however, it can also give the physician a great sense of gratification in providing support at a time of need.

DEALING WITH A CRISIS

In a neurological practice, a crisis can arise unpredictably while a patient's diagnosis is being discussed, in the course of ongoing treatment, or at the initial diagnostic visit. Having a well thought-out plan and trained office staff helps in dealing with such situations professionally and without panic. Such situations might be expressed as sudden uncontrollable crying at knowing a diagnosis such as MS or a brain tumor. It could also be the expression of suicidal ideation owing to increased stress of coping with lifelong diseases with increasing morbidity, violence in the context of TBI or dementia-related psychosis resulting in behavioral disturbance. Additionally, the family members of patients are often stressed as a result of the impact on their lives of an illness of a loved one and need help and support.

A crisis is defined as unusual stress that temporarily renders an individual ineffective in directing life successfully. As stress increases the usual coping mechanisms fail resulting in the individual experiencing extreme feelings of fear, anger, grief, hostility, hopelessness, helplessness, and alienation from self, loved ones, and society. The rule with crises is that they happen unexpectedly *(8,9)*. The aim of crises intervention is effective management of the problem and not resolution, the goal being short term focusing on the immediate future. Rosenbluh has described crises intervention as "emotional first aid" *(10)*.

Identification of the Crises-Prone Individual

An important first step is to have the capability of identifying the crises-prone individual such as those with low self-esteem, lack of lasting relationships and supports, those repeating the same mistakes, history of severe psychiatric illness, and those who have been unable to effectively resolve crises in the past.

Detection of Precipitants

In a neurological practice, the onset or detection of a severe debilitating illness such as MS, stroke, or brain tumor could result in a crisis. Other factors such as divorce, death in the family, change in living conditions, and impending loss of things of significance might also precipitate a crisis. On occasion, a very stressful situation might not lead to a crisis but a combination of multiple stressful events together might push the individual over the edge.

Recognizing an Individual in Crisis

The recognition of a crisis is dependent on paying attention to both verbal and nonverbal communication. Individuals indicate crises by various means such as crying, exploding, depression, withdrawal, or by verbalizing. Additional symptoms such as impaired concentration and confusion are also noted to occur. It is important to get collateral information from family and friends about the individual's pre-crisis behavior *(8)*. Knowing the profile of a crisis-prone person is helpful in early recognition.

Effective Intervention

To bring about effective intervention in the office there is need to take control of the situation to prevent the situation from getting out of hand. The response needs to be immediate to relieve anxiety and panic.

Evaluation of Risk to Self and Others

A quick evaluation of the situation should be conducted to assess suicide potential as well as the risk of harm to others. The patient should be asked "Do you feel down? " followed by "Have you lost interest?" A prior history of violence or suicide attempts, past history of mood disorder, family history of mood disorder, or completed suicide should be obtained. In addition, it is important to know if the patient has continuing sleep disturbance, inner tension or anxiety, and reasons to live. These are important indicators of suicide risk. The burden caused by suicide and the threat of suicide falls not only on the suicidal individual but also on those closest to them. It is important to know the demographics related to suicide. Having knowledge of the suicide demographics is helpful in assessment of suicide risk. (*See* Tables 1 and 2.)

The clinical situation in the office may require an oral/intramuscular administration of lorazepam to calm the patient. Patients considered a suicide risk or a risk to others should to be sent to the emergency room (ER) by a safe means of transportation utilizing a responsible relative orfriend, ambulance, or police. When trying to intervene in a crisis, it is important not to promise things that won't happen. A statement such as, "I would like hear what is upsetting to you so I can try to help" is helpful. It is important to listen actively to the individual's full message and to give full attention. It is important to determine which issue is of greatest concern and should be resolved first. Clarification techniques are helpful to ensure that the patient is understood. Repeating certain key words or phrases used by the patient is also helpful as this can help in obtaining more information. Knowledge of community resources is extremely helpful to get the individual linked for follow-up to prevent a recurrence. If the interview is focused on evaluation for suicide risk, one should not hesitate to ask a closed question such as "Do you have a suicide plan?". When asking questions, one should be careful so as not to increase the patient's stress level. If the patient is silent, one should be careful and be silent observing the patient's behavior and aiming to listen to what the patient is not saying. If the patient is being questioned about suicidal thoughts and he or she is silent, it indicates an increased risk *(8,9)*. When conducting a crisis intervention, one should come across as clear, confident, and capable.

ATTENTION TO CULTURAL ISSUES

To conduct effective crisis intervention it is important to be aware of any cultural issues that might have a bearing on better understanding of the situation. This helps in establishing rapport and extraction of important details and in understanding them. It is helpful to become aware of one's own cultural biases. It is also important to know that lack of knowledge about an individual's culture may increase stress within an intervention *(9)*. There is strong need to understand that one cannot change a person's cultural perspectives and that it is important to maintain objectivity. During an intervention it is key not to impose one's personal values, while clarifying any ambiguous statements made by the patient. The intervener should not take personally any communications from the individual in crisis, which may be insulting in the culture of the intervener. It is important not to judge a person from another culture by one's own cultural values unless one is familiar with the cultural values of the patient in crisis.

Table 1
Suicide Statistics

Years of age	Frequency per 100,000 population
15–24	12.8
25–34	14.8
35–44	19.9
45–54	15.5
55–64	17.8
65–74	19.9
75–84	29.2
85+	22.0

Table 2
Additional Suicide Statistics

- 15 to 19 Age group—Suicide second highest cause of death, car accidents are first.
- Three males to one female—Successfully complete suicide attempts.
- Three females to one male—Attempt suicides but are not successful.
- Psychiatrists have highest suicide rate per profession—Pediatricians have the lowest.
- In regard to psychiatric disorders—Most suicides occur within the first 3 months of improvement following depression.
- Of those diagnosed with affective disorder (major depression or bipolar disorder)—45% will attempt suicide and 15% will die.
- Among schizophrenics—25% will try, paranoids have the highest risk.
- Of those diagnosed with dysthymic disorder—25% will try, 12 out of 100,000 will succeed.
- Among alcoholics—25% to 30% will try suicide.

FAMILY IN CRISIS

In the office setting, a crisis involving an individual might ultimately result in a crisis for the entire family. The patient experiencing the crisis is usually considered the primary victim, whereas the significant others are considered the secondary victims. The family members of the individual in crisis experience their own crisis as they aim to fit what has happened in the life of the loved one into their own lives (8). In such crisis, it is important to pay attention to children of the patient as they have limited understanding compared to adults. The reality for children is often built by fantasy, partial truths, and the immature ability to discern what is happening in their surroundings. Family support may be provided through support groups or counseling referrals.

Case 1: Agitated Patient With Dementia

A 78-year-old female with a history of "memory problems" has been increasingly agitated with her husband. He has indicated to the family that she hit him because she thought he was stealing money out of her purse as well as having an affair with a neighbor. The woman was insisting that she should drive to the doctor's appointment despite some recent accidents resulting from poor judgment. Her husband indicated that she was wandering at night thinking there were strangers in her apartment, had been irritable, and had been keeping him awake at night. He reported that she forgets to wash her hands after visiting the restroom. He also reported that he had been doing the banking and has been watching after her as she left the stove on a number of times.

This patient has symptoms of psychosis consistent with those associated with Alzheimer's disease. In addition, she has poor judgment with regard to driving and banking. She is keeping her caregiver—

her husband—up at night, which increases his stress level causing him to burnout. Leaving the stove on is a potential fire hazard. This case represents a common emergency situation faced by the caregiver/family members of a patient with dementia living in the home. Most families prefer to keep the patient in the house as long as possible, often going through great hardship. A phone call received simulating this case should be answered promptly, the patient evaluated, and treatment started to avoid hospitalization. It is important to exclude infections such as urinary tract infection as a cause. Treatment can also be started empirically while waiting for the test results to come back. In this situation an antipsychotic medication such as risperidone (0.25 mg three times a day; maximum dose 2 mg per day), olanzapine (zydis 5 mg before sleep; maximum dose 10 mg per day), quetiapine (25 mg twice daily; maximum dose 200 mg per day), or aripiprazole (5 mg daily; maximum dose 15 mg daily) may be tried. The Food and Drug Administration (FDA) has issued a class warning with regard to the possible increased incidence of death in the elderly treated with antipsychotic agents. The possibility of a psychiatric consult can be considered for follow-up once treatment is started. In some cases, the situation is emergent, which requires calling the police (safe transportation) to get the patient to the nearest ER for an evaluation. In some situations, a psychiatric hospitalization may be required to stabilize the patient. During the hospitalization, a family meeting can be conducted to evaluate the ability of the patient to be cared for at home or in an assisted living/skilled nursing facility. When evaluating a patient with dementia-related behavioral disturbance, it is important to realize that one actually has two patients: the presenting patient and the caregiver who may be suffering from depression. It is important to consider increasing the supports in the home and to get the patient linked with the department of aging.

Case 2: Psychosis Associated With Parkinson's Disease

A 68-year-old, male with a history of Parkinson's disease (PD) was under care of a neurologist developed visual hallucinations which were frightening to him and his family was seen emergently in the office. The patient and family were concerned because the patient had never had such an experience in his life. An evaluation revealed that the patient's levodopa/carbidopa (sinemet) dosage was increased recently to better control his PD. Further evaluation revealed that he was irritable as well as having early memory impairment. The patient was unable to sleep because of fear, which kept his wife awake causing further crisis to the family system. His other medical conditions, which included hypertension, type 2 diabetes mellitus, and dyslipidemia were well controlled and he had been on a stable medication regimen for these illnesses for 1 year.

This patient clearly appears to have developed psychosis associated with the increase in antiparkinsonian medication as there is a temporal relationship between the two events. His other medications had not been adjusted in the past year. Visual hallucinations also are typical of such a problem. Other possibilities such as electrolyte disturbances and other possible causes of delirium need to be considered. In such a situation, with the patient in the office, it is important to reassure not only the patient but also the family regarding the cause of the psychosis and that it can be treated with medication. Quetiapine (seroquel) is the agent of choice because of its zero extrapyramidal symptoms extrapyramidal symptoms (EPS) profile (i.e., this second-generation (atypical) antipsychotic is not associated with neuroleptic-induced Parkinsonism).

This agent is started as low as 12.5 mg twice daily and titrated gradually to a maximum dosage of 200 mg daily in divided dosage. It is important to monitor fasting blood glucose as well as lipid profile with this class of drugs. The psychotic symptoms associated with this condition can be controlled with 5–7 days of therapy. If the agitation is severe and the patient is at home, one may suggest a safe mode of transportation to a nearby ER with the help of the local police department or ambulance service. In some towns, the local fire department helps with this function. If the family member feels comfortable transporting the patient to the nearest ER that can also be considered. Such decisions are to be made on a case-by-case basis.

If the patient is refusing medication, some of the atypical antipsychotics come in alternative formulations such as risperidone liquid and M tab (1–2 mg per day) or olanzapine zydis (5–10 mg per day), which dissolves rapidly in the patient's mouth. If the patient is seen in the office in this condition, any one of the atypical agents may be administered in the office. Talking with the patient slowly and in a calm tone can help. It is also important to decrease sensory stimulation from the environment. In such cases, quiet surroundings can be helpful.

Case 3: Suicidal Patient

The patient is a 55-year-old male with Huntington's disease (HD) and severe depression. He has had a progressive worsening of his choreiform movements, increased weight loss, and some early memory impairment. Specifically, he has difficulty remembering names as well as finding words and difficulties with calculation. His depression has worsened and during a routine neurological office visit for follow up of the HD he was noted to be weepy and reported that, "I don't feel like going on like this." On further questioning he indicated he had thoughts of overdosing on his pills and indicated his wife was capable of looking after the children alone. The wife, who was also present at the time of the interview, indicated that he had lost interest in activities such as playing with the grandchildren or even watching his favorite show on television and food did not taste good.

This patient has developed depressive symptoms as well as suicidal thoughts. He has HD resulting in increased functional limitations resulting in depression. As the patient has suicidal thoughts and appears to have a plan to possibly overdose on medication, his risk level is higher. He should be seen immediately for an emergency evaluation. The options would include getting him to an ER transported by a family member if considered reliable and the patient is willing. If the patient is unwilling and it is unclear whether the family member is able to handle the situation, the police should be called for safe transport to an ER with psychiatric evaluation capability. An alternative strategy would the ability to have a psychiatrist examine the patient immediately and determine the next course of action. It would also help to have the phone number for the local psychiatric crisis line (hot-line), which can be extremely beneficial in planning what to do. This may also serve as a resource for advice as well as consultation on how to get the emergency services activated.

ETHICAL ISSUES IN CRISIS INTERVENTION

Strong ethical practice should be followed, as patients are particularly vulnerable in times of crisis. It is important for the person conducting the crisis intervention to be aware of his or her own counter-transference issues (feelings a therapist or physician may develop toward a patient), which may be defined as an unconsciously determined attitudinal set held by the person conducting an intervention that interferes with work. The recognition of these feelings is important so that they can be dealt with appropriately in another setting such as personal therapy *(9)*.

Dual relationships are prohibited. These include sexual, social, employee, or financial. Hence, in the office setting, it is important to recognize the crisis and be alert to any of these factors so one can quickly get the patient to a safe and effective therapeutic setting. This is important because there is an enormous power differential between the person conducting the intervention and the patient.

Confidentiality is an important aspect of the ethical code for medical and paramedical personnel and is now protected by the Health Information Protection and Portability Act *(11)*. The communication is considered privileged unless agreed to by the patient to be given to another party. It is important to safeguard the patient from unauthorized disclosures. There are exceptions in certain crisis situations. Patients may be asked to give consent so information may be shared with another professional (e.g., such as the therapist where the patient will have follow-up after crisis intervention). Other examples include court testimony, health insurance claims, and to provide for supervision. Confidentiality may be broken in cases of child or elder abuse, when the patient is gravely disabled, and when the patient is in danger of harming self or others *(12)*. If the patient is gravely disabled or unable to take care of him or herself the helper may breach confidentiality to protect the patient. It is best to check the local laws of the state where practice is located. In many states, the knowledge of child or elder abuse should be reported to the appropriate social agency. It is also important to warn the intended victim and the police if a patient was making specific threats (The Tarasoff Case). If such a situation arises in the neurological office it is best to have the patient escorted safely (by the police) to the nearest ER, where a thorough psychiatric evaluation can be conducted, informing the evaluating agency by phone and in writing about the specific threat, including the nature of the threat and the person being threatened.

INFORMED CONSENT

It is important to obtain consent from the patient before the administration of medication or other therapeutic intervention. In a situation where the patient is clearly in danger of hurting him or herself or others, or the patient is gravely disabled, this requirement may be overridden. An essential element of informed consent is a determination that the patient is able to comprehend what is being said in addition to the benefits and risks of treatment and also to no treatment. If a patient does not have the capacity to give consent it should be obtained from the legally authorized representative, the definition of which may vary from state to state.

TRAUMATIC BRAIN INJURY

This diagnostic category refers to patients that have suffered brain contusion. The sequelae of TBI commonly include physical, cognitive, affective, and behavioral impairments. Each TBI patient brings to the situation his or her unique set of pre-injury intellectual skills, personality, emotional makeup, social relationships, and economic vocational, and/or academic roles. Character traits are commonly exacerbated after TBI. Substance abuse is more common among those who sustain TBI. Behavioral disturbances in this group of patients is determined by multiple factors including the location of the injury, the premorbid personality style, family supports, use of alcohol and drugs, other co-morbid illnesses, presence of pain, as well as the extent of the recovery process. Irritability, low frustration tolerance, rage, and impulsive aggression are noted in this group of patients. Behavioral symptoms such as aggressive or violent outbursts interfere with rehabilitation and also put the patient and caregiver at risk for physical injury. Such symptoms could result in a behavioral emergency. Antidepressants, antipsychotics, anticonvulsants, and antihypertensives have all been tried to treat the behavioral symptoms in TBI patients. There is a lack of controlled randomized clinical trials evaluating various medications to treat such problems. Most of the data is based on anecdotal case reports, retrospective reports, and open case series. The treatment of TBI patients with psychiatric issues, which includes the major psychiatric disorders such as mania, depression, psychosis as well as behavioral disturbances including aggression is largely off-label use of medicines.

Anticonvulsants in Traumatic Brain Injury

The anticonvulsant drugs are frequently prescribed for patients with TBI because of their membrane-stabilizing effect, the seizure risk in these patients, and their demonstrated utility in mood stabilization in brain injury-related and other neuropsychiatric illnesses such as bipolar disorder *(13)*. The use of anticonvulsants in TBI patients is entirely off-label as none have been approved by the Food and Drug Administration for TBI. Phenytoin has been used to treat aggressive behavior, however, the results have been equivocal. There has been criticism of the methodology of older studies with regard to drug dosing and experimental design. In the case of other anticonvulsants there is no supportive evidence from comparative controlled clinical trials (mostly open design), however, they are used because of the increased risk of posttraumatic epilepsy in these patients. It is difficult to extrapolate from their use in epilepsy studies because of underlying differences in the two populations. The anticonvulsants as a group exert an effect on the cognitive and motor functions in epileptic patients, the impairments worsening with increases in serum level of the drug. In a seizure prevention trial in post-TBI patients, no differences in efficacy were found between phenytoin, carbamezapine, and divalproex in the prevention of short-term seizures. None of the treatments were found to be effective in the prevention of long-term seizures *(13)*. The literature in TBI patients is scanty.

Divalproex

The literature associated with the use of this agent consists mostly of open studies and case series. One series was a retrospective chart review of 11 patients with a history of brain injury referred for psychiatric treatment who were treated with divalproex (mean dose 1818 mg per day; serum divalproex level of 85.6 µg/mL) alone or in combination with other medications *(14)*. This is one of the largest post-acute series, which demonstrated divalproex sodium to be well tolerated and efficacious in reducing a variety of neurobehavioral symptoms. The largest case series ($N = 29$) of patients being treated with divalproex revealed this agent to be effective in 90% of the sample within 7 days after a typical 1250 mg per day dosage *(15)*.

Studies report that divalproex lacks sedation and causes less cognitive impairment. Behaviors within the affective spectrum from depression to dysphoric mania may be amenable to divalproex. The lower sedation helps the patients participate in rehabilitation. Divalproex can also be combined with any of the atypical antipsychotics, which is an off-label use of this drug. In some cases, partial responders at adequate serum divalproex levels may have further improvement in target symptoms of aggression and violent behavior following the addition of an atypical agent.

In the hospitalized patient with TBI, intravenous valproate (Depacon) may be considered. Although a loading dose is not necessary for the initiation of therapy it has been reported in the literature. This intravenous formulation is administered as a 60 minutes infusion (not more than 20 mg per minute). A rapid infusion over 5–10 minutes has been performed using 15 mg/kg with a mean dosage of 1184 mg, which was well tolerated. In a safety study, 25 patients (aged 4–39 years) were given intravenous valproate to achieve a serum concentration of at least 100 µg/mL within 1 hour. No electrocardiogram abnormalities, injection site irritation, or significant changes in vital signs were observed. One patient had sedation (serum level 200 µg/mL), while the serum concentrations measured 10 minutes after the infusion ranged from 71–277 µg/mL *(16,17)*. The authors estimate that a loading dose of 25 mg/kg infused over 60 minutes should achieve a concentration of 100–150 µg/mL 10 minutes after the infusion. Most of the data with intravenous valproate is in epilepsy patients.

Case 4: TBI and Aggression

A 43-year-old male with TBI as a result of a motor vehicle accident in which he lost his fiancée and her two children was seen in psychiatric consultation as a result of increased irritability, depression (20-pound weight loss), and aggression. His cognition was impaired as determined by impaired recall, mathematical ability, as well as inability to do the clock test or copy intersecting polygons correctly. He was on 50 mg of desipramine daily, 450 mg of valproic acid daily in divided dosage, 50 mg of trazodone at bedtime, as well as vitamin supplements. The deispramine was stopped and he was started on sertraline, a selective serotonin reuptake inhibitor (SSRI) at 50 mg daily and titrated to 150 mg daily, and the divalproex was increased to a 1000 mg daily with much noted improvement in symptoms. In this case, the SSRI was started to reduce impulsivity as well as irritability. Noradrenergic agents may increase irritability. The divalproex dosage was increased to achieve better serum levels as well as decrease in aggression. This patient did not have clear psychotic symptoms and had been on divalproex that was then adjusted.

Other Anticonvulsants

There are only case series with the other agents. Pachet et al. reported a single case of a 40-year-old male with severe TBI resulting from being struck by a motor vehicle while crossing the street. In this case, there was lack of response to a combination of risperidone, trazadone, carbamezapine, and adjunctive lorazepam. The patient was continued on carbamezapine, paroxetine was added and increased to 40 mg daily, and subsequently lamotrigine was added at 25 mg daily and increased to 50 mg daily with significant reduction in aggression. The carbamezpine dosage was adjusted down to 800 mg daily from 1600 mg daily *(18)*. The patient did not require any supplemental lorazepam at the end of 6 months. The process took approx 6 months.

Antidepressants in Traumatic Brain Injury Patients

Patients with TBI may have dysphoria as they develop insight into their functional limitations and may have affective changes as a primary effect of their brain damage. This group of individuals may benefit from antidepressant therapy. The data is extremely limited by lack of randomized placebo-controlled trials.

Antipsychotics in Traumatic Brain Injury

The use of these agents in TBI patients is clearly based on clinical experience and not evidence based. Posttraumatic agitation has a prevalence of 11–50% *(19–21)*. Agitation may delay the rehabilitative process. The pathological bases, neuroanatomic, and physiological underpinnings are not well understood and vary from patient to patient. The use of antipsychotics in TBI patients is entirely off-label and controversial. Animal studies suggest that motor recovery after experimental brain injury is negatively affected by medications such as haloperidol. Primate work has revealed that cognitive benefits facilitated by catecholaminergic treatment are inhibited by haloperidol. Limited human studies suggest a negative impact of antipsychotics on recovery after stroke and TBI, specifically resulting in prolongation of amnesia *(22–24)*. Some of the literature is confounded because the patients were on multiple agents, antipsychotics being one of them. Comparison of the atypical agents to the typical agents is difficult to do as data are lacking. There are clinical scenarios when these agents need to be used. The literature suggests the following indications: (a) extreme agitation with or without accompanied psychotic symptomatology, (b) severe aggression or rage, and (c) acute mania associated with TBI. The presence of thought disorder premorbidly or after TBI is another possible indication *(25)*.

The typical (conventional/first-generation) agents were first introduced in 1950s starting with chlorpromazine and are known to be potent antagonists at the D2 receptor. These agents have a side-effect profile characterized by EPS and prolactin elevation *(25)*. The atypical agents (second-generation agents) have a lower affinity for the D2 receptor, however, have significant activity at various serotonergic receptor sites, and the α1 receptors. The 5HT2a : D2 ratio reflects the differences among these agents. These properties translate into a lower incidence of EPS as well as tardive dyskinesia *(25)*.

Clozapine

There are no controlled data using clozapine in TBI, however, there is an open trial of nine TBI patients. There was substantial benefit in three, modest benefit in three, but two patients suffered seizures on the drug. It is important to remember that patients on clozapine need weekly monitoring of their white cell count for the first 6 months of treatment and every 2 weeks subsequently *(25)*.

Risperidone

There are only two published case reports using risperidone in TBI patients *(25)*. The maximum reported dosage used appears to be 16 mg daily, although the utility of dosage above 6 mg is questionable because of increased risk of neuroleptic-induced Parkinsonism. In elderly and frail patients, the starting dosage suggested has been 0.5 mg, whereas the maximum dosage is 2 mg in dementia patients. In addition, in the dementia studies a statistically higher incidence of stroke was noted in the risperidone group compared with the placebo group, although the actual numbers were small *(26)*. There are no guidelines for TBI patients. The advantages of risperidone include multiple dosage forms such as liquid concentrate, dissolvable M-tab, and a long-acting depot injection (risperidal consta). These formulations are helpful in noncompliant patients or those unable to swallow tablets. There is no rapidly acting intramuscular injectable form available as yet.

Case 5: TBI With Psychosis

This case involved a 34-year-old male who suffered a TBI in 2001 following a motorcycle accident. He had surgery and a titanium plate was placed to reconstruct his skull. He was seen in consultation because of increased fear, marked irritability, as well as depression. He was disoriented, as he was unable to tell the year, month, and date. He was also severely cognitively impaired and was noted to be paranoid. He was unable to do serial sevens and recall was impaired. He was on 150 mg of sertraline per daily, oxycarbamezapine (600 mg in the morning, 600 mg at noon, and 900 mg in the evening). He was also on 50 mg of trazadone at bedtime for insomnia. There was no suicidal or homicidal ideation. He was treated with 1 mg of risperidone at bedtime to help with paranoid ideation. The sertraline was increased to 200 mg daily. The risperidone was increased to a maximum of 3 mg at bedtime with remission of psychosis. The patient was subsequently referred back to his primary care physician. There were no EPS noted.

Olanzapine

This agent separates from the others because of the beneficial effects on both depression and mania. This agent can be sedating and is effective in managing aggression and excitement. The stroke warning with risperidone applies to olanzapine also *(27)*. There is one case in the literature documenting the effectiveness of olanzapine in a patient with post-TBI delusions.

Olanzapine is now available in the zydis (rapidly disintegrating wafer), which is helpful for noncompliant patients (strengths 5 mg, 10 mg, 15 mg, 20 mg). This is useful for noncompliant individuals or those who can't swallow. Olanzapine is also available in a rapidly acting injection preparation.

Case 6: TBI With Psychosis

A 47-year-old male was referred by a neurologist because of auditory as well as visual hallucinations. On evaluation, the information obtained from the patient as well as his wife indicated he was suspicious as well as withdrawn, was worrying about minor matters, and had loss of interest. His wife also noted that he had been aggressive. Additionally, the patient had cognitive impairment. The patient had undergone removal of a brain tumor in 1979 and also had a seizure disorder in addition to dyslipidemia. He was on divalproex (2500 mg daily in divided doses, primidone 25 mg daily, as well as lamotrigine 100 mg twice daily). The patient was started on 10 mg of olanzapine at bedtime to reduce psychosis, aggression, and improve sleep. In addition buproprion was titrated to 300 mg daily in divided doses. Over the course of next 2 years, the lamotrigine was tapered to a stop while maintaining other mediciations. The patient's psychosis, as well as aggression, were well controlled and he was referred back to his physician with the olanzapine at a maintenance dosage of 5 mg at bed-time while continuing all other medications at the previous dosages. The aggression and irritability were well controlled along with improved mood.

There are no data on the use of aripiprazole or quetiapine in TBI patients. Despite the bias against antipsychotic agents in TBI patients, the atypical antipsychotic agents should be used judiciously, as control of aggression and agitation is critical for rehabilitation of TBI patients to proceed smoothly. To control an agitated patient, a sedating agent with multiple dosage forms would be preferred. Patients treated with these agents should have their weight as well as blood glucose and lipid profile monitored at baseline and periodically (3–6 months thereafter). The guidelines developed jointly by the American Diabetic Association and the American Psychiatric Association suggest that clozapine and olanzapine may have a greater weight-gain risk and highest occurrence of diabetes and dyslipidemia compared with ziprasidone and aripiprazole, which have the least *(28–30)*. Risperidone and quetiapine are suggested to have intermediate effects. It should also be noted that ziprasidone and aripiprazole have not been as extensively studied as other agents. In controlling aggression in TBI patients, one should aim to use a sedating agent to bring symptoms under control rapidly.

CONCLUSION

It is important to be able to pick up and address any psychiatric issues in patients with neurological illnesses. More importantly, psychiatric emergencies need to be dealt with confidently and adequately to reduce overall morbidity and mortality.

REFERENCES

1. Jones WH. Hippocrates. Decorum XVI. In: Jones WH, ed. Hippocrates with an English Translation, Vol. 2. London: Heinemann; 1923.
2. Vandekieft GK. Breaking bad news. Am Fam Physician 2001;64:1975–1978.
3. Creagan ET. How to break bad news-and not devastate the patient. Mayo Clin Proc 1994;69:1015–1017.
4. Tipper L, Bonas S, Fisher J, Barnett M. Female doctors break bad news best. E-Bulletin: University of Leicester: England; 2003.
5. Buckman R. Breaking bad news: why is it so difficult? Br Med J 1984;288:1597–1599.
6. Ley P. Giving information to patients. In: Eiser JR, ed. Social Psychology and Behavioral Medicine. New York: Wiley; 1982:353.
7. Rabow MW, McPhee SJ. Beyond breaking news. How to help patients who suffer. West J Med 1999;48:260–263.
8. Greenstine JL, Leviton SC. Elements of Crisis Intervention: Crises and How to Respond to Them, Second Edition. Pacific Grove, CA: Brooks/Cole; 2002.
9. Kanel K. A Guide to Crisis Intervention, Second Edition. Pacific Grove, CA: Brooks/Cole; 2002.
10. Rosenbluh ES. Emotional First Aid. Louisville, KY: American academy of crisis interveners; 1981.
11. Department of Health and Human Services. Office of Civil Rights (OCR). Health Information Portability and Accountability Act. www.hhs.gov/ocr/hippa/. Accessed April 24, 2005.
12. Tarasoff vs Regents of University of California. 551 P.2d 334. California; 1976.
13. Temkin NR, Dikmen SS, Anderson GD, et al. Valproate therapy for prevention of post-traumatic seizures. J Neurosurg 1999;91:595–600.
14. Kim E, Humaran TJ. Divalproex in the management of neuropsychiatric complications of remote acquired brain injury. J Neuropsychiatry Clin Neurosci 2002;14:202–205.
15. Chatham-Showalter PE. Agitated symptom response to divalproex following acute brain injury. J Neuropsychiatry Clin Neurosci 2000;12:395–397.
16. Venkataraman V, Wheless JW. Safety of rapid intravenous valproate loading doses in epilepsy patients. Epilepsy Res 1999; 35:147–153.
17. Wheless JW, Venkataraman V. Safety of high intravenous valproate loading doses in epilepsy. J Epilepsy 1998;11:319–324.
18. Pachet A, Friesen S, Winkelaar D, Gray S. Beneficial effects of lamotrigine in traumatic brain injury. Brain Inj 2003; 17:715–722.
19. Levin HS, Grossman RG. Behavioral sequelae of closed head injury. A quantitative study. Arch Neurol 1978;35:720–727.
20. Reyes RI, Bhattacharya AK, Heller D. Traumatic head injury: restlessness and agitation as prognosticators of physical and psychological improvement in patients. Arch Phys Med Rehabil 1981;62:20–23.
21. Brooke MM, Questad KA, Patterson DR, Bashak KJ. Agitation and restlessness after closed head injury: a prospective study of 100 consecutive admissions. Arch Phys Med Rehabil 1992 73:320–323.
22. Freeney DM, Gonzalez A. Amphetamine, haloperidol, and experience interact to affect rate of recovery after motor cortex injury. Science 1982; 217:855–857.
23. Feeney DM, Westerberg VS. Norepinephrine and brain damage: alpha noradrenergic pharmacology alters functional recovery after cortical trauma. Can J Psychol 1990;44:233–252.
24. Goldstein LB, Hovda DA. Basic and clinical studies of pharmacological effects on recovery from brain injury. J Neural Transplant Plast 1993;4:175–192.
25. Elovic EP, Lansang R, Li Y, Ricker JH. The use of atypical antipsychotics in traumatic brain injury. J Head Trauma Rehabil 2003;18:177–195.
26. Brodaty H, Ames D, Snowdon J, et al. A randomized placebo-controlled trial of risperidone for the treatment of aggression, agitation, and psychosis of dementia. J Clin Psychiatry 2003;64:134–143.
27. Folsom DP, Nayak GV, Jeste DV. Antipsychotic medications and the elderly. Primary Psychiatry 2004;11:47–50.
28. American Diabetes Association. Consensus development conference on antipsychotic drugs and obesity and diabetes. Diabetes Care 2004;27:596–601.
29. Allison DB, Casey DE. Antipsychotic-induced weight gain: a review of the literature. J Clin Psychiatry 2001;62:22–31.
30. Masand PS, Gupta S. Long-term adverse effects of atypical antipsychotics. J Psychiatr Pract 2000;6:299–309.

29

Informed Consent and Competency

Legal and Ethical Issues

David Naimark, Laura Dunn, Ansar Haroun, and Grant Morris

INTRODUCTION

Clinical issues related to informed consent and competency are present in all areas of medicine and are, quite possibly, the most relevant in the disciplines of psychiatry and neurology. The very nature of the specialty (involving disease of mind or brain) often calls into question the ability of the patient to understand the medical procedures or treatment that are being proposed.

In this chapter, we begin with an exploration of the legal aspects of informed consent and competency in order to give the reader an underpinning of the basic concepts, and then proceed to a "how-to" guide for accomplishing the medical task of assessment.

LEGAL ASPECTS OF INFORMED CONSENT AND COMPETENCY

The Doctrine of Informed Consent

The Tort of Battery

In 1914, Justice Benjamin Cardozo, writing for the New York Court of Appeals in *Schloendorff vs Society of New York Hospital (1)* declared, "Every human being of adult years and sound mind has a right to determine what shall be done with his own body; and a surgeon who performs an operation without his patient's consent commits [the tort of battery], for which he is liable in damages" *(1)*. This early 20th-century quotation is often cited as the starting point for the law's recognition of the patient's right to medical self-determination.

It is easy to understand why battery was the tort first chosen to champion the patient's right to control physician decision making. Early 20th-century cases typically involved fact situations in which the patient either specifically prohibited any operation, or authorized an operation different than the one performed by the surgeon. Under such circumstances, it was easy for the courts to find that the tort of battery had been committed. That tort protects the inviolability of one's person, described by writers as the first and greatest right of a free citizen, one that underlies all other rights. An operation performed without permission on an anesthetized patient violates that patient's bodily integrity. The tort is committed by the unauthorized contact, no matter how medically appropriate the surgery and no matter how skillfully it is performed. Neither an intent to harm the patient, nor negligence in performing the operation itself, are required for the tort of battery, only knowledge that the contact is made without the patient's consent. Actual physical harm to the patient is not a prerequisite for tort liability; battery is a dignitary tort, protecting individuals from offensive as well as harmful contact.

From: *Current Clinical Neurology: Psychiatry for Neurologists*
Edited by: D.V. Jeste and J.H. Friedman © Humana Press Inc., Totowa, NJ

When the operation, or other touching of the patient's body, was performed without any consent, the tort of battery was, and continues to be, well suited to protect the patient's autonomy interest. Over the years, however, patients demanded more for their autonomy right. Self-determination meant more than simply accepting or rejecting the doctor's decision; it meant the right for patients to make the decision themselves. And to make those decisions, patients needed the information about the proposed treatment or surgery that only their doctors could provide to them. But courts were far more reluctant to characterize as batteries treatments or operations that were performed with the patient's consent but without an adequate disclosure by the surgeon of the risks, benefits, and alternatives to the agreed upon procedure. The tort of battery was relegated to cases in which the physician either operated without obtaining any consent from the patient or the patient specifically declined the operation. In developing a duty of disclosure a half century after *Schloendorff*, courts distinguished between "real" or "basic" consent, necessary to avoid liability for battery, and failure to obtain the patient's "informed" consent, which most courts characterized as the tort of negligence.

The Tort of Negligence

A plaintiff claiming negligence must prove that the defendant breached a duty that was owed to the plaintiff and that the breach caused an injury to the plaintiff. The term "informed consent" was first mentioned in 1957 in a California Court of Appeal decision. That court embraced the principle of patient medical self-determination, declaring, "a physician violates his duty to his patient and subjects himself to liability if he withholds any facts which are necessary to form the basis of an intelligent consent by the patient to the proposed treatment" *(2)*. The physician's disclosure duty requires an explanation of the nature of the treatment or procedure that is being proposed by the physician, the possible alternatives to that treatment or procedure, and the material risks and anticipated benefits of the treatment or procedure.

The physician's disclosure duty, however, is not absolute. In *Natanson vs Kline*, the Kansas Supreme Court acknowledged that a physician probably has a therapeutic privilege to withhold a diagnosis of cancer or other dread disease from an unstable, temperamental, or severely depressed patient when disclosure would seriously jeopardize the patient's recovery. The court noted, however, that suppression of facts would not be warranted in the ordinary case. Merely because the physician believes that the patient may decline a procedure or operation if the risks are explained to him or her does not excuse the physician's failure to divulge those risks.

Although physicians are not permitted to deceive patients in order to substitute their own judgment for that of their patients, the *Natanson* court ruled that the physician's duty to disclose "is limited to those disclosures which a reasonable medical practitioner would make under the same or similar circumstances" *(3)*. In essence, the court engrafted onto the disclosure requirement the medical custom standard of care that is used to determine professional malpractice. As long as the defendant conformed to the level of disclosure of other physicians in good standing, and the defendant is presumed to have conformed in the absence of expert medical testimony to the contrary, no breach of the disclosure duty would be found.

The medical custom standard is used today by a majority of states to measure whether the physician's disclosure duty has been breached. In part, the dominance of this standard was assured by the legislative response to the perceived medical malpractice crisis of the mid-1970s. As one "reform" to reduce physician liability and malpractice insurance costs, several states enacted legislation adopting the medical custom standard to measure breach of the physician's disclosure duty.

Not all jurisdictions, however, allow physicians to establish their own standard for measuring disclosure. In *Canterbury vs Spence*, the US Court of Appeals for the District of Columbia Circuit rejected the medical custom approach, asserting, "[i]t is the prerogative of the patient, not the physician, to determine for himself the direction in which his interests seem to lie" *(4)*. "In our view," wrote the court, "the patient's right of self-decision shapes the boundaries of the duty to reveal." The adequacy of the physician's disclosures to the patient "must be measured by the patient's need, and that need is the information material to the decision: all risks potentially affecting the decision must be unmasked."

Concerned that physicians might not know what risks would be material to their patients, the *Canterbury* court defined "material risks" as those risks that a reasonable person in the patient's position would be likely to consider significant. Although the court acknowledged that "orthodox negligence doctrine" measures "the reasonableness of the physician's divulgence in terms of what he knows or should know to be *the patient's* informational needs," the court transformed the individual patient's informational needs into those of the hypothetical, reasonable patient.

The patient, the court acknowledged, has no duty to ask for information from the physician. The physician is obligated, despite the patient's silence, to volunteer information that the patient needs to make his or her decision. "Caveat emptor is not the norm for the consumer of medical services," says the court. But the *Canterbury* court did not require the physician to inquire of the silent patient whether there was anything he or she would like to know (i.e., what is important to that patient's decision making). And yet, by not obligating physicians to ask their patients what their concerns are, and then to respond to those concerns, the *Canterbury* court, in reality, ruled that the physician's disclosure duty is owed, not to his or her patient, but only to the reasonable patient. By homogenizing all patients into reasonable patients, the court perverted the very principle it proclaimed.

The *Canterbury* court erected other barriers to the patient's right to self-determination. If the physician fails to reveal the risks and alternatives that a reasonable patient would consider material to his or her judgment, negligence law requires the patient to prove that this breach of duty caused harm. The harm requirement is satisfied, said the court, only if an unrevealed risk that the physician was obligated to disclose, materializes, and the causation requirement is satisfied only if a reasonable person in the patient's position would have declined the treatment if the risk had been revealed.

Harm, according to the court, is limited to the patient's interest in his or her physical well-being (i.e., was the patient physically injured by the physician's breach of the disclosure duty?) The court assures us that "[t]he patient obviously has no complaint if he would have submitted to the therapy notwithstanding awareness that the risk was one of its perils." The patient, however, does have a complaint. The patient has been deprived of the right to decide. That loss of individual autonomy, in and of itself, is an injury Nevertheless, this dignitary loss, the right to make one's own choice as to what shall be done to one's own body, is not compensable. For the patient to succeed in a negligence claim against the physician, *Canterbury* requires that the plaintiff suffer a physical injury from the physician's breach of the disclosure duty.

The *Canterbury* court's analysis of the causation requirement is even more dubious. If the physician does not breach the disclosure duty, the patient's decision to accept or reject the proposed treatment or surgery will not be disturbed. "The patient," the court tells us, "is free to decide for any reason that appeals to him." But if the physician breaches the disclosure duty, depriving the patient of his or her right to decide, for any reason that appeals to him or her, then causation of harm will not be measured by what he or she would have decided, but rather, by what a reasonable person in the patient's position would have decided. The causation requirement is no longer an inquiry about what the patient would have decided if he or she had not been deprived of information material to his or her judgment. The patient who has been wronged by the physician's nondisclosure is permitted to win only if he or she would have made a decision that the jury considers to be reasonable.

Despite its doctrinal deficiencies, *Canterbury's* reasonable patient test—for measuring both breach of the disclosure duty and causation—has become *the* "liberal" alternative to the conservative reasonable doctor test. For nearly half the states, Canterbury did not become a new point of departure; it became a final destination.

Expanding the Definition of "Material Risks" That Must Be Disclosed

Suppose a physician informs the patient of the risks of and alternatives to procedures and diagnostic tests that the physician proposes, and the patient declines the proposed treatment. To fulfill his or her disclosure duty, must the physician also disclose to the patient the risks of patient's decision to refuse treatment? Some courts have responded in the affirmative. The California Supreme Court, for example, has ruled that this broadened disclosure obligation is needed to assure not only that the patient gives an informed *consent* to treatment, but also to assure that the patient's *refusal* of treatment is also informed. "The duty to disclose was imposed," said the California Supreme Court, "so that patients might meaningfully exercise their right to make decisions about their own bodies" *(5).*

But suppose, for example, that after evaluating a patient, the physician's proposed course of action is no action. The physician decides not to order additional laboratory tests to better diagnose a patient's medical condition, or simply decides to monitor the patient's condition but not to administer any treatment, or decides to terminate treatment because, in the physician's judgment, a successful outcome has been achieved. Must the physician disclose the risks of and alternatives to the nontreatment option that the physician has selected? Because the tort of battery requires unpermitted physical contact with the patient, that tort is not committed by physician's decision to select the "no-treatment" option.

But does a negligence-based informed consent doctrine require the physician to disclose the risks and alternatives of these nontreatment options, at least if a reasonable physician would disclose them or if a reasonable patient would find them material to his or her decision making? After all, the absence of treatment can result in physical injury to the patient just as assuredly as can active mistreatment. In an era of managed care, cost containment, and the rationing of medical services, this question is a serious concern for patients. It is also a serious concern for physicians who must comply with their disclosure duty under the doctrine of informed consent and who know that their patients are likely to demand affirmative, and costly, treatment options if they are informed of them.

Some courts have imposed a duty to disclose. For example, in *Matthies vs Mastromonaco (6)* the New Jersey Supreme Court was unwilling to limit a negligence-based informed consent doctrine to a nonconsensual touching proposed, but not adequately explained, by the physician. The court specifically upheld the patient's right to make an informed *decision* about medically reasonable alternatives, not merely to give an informed *consent* to the alternative that the physician recommends. The court would not allow the physician to, in essence, decide for the patient by discussing only the physician's treatment (or nontreatment) of choice. As the court stated, "physicians may neither impose their values on their patients nor substitute their level of risk aversion for that of their patients. . . . By not telling the patient of all medically reasonable alternatives, the physician breaches the patient's right to make an informed choice." Although the physician's choice might be medically appropriate and conform to the physician's standard of care, nevertheless, it might not be the choice that the patient would make. The absence of malpractice does not assure the presence of the patient's informed choice.

Other courts, however, disagree, limiting a patient's right to make decisions about his or her own body to situations in which the treating physician is proposing some affirmative course of action. These decisions appear erroneous. Under a negligence theory, the disclosure duty is imposed not to protect the patient from a nonconsensual touching, but rather, to protect the patient's right to medical self-determination. To make decisions about what shall be done and what shall not be done to their bodies, patients need information on the risks of and alternatives to the nontreatment option. They need that information, not only when they refuse a treatment proposed by the physician, but also when the physician proposes no treatment.

Although a physician's "decision" to prescribe bed rest instead of surgery or to order some diagnostic tests but not others may conform to acceptable medical practice and thus not constitute malpractice, the physician's professional duties to the patient are not circumscribed by his or her clinical judgment calls. The physician also owes the patient an independent duty of disclosure. If, as the *Canterbury* court announced, and numerous other courts echoed, "the patient's right of self-decision shapes the boundaries of the duty to reveal," the physician should be obligated to disclose information about alternative treatment options—including surgery and diagnostic testing—that the physician is not recommending. That information is not only material to the patient's decision, it is often critical to that decision. The decision on what treatment, or nontreatment, is acceptable belongs to the patient whose life will be affected by that decision, not to the physician who can only recommend options based on his or her professional expertise. Because the patient is entitled to make the decision, the physician should be obligated to disclose the information that the patient needs to make that decision.

In recent years, some courts have defined "material risks" broadly, requiring physicians to disclose not merely the risks and alternatives inherent in medical procedures that the physician might not recommend but that the patient might want to consider, but, in addition, other risks that emanate directly from the physician. For example, some courts have required surgeons to inform patients of the physician's chronic alcohol abuse or HIV-positive status. These physical infirmities may increase the risk of harm to the patient and must be disclosed as material to the patient's judgment to accept or reject treatment from that surgeon. Other physician-specific factors raise a similar concern. In one case, a patient consented to basilar bifurcation aneurysm surgery (a clipping of an aneurysm at the rear of the plaintiff's brain) and was rendered an incomplete quadriplegic. The Supreme Court of Wisconsin ruled that information about the neurosurgeon's limited experience in performing such surgery and the difficulty of the operation should have been disclosed because it was material and would have been considered by the reasonable patient *(7)*.

In *Moore vs Regents of University of California (8)*, the California Supreme Court held that to obtain a patient's informed consent, the physician must also disclose any financial or other interest that the physician has that conflicts with, or even potentially conflicts with the physician's fiduciary duty to that patient. In deciding whether to consent to proposed treatment, a patient would want to know of any research or economic interest extraneous to the patient's health that may have affected the physician's judgment to recommend that treatment, even if that conflicting interest was not consciously considered. In *Moore*, for example, the plaintiff alleged that the surgeon's research interest in the patient's rare blood and the surgeon's economic interest in patenting a cell line from the plaintiff's cells may well have influenced the surgeon to recommend a splenectomy, the surgical removal of the plaintiff's spleen.

A federal appeals court, applying Minnesota law, went one step further. The court imposed a duty on physicians to disclose conflicting loyalties even when they do not recommend any affirmative course of treatment. In *Shea vs Esenstein (Shea II) (9)*, a 40-year-old patient was experiencing symptoms of heart disease. His family doctors did not refer him to a cardiologist. When the patient's symptoms did not improve, the patient offered to pay for the referral, but "his physicians persuaded him to trust their judgment that neither his age nor his symptoms justified a visit to a cardiologist." The patient suffered a heart attack and died. In a wrongful death suit, the plaintiff alleged that the physicians failed to disclose financial incentives in the health maintenance organization (HMO) contract designed to minimize referrals to specialists and that if the patient had known of those incentives, he would not have trusted the physicians' medical advice but instead would have obtained the opinion of a specialist at his own expense. Even though the jury found that the physicians had not committed malpractice in the care and treatment of the patient, the court upheld the plaintiff's separate claim for the tort of negligent misrepresentation. Under Minnesota law, physicians have a state-imposed ethical duty to disclose conflicts of interests to their patients. Self-serving financial incentives, such as those found in an HMO contract, conflict with the physician's duty of loyalty to the patient's medical welfare, and must be revealed.

Although these case precedents for an expanded disclosure duty are important forays for future development of the law, they have not been universally, or even generally, accepted in American jurisprudence. For each case discussed here, there are others, often numerous others, that have reached a contrary result. Some courts have ruled that a physician's medical condition, including his or her addiction to alcoholism or drugs, or the physician's HIV-positive status, need not be disclosed. Some courts have held that a physician's inexperience in performing the particular surgery proposed to the patient need not be disclosed.

Courts that restrict the physician's disclosure duty to the risks inherent in the physician's proposed procedure deny patients the information they need, and, in fact, must have, in order to decide whether to trust their doctor. A patient's trust cannot be purchased with concealment or subterfuge. It can only be developed through honest communication. "[D]isclosure and consent," wrote Dr. Jay Katz, "do not abolish trust. Disclosure and consent only banish unilateral, blind trust; they make mutual trust possible for the first time" *(10)*. When courts do not require that communication, their narrowly crafted informed consent doctrine does not shield patients from their doctors' deceptions; it leaves them naked and exposed.

Competency

Competency as a Requirement for Giving or Withholding Informed Consent

A patient's informed consent to treatment is not required if an emergency arises that requires immediate medical attention and the patient is not competent to give or withhold consent to that treatment. For example, if at the scene of an auto accident, a person lays unconscious and bleeding to death, the law presumes that the person would consent to treatment necessary to save his or her life. The law makes this presumption because a reasonable person faced with the need for immediate life-saving treatment would authorize that treatment if the person were competent to make the decision at the time. The law protects the physician who acts in an emergency to save a life, even if subsequently facts become known that indicate that the unconscious person would not have consented to medical treatment.

Incompetence, however, is not limited to unconscious adults. Children, because of their youth and inexperience, are considered mentally unable to make treatment decisions, and in the absence of a life-threatening emergency, informed consent of a parent or legally responsible guardian is required for the physician to act. The parent or guardian makes a substituted judgment for the child, either accepting or rejecting treatment on the child's behalf. Adults, too, especially if they suffer from a severe mental disorder, may be incompetent to make a treatment decision. If the condition is likely to be of a lengthy duration, the court may appoint a guardian for the person with authority to make decisions for him or her. In essence, the guardian of the adult acts in the capacity of a parent for a child, until such time as the ward is restored to competency.

Civil Commitment of Mentally Disordered Persons and the Right to Refuse Treatment

When a person with a severe mental disorder is so incapacitated that he or she is either dangerous to himor herself or to others, or is unable to provide for the basic necessities of life, such as food, clothing, and shelter, that person may be civilly committed and placed in a mental hospital. Can the treating physician require the civilly committed person to take psychotropic medication to eliminate symptoms and improve the patient's condition or does the patient, relying on the doctrine of informed consent, have a right to refuse its administration? The issue has generated great controversy between psychiatrists and lawyers. Psychiatrists assert that the very purpose of placing the involuntarily committed person in a mental hospital is to treat the person's mental disorder so that the person's freedom can be restored. Lawyers contend that even involuntarily committed mental patients retain rights, including the right to refuse treatment, that should not be infringed on without proof of the necessity to do so.

Dr. Alan Stone, noted Harvard psychiatrist and former president of the American Psychiatric Association, has acknowledged that the legal justifications for the right to refuse treatment are so "clear and compelling" that psychiatrists should accept the right's existence *(11)*. Dr. Stone conceded that a mentally disordered person's refusal of psychotropic medication is merely one example of refusal of medical treatment by any ill person. In a treatment refusal situation, the doctrine of informed consent restricts the state's authority to intrude on the individual's autonomy. Only when the individual, whether from mental disorder or other cause, is unable to make competent decisions, may another's judgment be substituted. Although incompetence negates autonomous decision making, incompetence is not established solely by proof of mental disorder or proof that treatment is clinically indicated.

Similarly, incompetence is not established by proof that the mentally disordered individual meets the civil commitment criteria and is subject to involuntary detention. In most states, the laws do not presume or require incompetence as a criterion for civil commitment. The mentally disordered person's dangerousness to self or others, or inability to provide for basic necessities, justifies a deprivation of liberty but does not justify a deprivation of the patient's right to refuse treatment or other rights. A person may be incompetent to provide for basic necessities, but be competent to understand the risks and benefits of medication that is proposed to treat his or her condition. In other words, incompetence for one purpose does not equal incompetence for another. Only when a person's incompetence to make the treatment decision is established can another's judgment be substituted.

Most states have recognized the right of competent, though involuntarily committed, patients to refuse treatment. The United States Supreme Court has acknowledged that even mentally ill *prisoners* have a "significant liberty interest in avoiding the unwanted administration of antipsychotic drugs" *(12)*. The states, however, have divided almost equally on the question of procedural protections necessary to enforce that right. Some states use a medical decision-maker model, allowing a staff psychiatrist or hospital committee to make an informal decision of the patient's competence. Others, including the nation's five most populous states (California, Texas, New York, Florida, and Illinois), require a formal hearing on the patient's competence before a judge or other independent, law-trained decision maker. In these states, neither mental disorder alone, nor a decision to civilly commit the person, equates to a finding of incompetence to make treatment decisions. Before treatment may be imposed over the objection of a patient, even an involuntarily civilly committed mental patient, the judge must find that the patient lacks the mental capacity to make treatment decisions (i.e., to weigh the risks, benefits, and alternatives to the proposed medication).

Competent civilly committed patients, however, do not have an absolute right to refuse antipsychotic medication. The state does have a legitimate interest in protecting other patients and staff from dangerous mental patients. Hospital staff may respond to threatening situations by segregating the potentially dangerous patient or using physical restraints. In an emergency situation, when the patient presents an immediate danger to him or herself or to others, the patient may be involuntarily sedated. Nevertheless, this exercise of the state's police power must end when the emergency that warranted this exercise of authority ends. If a person's "significant liberty interest in avoiding the unwanted administration of antipsychotic drugs" is to have any meaning at all, an assertion that the patient was civilly committed as being too dangerous to live in society, or that he or she presents a generalized danger to other patients or staff in the institution, does not justify nonemergency, coerced treatment of a competent civil patient.

Assessing the Competence of Civilly Committed Mental Patients to Refuse Psychotropic Medication

In *Reise vs St. Mary's Hospital and Medical Center (13)*, the California Court of Appeal added California to the list of states that recognize the right of a competent, but involuntarily committed mental patient to refuse psychotropic medication in nonemergency situations and require a formal court hearing to determine if the patient is incompetent. The facts of the case demonstrate why the court rejected the medical decision maker model as an inadequate protection of the competent patient's right to refuse. Eleanor Riese was admitted to St. Mary's Hospital as a voluntary patient. Previously, she had been treated for chronic schizophrenia with Mellaril®, a psychotropic medication. As a result of that earlier treatment, her bladder had been severely damaged. Nevertheless, the treating physician prescribed Mellaril, and she consented to its use. Although she complained of dizziness and dry mouth and stated that she was receiving too much medication, her concerns were ignored and the dosage was not reduced. When she protested and refused medication, she was forcibly injected and committed as an involuntary patient. Ms. Riese brought a class action on behalf of patients involuntarily committed under California's 72-hour treatment and evaluation detention and its 14-day intensive treatment certification.

In upholding the right of involuntary civil patients to exercise informed consent, the *Reise* court, borrowing liberally from a text for psychiatrists prepared by Drs. Thomas Gutheil and Paul Appelbaum

(14) that identified three factors that judges should consider in assessing the competence of a patient's medication refusal. First, the judge should consider "whether the patient is aware of his or her situation." The court offered one example of such awareness: if the judge believes that the patient is psychotic, does the patient acknowledge the psychosis? The court's singular example seems unfortunate. A doctor, who has diagnosed a patient's mental disorder and made a clinical judgment on what medication is appropriate to treat that disorder, may view the law's requirement of obtaining a patient's informed consent as an unwelcome and unnecessary impediment to the doctor's authority to make the treatment decision. If the patient does not readily acknowledge that he or she has a mental disorder and acquiesce in the doctor's recommendation, the doctor may quickly decide, perhaps too quickly, that the patient is incompetent to make the treatment decision. After all, the doctor may assert, a patient who does not acknowledge having a mental disorder is unable to appreciate the benefits of the medication prescribed to treat that disorder.

Although denial of mental disorder may be a factor in assessing a person's awareness of the situation, it is certainly not the exclusive measure. Even if a person denies having a mental disorder, he or she is aware of the situation if the person knows that he or she is involuntarily confined in a mental hospital, that the doctor has diagnosed the person as having a mental disorder, that the doctor has prescribed psychotropic medication to treat the disorder, that the doctor believes the medication will benefit the person by relieving symptoms, and that the person is refusing the medication because of concern about medication side effects that have been previously experienced. Additionally, a person who denies having a mental disorder may be willing and able to acknowledge having a problem in "nonmedical" terms. The person, for example, may be denying a mental disorder in order to maintain control over his or her life and to avoid being thrust into the dependent role of a mental patient. The person may be denying mental illness in an attempt to avoid a catch-22 situation (i.e., by admitting mental disorder the patient strengthens the psychiatrist's assertion that the prescribed medication is the appropriate remedy). Denial of mental illness may be a rational, although hostile, reaction to the family members or the police who initiated the involuntarily commitment process, to the judge who ordered the patient committed, or to the psychiatrist who now seeks to impose treatment over the patient's objection.

Second, the judge should consider "whether the patient is able to understand the benefits and the risks of, as well as the alternatives to, the proposed intervention." Here, too, the *Riese* court gave an example. Even if the patient is acutely psychotic, the patient should understand that dystonic reactions are a risk, that resolution of the psychotic episode is a benefit, and that psychotherapy, milieu therapy, and possibly electroconvulsive therapy are alternatives. This example, suggested by Drs. Gutheil and Appelbaum, appears helpful. Nevertheless, one can question whether treating physicians typically consider alternative therapies as viable substitutes for psychotropic medication. In their eagerness to impose their treatment preference, physicians may be unwilling to consider patient objections to that choice and to suggest other alternatives that might be acceptable to their patients.

Third, the judge should assess the patient's ability "to understand and to knowingly and intelligently evaluate the information required to be given patients whose informed consent is sought (§ 5326.2) and otherwise participate in the treatment decision by means of rational thought processes." The court cited with approval a suggestion offered by Drs. Gutheil and Appelbaum that the patient should be assumed to be utilizing rational thought processes in the absence of proof clearly linking delusional or hallucinatory perceptions to the individual's ultimate decision. An assessment of a patient's ability to understand information begins with the information that the patient has been given. Although the *Riese* court did not itself discuss what information must be provided, it incorporated, by specific reference, California Welfare and Institutions Code section 5326.2. That statute itemizes information that must be given to the patient in a clear and explicit manner in order to obtain a voluntary and informed consent to treatment. Among the required disclosures are the following:

1. The nature and seriousness of the patient's mental disorder that serves as a reason for treatment.
2. The nature of the proposed treatment, including probable frequency and duration.

3. The degree and duration of improvement or remission anticipated with or without such treatment.
4. The nature, degree, duration, and the probability of side effects and significant risks of the proposed treatment and how and to what extent they may be controlled, if at all.
5. The reasonable alternative treatments, and why the physician is recommending this particular treatment.
6. The patient has the right to accept or refuse the proposed treatment, and if the patient consents, he or she has the right to revoke the consent for any reason and at any time prior to or between treatments.

A study of competency hearings *(15)* reveals that often, psychiatrists do not disclose to patients the information that the law requires them to disclose. Often, psychiatrists only inform patients about medication benefits. Even when they disclose risks, psychiatrists do not divulge "all information relevant to a meaningful decisional process"—the test of disclosure required to obtain a patient's informed consent. Sometimes psychiatrists speak about risks in general terms, informing the patient that any medication can have detrimental as well as beneficial effects. Of course, they will assert, the medication is being prescribed for its beneficial effects. At times, psychiatrists discuss some side effects but not others. Typically, a psychiatrist will inform the patient of non-neurological side effects, such as sedation or anticholinergic side effects, such as dry mouth, blurred vision, urinary retention, and constipation, but will omit any discussion of neurological side effects such as dystonia, Parkinsonism, akathisia, akinesia, and tardive dyskinesia. Obviously, if the risk of non-neurological side effects is material to a patient's decision, the risk of neurological side effects is likely to be even more so. The study concluded, "the failure of psychiatrists to inform patients adequately of medication risks and alternatives was not limited to a few isolated incidents. It was pervasive."

The author of the competency study suggested that in a proceeding to consider whether the patient is competent to refuse psychotropic medication, the judge can and should appropriately respond to psychiatrist nondisclosure by finding the patient competent. By failing to inform the patient, and failing to provide the judge with evidence that the patient is unable to understand and to evaluate that information, the psychiatrist has not sustained the burden of proving by clear and convincing evidence that the patient is incompetent. If the patient is found competent, then under traditional legal principles, the psychiatrist commits the tort of battery if he or she administers psychotropic medication over the patient's objection, and the psychiatrist can be held liable for punitive as well as compensatory damages. Liability for the tort of negligence is limited to situations in which a competent patient consents to the administration of psychotropic medication but suffers an injury from a risk of the drug that was not explained to him or her.

MEDICAL ASPECTS OF INFORMED CONSENT AND COMPETENCY

Informed Consent

In clinical as well as research settings, informed consent is one of the cornerstones of ethical practice *(16,17)*. The consent process epitomizes professional ideals and protects individual rights. Too often, however, in part due to the many competing demands of medical care and research, the informed consent discussion "morphs" into a procedure done *to* the patient or research participant (i.e., "consenting" the patient). This phrasing implies that the patient is a passive recipient of information who then acquiesces to the proposed test, treatment, or research protocol. Viewed through a different lens, however, the informed consent process presents an ideal opportunity for the patient and the physician or investigator to participate in a meaningful discussion of alternatives and their potential risks and benefits. In this process, the patient or participant becomes more of a partner with the physician in management of his or her own care. In addition to providing information, the overall process then serves as an optimal context for clarifying patient preferences and values, which leads to authentic decision-making. Ultimately, it is the patient who is the final decision maker.

In the research context, informed consent also embodies the careful attention of investigators and ethics review boards to address concerns about research with human subjects. The need to protect and respect human subjects by obtaining informed consent is not merely an historical artifact related to past abuses. There are many recent instances in which ethical questions about human research have turned on the question of whether informed consent was properly obtained. In addition, concerns have emerged relative to the capacity of some subjects to give their consent. In fact, some institutional review boards require that researchers who plan "to recruit from populations with disorders known to be associated with impairment of decision-making capacity" have a specific plan to ensure that decisional capacity is addressed at the earliest stages of the study *(18)*.

The doctrine of informed consent holds that three components are necessary for valid consent *(19,20)*. The consent must be based on full and relevant information, must be given voluntarily, and must derive from a capable/competent decision maker. (We use the term *capacity* here in distinction from the legal term *competency*, because physicians are asked to assess decision-making capacity in the clinical setting, whereas a judge must make a determination of legal competency.) We discuss each of these components separately.

Information Provision

For patient autonomy to be promoted and respected, at a minimum, physicians should disclose what a "reasonable person" would want to know about the recommended treatment or procedure, its risks and benefits, as well as treatment alternatives and their attendant risks and benefits. The alternative of no treatment should be discussed as well (whether or not this is the physician's recommendation), so that a patient's decision to accept or reject treatment is based on an understanding of its likely consequences.

Shared decision making involves going a step further, beyond the "reasonable person" standard. Asking patients open-ended questions about what other information they may need in order to make the decision is a simple way to address this. The presentation of the information must be done in such a way as to optimize the patient's understanding. When done in a hurry or without concern for whether the patient has actually understood the information, the disclosure process is unlikely to meet ethical standards (and undermines patient autonomy). Testing for comprehension can be done fairly quickly and efficiently using open-ended questions followed by closed-ended questions. When doubt exists about the adequacy of decision-making capacity, numerous instruments exist to assist with the capacity assessment; these are described in more detail below.

Voluntariness

The second requirement for informed consent mandates that the decision maker give consent voluntarily and free from coercion. This does not mean that physicians cannot provide treatment recommendations, patients legitimately rely on physicians to help sort through decisions. Encouragement to follow a particular course of treatment is also ethically acceptable so long as there is no coercion *(16)*. (For a summary of potential influences on voluntarism, the reader is referred to Roberts' conceptual framework *[21]*.)

Decision-Making Capacity

Decision-making capacity is widely considered by experts to consist of four abilities: (a) understanding (or comprehension) of the disclosed information, (b) appreciation (the ability to apply the information to one's situation), (c) reasoning (weighing options, including risks and benefits), and (d) expression of a stable choice *(16,22)*.

Each of these abilities has been used, in different instances, as the legal standard for determination of capacity, with different jurisdictions applying different standards. Requiring that all four abilities be intact is the most stringent standard. There is no consensus regarding the degree of impairment that should be considered to represent a lack of capacity. The choice of standard directly affects the proportion of patients who will be found to be impaired. Although expression of a stable choice is viewed as the least stringent of these standards, research into decisional abilities of patients with both psychiatric and medical disorders has not consistently demonstrated a "hierarchy of rigorousness" among these abilities in patients *(22)*. In other words, demonstration of intact reasoning and appreciation does not necessarily mean that the patient has understood the information, and vice versa. It is important for the physician to be cognizant of differing state laws regarding the level of ability that is required for the patient to retain mental capacity, even if there is some level of impairment.

As a way of illustrating the differences among these ability areas, consider a patient with schizophrenia who lacks insight into having the illness. The patient believes that agents of the government have implanted a "scanning chip" in his brain for the purpose of tracking his thoughts, behavior, and movements. The patient has been diagnosed with colon cancer and is refusing what his doctors consider a medically necessary surgical procedure.

The patient's capacity is assessed in order to determine if he can provide meaningful informed consent. The patient is provided with information about the recommended treatment, the reasons why the doctor is recommending it, its possible risks and discomforts, and the likely benefits. He is also told that, without the surgery, his chance of surviving the cancer is slim. The patient is able to paraphrase the information disclosed to him about the procedure's purpose, risks, and benefits (thus evidencing adequate understanding). However, when asked specifically whether he believes this information applies to his own case, he talks about the government trying to force him to have the procedure because "they want to put me under the knife" (in order to implant more devices in him). He believes that the cancer diagnosis is being invented to fool him into having surgery (thus he does not appreciate the situation adequately). When asked to discuss how he arrived at his decision to refuse the surgery, he states that because the government is trying to force him to do it, he doesn't want to have the surgery (thus his reasoning is also affected by the delusional system).

In this example, the patient's understanding and expression of a choice seem adequate, yet his appreciation and reasoning appear to be driven by delusional thinking. Thus, the patient has impairments in some, but not all, of the aspects of decisional capacity. Most experts would agree that the patient's capacity is diminished. If at all possible, the reason for his diminished capacity (delusional thinking) should be addressed (by optimizing the patient's antipsychotic regimen), with the goal of allowing the patient to make the decision himself, based on rational reasons and genuine appreciation. Ultimately, a court may have to decide whether treatment may or may not be forced on him.

Competency

The purpose in this section is to provide guidance on performing capacity assessments when there is a need to determine whether the patient is legally competent. Although any physician can assess decision-making capacity, a formal consult by an expert is sometimes desirable.

When Capacity Should Be Assessed

Patient capacity for medical decision making may be affected by many different factors, including medical and neuropsychiatric disorders. The most common reason for consultations regarding decisional capacity is a patients' refusal of recommended treatment. Such refusal does not in and of itself indicate impaired capacity. It is reasonable, however, to be concerned about patient capacity when treatment refusal would jeopardize the patient's health or well-being or seems to be irrational. Empirical data indicate that most refusals are, in fact, related to impaired decision-making capacity *(16)*. The most important point regarding capacity assessment is to determine the reasons for the patient's refusal and whether these reasons may represent impaired capacity. (This is addressed further below.)

Many clinicians are particularly concerned about decision-making capacity in patients with psychiatric disorders. Research in this area reveals a subtle picture. Although patients with schizophrenia have higher rates of impaired decision-making capacity, they cannot be assumed to lack capacity *(23)*. A number of studies have demonstrated that psychiatrically ill patients show a great deal of heterogeneity of performance, with most *not* performing in the impaired range *(24)*. The research cited above was conducted with psychiatric inpatients, a group tending to be more severely ill than psychiatric outpatients. In a study of decision-making capacity for research in outpatients with major depression, for example, study participants performed quite well on measures of understanding, appreciation, and reasoning *(25)*.

Not surprisingly, a number of studies have shown that dementia is associated with a high rate of impaired decision-making capacity *(26–28)*. Yet, even a diagnosis of dementia does not inevitably mean that patients do not retain some abilities to decide for themselves. It is worth emphasizing that impairment in decision-making capacity does not necessarily equate to legal incompetence to make the decision. It has been demonstrated, for instance, that patients with mild dementia may continue to possess some decision-making abilities *(27,28)*. It is also not known to what degree mild cognitive impairment may compromise decisional abilities for medical or research-related decision making, as there is scant research in this area.

Steps in Assessing Capacity

The first step in assessment of capacity is to ensure that the patient has been provided with the relevant information necessary to make the decision. Provision of information, as described above, should entail using whatever formats will optimize the patient's understanding. Next, it is important to ask the patient if he or she has any questions about what has just been disclosed. During the actual capacity assessment, the goal should be to determine whether the patient has actually comprehended the information, not just whether he or she can repeat back the information. Therefore, open-ended questions should be used initially (i.e., "Can you tell me in your own words about the treatment [test, procedure, study] that I've just described to you?"). Questions should cover the nature and purpose of the procedure, test, treatment, or research protocol, the potential risks, the possible and/or likely benefits, as well as alternatives to the recommended treatment (including no treatment) and the risks and benefits of these alternatives. Risks may be construed not simply as possible negative outcomes, but also as discomforts and consequences. Risks of foregoing a treatment option should also be disclosed and discussed.

If a patient does not appear to understand any of these aspects of the treatment, the information should be provided again (re-disclosure) and the patient should be given at least a second opportunity to demonstrate understanding. In some cases (e.g., in a patient experiencing delirium), attention deficits may be worse at certain times than at others; thus, multiple attempts to test comprehension may be necessary if a patient does not initially grasp the information. In other cases (e.g., advanced dementia), memory for the disclosed information is extremely unlikely to improve upon retesting, so poor understanding can usually be assumed to represent a stable deficit.

Appreciation, the next element of decision-making capacity, can be assessed by asking the patient to apply the disclosed information to his or her own situation. This is best achieved by disclosing, again, what the doctors think is wrong and subsequently asking the patient if he or she believes this to be the case. Patients who possess appreciation can acknowledge: (a) that they are ill (acknowledgement of disorder), and (b) that treatment may be effective. A disbelief in either of these should be explored to determine why the patient does not believe it. The crucial distinction to make in ascertaining appreciation is whether a belief that one is not ill or that treatment is unlikely to be effective is based on realistic versus delusional thinking (or other illness-based impaired thinking, such as hopelessness as may be seen in severe depression) *(16)*. Refusal to acknowledge a disorder does not, however, necessarily equate to lack of appreciation—the patient still may comprehend the risks, benefits, and alternatives as they relate to him or her.

Assessment of reasoning can be done in conjunction with assessment of whether the patient can express a stable choice. A treatment decision that fluctuates, with the patient changing his or her mind over time, cannot be considered to be a consistent choice. The patient should be asked what choice is being considered, and the reasons underlying this choice should be explored. Intact reasoning should consist of the patient being able to compare alternatives (comparative reasoning) and generate potential consequences of the various options (consequential reasoning), such as how different choices would affect his or her everyday life or activities *(16)*.

Instruments

Several instruments have been designed to assess decision-making capacity for treatment and research. Of these, the most thoroughly studied have been the MacArthur Competence Assessment Tools (the MacCAT-T for treatment and MacCAT-CR for clinical research). These instruments were derived from a large study of patients with schizophrenia, depression, and medical illness (ischemic heart disease), as well as healthy community controls *(24)*. The instruments have demonstrated excellent reliability and validity in multiple populations. The MacCAT-T and MacCAT-CR have become as close to a "gold standard" as exists in capacity assessment, although this by no means implies that there are not other valid scales and ways to assess capacity. In part, the need for standardized instruments stems from the unreliability of using "expert" judgments of capacity *(29)*. Medical students and residents are not routinely trained in capacity assessment, and even physicians experienced in capacity assessment use widely varying methods to assess capacity, often coming to different conclusions in their judgments of capacity *(30)*. The MacArthur instruments provide a semi-structured interview for evaluating the four widely accepted aspects of decision-making capacity: understanding, appreciation, reasoning, and expression of a choice *(31,32)*. Each of the four components is rated on a subscale; no total score is derived.

Cognitive screening instruments (e.g., the Mini-Mental State Examination) and other neuropsychological tests do not demonstrate enough sensitivity or specificity to serve as substitutes for direct assessment of capacity for the decision at hand *(26,33–38)*. Decision-making capacity is domain-specific: individuals may be unable to manage certain functions in their daily lives, but may still retain sufficient abilities to decide about their own treatment. In our autonomy-protective society, this means that decision-making capacity cannot be assumed to be lacking simply because impairments exist in other functional domains.

CONCLUSIONS

In 20th-century American society, courts could not ignore or deny patients' demands for self-determination in medical decisions that affect their own bodies and their own lives. However, courts fashioned an informed consent doctrine that limits the information that physicians must disclose about the procedures they propose. Even as that doctrine has been most liberally formulated, patients do not receive the information they need to make medical decisions, but rather, only receive the information that reasonable patients would need. When physicians wrongfully deprive their patients of this information, the law places no monetary value on the loss of patients' legal right to make their own decisions. To succeed in an informed consent claim against their physicians, patients must prove that the breach of the disclosure duty caused them physical injury. Typically, however, causation is not measured by a true test of causation. The law does not ask whether the patients would have consented if the doctor had not breached the disclosure duty, but rather, whether reasonable patients would have consented. Despite these limitations on the doctrine of informed consent, some courts have recently expanded the definition of "material risks" that the physician is required to disclose to the patient. These courts have held that physicians must reveal their physical infirmities, inexperience in performing the procedure or surgery, and any financial or any other interest that potentially conflicts with their fiduciary duty as physicians to their patients.

The law does not require a physician to obtain informed consent from a patient who is incompetent to give or withhold consent. If a person is unconscious and emergency treatment is needed to preserve his or her life, the law presumes the consent of the patient. The parent of a child, or the legal guardian of an incompetent ward, may consent for the patient. Mental disorder, however, does not *per se* equate with incompetence to make treatment decisions. Even if the mentally disordered person is involuntarily civilly committed, in most states, the commitment order does not *per se* equate with incompetence to make treatment decisions. Court decisions and legislation in many states specifically uphold the right of involuntarily committed mental patients to refuse psychotropic medication in nonemergency situations. In essence, unless a court specifically finds that these patients are incompetent to make the treatment decision (i.e., unless they are unable to understand the risks, benefits, and alternatives to the proposed therapy) thenthey are entitled to give or withhold their consent. Because the decision belongs to the patient, not the doctor, the failure of the treating physician to provide the information necessary for the patient to make an informed decision cannot be countenanced.

REFERENCES

1. Schloendorff vs Society of New York Hospital, 105 N.E. 92. New York; 1914.
2. Salgo vs Leland Stanford Jr. University Board of Trustees, 317 P.2d 170. California; 1957.
3. Natanson vs Klein, 350 P.2d 1093. Kanas; 1960.
4. Canterbury vs Spence, 464 F.2d 772. Washington DC; 1972.
5. Truman vs Thomas, 611 P.2d 902. California; 1980.
6. Matthies vs Mastromonaco, 733 A.2d 456. (New Jersey; 1999.
7. Johnson vs Kokemoor, 545 N.W.2d 495. Wisconsin; 1996.
8. Moore vs. Regents of University of California, 793 P.2d 479 (California; 1990.
9. Shea vs. Esenstein (Shea II), 208 F.3d 712. Eighth Circuit; 2000.
10. Katz J. The Silent World of Doctor and Patient. New York: Free Press; 1984:xvi.
11. Stone AA. The right to refuse treatment: why psychiatrists should and can make it work. Arch Gen Psychiatry 1981;38: 358–362.
12. Washington vs. Harper, 494 U.S. 210. Washington; 1990.
13. Riese vs. St. Mary's Hospital and Medical Center, 271 Cal. Rptr. 199. California;1987.
14. Gutheil TG, Appelbaum PS. Clinical Handbook of Psychiatry and the Law. New York: McGraw-Hill; 1982:219–220.
15. Morris GH. Judging judgment: assessing the competence of mental patients to refuse treatment. San Diego L Rev 1995;32: 343–435.
16. Grisso T, Appelbaum PS. Assessing Competence to Consent to Treatment: A Guide for Physicians and Other Health Professionals. New York:Oxford University Press;1998.
17. Emanuel EJ, Wendler D, Grady C. What makes clinical research ethical? JAMA 2000;283:2701–2711.
18. (2004) http://irb.ucsd.edu/decisional.shtml.
19. Faden RR, Beauchamp TL, King NMP. A History and Theory of Informed Consent. New York: Oxford University Press; 1986.
20. Meisel A, Roth L, Lidz C. Toward a model of the legal doctrine of informed consent. Am J Psychiatry 1977;134:285–289.
21. Roberts LW. Informed consent and the capacity for voluntarism. Am J Psychiatry 2002;159:705–712.
22. Grisso T, Appelbaum PS. Comparison of standards for assessing patients' capacities to make treatment decisions. Am J Psychiatry 1995;152:1033–1037.
23. Carpenter WT, Conley RR. Sense and nonsense: an essay on schizophrenia research ethics. Schizophr Res 1999;35: 219–225.
24. Appelbaum PS, Grisso T. The MacArthur treatment competence study. I. Mental illness and competence to consent to treatment. Law Human Beh 1995;19:105–126.
25. Appelbaum PS, Grisso T, Frank E, O'Donnell S, Kupfer DJ. Competence of depressed patients to consent to research. Am J Psychiatry 1999;156:1380–1384.
26. Marson DC, Schmitt FA, Ingram KK, Harrell L. Determining the competency of Alzheimer patients to consent to treatment and research. Alzheimer Dis Assoc Disord 1994;8:5–18.
27. Kim SY, Caine ED, Currier GW, Leibovici A, Ryan JM. Assessing the competence of persons with Alzheimer's disease in providing informed consent for participation in research. Am J Psychiatry 2001;158:712–717.
28. Karlawish JHT, Casarett D, James B. Alzheimer's disease patients' and caregivers' capacity, competency, and reasons to enroll in an early-phase Alzheimer's disease clinical trial. J Am Geriatr Soc 2002;50:2019–2024.
29. Marson DC, Ingram KK. Commentary: competency to consent to treatment: a growing field of research. J Ethics Law Aging 1996;2:59–63.
30. Marson DC, McInturff B, Hawkins L, Bartolucci A, Harrell LE. Consistency of physician judgments of capacity to consent in mild Alzheimer's disease. J Am Geriatr Soc 1997;45:453–457.
31. Appelbaum PS, Grisso T. MacCAT-CR: MacArthur Competence Assessment Tool for Clinical Research. Sarasota, FL: Professional Resource Press; 2001.
32. Grisso T, Appelbaum PS, Hill-Fotouhi C. The MacCAT-T: a clinical tool to assess patients' capacities to make treatment decisions. Psychiatr Serv 1997;48:1415-1419.
33. Kim SY, Caine ED. Utility and limits of the Mini Mental State Examination in evaluating consent capacity in Alzheimer's Disease. Psychiatr Serv 2002;53:1322–1324.
34. Marson DC. Loss of competency in Alzheimer's disease: conceptual and psychometric approaches. Int J Law Psychiatry 2001;24:267–283.

35. Janofsky JS, McCarthy RJ, Folstein MF. The Hopkins Competency Assessment Test: a brief method for evaluating patients' capacity to give informed consent. Hosp Community Psychiatry 1992;43:132–136.
36. Glass KC. Refining definitions and devising instruments: Two decades of assessing mental competence. Int J Law Psychiatry 1997;20:5–33.
37. Fitten LJ, Lusky R, Hamann C. Assessing treatment decision-making capacity in elderly nursing home residents. J Am Geriatr Soc 1990;38:1097–1104.
38. Marson D, Cody HA, Ingram KK, Harrell LE. Neuropsychological predictors of competency in Alzheimer's disease using a rational reasons legal standard. Arch Neurol 1995;52:955–959.

Index